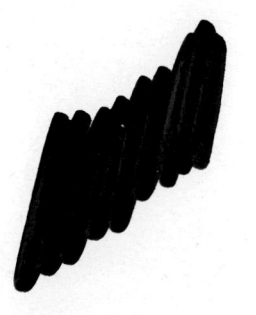

Essentials of
Obstetrics

Essentials of *Obstetrics*

Editors

Sabaratnam Arulkumaran
DCH FRCS FRCOG FAMS MD PhD
Hon: FACOG FSLCOG FSOGC
Professor and Head, Division of Obstetrics and Gynaecology
St. George's Hospital Medical School, London, UK

V Sivanesaratnam
MBBS (S'pore) FRCOG FICS FACS FAMM
Professor, Department of Obstetrics and Gynaecology
Faculty of Medicine, University of Malaya, Kuala Lumpur, Malaysia

Alokendu Chatterjee
FRCOG FICS
Formerly, Professor and Head, Department of Obstetrics and Gynaecology
NRS Medical College and Hospital, Kolkata

Pratap Kumar
MD DGO FICS FICOG FICMCH
Professor and Head, Department of Obstetrics and Gynaecology
Kasturba Medical College, Manipal

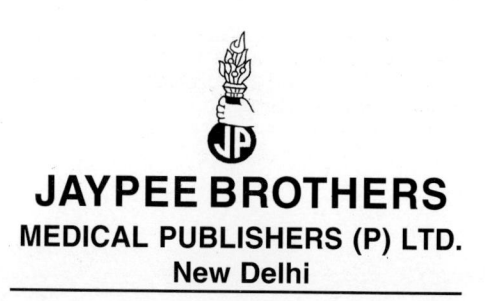

JAYPEE BROTHERS
MEDICAL PUBLISHERS (P) LTD.
New Delhi

Published by
Jitendar P Vij
Jaypee Brothers Medical Publishers (P) Ltd
EMCA House, 23/23B Ansari Road, Daryaganj
New Delhi 110 002, India
Phones: 23272143, 23272703, 23282021, 23245672
Fax: 91-11-23276490, 23245683
e-mail: jpmedpub@del2.vsnl.net.in
Visit our website: www.jaypeebrothers.com

Branches

- 202 Batavia Chambers, 8 Kumara Krupa Road, Kumara Park East,
  Bangalore 560 001, Phones: 2285971, 2382956 Tele Fax: 2281761
  e-mail: jaypeebc@bgl.vsnl.net.in

- 282 IIIrd Floor, Khaleel Shirazi Estate, Fountain Plaza
  Pantheon Road, **Chennai** 600 008, Phone: 28262665 Fax: 28262331
  e-mail: jpmedpub@md3.vsnl.net.in

- 4-2-1067/1-3, Ist Floor, Balaji Building, Ramkote Cross Road, **Hyderabad** 500 095
  Phones: 55610020, 24758498 Fax: 24758499 e-mail: hyd2_jpmedpub@sancharnet.in

- 1A Indian Mirror Street, Wellington Square
  Kolkata 700 013, Phone: 22451926 Fax: 22456075
  e-mail: jpbcal@cal.vsnl.net.in

- 106 Amit Industrial Estate, 61 Dr SS Rao Road, Near MGM Hospital
  Parel, **Mumbai** 400 012, Phones: 24124863, 24104532 Fax: 24160828
  e-mail: jpmedpub@bom7.vsnl.net.in

Essentials of Obstetrics

© 2004, Editors

All rights reserved. No part of this publication and CD ROM of illustrations should be reproduced, stored in a retrieval system, or transmitted in any form or by any means: electronic, mechanical, photocopying, recording, or otherwise, without the prior written permission of the editors and the publisher.

This book has been published in good faith that the material provided by contributors is original. Every effort is made to ensure accuracy of material, but the publisher, printer and editors will not be held responsible for any inadvertent error(s). In case of any dispute, all legal matters to be settled under Delhi jurisdiction only.

First Edition: **2004**

ISBN 81-8061-362-3

Typeset at JPBMP typesetting unit
Printed at Sanat Printer.

Contributors

Sabaratnam Arulkumaran
DCH, FRCS, FRCOG, FAMS, MD, PhD
Hon: FACOG, FSLCOG, FSOGC
Professor and Head
Division of Obstetrics and Gynaecology
St George's Hospital Medical School
London, United Kingdom
Chapters: 2, 3, 9, 13, 15, 24, 31, 32, 34

Gita Basu (Banerjee) DGO, MD (G & O), DNB, MRCOG,
R.M.O./Clinical Tutor,
NRS Medical College and Hospital
Kolkata, India
Chapter: 23

Rajesh Bhakta MD
Assistant Professor
Department of Obstetrics and Gynecology
Kasturba Medical College
Manipal, India
Chapter: 4

Sudip Chakravarti FRCOG, FRCS, FICOG
Professor
Dept. of Obstetrics and Gynaecology
Vivekananda Institute of Medical Sciences
Kolkata, India
Chapters: 38, 46

BN Chakravarty MD, FRCOG, DSc (Hon)
Professor
Institute of Reproductive Medicine
Salt Lake City
Kolkata, India
Chapter: 1

Alokendu Chatterjee FRCOG, FICS
Formerly Professor and Head
Dept. of Obstetrics and Gynaecology
NRS Medical College and Hospital, Kolkata, India
Chapters: 12, 23, 35

Tan Peng Chiong
MBBS (Lond), MRCOG, CCST (O & G UK)
Lecturer in Obstetrics and Gynaecology
Department of Obstetrics and Gynaecology
University of Malaya
Kuala Lumpur, Malaysia
Chapter: 26

Teresa WP Chow MRCOG
Department of Obstetrics and Gynaecology
University of Malaya Medical Centre
Kuala Lumpur
Malaysia
Chapter: 17

NN Roy Chowdhury
MD, PhD, FRCS, FRCOG, FACS, FAMS, FICOG
Ex-Professor of Obstetrics and Gynaecology
Medical College
Kolkata, India
Chapter: 20

S Dasgupta FRCS, FRCOG, FICOG
Formerly Professor of Obstetrics and Gynaecology
Jamshedpur Medical College
Jamshedpur
India
Chapter: 6

Sajal Datta MBBS, MD, DNB
Reader
Dept. of Obstetrics and Gynaecology
Vivekananda Institute of Medical Sciences
Kolkata, India
Chapters: 38, 46

Pankaj Desai MD, FICOG, FICMCH
A. Professor and Head
Dept. of Obstetrics and Gynaecology
Medical College and SSG Hospital
Baroda, India
Chapter: 21

KK Diwakar MD
Head, Neonatal Division
Professor, Department of Pediatrics
Malankara Orthodox Syrian Church Medical College
Kolenchery, Kochi, Kerala, India
Chapter: 43

Suku Mathew George MD, DNB
Assistant Professor
Department of Obstetrics and Gynaecology
Kasturba Medical College
Manipal, India
Chapter: 10

Krishnendu Gupta MBBS, DGO, MD, FICMCH, FICOG
Professor
Dept. of Obstetrics and Gynaecology
Vivekananda Institute of Medical Sciences
Kolkata, India
Chapters: 38, 46

Samiksha Gupta
Malhotra Nursing and Maternity Home (P) Ltd
Agra, India
Chapter: 33

Jamiyah Hassan MBBS (UM), MMed (O & G)
Associate Professor and Consultant
Department of Obstetrics and Gynaecology
University of Malaya Medical Centre
Kuala Lumpur
Malaysia
Chapters: 16, 29

Shripad Hebbar MD
Associate Professor of O & G
Kasturba Medical College
Manipal
India
Chapter: 18

Thaneemalai Jeganathan MBBS, MOG
Dept. of Obstetrics and Gynecology
University of Malaya Medical Centre
Kuala Lumpur
Malaysia
Chapter: 44

Devendra Kanagalingam
Locum Lecturer in Obstetrics and Gynaecology
St. George's Hospital Medical School
London
United Kingdom
Chapters: 9, 32

Hira Lal Konar MBBS, MD, DNB, MRCOG
Assistant Professor
Department of Obstetrics and Gynaecology
NRS Medical College
Kolkata, India
Chapter: 30

Eugene Leong Weng Kong
Lecturer
Department of Obstetrics and Gynaecology
University of Malaya Medical Centre
Kuala Lumpur
Malaysia
Chapter: 22

Chan Yoo Kuen MBBS (Mal), FFARCS (Ireland)
Professor
Department of Anaesthesiology
Faculty of Medicine
University of Malaya
Kuala Lumpur
Malaysia
Chapter: 37

Pratap Kumar MD, DGO, FICS, FICOG, FICMCH
Professor and Head
Department of Obstetrics and Gynecology
Kasturba Medical College
Manipal
India
Chapters: 4, 8, 10

Jaideep Malhotra
Malhotra Nursing and Maternity Home (P) Ltd
Agra
India
Chapter: 33

Narendra Malhotra
Malhotra Nursing and Maternity Home (P) Ltd
Agra
India
Chapter: 33

Matthews Mathai MD, MObstet, PhD
Professor of Obstetrics and Gynaecology
Christian Medical College and Hospital
Vellore, India
Chapter: 28

Vanaj Mathur
Malhotra Nursing and Maternity Home (P) Ltd
Agra, India
Chapter: 33

Wong Yat May MRCOG, MBChB
Lecturer
Department of Obstetrics and Gynaecology
University of Malaya Medical Centre
Kuala Lumpur
Malaysia
Chapter: 5

Idora Mohamed MBBS (Mal) MMed (O & G) (Mal)
Lecturer
Department of Obstetrics and Gynaecology
University of Malaya Medical Centre
Kuala Lumpur
Malaysia
Chapter: 11

CONTRIBUTORS

Joydev Mukherji MD (Gynae and Obst)
Associate Professor
Dept. of Gynaecology and Obstetrics
North Bengal Medical College
West Bengal
India
Chapter: 41

Gautam Mukhopadhyay MD, DNB
Dept. of Obstetrics and Gynaecology
NRS Medical College and Hospital, Kolkata
Salt Lake City
Kolkata
India
Chapter: 12

Partha Mukhopadhyay MBBS, DGO, MD
Assistant Professor
Department of Obstetrics and Gynaecology
NRS Medical College
Kolkata
India
Chapter: 40

Sambit Mukhopadhyay
Consultant
Department of Obstetrics and Gynaecology
Norfolk and Norwich University Hospital NHS Trust
Norwich
United Kingdom
Chapters: 2, 3, 24, 34

Muralidhar V Pai
Associate Professor
Dept. of Obstetrics and Gynaecology
Kasturba Medical College
Manipal
India
Chapter: 27

Suchitra N Pandit
BPharm, MD, DNBE, DGO, DFP, MRCOG (UK), MICOG
Associate Professor and Head of Unit
Department of Obstetrics and Gynaecology
LT Medical College and
LT Municipal General Hospital
Mumbai
India
Chapter: 25

Sukhpreet Patel MD, DNB, FCPS, DGO
Mumbai
India
Chapter: 14

Lavanya Rai MD, DGO
Department of Obstetrics and Gynecology
Kasturba Medical College Hospital
Manipal, Karnataka, India
Chapter: 19

A Padma Rao MD, DGO
Emeritus Professor and Retired Head and
Director of Postgraduate Studies
Department of Obstetrics and Gynaecology
Kasturba Medical College, Manipal, Karnataka
India
Chapter: 7

Sanjay B Rao MD, DNBE, DGO, DFP, FCPS, DICOG
Lecturer
Department of Obstetrics and Gynaecology
LT Medical College and LT Municipal General Hospital
Mumbai, India
Chapter: 25

Charu Rawat MD (O & G)
Department of Obstetrics and Gynaecology
Medical College and SSG Hospital, Baroda
India
Chapter: 21

Silvam Sellappan MBBS (Mal.), MOG (Mal)
Department of Obstetrics and Gynaecology
Faculty of Medicine
University of Malaya
Kuala Lumpur
Malaysia
Chapter: 39

Duru Shah MD, FCPS, FICS, FICOG, DGO, DFP, FICMCH
Consultant Obstetrician and Gynaecologist
Breach Candy Hospital, Jaslok Hospital,
Sir Hurkisonadas Hospital
Mumbai, India
Chapter: 14

Jyothi Shetty MD
Associate Professor
Dept. of Obstetrics and Gynaecology
Kasturba Medical College
Manipal, India
Chapter: 45

Kamala Sikdar MD, FRCOG, MNAMS, PhD, FACS
Professor and Head
Department of Obstetrics and Gynaecology
NRS Medical College and Hospital
Kolkata, India
Chapter: 35

Amita Singh
Malhotra Nursing and Maternity Home (P) Ltd
Agra, India
Chapter: 33

V Sivanesaratnam MBBS (S'pore), FRCOG, FICS, FACS, FAMM
Professor
Department of Obstetrics and Gynaecology
Faculty of Medicine, University of Malaya
Kuala Lumpur, Malaysia
Chapters: 39, 44

B Subhasri MD
Lecturer in Obstetrics and Gynaecology
Christian Medical College and Hospital
Vellore, India
Chapter: 28

K Sujata MD
Obstetrics and Gynecology
Kasturba Medical College, Manipal
Chapter: 36

Sofiah Sulaiman MBBcH, MMed (O & G)
Lecturer
Department of Obstetrics and Gynaecology
University of Malaya Medical Centre
Kuala Lumpur, Malaysia
Chapters: 16, 29

Onnig Tamizian
Specialist Registrar
Department of Obstetrics and Gynaecology
Kings Mill Hospital
Nottingham
United Kingdom
Chapters: 13, 15, 31

Lim Chin Theam
MBBS, FRCP (Lond), FRCP (Edin), FAMM (Fellow Academy of Medicine Malaysia)
Professor and Senior Consultant Neonatologist
Department of Paediatrics
University of Malaya Medical Centre
Kuala Lumpur
Malaysia
Chapter: 42

Anita Thomas MD
Assistant Professor
Department of Obstetrics and Gynaecology
Kasturba Medical College
Manipal, India
Chapter: 8

Foreword

This book rightly focuses on undergraduates since the future truly rests on them.

We live in an era of hope with awesome scientific advances, with an ever-growing need to identify fetal well-being and obstetric aberrations. This book is truly the work of select obstetricians who have a deep concern for women's health and in these chapters, they have dealt with practical aspects, with utmost care to provide a crystal clear pathway to obstetric management for the undergraduates.

The greatest benchmark for the disparity in medical care between rich and poor countries is their obstetric outcome—their reproductive status. The Editors' deep concern for this problem is easily visualized through a comprehensive chapter on Safe Motherhood and the emphasis on fundamentals of reproduction as an opening chapter, at the same time not ignoring important players like endocrinal and immunological components.

I feel privileged and happy to welcome this addition to our literature and look forward to it becoming a boon to all hues of Obs-Gyn. practitioners. Its rich contents should please every undergraduate as well as his teachers.

Shirish S Sheth
Past President
FIGO

27th April, 2004

Preface

The knowledge in obstetrics is expanding and one finds it difficult to keep pace with recent research. Research findings of today form the basis of practice in years to come. The core knowledge keeps changing and forms the basis of understanding of the disease process and management and is covered in this book. One may think of obstetrics as childbirth and its complications, but the expansion of knowledge in this area is exemplified by 46 chapters under 2 subsections. The book starts with issues related to conception, implantation and growth of the fetus and placenta. From this point, it expands to the knowledge needed for prenatal care followed by normal pregnancy and childbirth. The various obstetric and medical complications in the antenatal period are covered followed by normal and abnormal labor including operative deliveries. It ends with normal and complicated puerperium.

This book is multi-authored and hence the tendency for some overlap and repetition of knowledge. The editors have taken great effort in avoiding such duplications, but where it is felt that it may enhance continuity of reading an individual chapter, little change has been made. The authors have been selected based on their individual expertise, which has been useful to provide the best knowledge. This has led to the standards set high for many chapters. The knowledge provided straddles between what is needed for an undergraduate and a postgraduate. The editors had the difficult task of trimming down many chapters to make this book a reference source for undergraduates. In addition, it will form a basic reading book for postgraduates. The authors are from a variety of backgrounds and countries. This has led to some differences in the style and reporting of incidence of disease, but it does not alter the subject material.

We believe that this will be a good reference source for undergraduates and would welcome any comments or criticism that will help us to make this book better in the next edition. Your suggestions can be sent to any one of the editors or the publishers.

Sabaratnam Arulkumaran
V Sivanesaratnam
Alokendu Chatterjee
Pratap Kumar

Acknowledgements

The editors would like to sincerely thank the contributors to this book. It had a long conception period due to some chapters arriving late and the need to have an extensive editorial process to make the chapters uniform, avoid duplication and step down postgraduate into undergraduate knowledge. The latter process has made some chapters so different from the original submission by authors. We ask the authors for their understanding and acceptance of this process. The principal editor collated the chapters from the other editors to streamline the publication and would like to acknowledge the help and advice provided by Mrs. Sue Cunningham at St. George's Hospital Medical School, University of London. We are grateful to the authors and publishers for their patience in the production of this book. Mr. JP Vij, Chairman and Managing Director and his team from Jaypee Brothers Medical Publishers (P) Ltd. need special commendation for the constant encouragement, in-house editorial work and production of the vast number of figures in the book. We would like to thank Dr. Shirish Sheth, past President of FIGO and an internationally renowned Obstetrician and Gynaecologist for writing the foreword for this book.

Contents

Part 1: Introduction

1. **Fundamentals of Reproduction** 1
   BN Chakravarty

2. **Anatomy of Female Reproductive Organs** 19
   Sambit Mukhopadhyay, Sabaratnam Arulkumaran

3. **Anatomy of the Female Pelvis** 25
   Sambit Mukhopadhyay, Sabaratnam Arulkumaran

4. **Diagnosis of Pregnancy** 33
   Rajesh Bhakta, Pratap Kumar

5. **Physiological Changes in Pregnancy** 41
   Wong Yat May

6. **Endocrinology of Pregnancy and Labor** 50
   S Dasgupta

7. **Immunology of Pregnancy** 57
   A Padma Rao

8. **Fetus, Placenta and Membranes** 64
   Anita Thomas, Pratap Kumar

9. **History and Examination of a Pregnant Mother** 72
   Devendra Kanagalingam, Sabaratnam Arulkumaran

10. **Miscarriage** 80
    Suku Mathew George, Pratap Kumar

11. **Ectopic Pregnancy** 88
    Idora Mohamed

12. **Safe Motherhood** 95
    Alokendu Chatterjee, Gautam Mukhopadhyay

Part 2: Feto-maternal Medicine

13. **Antenatal Care** 102
    Onnig Tamizian, Sabaratnam Arulkumaran

14. **Hyperemesis Gravidarum** 108
    Duru Shah, Sukhpreet Patel

15. **Minor Disorders of Pregnancy** 115
    Onnig Tamizian, Sabaratnam Arulkumaran

16. **Basic Ultrasonography in Pregnancy** 118
    Jamiyah Hassan, Sofiah Sulaiman

17. **Prenatal Diagnosis** 125
    Teresa WP Chow

18. **Anemia in Pregnancy** 138
    Shripad Hebbar

19. **Diabetes in Pregnancy** 147
    Lavanya Rai

20. **Tropical Diseases in Pregnancy** 156
    NN Roy Chowdhury

21. **Infections and Immunization in Pregnancy** 165
    Pankaj Desai, Charu Rawat

22. **Antepartum Hemorrhage** 176
    Eugene Leong Weng Kong

23. **Hypertensive Disorders in Pregnancy** 186
    Alokendu Chatterjee, Gita Basu (Banerjee)

24. **Gynecological Disorders in Pregnancy** 199
    Sambit Mukhopadhyay, Sabaratnam Arulkumaran

25. **Multiple Pregnancy and Polyhydramnios** 203
    Suchitra N Pandit, Sanjay B Rao

26. **Preterm Labor and Prelabor Rupture of Membranes** 213
    Tan Peng Chiong

27. **Intrauterine Growth Restriction** 227
    Muralidhar V Pai

28. **Prolonged Pregnancy** 234
    Matthews Mathai, B Subhasri

29. **Thalassemia and Rhesus Isoimmunization** 239
    Jamiyah Hassan, Sofiah Sulaiman

30. **Medical Disorders in Pregnancy (Cardiac, Respiratory and Endocrine Disorders)** 244
    Hira Lal Konar

31. **Principles of Drug Use in Pregnancy** 250
    Onnig Tamizian, Sabaratnam Arulkumaran

32. **Acute Abdomen in Pregnancy** 258
    Devendra Kanagalingam, Sabaratnam Arulkumaran

33. **Antenatal Assessment of Fetal Wellbeing** 264
    Narendra Malhotra, Jaideep Malhotra, Amita Singh, Vanaj Mathur, Samiksha Gupta

34. Induction of Labor **274**
Sambit Mukhopadhyay, Sabaratnam Arulkumaran

35. Mechanism of Labor **283**
Kamala Sikdar, Alokendu Chatterjee

36. Normal Labor **291**
K Sujata

37. Obstetric Analgesia and Anesthesia **301**
Chan Yoo Kuen

38. Malposition, Malpresentations and Cord Prolapse **306**
Sudip Chakravarti, Krishnendu Gupta, Sajal Datta

39. Operative Obstetrics **330**
Silvam Sellappan, V Sivanesaratnam

40. Injuries to Birth Canal **338**
Partha Mukhopadhyay

41. Prolonged and Obstructed Labor **345**
Joydev Mukherji

42. Resuscitation of the Newborn **351**
Lim Chin Theam

43. Diseases of the Newborn **357**
KK Diwakar

44. Complications of Third Stage of Labor **364**
Thaneemalai Jeganathan, V Sivanesaratnam

45. Normal Puerperium **373**
Jyothi Shetty

46. Abnormalities of Puerperium **378**
Krishnendu Gupta, Sajal Datta, Sudip Chakravarti

Index *387*

PLATE 1

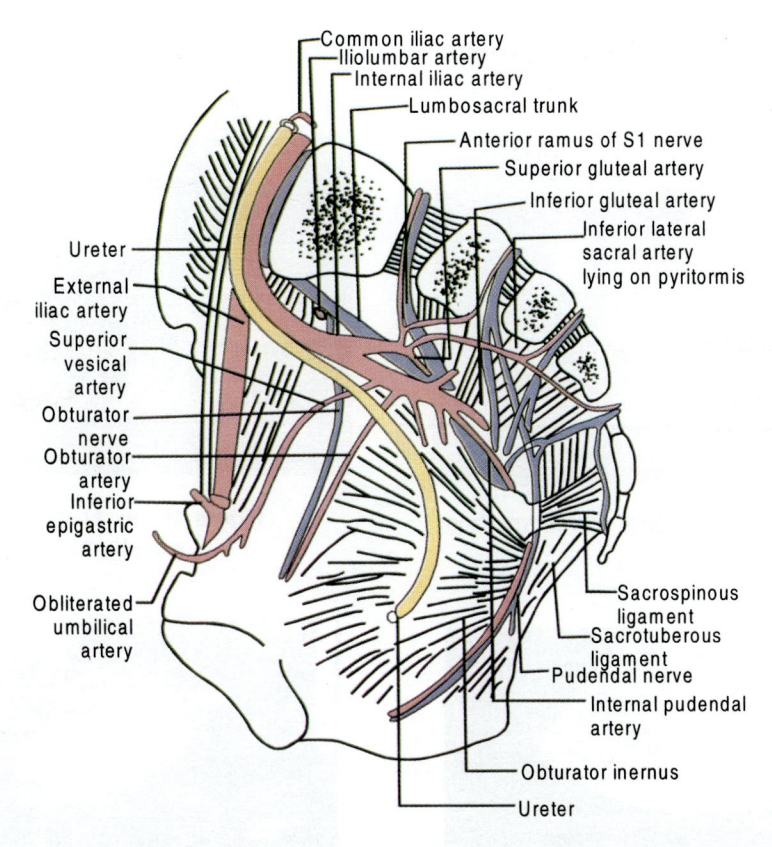

Figure 2.2: Sagittal section of right half of the pelvis showing vessels and nerves

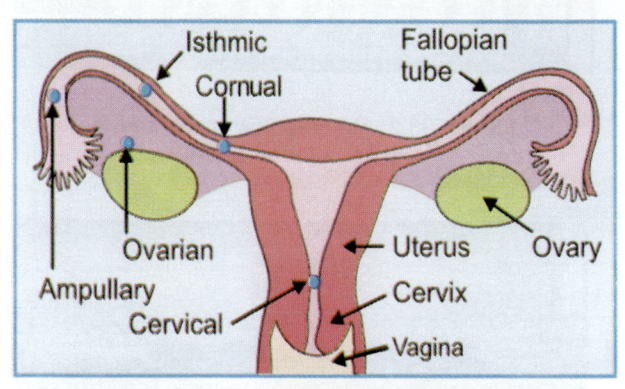

Figure 11.1: The sites of ectopic pregnancy

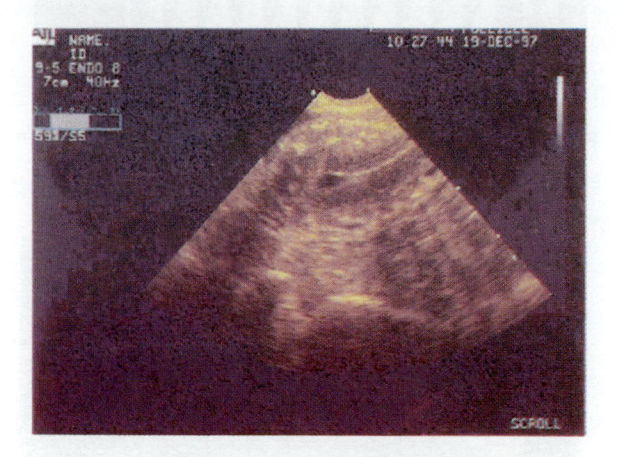

Figure 16.1: Gestational sac

PLATE 2

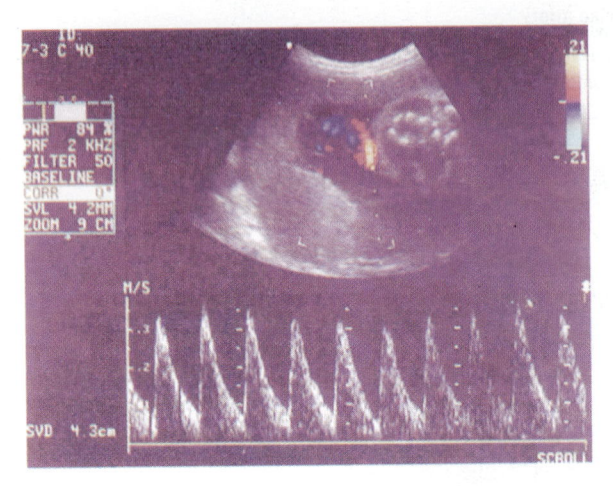

Figure 16.17: Normal flow velocity waveforms from umbilical artery

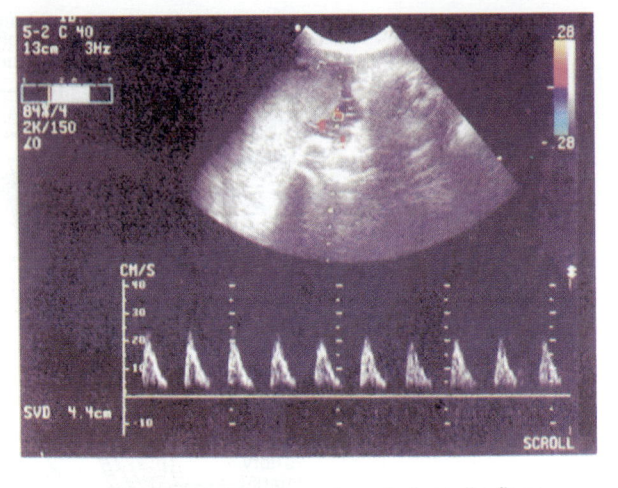

Figure 16.18: Absent end diastolic flow waveforms—pathological

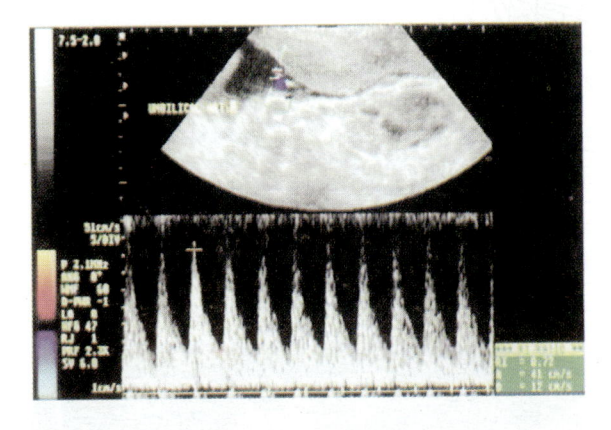

Figure 33.1: Doppler flow measured in umbilical artery

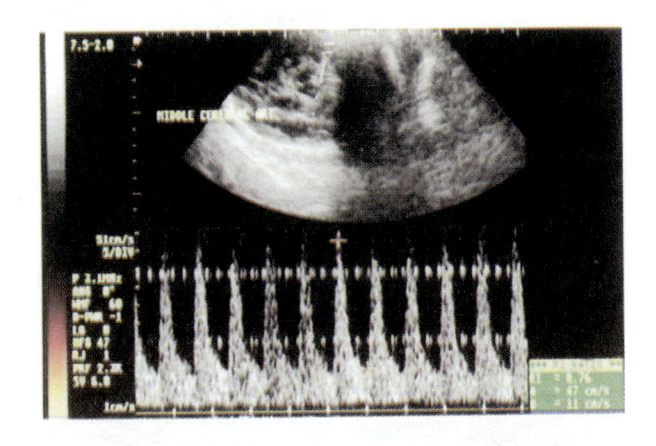

Figure 33.2: Doppler flow measured in middle cerebral artery

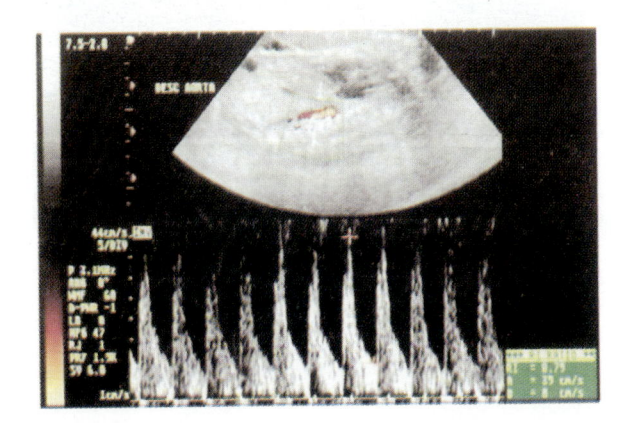

Figure 33.3: Doppler flow measured in descending aorta

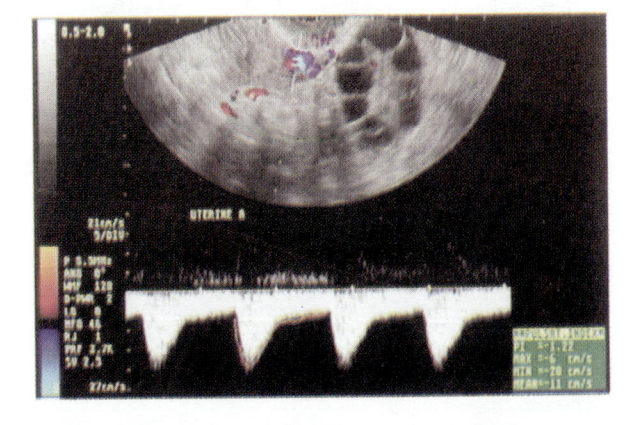

Figure 33.4: Doppler flow measured in uterine artery

PLATE 3

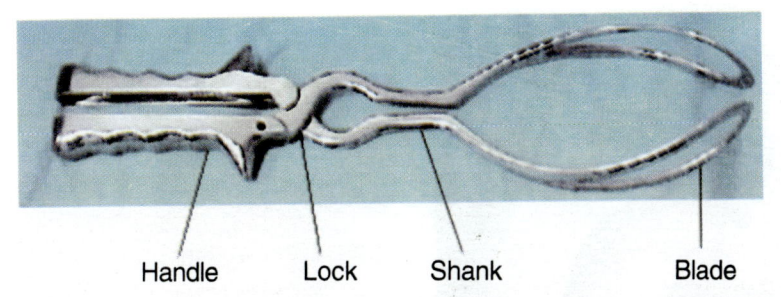

Figure 39.1: Anatomy of classic obstetric forceps (Neville-Barnes forceps)

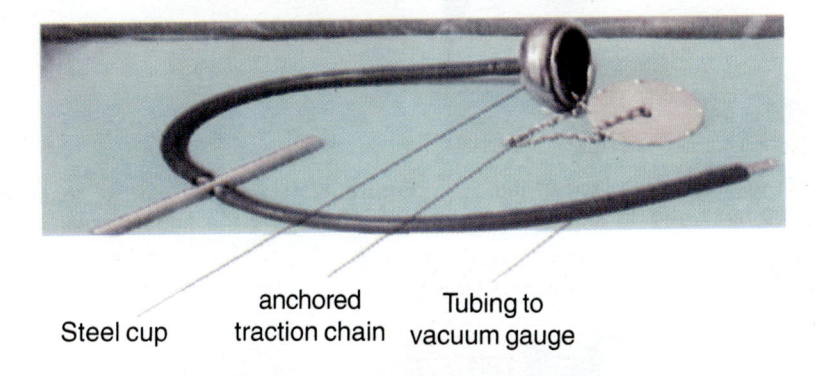

Handle   Lock   Shank   Blade

Figure 39.2: Malmstrom vacuum extractor

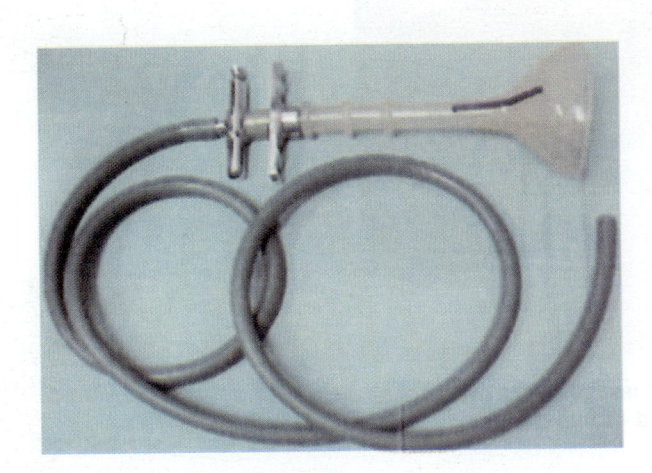

Steel cup   anchored traction chain   Tubing to vacuum gauge

Figure 39.3A: Kobayashi soft cup unit

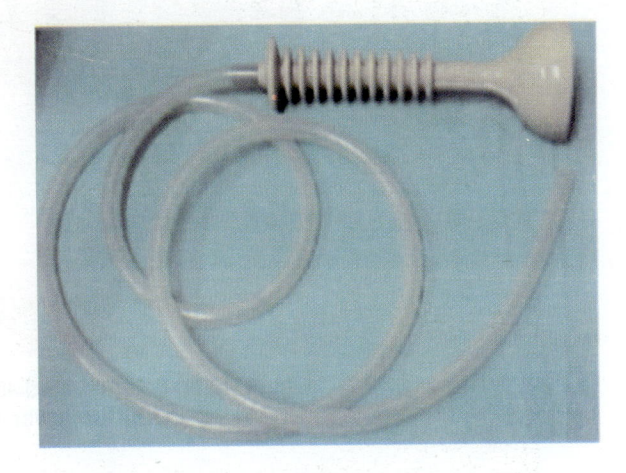

Figure 39.3B: Modified silastic soft cup unit

PLATE 4

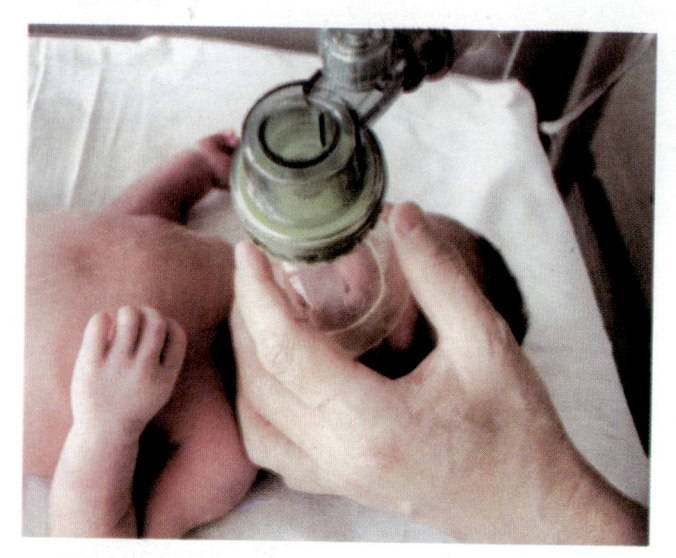

Figure 42.2: Face mask applied to the face of the newborn – covering the nose, mouth and chin

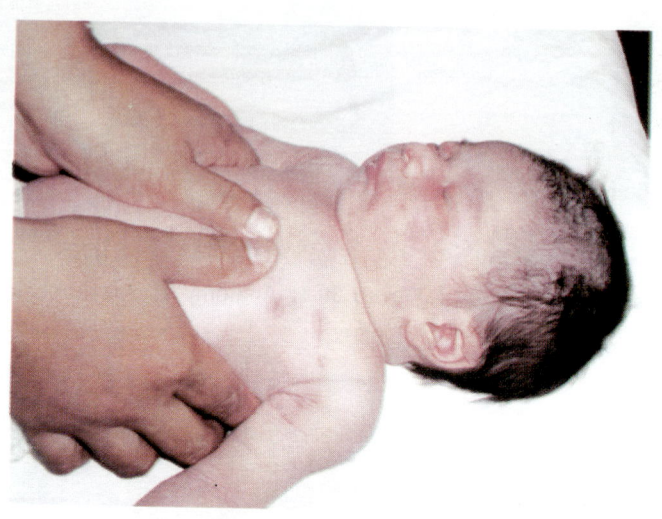

Figure 42.4: External cardiac massage using two thumbs while the fingers encircling the chest

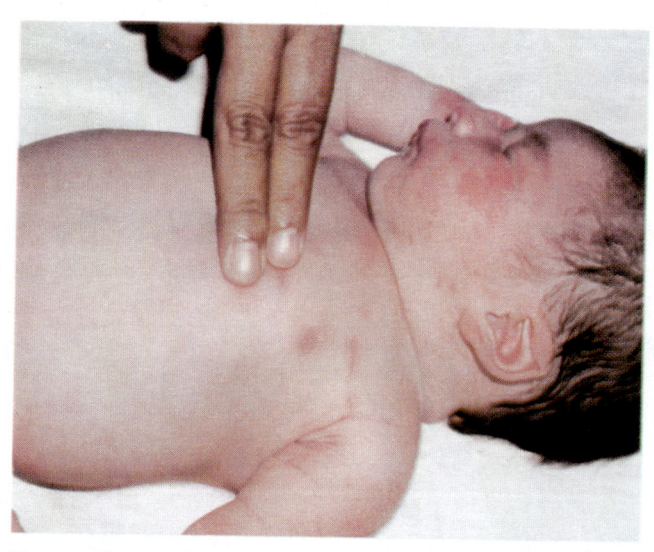

Figure 42.5: External cardiac massage using two fingers placed at the lower third of the sternum

1. Fundamentals of Reproduction

BN Chakravarty

PART One — Introduction

INTRODUCTION

Reproduction is the creation of a new individual or individuals from previously existing individuals. The union of sperm and egg is the essential step in the process of reproduction.

In the historical milestones, the factors involved in reproduction remained a mystery till the earlier part of seventeenth century. Leeuwenhock of Holland for the first time in 1677, with his home-made microscope described fairly accurately the anatomy of the sperm. Thereafter in the 18th century, there was insignificant progress in the knowledge of biology. In 1822, Karl Dernt von Baer "Father of Modern Embryology" documented observation on eggs and their developmental stages. It was Oscar Hertwig in Germany who first demonstrated in 1875 by his observation on sea urchins that the union of sperm and egg was the essential step for reproduction. However, in humans, the remote site of these events and the secluded place of origin of the participants (gametes) made fertilization a difficult subject for study. Most of the knowledge about human reproduction was achieved through experiments in animal species. Scope of study directly in humans has only been possible following the advent of Assisted Reproduction. The understanding of the process of gametogenesis, their maturation, sperm-egg interaction, fertilization and implantation is one of the many major benefits that have been derived through clinical application of the Assisted Reproductive Technologies. Some of the information about the basics of human reproduction gathered so far through these technologies backed up by studies on animal models will be discussed in this chapter.

CLASSIFICATION

Fundamental requirements for sexual reproduction can be classified under three broad groups:
1. Development of morphologically and functionally competent gametes (oocytes and spermatozoa).
2. Existence of anatomically and physiologically normal male and female reproductive organs.
3. Delicately balanced intricate interactive events leading to release of gametes (male and female), their transport, fusion and fertilization, cleavage and implantation.

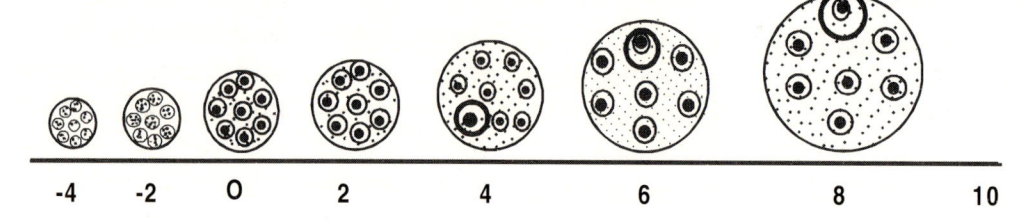

Figure 1.3: Folliculogenesis and selection of dominant follicle

4. *Late follicular phase and periovulatory events:* FSH in the early and mid-follicular phase has already produced receptors for LH in the dominant follicle. Under the influence of rising LH, the dominant follicle continues to grow. The remaining follicles become atretic. There is luteinization of granulosa cells with release of small amount of progesterone (0.8 to 1.8 ng/ml). This will lead to oocyte maturation by completing the first meiotic division. Before the FSH starts declining in the later part of mid-follicular phase, the estradiol has reached the peak (around 100 pg/ml). This peak level is maintained for about 48 hours (plateau). Estradiol at this peak and pleateu level exerts negative 'feedback' effect on the pituitary for which FSH declines and LH starts rising. At the same time, the rise of estradiol finally exerts a positive feedback effect on hypothalamus for which a bolus of GnRH is released. Pulsatile rise of GnRH stimulates the pituitary to release a bolus amount of LH (about 75 to 90 mIU/ml) which is known as ovulatory "LH surge". The follicle ruptures with release of mature oocyte. This is known as ovulation. Besides the dynamic event of ovulatory LH surge, intrafollicular prostaglandin and an enzyme collagenase, generated by plasminogen activator, plasmin are also involved in the mechanism of follicular rupture. The liberated mature oocyte is picked up by fimbria of the fallopian tube and proceeds toward ampulla, which is now ready to be fertilized if a mature sperm is available.

The entire mechanism of ovulatory menstrual cycle may be schematically represented in Table 1.1.

Endocrine events and folliculogenesis in ovulatory menstrual cycle have been diagrammatically represented in Figures 1.3 to 1.5.

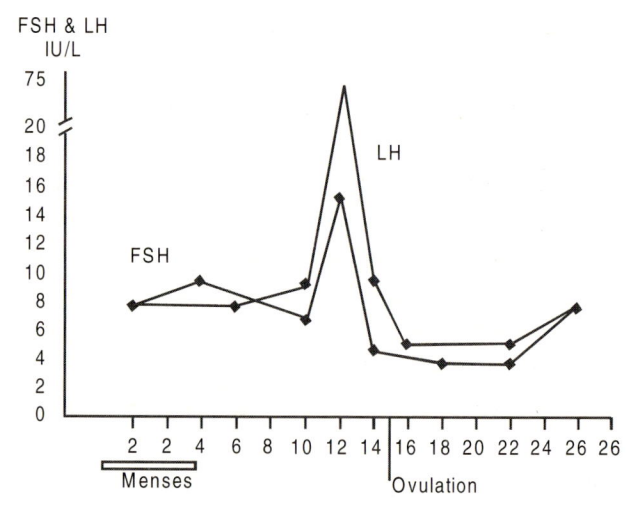

Figure 1.4: Endocrine control of ovulatory menstrual cycle (FSH and LH Pattern)

Table 1.1: Main events in normal ovulatory menstrual cycle

Late luteal phase	Menstrual and early follicular phase	Mid-follicular phase	Periovulatory events
• E_2 and inhibin-B declines • FSH starts rising • Fresh batch of follicles recruited	• FSH continues to rise • Follicular growth continues (multiplication of granulosa cells) • E_2 starts increasing	• Dominant follicle selected • E_2 continues to rise • FSH starts declining • LH starts rising	• Luteinization of granulosa cells • 1st meiotic division of oocyte is completed • LH surge • Ovulation

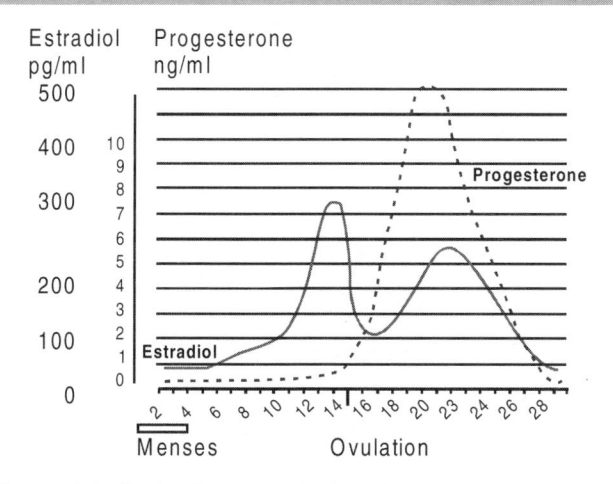

Figure 1.5: Endocrine control of ovulatory menstrual cycle (Estradiol and progesterone pattern)

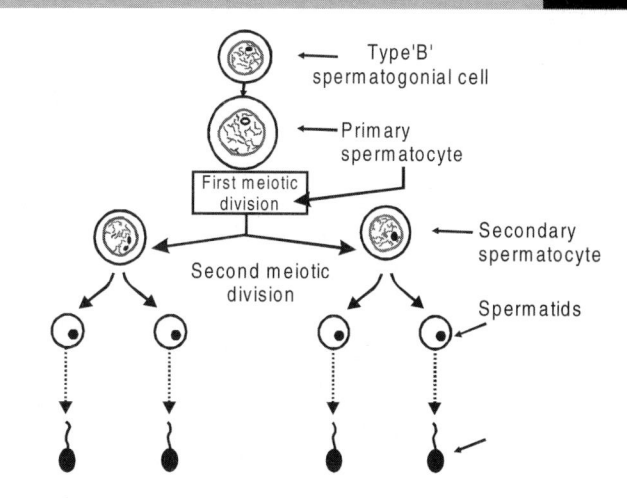

Figure 1.6: Maturational changes of spermatozoa

Spermatogenesis

In the testes two types of spermatogonial cells (germ cells) have been recognized: Type-A and Type-B cells. All Type-A spermatogonia have been considered to play a stem cell role. Some of the A-type spermatogonia act, as reserve stem cells while others are active stem cells. From these active stem cells Type -B Spermatogonia are produced which ultimately lead to the development of spermatocytes.[10] The reserve Type-A stem cells lie dormant and become active on demand.

These germ cells are scattered between radially directed supporting cells called Sertoli cells. The Sertoli cells lie within the seminiferous tubules. By forming tight junctions with each other, the Sertoli cells divide seminiferous tubules into two compartments called the basal and the adluminal compartment. Sertoli cells produce inhibin and a protein known as androgen binding globulin (ABG). Androgen binding globulin transports the androgens produced by Leydig cells (which lie outside the seminiferous tubules) into the basal compartment for completing the maturational changes of the spermatozoa. Maturational changes of spermatozoa occur in four stages (Figure 1.6).

Type-B spermatogonia differentiate into primary spermatocyte.

By first meiotic division one primary spermatocyte divides into two secondary spermatocytes.

By second meiotic division two secondary spermatocytes will further divide into four spermatids.

Maturational changes upto this stage occurs within the seminiferous tubules. Finally, adult spermatozoa are formed which by this time has reached the caudal epididymis. The sperms reach the caudal epididymis approximately 72 days after the initiation of spermatogenesis. The sperms are stored in the caudal epididymis for final ejaculation. During the maturation of spermatids to spermatozoa, several events occur, including formation of acrosome, changes in nuclear morphology and formation of the flagellum.

The sperm functions are preserved during this period of storage by adequate amount of circulating plasma testosterone.

Anatomy of Human Spermatozoa

A normal spermatozoon is 60 μm in length. The different parts of spermatozoa are: (a) head, (b) neck (also known as connecting piece) and (c) tail. The tail is subdivided into three segments viz. midpiece, principal piece and end piece. The sperm head is the part-containing nucleus, covered in its anterior aspect by the acrosomal cap. The acrosomal cap has two layers—outer acrosomal and inner acrosomal layer. The acrosomal cap contains various types of enzymes of which two are significant, namely acrosin and hyaluronidase. Covering the outer acrosomal layer is the plasma membrane, which is the outermost layer of the sperm head.

The neck contains proximal centriole and the remnants of the distal centriole. Sperm centriole has an important function during fertilization. Following entry of sperm head into the oocyte, sperm centriole triggers up formation of female pronucleus inside the ooplasm. This area has been termed as the 'black box' (preserving all the informations for fertilization) of the spermatozoa (Figure 1.7).

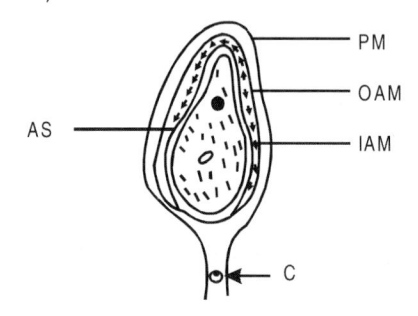

Figure 1.7: "Biochemical anatomy of sperm head and neck"
PM — Plasma membrane
OAM — Outer acrosomal membrane
IAM — Inner acrosomal membrane
AS — Acrosomal sac containing enzymes; acrosin and hyaluronidase
C — Centriole

Tail has the important function as it provides energy for the sperms to move. Presence of dyenin bands (a type of protein) in the tail is the source of energy and motility of sperm. Absence of dyenin or deformity of tail is the factors for sperm immotility.

Endocrine Regulation of Spermatogenesis

Like ovulatory control, endocrine regulation of spermatogenesis depends on 'two gonadotropin-two cell' system. There is a regulatory 'feedback' mechanism in the hypothalamic-pituitary-testicular axis. Spermatogenesis is a continuous process. Hence, unlike ovulatory cycles, 'feedback' mechanism in the hypothalamic-pituitary-testicular axis in spermatogenesis has no specific cyclicity.

The endocrine regulation of spermatogenesis has been diagrammatically represented in Figure 1.8.

Under the influence of GnRH stimulation released by hypothalamus, pituitary produces two gonadotropins, viz. follicle stimulating hormone (FSH) and luteinizing hormone LH. LH stimulates the Leydig cells of the testes to generate adequate amount of testosterone. Leydig cells also produce some amount of estradiol. Leydig cells lie outside the lumen of the seminiferous tubules. Hence, testosterone production is extraluminal.

FSH secreted by anterior pituitary will stimulate the Sertoli cells to produce inhibin and another peptide known as androgen binding globulin (ABG). Androgen binding globulin produced by Sertoli cells has the capability of carrying extraluminally produced androgen inside the lumen of the seminiferous tubules. Androgens now within the lumen of the seminiferous tubules will help in the maturational changes of the spermatozoa.

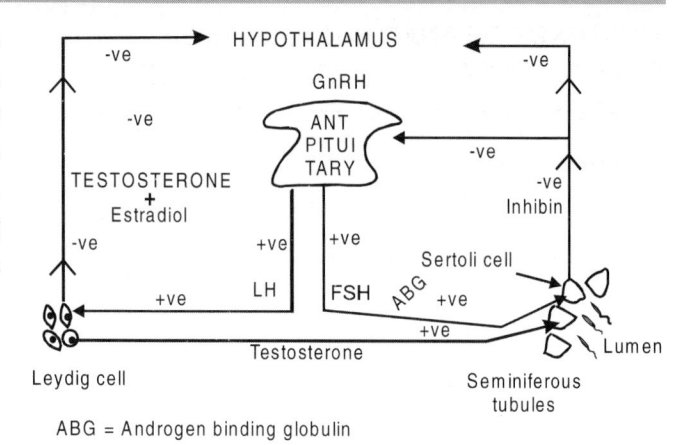

Figure 1.8: Endocrine regulation of spermatogenesis
ABG = Androgen binding globulin

KEY POINTS

- Oocytes and spermatocytes originate from germ cells developing in the embryonic hind gut and yolk sac
- Thereafter they migrate and settle in genital ridge which will develop into either testes or ovary
- The sex differentiation of the gonad will depend on chromosomal complement of embryo
- Maturational changes of spermatocyte (two meiotic divisions) are completed within the testes while for oocytes, this is completed at the time of fertilization
- Maturational changes are influenced by genetic, endocrine, autocrine and paracrine factors.

EXISTENCE OF ANATOMICALLY AND PHYSIOLOGICALLY NORMAL MALE AND FEMALE REPRODUCTIVE ORGANS

Embryogenesis

The wolffian (mesonephric) and mullerian (paramesonephric) ducts develop during the ambisexual period of embryonic development (upto 8 weeks). Thereafter one duct will persist and give rise to sex-specific internal and external genital organs and the other will disappear by the third fetal month except for rudimentary vestiges.

The crucial factor which will determine as which duct will persist or regress is the presence or absence of antimullerian hormone (AMH) secreted by the testes. If antimullerian hormone is present, paramesonephric duct will disappear and wolffian duct will start developing. On the other hand, in the absence of antimullerian hormone, the paramesonephric ducts will develop and wolffian duct will disappear.

Internal genital organs have the intrinsic tendency to feminize. In the absence of a Y-chromosome, a functional testes and antimullerian hormone, the mullerian system will develop into fallopian tubes, uterus and upper vagina. Therefore, development of female reproductive organ is passive and does not require an active stimulus.

On the other hand, differentiation of wolffian system requires active stimulation through testosterone production by testes.

Developmental Anatomy of Female Reproductive Organs

In the absence of antimullerian hormone, the two paramesonephric ducts come into contact in the midline to form a Y-shaped structure, which will form the uterus, tubes and upper part vagina.[11] The fallopian tubes, uterus and the upper portion of the vagina are created by fusion of the mullerian ducts by 10th week of gestation. By 22nd week of gestation, canalization of the uterine cavity, cervix and vagina is completed. Smooth muscle cells and uterine stroma will originate from the mesenchymal tissue underneath the epithelium. By 20th week, uterine mucosa has differentiated into the endometrium. Endometrium, one of the most complex tissues of the human body is essential for reproduction. Endometrium is cyclically changing in response to estrogen and progesterone of the ovulatory menstrual cycle and to a complex interaction among its own autocrine and paracrine factors.

Functional Anatomy of Male Reproductive Organs

Male reproductive organs consist of: (a) testes, (b) epididymis, (c) vas deferens, (d) ampulla of vas, (e) seminal vesicles, (f) prostate, (g) Cowper's and urethral glands, (h) penis (Figure 1.9).

Testes

Human testes is ovoid in shape and is located within the scrotal sac. The length and weight are approximately 4.5 cm and 34 to 45 gm respectively. The reproductive components within the testes are: (a) Leydig cells, (b) seminiferous tubules, (c) Sertoli cells.

Leydig cells are found in clusters and form about 5 to 15 percent of the total volume of testes. They lie outside the lumen of seminiferous tubules and are the source of androgen production. The number of Leydig cells in both testes in a 20-year-old male is 700 million and diminishes by one-half by the age of 60.

Seminiferous Tubules

Seminiferous tubules are the sites of spermatogenesis. They are long, loop-like convoluted ducts with both ends terminating in the rete testes. The number of seminiferous tubules is 600 to 1200 with an estimated total length of 250 m.[12] Spermatozoa and fluid originating in the tubules are transported to the rete testes and then to the epididymis. Rete testes acts as a valve that controls the flow.[13]

Sertoli Cells

Sertoli cells line the inner aspect of the basement membrane of seminiferous tubules. The germinal cells are arranged and scattered inbetween the Sertoli cells. The undifferentiated spermatogonia are located near the basement membrane, and the more advanced forms are arranged successively at higher levels of Sertoli cells

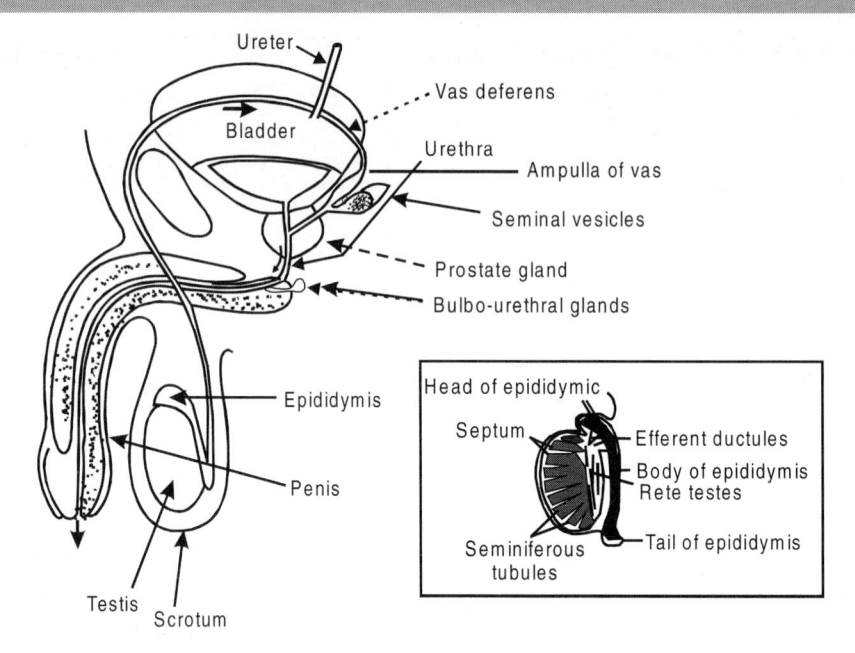

Figure 1.9: Male reproductive organs and tract

near the tubular lumen. Sertoli cells are more than nursing cells to the adjacent germinal cell. The adjacent Sertoli cells are joined to one another by inter-Sertoli 'tight' junctions. Sertoli-cell 'tight' junctions subdivide the seminiferous tubules longitudinally into basal and adluminal compartments. These tight junctions of the adjacent Sertoli cells form an impermeable "blood testes" barrier. Germ cells develop upto the stage of primary spermatocytes within the basal compartment which has free access to the extratubular environment. Secondary spermatocytes continue their development in the adluminal compartment. Because of the blood-testes barrier, any factor influencing the latter stages of spermatogenesis must be mediated through the Sertoli cells.

Epididymis

Epididymis is an elongated structure which extends from cranial to caudal pole of testes. It begins from efferent ducts and continues upto vas deferens. The epididymis consists of three parts: caput, corpus and cauda. Coiled efferent ducts emerge from the rete testes and constitute most of the caput epididymis. The length of epididymis has been measured to be 5-6 m. Epididymis synthesizes certain compounds that are secreted into the lumen of the canal. These include protein, carnitine, lipids, glycerophosphoryl choline (GPC), carbohydrates, steroids and other small molecules. Carnitine is an epididymal marker and helps in preserving sperm viability and stimulating motility after ejaculation.

Vas deferens

Vas deferens is a tube, 35 to 45 cm long with a diameter of 0.85 ± 0.7 mm. It extends from the tail of the epididymis, runs along the medial side of the spermatic cord, through the inguinal canal and ends in a glandular enlargement on the medial side of the seminal vesicle. This terminal glandular enlarged portion is known as ampulla of vas. Ampulla of the vas finally fuses with the neck of the seminal vesicle to form the ejaculatory duct. Ejaculatory duct passes through the prostate and opens into the floor of prostatic urethra at the level of verumontanum. Ampulla of vas helps in continuous maturation process of spermatozoa which has started in the epididymis.

Prostate

Prostate is the largest accessory male sex gland. In young and middle aged adults, the gland is 3 to 4 cm in diameter and approximately 20 gm in weight. The two ejaculatory ducts pierce the prostate obliquely and pass into the interior of the gland. Within the prostate, they converge, decrease in diameter and terminate in the floor of the prostatic urethra, in the region known as verumontanum.

Prostate fluid accounts for 15-30 percent of the total ejaculate volume. Prostatic fluid contains a number of constituents of which acid phosphatase, plasminogen activator, seminin, zinc, magnesium and calcium are significant. Plasminogen activator and seminin cause lysis of seminal clot. Acid phosphatase can be used as prostatic marker.

Seminal Vesicles

Seminal vesicles are paired, highly convoluted pyriform glands. Each vesicle is 5-6 cm long and 1-2 cm wide. They lie lateral to ampulla of vas deferens, posterior to urinary bladder and superior to prostate. About 70 percent ejaculate originate in seminal vesicles.

Of the various secretion of seminal vesicles, fructose and prostaglandins are important. Though constituents of seminal plasma are not absolutely essential for fertilization, the secretion may optimize conditions for sperm motility, survival and transport in both the seminal pathway and the female reproductive tract.

Cowper's (Bulbourethral) and Urethral Glands

Cowper's glands are paired bodies 3-5 mm in diameter which are homologous to Bartholin's glands in the female. They secrete droplets of mucin which help in urethral lubrication. Scattered accessory glands can be found throughout the male reproductive tract.

Penis

Penis is composed of three cylindrical masses of erectile cavernous tissue, blood vessels, lymph and nerves. The erectile tissue within the penis is a labyrinth of irregular blood sinus and spaces. Male sexual function consists of: (a) erection: this is both reflexogenic and psychogenic, (b) accessory glandular secretion and seminal emission and (c) ejaculation.

KEY POINTS

- The male and female reproductive organs predominantly develop from wolffian (mesonephric) and mullerian (paramesonephric) ducts. Lower part of urogenital sinus contributes to the development of membranous part of urethra in male and in female, the vestibule and perhaps the lower part of vagina.
- The development of male reproductive accessory organs, viz. epididymis, vas deferens, seminal vesicles and prostate will require the presence of testosterone and antimullerian hormone synthesized and released by testes.
- Whereas the female reproductive organs will develop in the absence of Y-chromosome, a functional testes and antimullerian hormone.
- Internal genital organs have the intrinsic tendency to feminize. Positive influence of ovarian hormones is not essential.
- The accessory male sex organ secretions through their biochemical constituents enhance the fertilizing potential of spermatozoa.

EVENTS LEADING TO RELEASE OF GAMETES, THEIR TRANSPORT, FUSION AND FERTILIZATION, CLEAVAGE AND IMPLANTATION

Egg Release and Transport

Prior to ovulation, the oocyte completes its first meiotic division under the influence of midcycle 'surge' of LH. Thereafter, it enters into second meiotic division and is arrested at second metaphase. The dominant follicle gradually moves up to the surface of the ovary. After follicular rupture, the ovum is picked up by fimbriated end of the fallopian tube by sweeping movement. Entry into the tube is facilitated by muscular movements that bring the fimbriae into contact with the surface of the ovary. Variations in the method of ovum pick up surely exist, because women may achieve pregnancy even with one ovary and a single tube located on contralateral side. Furthermore, pregnancies have been recorded following direct intraperitoneal insemination (DIPI).[14]

Egg and subsequently, zygote and embryo transport involves the time that elapses from ovulation up to the time of entry of compacted morula into the uterus. The egg is fertilized in the ampulla of the fallopian tube.

The epithelium of fallopian tube consists of two types of cells—ciliated and non-ciliated. They undergo cyclic changes of the menstrual cycle.[15] The non-ciliated cells secrete cytoplasmic components during passage of the egg or embryo providing important metabolic factors for transport and implantation. Ciliary movement and tubal muscular contractions are both involved for transport of egg from ampulla toward the uterus.

Following ovulation, the egg is inside the ampulla within 2-3 minutes. The transport time from ampulla to uterus for the fertilized oocyte is approximately 3 days. In human, 80 percent of this time, period are spent in the ampulla (Figure 1.10).

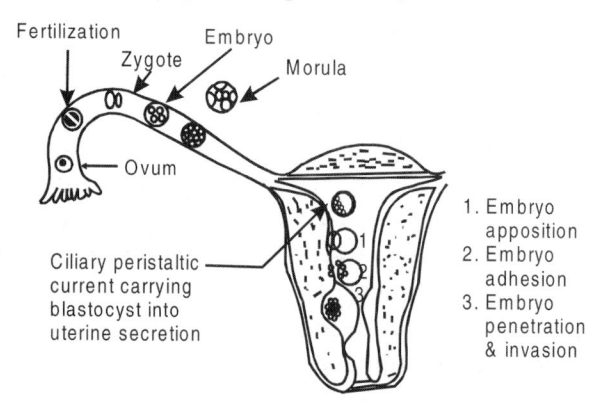

Figure 1.10: Gamete transport, fertilization cleavage, implantation

In most species, the fallopian tube appears to be essential for full development of embryos, because uterine fluid during the first 48 hours following ovulation remains toxic to the egg. In humans also, if the endometrium is in the reduced or advanced stage of development compared with the developmental stage of the fertilized egg, implantation may fail. This may not be always true. Because, pregnancies have been recorded following Estes operation where the eggs are ovulated directly inside the uterine cavity. Moreover, when fertilized donor eggs are transferred to women, who are receiving hormone supplementation, a larger implantation window is created in the endometrium when the blastocyst will implant. Hence, a perfect synchrony between the incoming embryo and developing endometrium is not absolutely essential.

Sperm Release and Transport

The sperms reach caudal epididymis approximately 72 days after initiation of spermatogenesis. The caudal epididymis is the storehouse of the sperms, which should be available for ejaculation. Semen coagulates immediately following ejaculation. But this is liquefied in 20 to 30 minutes following ejaculation by an enzyme derived from prostate gland. Most of the sperms become immotile in the acid pH of vaginal secretion. The alkaline pH of semen offers some transient protection for the spermatozoa to survive but majority of sperms are immobilized within 2 hours. The more active sperms by their own motility enter into the cervical canal and then into the uterine cavity. It is generally believed that cervical mucus has a filtering action. Sperm antibodies on the sperm head interacts with cervical mucus and inhibits sperm motility and entry into uterine cavity. Similarly, less active sperms are unable to swim up into the uterine cavity. The number of active sperms remaining within the cervical mucus remains constant for 24 hours and after 48 hours only few sperms are left behind in the cervical canal.[16] In many animals isthmus of the fallopian tube is believed to be the storehouse of sperms but in humans, cervical mucus rather than fallopian tube seems to be the reservoir of sperms.[17] Approximately 80 to 100 million sperms are deposited in the vagina and out of these, only a few are able to achieve proximity of the egg in the ampulla.[17] Majority of sperms are lost in the vagina either by enzymatic digestion or by phagocytosis.

In the uterus and in the fallopian tube, the sperms acquire two very important functions, viz. capacitation and hyperactivated motility.

Capacitation and Hyperactivation

While in the female genital tract (cervix, uterus or in the fallopian tube) the sperms undergo some physiobiochemical modifications which is called "Capacitation".[18] Capacitation involves removal of seminal plasma factors coating the surface of the sperm, and modification of some biochemical properties of the sperm head membrane. Capacitation will help in acrosome reaction and acquisition of hypermotility; further requirements for sperm penetration through cumulus cells and zona pellucida; the outer vestments surrounding the oocyte.

Preparatory Changes in Gametes before Fertilization

Further Sperm Maturation (Acrosome Reaction)

The fusion of plasma membrane with outer acrosomal layer followed by breakdown of the membranes to allow escape of acrosome cap contents is known as 'acrosome reaction'.[19] Sperm capacitation is a prerequisite change for acrosome reaction. While passing through cumulus the sperms do not release acrosin.[20] The acrosome cap contains enzymes—the important ones are hyaluronidase and acrosin. Hyaluronidase digests the cumulus cells (Figure 1.11) and acrosin helps penetration of zona pellucida. Sperm hypermotility induced by capacitation is also an essential step for rapid sperm entry through zona pellucida.

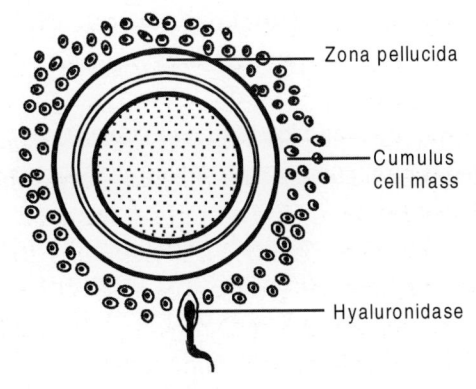

Figure 1.11: Sperm penetration through cumulus matrix

Further Oocyte Maturation

Apart from meiotic divisions of the oocytes, there is an influx of extracellular calcium in response to estradiol which improves the chances of fertilization. This is followed by secondary rise in calcium ions from intracellular stores. This is characterized by wavelike oscillations within the ooplasm.[21] This transient increase in intracellular calcium, which is estrogen dependant, improves quality of oocyte and increases the chances of fertilization. These events are not related to oocyte meiosis. However, improved fertilization following estradiol induced calcium increases indicates the important role of intrafollicular estradiol for overall oocyte maturation.

Fertilization

Fertilizable life span of oocyte ranges between 12 and 24 hours. Similarly, fertilizable life period of the spermatozoa ranges between 48 and 72 hours. Majority of pregnancies occur when coitus takes place within 3 days prior to ovulation.[22] The process of fertilization consists of series of events occurring in both sperms and eggs. Contact of a single sperm with egg is due to chemotactic activity exerted by the egg on the sperm (Figure 1.12).

Events in Sperm-egg Interaction

There are three types of glycoproteins in zona pellucida. These are known as ZP_1, ZP_2 and ZP_3 of which ZP_3 is most abundant.[23] ZP_3 is the primary ligand for the sperm and ZP_2 is responsible for zona reaction following sperm penetration to prevent polyspermy. Penetration through

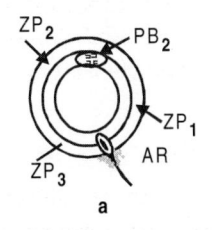

a
- Acrosome reaction (AR)
- Sperm entering through zona pellucida (ZP_3)

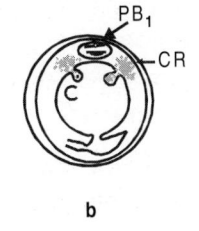

b
- Sperm oelema fusion
- Cortical granules (C)
- Cortical reaction (CR)

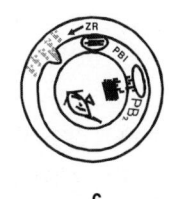

c
- Nuclear decondensation
- Extrusion of 2nd polar body (PB_2)
- Zona reaction (ZR)

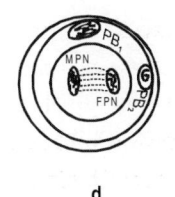

d
- Pronucleus formation (male, MPN; female, FPN)
- Limiting membrane breaks down
- Exchange of chromosomes. (Syngamy)

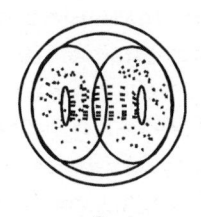

e
- Organised for cell division by mitosis and formation of zygote

Figure 1.12: Events at fertilization

the zona is rapid and mediated by acrosin, a trypsin like proteinase.[24]

Spermatozoa enters perivitelline space at an angle. Then there is binding between inner acrosomal membrane of the sperm head and oelema (the outer membrane of ooplasm). This induces cortical and zona reactions which prevent entry of further spermatozoa into the oocyte, thereby blocking polyspermy.

Pronucleus Formation-syngamy-embryonic Cleavage

Approximately, 3 hours after entry of sperm head in the oocyte, the second meiotic division is completed and the second polar body is released with a haploid complement of chromosomes. The remaining haploid number of chromosomes in the oocyte will form the female pronucleus. The nucleus of the sperm head undergoes decondensation and the male pronucleus is formed. The male and female pronuclei migrate toward each other. When they come in close proximity, the limiting membranes break down. There is exchange of chromosome material between the male and female pronucleus. The process is known as syngamy. A spindle is formed on which chromosomes become arranged. The stage for first mitotic cell division has now been organized and with first cell division a zygote is formed. Embryonic-genomic activity starts between 4 to 8 cell stages of cleavage, 2-3 days after fertilization.[25] Normal embryonic-genomic activity will now control further cell division into morula and blastocyst.

Preimplantation Preparatory Changes

Prior to implantation both incoming embryo and developing endometrium and incoming embryo undergo some preparatory changes.

Endometrial Preparation for Implantation

Endometrial preparation for implantation involves: (a) histologic changes, (b) synthesis of PGE_2 and (c) production of many cytokines, peptides, and lipids.

Preparatory histologic changes in the endometrium: After ovulation, the endometrial growth is under the influence of estrogen and progesterone. The striking feature is that height of endometrial growth is fixed initially at its preovulatory extent inspite of continued availability of estrogen. Epithelial proliferation is inhibited and this is brought about by progesterone. Though epithelial proliferation is restricted, the growth of individual components of the endometrium continued by edema and swelling under the influence of progesterone and prostaglandins. But confinement in a fixed structure leads to progressive tortuosity of glands and coiling of spiral vessels. Subnuclear vacuoles appear in the cells lining the glands. They contain glycogen and mucin. The cells being distended finally rupture pouring their contents into the gland lumen. Stroma becomes increasingly edematous and spiral vessels are prominent and densely coiled. By day 3 post-ovulation, the endometrium by these secretory changes is differentiated into three distinct zones viz., the innermost zone known as stratum basalis (less than twenty-five percent thickness; not affected by hormones); the stratum spongiosum, the middle zone of the endometrium (comprising at least 50 % of thickness) and stratum compactum, the outer layer (about 25% of the thickness). At the time of implantation the main endometrial change is stromal edema with increased vascularity induced by estrogen-progesterone and increase in prostaglandin production (mainly PGE_2) by the endometrium.

The 'window' of endometrial implantation is restricted to days 16-22 of 28 day normal cycle and day 16-19 of cycles stimulated with exogenous gonadotropins.[26, 27]

During the peak secretory phase of endometrium 'pinopodes' form on the surface epithelium. Pinpodes form as a result of cystic change in the surface epithelial microvilli. Pinpodes serve to absorb uterine fluid from the uterine cavity forcing the blastocyst to be in contact with the endometrial epithelium.

Origin and role of prostaglandins in the endometrial preparatory process:

Apart from estrogen-progesterone stimulation, prostaglandin synthesis at the implantation site increases in response to blastocyst factors like platelet activating factor (PAF). The increase in prostaglandin concentration involves prostaglandin E_2 component and not $PGF_2-\infty$. While PGE_2 is essential at the implantation site, decidual synthesis of prostaglandin in general is reduced, apparently a direct effect of progesterone and perhaps a requirement in order to maintain pregnancy.[28]

Role of endometrial cytokines and growth factors in the process of implantation:
Numerous members in the cytokine family and various growth factors have been identified in all tissues associated with implantation. They are believed to be the biochemical vehicles through which the physical process of embryonic apposition, adhesion, penetration and trophoblastic invasion are completed. Of various types of molecules (proteins) identified, some will help in adhesion (adhesive molecules), others will prevent adhesion (e.g. some members in the family of cytokines, e.g. human IL-1 receptor antagonists). Antiadhesive molecules are commonly found on tubal epithelium. If they are deficient in tubal epithelium, ectopic pregnancy might result.

The important adhesion molecules include integrin, immunoglobulin superfamily, selection and caderhins—which are expressed on epithelial cell surface and help in attachment and adhesion of the embryo. Basement membrane and matrix substrates include collagen, fibronectin, laminin, enactin and tenascin which help to guide the trophoblast through basement membrane and stromal matrix for anchorage on maternal decidua.

Embryonic Preparation for Implantation and Preimplantation Signals

Signals: Embryo while still in the fallopian tube signals to the mother as it prepares for implantation. In response to this signal, mother produces early pregnancy factor (EPF).[29] EPF has immunosuppressive property and is associated with cell proliferation and growth.

After reaching the uterine cavity in the compacted morula or blastocyst stage, the embryo produces βhCG which is essential for embryo hatching and embryonic implantation. hCG liberated by the embryo (even before implantation) will signal the corpus luteum to secrete higher level of estradiol and progesterone which can be detected in the maternal serum.[30] Function of corpus luteum is essential for endometrial bed preparation, implantation and maintenance of pregnancy daring the first 9 to 10 weeks of gestation.

Embryo Hatching

A prerequisite change for the embryo is embryo hatching. After its entry into the uterine cavity in the morula (16 to 64 cells) or blastocyst stage (30 to 200 cells), it remains in the uterine cavity for 2-4 days still encapsulated by zona pellucida. Zona must be lysed before the embryo can attach to the maternal decidua. Lysis of zona and escape of embryo is known as zona hatching. Zona hatching is accomplished by components of uterine fluid as well as by blastocyst movement. By this time, blastocyst has differentiated into inner cell mass (embryo) at one pole and trophectoderm (placenta) at the other pole with a cystic cavity (blastocele) inbetween. Zona pellucida becomes thin and ultimately disrupts through which the inner cell mass wriggles out to differentiate into three primitive layers of future fetus, namely ectoderm, mesoderm and endoderm. Initially, primitive embryonic plate is bilaminar consisting of ectoderm and endoderm. After certain period of growth, a third layer, mesoderm originating from ectoderm insinuates between ectoderm and endoderm so that embryonic plate now becomes trilaminar. All tissues and organs of the growing fetus will develop from these three layers. Trophoectoderm and inner cell mass are essential for implantation. Even if the endometrial preparation is adequate for implantation, this may not occur if the embryo is not at the proper stage of development. This disparity is often observed in *in vitro* fertilization procedure when there is a risk of failure of zona hatching after the embryo has been transferred into the uterine cavity. In *in vitro* procedure the zona may become hard because of its exposure to culture medium. However, under favourable circumstances, the process of implantation starts with embryo-endometrial contact.

Implantation

Implantation occurs in four stages: apposition, adhesion penetration and invasion (Figure 1.13).

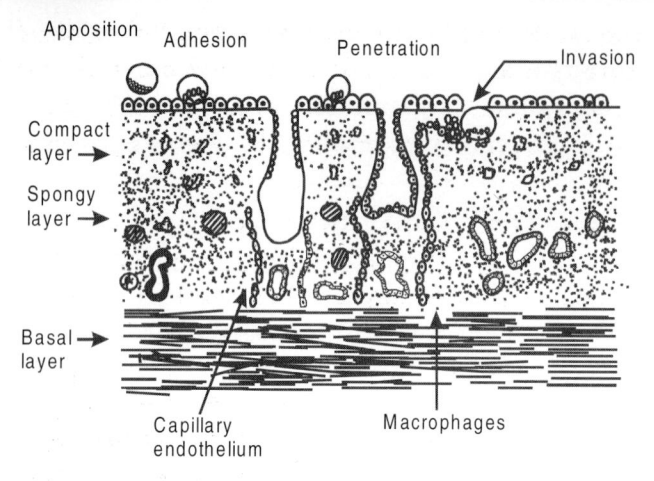

Figure 1.13: Different phases of embryonic implantation

Embryo-Endometrial Contact

Apposition and adhesion: As the blastocyst comes into close contact with the endometrium, the microvilli on the surface of the trophectoderm will interdigitate with those on the luminal surface of the decidual epithelial cells. At this stage, the cell membranes are in close contact and junctional complexes have been formed. Thereafter the early embryo cannot be easily dislodged.

Penetration and invasion (anchorage and placentation): Trophoblast is invasive in nature. The early embryo secretes a variety of enzymes (e.g. collagenase and plasminogen activators) and these are important for digesting the intracellular matrix that holds the decidual cells together. This highly proliferative phase of trophoblast in early embryogenesis is regulated by many growth factors and cytokines produced in both fetal and maternal tissues. This is essential for effective anchorage and at the same time limiting the extent of trophoblastic invasion of maternal decidual tissue. Invasion requires the expression of integrins stimulated by insulin like growth factor II and inhibited by transforming growth factor-2.[31]

The trophoblast differentiates into two layers—cytotrophoblast (the cellular layer) and the syncytiotrophoblast (the acellular layer). Cytotrophoblast invades the uterine spiral anterioles and allows the maternal blood to enter into the decidual lacunae created by trophoblastic invasion. These lacunae are built up by cytotrophoblastic cells which remain in contact and constantly bathed by maternal blood for fetal nutrition and exchange of gaseous materials.

Penetration of the maternal decidua will depend on factors which are capable of suppressing the maternal immune response to paternal antigens. The endometrial tissue is responsible for immune suppression by synthesizing proteins in response to the blastocyst even before implantation.[32] Usually the genetically abnormal embryos are rejected by the decidua. It may be possible that the abnormal embryo cannot produce a signal in early pregnancy that can be recognized by the mother.

KEY POINTS

- The spermatozoon travels a long way before meeting the oocyte for fertilization. The biochemical constituents of the male accessory sex gland secretions supply the energy during transport, while the significant transformation for final fertilization will be completed in the female genital tract by capacitation and hyperactivation. Intracellular calcium influx will add to fertilizing potential of the oocyte.
- Capacitated sperm undergoes acrosome reaction which induces sperm-ovum interaction.
- Following zona penetration, there is zona reaction which blocks polyspermy.
- The oocyte completes the second meiotic division; and male and female pronuclei are formed.
- This is followed by syngamy and mitotic cleavage into a two-celled zygote.
- Zygote sends signals to maternal host who now prepares to receive the incoming embryo for implantation.
- Implantation occurs in 4 stages namely: attachment, adhesion, penetration and invasion. Apart from steroid hormones, endometrial cytokine family and growth factors play active role in helping and restricting trophoblastic proliferation and invasion.

CONCLUSION

The fundamentals of normal reproduction involves the fulfilment of three basic requirements. These are: availability of male and female gametes, anatomically and functionally competent reproductive organs of both the partners and the ability of the gametes to achieve biological competence for fertilization and implantation in the female genital tract. The gametes, originating as germ cells in the hind gut and yolk sac, migrate to the genital ridge (future gonad) to become either oocyte or spermatocyte. Genital ridge differentiates into ovary or testes in response to chromosomal complement of the embryo. For spermatocyte, the maturational changes are nearly completed within the testes as the diploid spermatogenia are reduced to haploid before leaving the testes. In case of oocytes the first meiotic division which starts in the intrauterine life remains arrested at prophase and is completed before ovulation. The maturational changes of gametes and their periodic release from testes and ovary are influenced by endocrine, autocrine and paracrine factors. DNA in the nucleus of the sperm head, centriole in the neck and release of mature haploid oocyte from the dominant follicle are the vital segments of gametes which are actively involved for successful fertilization.

Anatomically normal and physiologically active male and female reproductive organs are essential for further maturation and for accelerating fertilizing potential of the gametes. For this, sperm requires additional energy because it has to travel a long distance to penetrate the outer vestments of the oocyte, namely the cumulus matrix and zona pellucida. The additional energy is acquired by the sperm in different phases. As it travels through the seminal pathway in the male genital tract, sperm acquires motility and other biochemical back up from secretion of epididymis, vas deferens, seminal vesicles and prostate. In the female genital tract climax fertilizing potential of the sperm is completed by two very significant changes, namely capacitation and hyperactivation. Oocyte after ovulation, travels relatively a shorter distance before it reaches the sperm for sperm-ovum interaction. During this short journey, there is intracellular influx of calcium which accelerates its fertilizing potential.

The biological competence of gametes induces sperm-ovum interaction, fertilization, formation of pronucleus and cleavage into a two-celled zygote. Zygote sends signals to the maternal tissues which now prepare to receive the incoming embryo for implantation.

Implantation occurs in four stages, namely attachment, adhesion, penetration and anchorage. Besides endometrial bed preparation under the influence of steroid hormones and prostaglandins (PGE$_2$) the process of implantation is additionally controlled by various members of the endometrial cytokine family and growth factors. These cytokines and growth factors are the biochemical vehicles through which the various phases of embryonic adhesion, trophoblastic invasion and placentation are completed.

REFERENCES

1. Yoshinaga K, Hess DL, Hebdrucjt AG, Zamboni L: The development of the sexually indifferent gonad in the prosimian, Galago crassicaudatus. *Am J Anat* **181**: 89, 1998.
2. Baker TG: A quantitative and cytological study of germ cells in human ovaries. *Prac Roy Sec land* **158**: 417, 1963.
3. Motla PN, Makabe S, Nottola SA: The Ultrastructure of human reproduction, I. The natural history of the female germ cell: Origin, migration and differentiation inside the developing ovary. *Hum Reprod Update* **3**: 281, 1997.
4. Jost A, Vigier B, Prepia J, Perchellet JP: Studies on sex differentiation in mammals. *Recent Prac. Hormone Res* **29**: 1, 1973.
5. Gondos B, Bhiraleus P, Hobee C: Ultrastructural observation on germ cells in human fetal ovaries. *Am J Obstet Gynecol* **110**: 644, 1971.
6. Gondos B, Westergard L, Byskov A. Initiation of oogenesis in the human fetal ovary: Ultrastructural and squash preparation study. *Am J Obstet Gynecol* **155**: 189, 1986.
7. Thomas GB, Meweilly AS, Gibson F, Brooks AN: Effects of pituitary-gonadal suppression with a gonadotrophin-releasing hormone agonist on fetal gonadotrophin secretion, fetal gonadal development and maternal sternid secretion in the sheep. *J Endocrinal* **141**: 317, 1997.
8. Robinovici J, Jaffe RB: Development and Regulation of growth and differentiated function of human and subhuman primate fetal gonads. *Endocr Rev* **11**: 532, 1990.
9. Gougeon A: Dynamics of follicular growth in the human: A model from preliminary results. *Hum Reprod* **1**: 81, 1986.
10. Clermont Y, Antar M: Duration of the cycle of the seminiferous epithelium and the spermatogonial renewal in the monkey Macca Auctoides. *Am J Anat* **136**: 153, 1973.
11. Acien P: Embryological observations on the female genital tract. *Hum Reprod* **7**: 437, 1992.
12. Lennox B, Ahmad KN: The total length of tubules in the human testes. *J Anat* **107**: 191, 1970.

13. Roosen-Runge EC, Holstein AF: The human rete testes. *Cell Tissue Res* **189:** 409, 1987.
14. Sharma V, Mason B, Riddle A, Campbell S: Peritoneal oocyte and sperm transfer. *Filth World Congress on in vitro Fertilisation and Embryo Transfer*, Norfolk, Virginia, 1987.
15. Crow J. Amso NN, Lewin J, Shaw RW: Morphology and Ultrastructure of fallopian tube epithelium at different stages of the menstrual cycle and menopause. *Hum Reprod* **9:** 2224, 1994.
16. Perloff WH, Steinberger E: *In vivo* survival of spermatozoa in cervical mucus. *Am J Obstet Gynecol* **88:** 439, 1964.
17. Williams M, Hill CJ, Seudamore I, Denphy B, Cooke ID, Barratt CLR: Sperm numbers and distribution within the human fallopian tube around ovulation. *Human Reprod* **8:** 2019, 1993.
18. Chang MC: Fertilising capacity of spermatozoa deposited into the fallopian tubes. *Nature* **168:** 696, 1951.
19. Yanagimachi R: Capacitation and the acrosome reaction. In Asch R Balmaceda JP, Johnston I (Eds): *Gamete Physiology, Seronosymposia*, Norewell, Massachusets, 31, 1990.
20. Talbot P: Sperm penetration through oocytes investments in mammals. *Am J Anat* **174:** 331, 1985.
21. Tasarik J, Mendoza C: Nongenomic effects of 17-β-estradiol on maturing human oocytes: Relationship to oocytes developmental potential. *J Clin Endocrinol Metab* **1438:** 80, 1995.
22. Wilcox AJ, Weinberg CR, Baird DD: Timing of sexual intercourse in relation to ovulation in the probability of conception, survival of the pregnancy and sex of the baby. *New Engl J Med* **833:** 1517, 1995.
23. Shabanowitz RB, Orand MG: Characterization of the human zona pellucida from fertilized and unfertilized eggs. *J Reprod Fertil* **82:** 151, 1988.
24. Zaneveld LJD, Polakoski KL, Williams WL: Properties of a proteolytic enzyme from rabbit sperm acrosome. *Biol Reprod* **6:** 30, 1972.
25. Brande P, Bolaton V, Moore S: Human gene expression first occurs between the four and eight cell stages of preimplantation development. *Nature* **332:** 459, 1988.
26. Rosenwaks Z: Donor eggs: their application in modern reproductive technologies. *Fertil Steril* **47:** 895, 1987.
27. Psychoyos A: Uterine receptivity for nidation. *Ann NY Acad Sci* **476:** 36m, 1986.
28. Vander Weiden RMF, Helmerhorst FM, Keirs: MJNC, Influence of prostaglandins and platelet activating factor on implantation. *Human Repord* **6:** 436, 1991.
29. Morton H, Raefe BE, Cavanagh AC: Early pregnancy factor, seminars. *Reprod Endocrinol* **10:** 72, 1992.
30. Stewart DR, Overstreet JW, Nakajima ST, Lasley BL: Enhanced ovarian sternit secretion before implantation in early human pregnancy. *J Clin Endocrinol Metab* **76:** 1470, 1993.
31. Irving JA, Tala PV: Functional role of cell surface integrins on human trophoblast cell migration: Regulation by TGF-β, IGF-II, and IGFBP-1. *Exp Cell Res* **217:** 419, 1995.
32. Clark DA, Slapsys RM, Croy BA, Kreck J, Rossant J: Local active suppression by suppressor cells in the deciduas: A review. *Am J Reprod Immunol* **6:** 78, 1984.

2.

Sambit Mukhopadhyay
Sabaratnam Arulkumaran

PART One

Anatomy of Female Reproductive Organs

Introduction

Sexual development depends initially on the arrangement of the sex chromosome. Normal men have XY chromosome complement and normal women have XX chromosome complement. Gonadal sex differentiation happens at the time of fertilization. Normally if two or more X chromosomes are present without Y chromosome ovaries develop in the embryo, there is a relationship between the differentiated gonad and the development of other genital organs. Briefly if testes form in the early embryo male genital organs develop. If the testes do not form the individual will form female genital organs whether ovaries are present or not. Therefore the sex chromosomes determine the nature of the gonads and these in turn determines the differentiation of the other genital organs. This basic principle of early development is important. It helps to understand the aberrations of function and anatomic abnormality.

OVARY

The primitive gonad is first evident in embryos of 5.5-7.5 mm crown rump length. Gonad is of triple origin from the celomic epithelium of the genital ridge, the underlying mesoderm and the primitive germ cells from extragenital source.

The size and the appearances of the ovaries depend on both age and the stage of menstrual cycle. In the young adult, they are almond shaped, solid and greyish pink in color; 3 cm long, 1.5 cm wide and about 1 cm thick. The ovary is the only intra-abdominal structure not to be covered by peritoneum. Each ovary is attached to the cornu of the uterus with ovarian ligament and at the hilum with broad ligament by the mesoovarium, which contains its supply of vessels and nerves. Laterally, each is attached to the pelvic wall by the infundibulopelvic ligament which is fold of peritoneum containing ovarian blood vessels from the abdominal aorta. The peritoneal fold becomes continuous with that over the psoas major.

Structure

The surface of the ovary is covered by a single layer of cuboidal cells known as the germinal epithelium. Beneath this is an ill-defined layer of thick connective tissue known as tunica albugenia. This increases in density with age. The inner medulla is vascular consisting of loose connective tissue containing many elastin fibers and non-striated muscle cells. There is no clear-cut demarcation between inner medulla and the outer cortex. Primordial follicles are mostly found in the cortex. The number of primordial follicles are maximum during intrauterine life and undergo steady state of atresia from 20 weeks of intrauterine life. With the onset of puberty primordial follicles form graafian follicles each month. Ovulation occurs with release of the ovum from a mature graafian follicle followed by formation of corpora lutea and ultimately atretic follicles, the corpora albicantes.

Embryological Remnants

The vestigial remnants of the mesonephric ducts and the tubules are often found in the adults. Clinically they can give rise to cyst formation and the patient can present with abdominal pain. The epoophoron, a series of parallel blind tubules, lie in the part of the broad ligament between the broad mesoovarium and the fallopian tube. The tubules run to rudimentary duct of epoophoron, which runs parallel to the fallopian tube. Occasionally rudimentary tubules called paroophoron can be seen between epoophoron and the uterus. In a few individuals the caudal part of the mesonephric duct is also well developed. This actually runs alongside the uterus upto the internal os. This structure is called Gartner's duct.

Blood Supply

The ovary is supplied by the ovarian artery. Ovarian artery is a branch of the abdominal aorta just below the renal artery. The vessel courses behind the peritoneum of the infracolic compartment and the colic vessels. It crosses the ureter obliquely before entering the pelvic brim. After crossing the pelvic brim it enters the suspensory ligament or more popularly known as the infundibulopelvic ligament at the lateral end of the broad ligament. It gives off a tubal branch, which runs parallel to the tube and anastomose with the uterine artery. The artery ends by entering into the ovary through the hilum of the ovary

The ovarian veins form a plexus in the mesoovarium. This plexus is equivalent to pampiniform plexus of the testes. The ovarian vein then enters the infundibulopelvic ligament and accompany the ovarian artery. The right ovarian vein drains into the inferior vena cava and the left into the left renal vein.

Lymph Drainage

The lymphatics of the ovary drain to the para-aortic nodes along side the origin of the ovarian artery.

Nerve Supply

Ovaries receive both sympathetic and parasympathetic innervations. Sympathetic is derived from the aortic plexus (T10 and 11). The parasympathetic is derived from the inferior hypogastric plexus via the uterine artery. Sensory nerve fibers accompany the sympathetic nerves and are referred around the umbilicus.

Changes with Age

During early fetal life the ovaries are situated in the lumbar region. They gradually descend into the lesser pelvis and during childhood they are small and situated near the pelvic brim. The ovary increases in size with the onset of puberty. Regular ovulation is established few years after menarche. The ovary atrophies after menopause. The fully involuted ovary of old age practically contains no germinal elements.

FALLOPIAN TUBE

The fallopian tubes are two oviducts originating at the cornu of the uterus. They are derived from the paramesonephric ducts. They run along the upper margin of the broad ligament and 10 cm in length. The abdominal opening is situated at the distal dilated portion of the tube known as infundibulum. This opening is fringed by a number of petals like processes, the fimbriae, one of which closely embraces the tubal end of the ovary. The fimbrial ends contain few smooth muscle fibers, which plays an important part in ovum pick-up. Medial to the infundibulum is the ampulla, which is thin walled and tortuous and comprises at least half the length of the tube. The medial third of the tube, the isthmus is relatively straight. The tube gets narrowed at this point and the final interstitial portion within the uterus is the narrowest.

Structure

The outer serosal layer consists of peritoneum and underlying areolar tissue. This covers the whole part of the tube apart from the fimbriae at one end and the interstitial portion at the other end. The middle muscular layer consists of inner circular and outer longitudinal fibers. The mucous membrane of the tube is the most delicate structure. The mucous membrane is thrown into several folds particularly near the fimbrial end. It is lined by columnar epithelium, much of which contains cilia. This ciliated columnar epithelium along with peristaltic action of the tube helps in transport of sperm and ovum. Secretory cells are also seen in the tubal mucous membrane.

UTERUS

The uterus is developed from fusion of the paramesonephric ducts at the midline.

In the non-pregnant state the uterus is situated entirely in the pelvis. It is a hollow inverted pear-shaped muscular organ. The maximal measurements are about 9 cm long, 6 cm wide and 4 cm thick. The upper part is known as body of the uterus. The area of insertion of the fallopian tube is known as cornu. The portion of the uterus above the cornu is known as fundus of the uterus. The uterus tapers to a small-constricted area known as isthmus. Inferiorly this is continuous with the cervix. The cervix projects obliquely into the vagina and can be divided into supravaginal and vaginal cervix (Figure 2.1).

The cavity of the uterus is actually in the shape of an inverted triangle. It is apposed anteroposteriorly. The cervix joins the uterus at the level of isthmus. This is known as anatomical internal os. Microscopically, the mucous membrane of the isthmus changes to that of the cervix at the level of histological internal os.

Structure

The uterus consists of three layers—the outer serous layers, the middle muscular layer and the inner mucous layer. The peritoneum covers the body of the uterus and posteriorly the supravaginal portion of the cervix. Anteriorly the peritoneum is reflected over the bladder creating the loose uterovesical fold of peritoneum. Laterally it spreads out to form the leaves of the broad ligament.

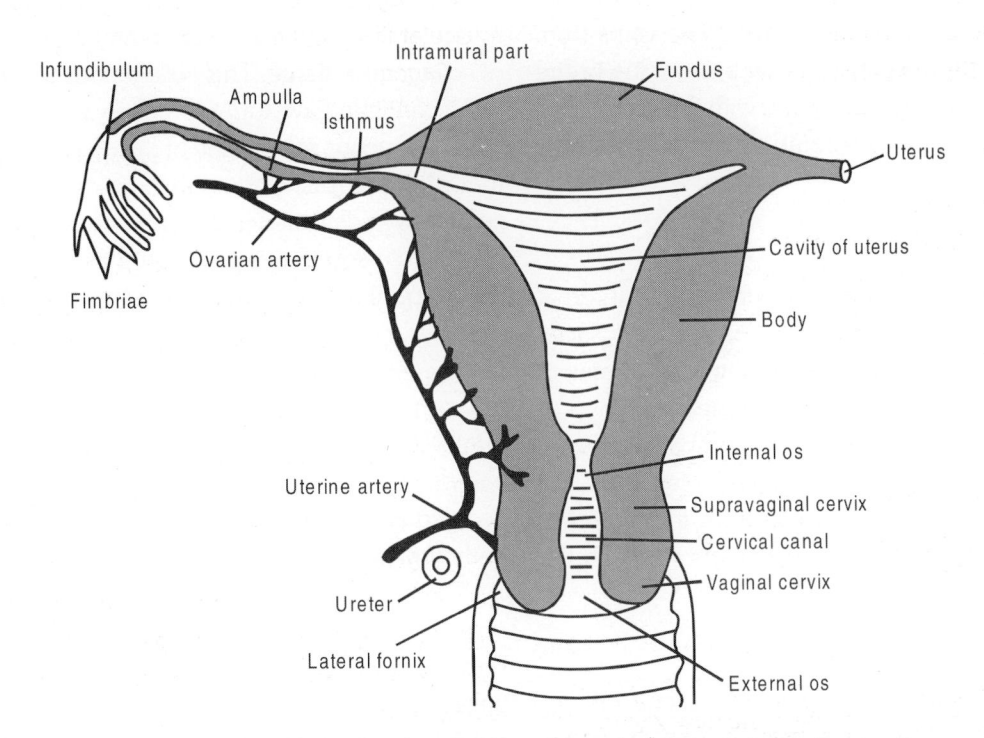

Figure 2.1: Different parts of the uterus, tube and cervix

The myometrium or the muscular layer contains outer longitudinal and oblique and inner longitudinal and circular fibers. They make up the main bulk of the uterus. The inner lining or the endometrium is not sharply separated from the myometrium. It is lined by a single layer of columnar epithelium. The stroma contains tubular glands, which often dip into the innermost muscle fibers. The endometrial lining is ciliated prior to puberty. The endometrium responds to gonadal steroids and undergoes cyclical histological changes during menstrual cycle. The thickness of the endometrium can vary from 2 to 10 mm.

Blood Supply of the Uterus and the Tube

The uterus is supplied by the uterine artery, a branch of the hypogastric artery. It passes medially across the pelvic floor in the base of the broad ligament, above the ureter. After reaching the lateral margin of supravaginal cervix it gives a branch to the cervix and the vagina and the vessel then turns upward alongside the uterus as far as the cornu. It gives off several branches, which penetrate the uterus and anastomose in the midline with the corresponding branches of the opposite artery. At the junction of the cornu the uterine artery anastomose with the tubal branch of the ovarian artery. The veins from the uterus often form a plexus in the base of the broad ligament. This plexus communicates with the vesical and the rectal plexus and finally drains into the internal iliac vein.

Lymphatic Drainage

Lymph from the cervix drains to external and internal iliac nodes and also to the sacral nodes via the uterosacral ligaments. The lower part of the uterine body drains to external iliac nodes. Lymphatics from the upper part of the body, the fundus and the tube accompany those of the ovaries to para-aortic lymph nodes. A few pass into the external iliac node and lymphs from the region of the cornu accompany the round ligament to reach the superficial inguinal lymph nodes.

Nerve Supply

The uterus is innervated from the branches of the inferior hypogastric plexus. The pain sensation from the cervix is carried by the pelvic splanchnic nerves, although sensation from the upper part of the cervix runs with the sympathetic nerves, as does the pain from the body of the uterus. The spinal cord segments concerned are T10–L1. In presacral neurectomy the hypogastric nerves are severed from the superior hypogastric plexus. It sometimes relieves dysmenorrhea but does not abolish the labor pains. Like any hollow viscera, distention cause pain but both the cervix and body of the uterus are relatively insensitive to cutting and burning; on the contrary the fallopian tube seems to be sensitive to diathermy and cutting.

CERVIX

The cervix is cylindrical in shape and 2-3 cm in length. It can be divided into supravaginal and the vaginal portion. The posterior aspect of the cervix is covered with the peritoneum of the pouch of Douglas. Anterior and lateral to the supravaginal cervix is parametrial tissue containing blood vessels and lymph nodes. The ureter runs very close to the cervix and is approximately 1-2 cm from the supravaginal cervix. The vaginal portion of the cervix projects inside the vagina to form the fornices.

The upper portion of the cervix contains some muscular fibers but the lower portion is mainly composed of collagenous tissue. This collagenous tissue undergoes significant changes during pregnancy and childbirth.

The mucous membrane of the cervix is different from that of the uterus. The epithelium of the endocervix is columnar and ciliated in the upper two-thirds. It changes to stratified squamous epithelium around the region of the external os. This change is abrupt or it may happen over a transitional area of 1 cm in width.

The long axis of the cervix is not in the same axis of the uterus. This is due to anteflexion or retroflexion. The uterus is flexed forward on itself at the isthmus, this is called anteflexion. Similarly when it is flexed backward it is called retroflexion. In most cases retroflexion is of no pathological significance.

The cervix is related to the bladder anteriorly and is separated from it by the uterovesical pouch of peritoneum. Posteriorly is the pouch of Douglas and coils of intestine, pelvic colon and the upper rectum. Laterally, the uterine artery and ureter are close to the supravaginal cervix.

Changes with Age

Before puberty the cervix is twice the length of the body of the uterus. After puberty the ratio reverses as the corpus grows much faster. After menopause the cervix and the uterus undergoes atrophy but is more marked in the cervix. The cervical lips often disappear and become flushed with the vault.

VAGINA

The vagina is derived partly from the fused mullerian ducts or the paramesonephric ducts and partly from the urogenital sinus (sinovaginal bulbs). It is a fibromuscular tube, which extends posterosuperiorly from the vestibule to the uterine cervix. It is longer in its posterior wall (9 cm) than anteriorly (7.5 cm). The vault of the vagina is divided into four fornices by the projection of the cervix. The posterior fornix is deeper. The lower portion of the vagina is H shaped in cross-section.

Anteriorly the upper vagina is in direct contact with the bladder base. The urethra is related to the lower half in the midline. The upper posterior vaginal walls form the anterior peritoneal reflection of the pouch of Douglas. The middle third is separated from rectum by pelvic fascia and the lower third is related to the perineal body.

Structure

The vagina is lined by stratified squamous epithelium. Vagina does not contain any glands but is lubricated by secretions from the cervix. The epithelium is thick and rich in glycogen. Lactobacilli break the glycogen in the vagina to form lactic acid. The pH of the vagina is around 4.5. This helps to protect against infection. The muscle layer consists of inner circular and outer longitudinal but these are not distinctly separate and are spirally arranged.

Hymen

The hymen is derived from the sinovaginal bulbs and therefore, epithelium of both surfaces of hymen is of urogenital sinus in origin. It has no known function but imperforate hymen can give rise to hematocolpos. Hymen is usually torn during first intercourse or during insertion of a tampon. It is certainly destroyed during vaginal delivery and only small tags remain. These are known as carunculae myritiformes.

Blood Supply

The vagina is supplied by the vaginal branch of the internal iliac artery. The uterine, middle rectal and inferior vesical vessels also supplement it. They freely anastomose in the vaginal walls. Veins drain to internal iliac vein (Figure 2.2, Plate 1).

Lymphatic Drainage

The lymphatics of the upper vagina, like those of the cervix drain into the external and internal iliac group of lymph nodes. The lymphatics from the lower vagina drain into the superficial inguinal nodes.

Changes with Age

The pH of the vagina changes with age. Few weeks after birth when maternal estrogens have cleared of the system, the pH rises to 7 and the epithelium atrophies. The situation reverses during puberty. The pH becomes acidic under the influence of estrogens and lactobacilli. At menopause the vagina tends to shrink and epithelium atrophies.

FEMALE EXTERNAL GENITALIA

Vulva

The female external genitalia commonly referred to as the vulva, include the mons pubis, labia majora, labia minora, clitoris, vestibule, bulb of the vestibule and greater vestibular glands. They are derived from the urogenital sinus. Developmentally the essential difference with the male anatomy is the failure of the midline fusion of the genital folds. The scrotum is represented by the labia majora, and the corpora spongiosum by the labia minora and the bulb of the vestibule with corresponding vessels and nerve.

Labia Majora

The labia majora are two prominent folds of skin with underlying adipose tissue. They contain numerous sebaceous glands. Anteriorly they fuse together over the symphysis pubis to form a mound called as mons pubis. Posteriorly they fuse at the perineum. From puberty onward, growth of pubic hair occurs at the lateral aspect of the labia majora and at the mons but the inner aspect remains smooth with numerous sweat glands.

Labia Minora

The labia minora are two small vascular folds of skin, containing sebaceous glands but devoid of any adipose tissue. Anteriorly they divide into two to form prepuce and frenulum of the clitoris. Posteriorly they fuse to form the fourchette. They are not well-developed before puberty and atrophies after menopause.

Clitoris

Clitoris is a small erectile structure homologous to penis but not containing the urethra. It is formed by two miniature corpora cavernosa without any corpus spongiosum. The two corpora cavernosa are attached to the pubic rami. Its free extremity, the *glans,* is highly sensitive to sexual stimuli and is usually overlapped by the prepuce.

Vestibule

Vestibule is the cleft between the labia minora and contains the external urethral meatus, the vaginal orifice and the ducts of greater vestibular (Bartholin's) glands. The vestibular bulbs are two masses of erectile tissue on either side of vaginal opening and contain rich plexus of veins within the bulbospongiosus muscle. The Bartholin's gland is the size of a pea and lies at the base of the each bulb. It opens to the vestibule through a small duct between the labia minora and the hymen. They produce copious amounts of mucus and help in lubrication particularly during sexual intercourse.

The lesser vestibular glands are very small mucous glands with minute openings between urethral and vaginal openings.

Blood Supply of the Vulva

Blood supply of the labial skin is from the superficial and deep pudendal arteries (from femoral arteries) and labial branches of the perineal artery (from internal pudendal). Clitoris is supplied by the dorsal artery of the clitoris, which is a branch of internal pudendal artery. Venous drainage is mainly by the external pudendal veins, superficial and deep, to the great saphenous vein.

Nerve Supply of the Vulva

The ilioinguinal nerves and the genital branch of genitofemoral nerves supply the anterior parts of the vulva. The posterior parts of the vulva are supplied by the perineal nerves and the posterior cutaneous nerves of the thigh.

Lymph Drainage

The skin of the vulva is drained into medial group of superficial inguinal lymph nodes.

KEY POINTS

- The ovarian arteries arise from the abdominal aorta. The right ovarian vein drains into the vena cava while the left usually drains into the left renal vein.
- The size and ratio of the cervix to uterus change with age and puberty.
- The ureter runs close (1.5 cm lateral) to the cervix, anterolateral to upper part of the vagina.

BIBLIOGRAPHY

1. Sinnatamby CS: Female internal genital organs. In Sinnatamby CS (Ed): *Last's Anatomy Regional and Applied.* Churchill Livingstone 293, 1999.
2. Vellacott I: Pelvic anatomy. In Shaw R, Soutter P, Stanton S (Eds): *Gynaecology.* Churchill Livingtone 23, 1992.

3. Anatomy of the Female Pelvis

Sambit Mukhopadhyay
Sabaratnam Arulkumaran

PART One — Introduction

BONY PELVIS

The pelvis is made up three bones. The two innominate bones and the sacrum. When articulated they enclose a cavity. The sacrum is wedged between the two innominate bones. Each innominate bone is made up of three parts—ilium, ischium and the pubis. The innominate bones are joined anteriorly at the symphysis pubis.

The pelvic brim is formed by the pubic crest, pectineal line of the pubis, arcuate line of the ilium, the alae of the sacrum and the promontory of the sacrum (Figure 3.1). The brim separates the false pelvis above from the true pelvis below. Inferiorly it is separated from the perinium by the urogenital diaphragm. The plane of the pelvis is at an angle of 55° with the horizontal. In an anatomical position the pelvic cavity projects backward from the pelvic brim. The upper border of the symphysis pubis, the ischial spines, tip of the coccyx, the head of the femur and the greater trochanter lie in the same plane. This can be reached by tip of the finger during vaginal examination.

Female pelvis differs from male pelvis. The basic differences are that female pelvis is broader than that of the male pelvis and the female pelvic bones including the neck of the femur are more slender than those of the male. The outline of the male pelvic brim is heart shaped and the brim is widest toward the back whereas in female pelvis the brim is transversely oval (widest further forward) due to less prominence of the sacral promontory. The female pelvis has evolutionally developed for childbirth; therefore, it is roomier. The outlet is also wider than the male pelvis. The subpubic angle in the male pelvis is acute like a Gothic arch whereas it is rounded like a Roman arch in a female pelvis.

The major obstetric interest in the bony pelvis is that it is not distensible; only minor degrees of movements are possible at the sacroiliac joints. Its dimensions are therefore critical at childbirth. The diameters of the pelvis vary at different parts of the pelvis. The normal diameters at different planes of the pelvis are as follows:

1. At the brim
   - Anteroposterior
     - 11.5 cm
   - Transverse
     - 13 cm
   - Oblique
     - 12 cm
2. Mid pelvis
   - All diameters
     - 12 cm
3. Outlet
   - Anteroposterior
     - 12 cm
   - Transverse (Bispinous)
     - 10.5 cm

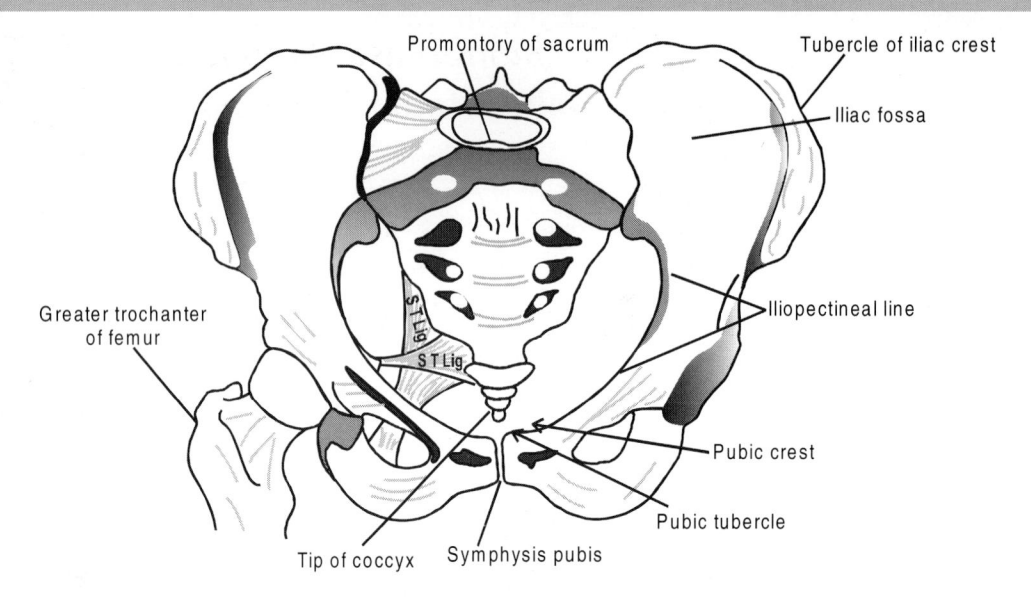

Figure 3.1: Female pelvis

However, it is the shape of the pelvis that determines the availability of pelvic diameters. There are four basic types:
- Gynaecoid type: The classical female pelvis the inlet transversely oval and roomier pelvic cavity
- Android type: The inlet is heart shaped. The cavity is funnel shaped with contracted outlet.
- Anthropoid type: It is due to high assimilation, i.e. the sacral body assimilated to the fifth lumbar vertebra. It is long narrow and oval in shape.
- Platypelloid type: This is a wide pelvis flattened at the brim with the promontory of the sacrum pushed forward.

Female pelvis contains the organs of reproduction, bladder and the rectum. Anatomy of the female reproductive organs is discussed in separate chapter and is therefore not repeated.

PELVIC WALLS

The inner aspect (cavity) of the pelvic bones is covered by muscles. Above the brim it is covered by iliacus and psoas. The sidewalls are clad with obturator internus and its fascia. The curved posterior wall is covered by the pyriformis, which courses laterally to the greater sciatic foramen. The levator ani and coccygeus with their opposite counterparts constitute the pelvic floor (Figure 3.2).

PYRIFORMIS

Pyriformis muscle is classed as muscle of the lower limb. It arises from the anterior aspect of the middle three pieces of the sacrum. It extends medially between the anterior sacral foramina. The sacral plexus and the nerves lie on the muscle. The muscle then traverses through the greater sciatic foramen and enters into the buttock where it converges into a tendon and is attached to the medial surface of the upper border of the greater trochanter. The pelvic surface of the muscle and the sacral nerve and plexus are covered with pelvic fascia, which is attached to the pelvic periosteum alongside the margin of the muscle.

OBTURATOR INTERNUS

The obturator foramen is covered with a membrane called the obturator membrane. A gap exists on the upper part of the membrane thereby converting the obturator notch into a canal for passage of obturator nerves and vessels. The obturator internus muscle takes origin from the whole membrane and from the adjacent bony margin of the foramen. The muscle takes its origin from the surface of the ischium near the greater sciatic notch and the falciform ridge of the ischial tuberosity. From its wide origin the muscle converges toward the lesser sciatic notch. It emerges through the lesser sciatic notch becomes tendinous and blends with superior and

ANATOMY OF THE FEMALE PELVIS

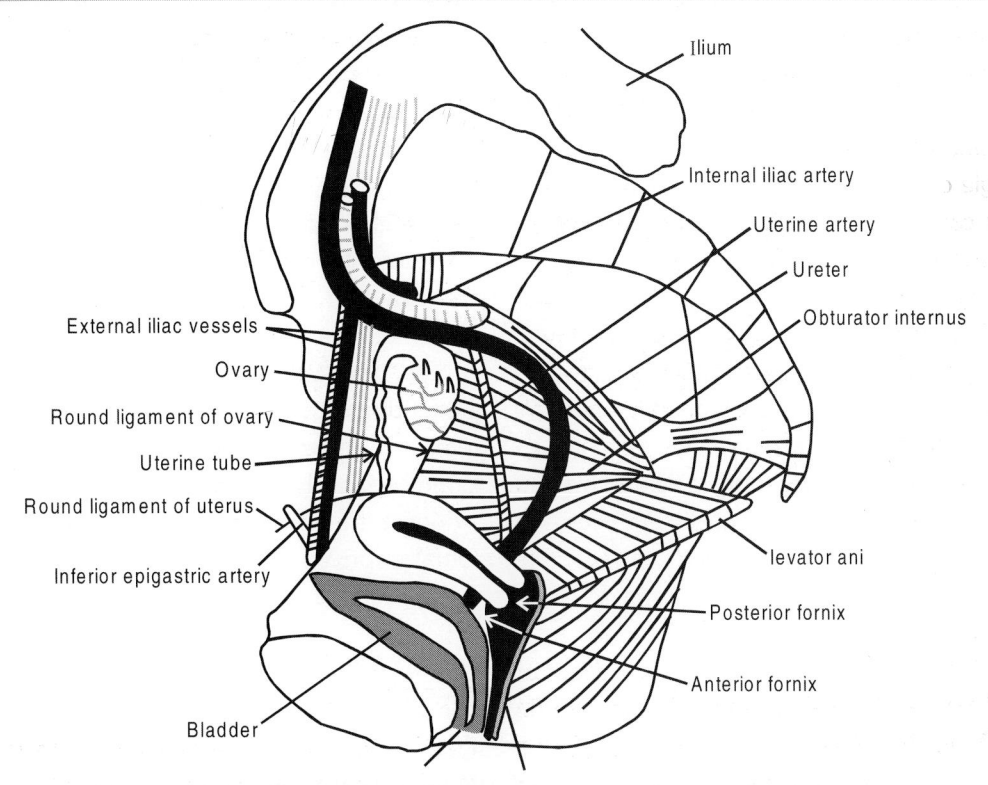

Figure 3.2: Sagittal section of the pelvis showing uterus in anteversion. Note the relationship of the ureter to the ovary and the uterine artery

inferior gamelli. It is then inserted to the medial surface of the greater trochanter above the trochanteric fossa. The muscle is covered with strong fascia called obturator fascia. This arises from the bony margin of the insertion of the muscle and fuses below with the falciform process of the sacrotuberous ligament on the ischial tuberosity. The levator ani (tendinous arch) slopes across this fascia.

Apart from major blood vessels the other most important structure in the pelvic wall is the ureter. The blood vessels are discussed under pelvic vessels. The ureter is described here.

URETER

The ureters are pair of tubes connecting the bladder and the kidneys. They are retroperitoneal and between 25 and 30 cm in length. Half of its course is in the abdomen over the psoas muscle the rest half is in the pelvis. Its diameter is around 3 mm and has three constrictions. These are at the pelviureteric junction, at the pelvic brim and as it passes through the bladder wall.

It passes down on the psoas muscle in front of the genitofemoral nerve and is crossed by the ovarian vessels. On the right, the upper part is behind the third part of the duodenum, while lower down it is crossed by the colic vessels and the root of the mesentery. On the left, it is lateral to the inferior mesenteric vessel and is crossed anteriorly by the left colic vessel and the apex of the sigmoid mesocolon.

The ureter enters the pelvis anterior to the sacroiliac joints and crosses the bifurcation of the common iliac artery (Figure 3.2). It adheres to the peritoneum of the posterior abdominal wall. It can be distinguished from blood vessels by its peristaltic action. It then passes along the posterior and lateral aspect of the pelvic wall, running in front of the internal iliac artery (and behind the ovary). In order from above downward it crosses the obturator nerve, superior vesical artery, obturator artery and vein. At the level of the ischial spines it turns forward and medially to enter the bladder. Here it lies at the base of the broad ligament where it is crossed above by the uterine artery. The ureter then traverses through the thick parametrial tissue and crosses the lateral vaginal fornix 1-2 cm from the cervix before entering into the bladder in front of the fornix. In the bladder it runs obliquely through the bladder wall for 1-2 cm before opening at the lateral angle of the trigone of the bladder.

The ureter can be damaged during gynaecological surgery at various points. It can be injured during clamping the infundibulopelvic vessels near the pelvic brim where it is adjacent to the ovarian vessels or lower during clamping of the uterine vessels where it is crossed by the uterine artery. The dangers are greater when the anatomy is distorted by fibroids or pelvic infection or endometriosis. Ischemic injury leading to fistula can also occur during extensive dissection particularly during pelvic lymphadenectomy.

PELVIC FLOOR

The pelvic floor is made up of gutter shaped sheet of muscles. It is higher posteriorly than anteriorly. The muscles of pelvic floor are the levator ani and the coccygeus and their covering fascia. They arise in continuity from the body of the pubis, from the tendinous arch over the obturator fascia and the ischial spines. They are inserted into the midline raphae or the anococcygeal raphae and the coccyx. The fibers slope downward and backward toward the midline from their origin, thereby producing a gutter, which slopes downward, and faces forward. It is incomplete anteriorly to allow for the passage of urethra and the vagina (Figure 3.3).

LEVATOR ANI

Levator ani consists of two main parts, iliococcygeus and pubococcygeus. In most mammals the levator ani arises from the pelvic brim but in human it has migrated down the sidewall of the pelvis from its original origin at the pelvic brim.

The *pubococcygeus* part of the levator ani arises from the anterior half of the tendinous arch and from the posterior surface of the body of the pubis. The bulk of the posterior fibers of the pubococcygeus are inserted into the tendinous plate or anococcygeal raphae in front of the coccyx. The fibers arising more anteriorly from the body of the pubis swing more medially and more inferiorly around the anorectal junction. It joins with the similar fibers of pubococcygeus of the opposite side and blends with the external anal sphincter. This part of the pubococcygeus is U shaped and is known as puborectalis sling of pubococcygeus. This helps to hold the anorectal junction forward. The most medial fibers pass backward along side the sphincter urethrae and insert into the perineal body. Some of the medial fibers are attached to the vaginal muscle and are called pubovaginalis.

The *iliococcygeus* arises from the posterior half of the tendinous arch and the pelvic surface of the ischial spines. It is inserted into the anococcygeal raphae and to the coccyx. The term iliococcygeus is a misnomer, as it does not arise from the ilium. However, the name is actually derived from its former origin on the iliac bone at the pelvic brim.

COCCYGEUS

Coccygeus arises from the tip of the ischial spine. Its fibers spread out and are attached to the side of the lowest piece of sacrum. Anteriorly it is overlapped by the iliococcygeus and posteriorly it lies edge to edge with the pyriformis. The gluteal surface has fibrous tendinous appearance and is known as the sacrotuberous ligament.

Nerve Supply

Branches of S3 and S4 from the sacral plexus mainly supply levator ani. Coccygeus is supplied by the perineal branches of S3 and S4.

PELVIC VESSELS

The thoracic aorta enters the abdomen between the crura of the diaphragm at the level of the 12th thoracic vertebra. The abdominal aorta then runs downward to the left of the midline along the front of the vertebral column and bifurcates at the level of the body of the fourth lumbar vertebra to right and left common iliac arteries. The inferior vena cava runs on its right. The lower part of the abdominal aorta give rise to several branches which supply pelvic organs. The ovarian and the inferior mesenteric artery arise from the front of the aorta while the median sacral and the lumbar artery arise from the dorsal aspect of the aorta.

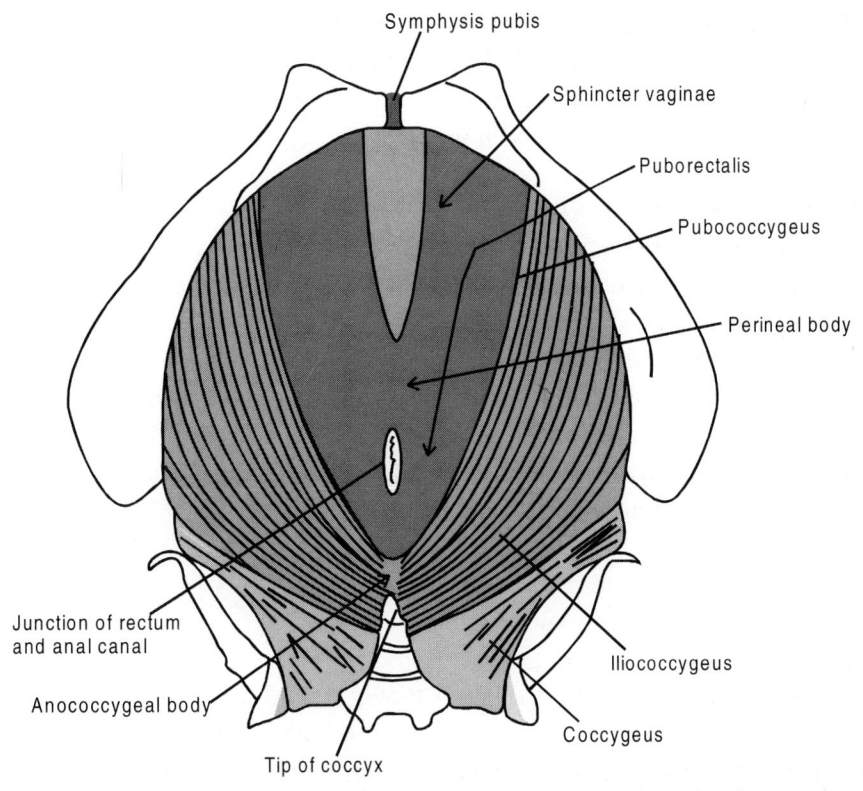

Figure 3.3: Muscles of the pelvic floor (as seen on their perineal aspect)

OVARIAN ARTERY

The ovarian arteries arise from the anterior aspect of the aorta just below the origin of the renal arteries. The right artery crosses the anterior surface of the vena cava, the lower part of the abdominal ureter and enters into the pelvis via the infundibulopelvic ligament. The left artery crosses the ureter after its origin and then courses lateral to it. It then crosses the bifurcation of the common iliac artery at the pelvic brim to enter the infundibulopelvic ligament. The ovarian arteries then divide into numerous branches supplying the ovaries and the fallopian tubes. Small branches also supply the ureter. A branch of ovarian artery supplies the cornu of the uterus and anastomoses with the branch of uterine artery.

The right ovarian vein drains into the inferior vena cava and the left usually into the left renal vein.

INFERIOR MESENTERIC ARTERY

The inferior mesenteric artery is the artery of the hindgut. It arises from the front of the aorta behind the behind the inferior border of the third part of the duodenum at the level of the L3 vertebra. It descends at first infront of the aorta and then left to it. It gives off the left colic and sigmoid arteries. It crosses the pelvic brim at the bifurcation of the left common iliac vessels over the sacroiliac joint, at which point it converges toward the ureter with inferior mesenteric vein lying in between them, at the apex of the ^-shaped attachment of the sigmoid mesocolon. The artery continues along the pelvic wall as superior rectal artery. It supplies the rectum and anastomoses with the middle and inferior rectal branches. Its anatomical relationship is of importance during para-aortic lymph node dissection as it can be severed. However, blood supply to the bowel is maintained as there exists anastomosis with the branches of the internal iliac arteries (inferior and middle rectal arteries).

COMMON ILIAC ARTERY

The common iliac arteries arise at the level of 4th lumbar vertebra from the bifurcation of the aorta. The bifurcation occurs to the left of the midline; therefore the right artery is longer than the left. It runs for a distance of 4-5 cm and again bifurcates into internal and external iliac arteries. This bifurcation takes place at the level of sacroiliac joints and the ureter lies in front of this bifurcation or very beginning of the external iliac. The left artery runs partly lateral and partly in front of the corresponding vein. The right artery runs in front of the lower most portion of the inferior vena cava and the terminations of two common iliac veins and then lateral to the right common iliac vein.

External Iliac Artery

The external iliac artery continues in the line of the common iliac artery along the pelvic brim over the psoas muscle and enters into the lower limb beneath the inguinal ligament. It lies in the femoral sheath beneath the inguinal ligament and is known as the femoral artery. It gives of two branches just above the inguinal ligament; they are inferior epigastric and deep circumflex iliac. The femoral artery gives off external pudendal artery, which supplies much of the skin of the vulva and anastomoses with the labial branches of the internal pudendal artery.

Internal Iliac Artery

The internal iliac artery and its branches mostly supply the pelvic organs and the walls. From the point of bifurcation of the common iliac artery at the level of the sacroiliac joint the internal iliac artery passes downward and divides into anterior and posterior division. The posterior division gives only parietal branches whereas the anterior division gives both parietal and visceral branches. The branches of the internal iliac artery are given in Table 3.1.

The internal pudendal artery descends anterior to the pyriformis and leaves the pelvis through the inferior aspect of the greater sciatic foramen below the pyriformis and crosses the gluteal aspect of the ischial spine and enters the perineum through the lesser sciatic foramen. It then runs in the pudendal canal accompanying the pudendal nerve about 4 cm above the ischial tuberosity. It then courses forward and divides into number of branches (Figure 3.2). The inferior rectal branch supplies the anus and anastomoses with the middle and superior rectal arteries. The perineal branch supplies much of the perineum and small branches supply the labia, vestibular bulbs and the vagina. The artery is continued as dorsal artery of the clitoris.

The inferior gluteal artery is the larger terminal trunk and runs backward through the pelvic fascia, passes below the S1 nerve root and leaves the pelvis through the greater sciatic foramen below the pyriformis and supplies much of the buttock and the back of the thigh.

Table 3.1: The branches of the internal iliac arteries

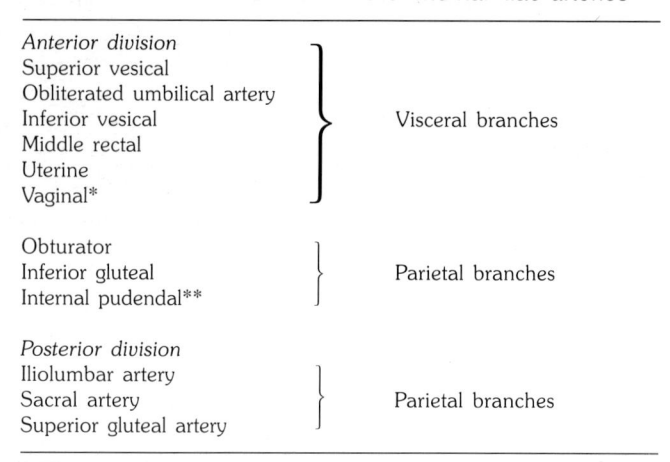

Anterior division Superior vesical Obliterated umbilical artery Inferior vesical Middle rectal Uterine Vaginal*	Visceral branches
Obturator Inferior gluteal Internal pudendal**	Parietal branches
Posterior division Iliolumbar artery Sacral artery Superior gluteal artery	Parietal branches

* The vaginal artery corresponds to the inferior vesical artery of the male. It supplies the upper part of the vagina. It may be a branch of the uterine artery.
**The internal pudendal and the inferior gluteal arteries are the terminal branches of the internal iliac.

PELVIC NERVES

Somatic Nerves

Lumbar Plexus

Lumbar plexus is formed within the substance of psoas muscle. It is formed by the anterior primary rami of the first three lumbar nerves and part of the fourth and a contribution from the 12th thoracic nerve (subcostal nerve). The plexus innervates part of the lower abdominal wall, but is chiefly concerned in supplying the muscle of the lower limb. Branches of the lumbar plexus are (Figure 3.4):

Iliohypogastric nerve and ilioinguinal nerve (L1): The former gives branches to the buttock while the latter supplies the skin of the mons pubis and the surrounding vulva.

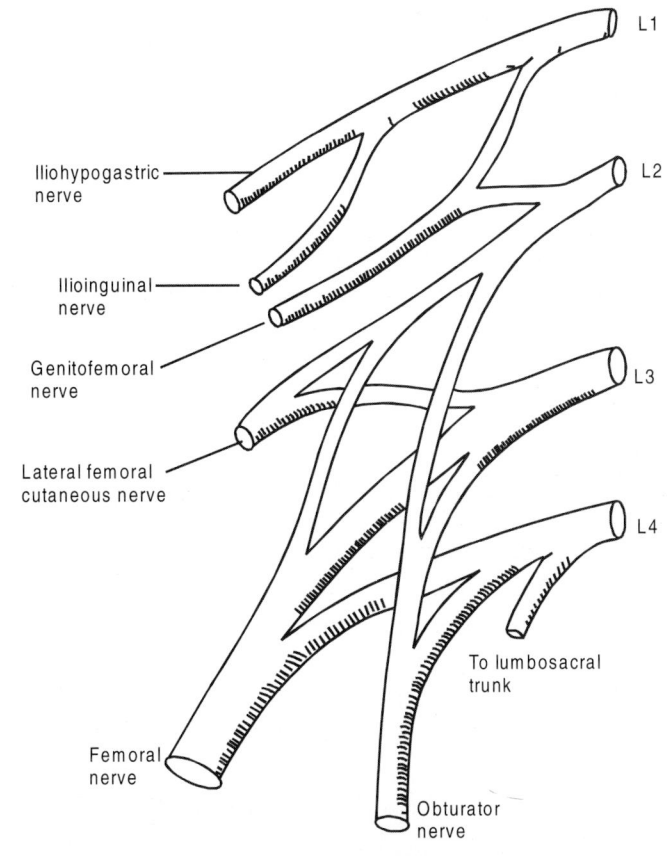

Figure 3.4: Lumbar plexus

Genitofemoral nerve (L1, 2): Femoral branch supplies the upper thigh and the genital branch supplies the skin of the labia majus.

Lateral femoral cutaneous nerve (L2, 3 posterior division): This nerve is purely sensory and supplies the peritoneum of the iliac fossa and to the lateral side of the thigh down to the knee.

Femoral nerve (L2, 3, 4 posterior division): This is the largest branch and descends in the groove between the psoas and iliacus muscle and enters the thigh deep to the inguinal ligament, lateral to the femoral sheath and supplies the flexors of the hip, extensors of the knee and numerous cutaneous branches including the saphenous nerve.

Obturator Nerve (L2, 3, 4 anterior division): The obturator nerve arises from the lumbar plexus and it lies within the substance of psoas major. It is formed from the anterior divisions of the anterior rami of second, third, fourth lumbar nerves. It is the nerve of the adductor compartment of the thigh. It reaches the adductor compartment by piercing the medial border of the psoas muscle and passing straight along the wall of the pelvis to the obturator foramen. It crosses the pelvic brim medial to the sacroiliac joint and in the ovarian fossa it is only separated from the normally situated ovary by the parietal peritoneum. Therefore pain from the ovary may be referred to the inner side of the thigh.

The obturator vessels converge into the obturator foramen with the nerve lying highest (Nerve Artery Vein—NAV) against the pubic bone. The nerve then divides in the foramen to anterior and posterior divisions. The posterior division pierces the obturator externus and descends vertically downward on the adductor magnus and supply the adductor compartment of the thigh. It also supplies the capsule of the knee joint. The anterior division supplies the obturator externus.

Sacral Plexus

Sacral plexus is formed out of the lumbosacral trunk (L4, 5) and the upper four sacral rami (anterior rami). The branches are:

Nerve to pyriformis (S1, 2): This is as follows:
Perforating cutaneous nerve (S2, 3): It perforates the sacrotuberous ligament and the fibers of gluteus maximus. It supplies the medial side of the buttock.

Posterior femoral cutaneous nerve (S1, 2, 3): It supplies the lateral part of the posterior two-thirds of labia majus.

The pelvic splanchic nerves (S2, 3, 4) constitute the sacral parasympathetic outflow. The fibers join the hypogastric plexus. In the pelvis they are motor to the bladder and cause clitoral erection. Afferent fibers of pelvic splanchic nerve carries sensation of distention and pain from the bladder, lower cervix, lower colon and rectum.

Pudendal nerve (S2, 3, 4): It is the nerve of the pelvic floor and the perineum. It leaves the pelvis between pyriformis and coccygeus and curls around the ischial spine to enter the pudendal canal through the lesser sciatic foramen. In the pudendal canal it lies on the lateral wall of the ischiorectal fossa and toward the end of the canal it gives the inferior rectal nerve the branches of which supply the external anal sphincter anal canal and the perianal skin (Inferior rectal nerve do not supply the rectum).

The perineal nerve is a terminal branch of the pudendal nerve. It supplies the posterior two-third of the vulva and the mucous membrane of the urethra and the vagina. It is motor to perineal muscle, bulbospongious and sphincter urethrae.

The other terminal branch of the pudendal nerve is the dorsal nerve of the clitoris.

- The muscular branches of the S3 and S4 supply levator ani and coccygeus at its pelvic surface.
- Perineal branch of S4 supplies the skin of the ischiorectal fossa.
- Nerve to obturator internus (L5, S1, 2)
- Nerve to quadratus femoris (L4, 5 S1)
- Superior gluteal nerve (L4, 5, S1)
- Inferior gluteal nerve (L5, S1, 2)

Sciatic Nerve (L4, 5 S1, 2—Common peroneal nerve; L4, 5, S1, 2, 3—Tibial nerve): It is the largest branch of the sacral plexus. It is formed at the lower margin of pyriformis by the union of the component nerves.

Autonomic Nerves

The pelvic organs are supplied by the sympathetic and the parasympathetic nervous system. The sympathetic components are derived from the superior hypogastric plexus via the hypogastric nerve and from the sacral sympathetic ganglion. The parasympathetic nerves enter the pelvis through the pelvic splanchnic nerves. The preganglionic fibers are distributed through the pelvic plexus and the parasympathetic ganglia are situated close to the walls of the viscera concerned. The ovaries and the fallopian tube are supplied directly by nerves from the pre-aortic plexus travelling by the ovarian vessels. Rest of the pelvic organs are supplied via the pelvic plexus. The pelvic parasympathetic fibers are motor to emptying the bladder and the rectum and secretomotor to the gut. The sympathetics are motor to the sphincter urethrae and anal sphincter.

PELVIC LYMPHATIC DRAINAGE

The lymph nodes in the pelvis are arranged along the major blood vessels. The *lateral aortic* lymph nodes lie on the either side of the aorta. From the aortic lymph nodes efferents form the lumbar trunk on either side. Lumbar trunks then terminate into cysterna chyli. The ovaries, fallopian tubes, upper ureter and the fundus of the uterus drain to the lateral aortic group of lymph nodes.

The other pelvic organs drain into the groups of lymph nodes associated with iliac vessels. The *common iliac* groups are grouped around the bifurcation of common iliac artery and can be divided into medial, lateral and intermediate chains. They receive afferents from external and internal iliac groups and in turn drain into the lateral aortic group of lymph nodes. The *external iliac* group of nodes lie along side of the external iliac vessels and can be grouped as lateral, medial and anterior. The cervix, upper vagina, bladder, and the lower abdominal wall drain into the external iliac lymph nodes. The *internal iliac* lymph nodes are situated around the internal iliac vessels and receive afferents from all the pelvic viscera, deeper perineum and muscle of the buttock.

The *inguinal group* of nodes is divided into superficial and deep group of nodes. The superficial lymph nodes radiate toward the saphenous opening and are arranged in the form of T. The horizontal arm of the T lies parallel to the inguinal ligament and can be divided into lateral and medial group. The group associated with terminal part of the saphenous vein makes up the stem of the T. The lateral members of the horizontal arm of the T receive afferents from the gluteal region and the adjoining portion of the abdominal wall muscle. The medial group receives afferents from the vulva, lower vagina, perineum and the lower portion of the anus and the adjoining abdominal wall. It also receives lymph vessels from the uterus through the round ligament. The lymphatics of either side of the vulva communicates but do not cross the labiocrural folds. The efferents from the superficial inguinal lymph nodes drain into the external iliac lymph nodes. The deep inguinal lymph nodes lie on the medial side of the femoral vein. They receive efferents from the superficial inguinal nodes and from the deep femoral vessels. One of the nodes, known as the node of Cloquet is thought to drain the clitoris. The deep nodes drain into the external iliac nodes through the femoral canal.

4. Diagnosis of Pregnancy

Rajesh Bhakta
Pratap Kumar

PART One

Introduction

INTRODUCTION

Pregnancy is a physiological state, but the importance of the diagnosis of pregnancy cannot be overstated. The diagnosis of pregnancy is not difficult in the majority of cases but is easily overlooked when the symptoms are atypical and when the patient tries to conceal it. Mistakes made in diagnosis of pregnancy are made most frequently in the first several weeks of pregnancy, while the uterus is still a pelvic organ.

The endocrinological, physiological and anatomical alterations that accompany pregnancy give rise to symptoms and signs that provide evidence that pregnancy exists. The subjective symptoms and objective signs of pregnancy vary with different trimester and may be described under three trimesters.

FIRST TRIMESTER (1-13 WEEKS)

Subjective Signs of Pregnancy

Cessation of Menstruation (Amenorrhea)

Amenorrhea is the earliest sign of pregnancy. In a healthy woman, whose menstrual periods were regular in her reproductive period, has a sudden cessation of her periods the presumption must always be that she is pregnant unless some other cause of the amenorrhea can be found. Apart from pregnancy, amenorrhea is seen in lactation, late teens, emotional disturbance, etc. Amenorrhea does neither have the same importance in the case of women whose periods were irregular, nor may it have any significance in menopausal age. Pregnancy has known to occur in young girls before menarche and during lactational amenorrhea.

Nausea with or without Vomiting

Nausea and vomiting are well known symptoms of pregnancy, also called as morning sickness. It is well recognized that such sickness occurs at any time of the day. It usually appears at the beginning of the second month and it varies greatly in severity. Majority of primi gravidae suffer from it, but in subsequent pregnancies it is frequently absent. Some pregnant women are seized with nausea, ending in vomiting, immediately on rising or after their first meal. Once the vomiting is over, there is no further discomfort or any loss of appetite during the rest of the day. Others are subject to nausea, without vomiting, which may last for several hours and is more troublesome than the previously mentioned variety. But in neither case is the general health affected. All gradations may be observed between this symptom and the serious disorder known as hyperemesis. Morning sickness in either of these common forms usually last only for few weeks, rarely more than three months.

Breast Discomfort

Feeling of fullness and tenderness in breast is evident as early as 6 to 8 weeks especially in primigravida.

Urinary Symptoms

Urinary symptoms are often present. The first symptom is usually frequency of micturition, which starts before long the increase in size of the uterus. This could be due to a higher progesterone level and increased vascularity. The women notice this at 8 to 10 weeks and it can be very disturbing. It usually subsides after the first trimester and reappears at the end of pregnancy.

Fatigue

Fatigue may also be present.

Objective Signs

During the first 4 weeks of pregnancy that is until the menstruation period is more than 2 weeks overdue, it is usually impossible to diagnose pregnancy on clinical examination. Indeed the diagnosis can rarely be made based on physical signs before 6 to 8 weeks of pregnancy.

Breast Changes

Anatomical changes in the breast that accompany pregnancy are quite characteristic in primigravida. The breasts of a primigravida may present recognizable indications of activity by 6 to 8 weeks, but frequently they show very little change the following month.

The earliest symptoms and signs—increased vascularity and a sensation of heaviness, appear at 6 weeks. The cutaneous veins over and between the breast are more noticeable. By 8 weeks the nipple and surrounding area, the primary areola have become more pigmented. Montgomery's tubercles—the sebaceous glands, become more prominent as raised pink red nodules on the areola. Some hypertrophy of the peripheral lobules of the glands is indicated by a nodular feel and slight tenderness may be apparent. Occasionally little clear secretion may be expressed by a gentle squeeze of the base of the gland toward the nipple. In multipara no importance can be given to the existence of these signs, as they frequently persist in a gland, which has previously passed through the phase of functional activity (Figure 4.1).

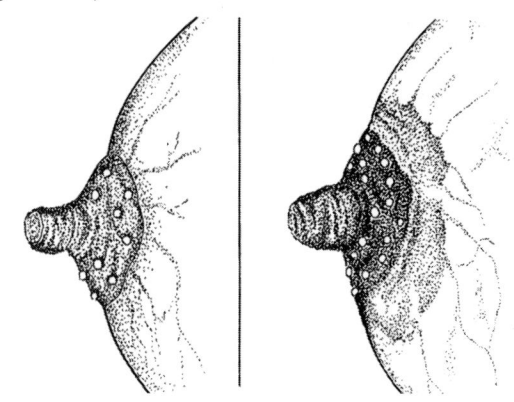

Figure 4.1: Breast changes in pregnancy

Pelvic Organ Changes

Abdominal examination: Abdominal examination is usually not helpful in early pregnancy. By the time uterus can be convincingly felt above the pubic symphysis, usually the pregnancy has advanced to 12 to 14 weeks. By then the diagnosis is usually made by other means, but changes in the uterus may be detected by a careful bimanual examination.

Vaginal examination: Examination with a speculum will show a cervix that has become typically blue or violet colored (Chadwick's sign). However, there is no reason for speculum examination at this stage and this sign is nonspecific.

Cervix: It becomes very soft changing in consistency from the fibrous feel of the nonpregnant uterus and cervix (Goodell's sign).

Uterus: If the abdominal wall is thin and lax, a gentle bimanual examination can detect the softness of the uterus by 6 to 8 weeks of pregnancy. The uterus may not be very enlarged but it feels much broader and globular. There may be irregularity in shape (Piskack's sign) or consistency of the uterus. Uterine contraction may be palpable (Palmer's sign). Pulsation of the vaginal and uterine arteries can be detected in the vaginal fornices (Osiander's sign). Because of the soft consistency of the uterus, on bimanual examination the abdominal and vaginal fingers seem to appose below the body of the uterus (Hegar's sign).

Hegar's sign can be elicited in women with a lax abdominal wall. Two fingers are introduced into vagina behind the cervix, while the fingers of the other hand are pressed down into the abdomen just above the pubic symphysis. The uterus can be felt above the apposing fingers of both hands. Because of the danger of causing an interruption to the pregnancy, these manipulations should be gentle and pressure over the body of uterus must be avoided. There is little need to elicit Hegar's sign after 12 weeks.

Investigations

Hormonal Tests of Pregnancy

Presence of human chorionic gonadotropin (hCG) in maternal plasma and its excretion in urine provides the basis for the endocrine test for pregnancy.

Human chorionic gonadotropin (hCG) is a glycoprotein with a and b subunits. hCG is produced in placenta exclusively by syncytiotrophoblast. The production of hCG in trophoblast begins very early in pregnancy, almost certainly by the day of implantation. Thereafter the level of hCG in maternal plasma and urine raises rapidly. The levels of hCG in blood and urine reach peak levels at about 60 to 70 days of pregnancy. The concentration of hCG declines slowly until a nadir is reached at about 100 to 130 days of pregnancy.

Methods: Different methods for hormonal tests of pregnancy are discussed as follows (Table 4.1).

1. Bioassay with animals (Obsolete)
   The earlier biological tests based on animals, e.g. Ascheim-Zondeck test are only of historical interest and are no longer in use.

Table 4.1: Summary of hormonal test for pregnancy

	Tests	Sensitivity	Time taken	Positive after days of LMP (mIU/ml)
1.	Biological test	3500	5-6 days	45
2.	Immunological test			
	a. Slide test	1500	2 min	44
	b. Using latex	500	2 min	34
3.	Home test kits	10-50	2 min	30
4.	Radioimmunoassay	0.1-0.3	3-4 hr	25

2. Immunological test:
   Modern sensitive immunological test for early diagnosis of pregnancy are based upon detection of beta subunit of hCG in maternal urine/serum (antigen-antibody test).

   Agglutination inhibition tests (Obsolete) are as follows:
   i. Slide test: not done as its sensitvity is 1500 IU/L.
   ii. Tube test: not done as its sensitvity is 750 IU/L.
   iii. Using latex agglutination inhibition (LAI) technique.
   iv. Direct agglutination test.

   Principle employed in immunological test to confirm pregnancy is shown in the flow chart (Figure 4.2).

   Absence of agglutination indicates presence of pregnancy.

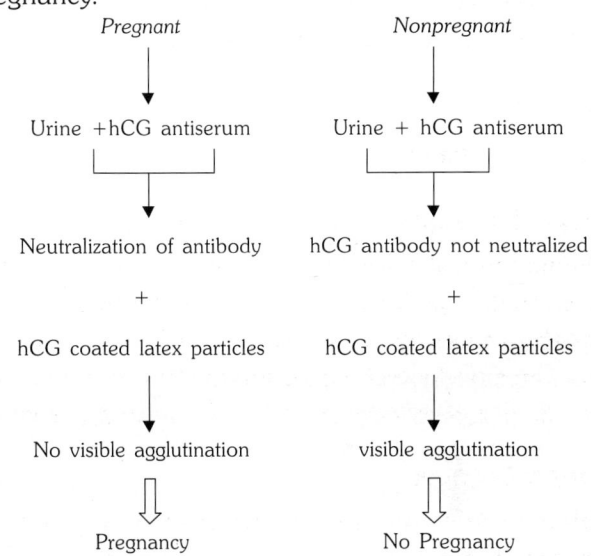

```
        Pregnant                      Nonpregnant
           ↓                              ↓
   Urine + hCG antiserum          Urine + hCG antiserum
           ↓                              ↓
 Neutralization of antibody      hCG antibody not neutralized
           +                              +
  hCG coated latex particles     hCG coated latex particles
           ↓                              ↓
    No visible agglutination       visible agglutination
           ⇓                              ⇓
        Pregnancy                    No Pregnancy
```

Figure 4.2: Flow chart showing principle employed in immunological test to confirm pregnancy

3. Home test (Do it yourself (DIY)) kits:
   Use enzyme immunometric/immunochromatographic method to detect hCG in urine. It is a rapid test and takes 2 to 5 minutes. Sensitivity ranges from 10 to 50 mIU/ml.

4. *Quantitative laboratory test kits:* Radioimmunoassay (RIA) and immunoassay can be used to detect hCG beta subunit 7 to 10 days after conception, even before the period has been missed. Assay for the detection of the beta subunit are much less likely to give false-positive results due to cross-reaction with

LH subunit. Radioimmunoassay are now replaced by the enzyme-linked immunosorbent assay (ELISA)

Note: It is important to remember that positive pregnancy test does not always mean that it is intrauterine pregnancy. Other abnormal conditions, in which the pregnancy test can be positive are ectopic pregnancy and vesicular mole.

Ultrasound

1. To confirm, it is intrauterine or extrauterine
2. To confirm that there is a fetal heartbeat.
3. To diagnose multiple pregnancy.
4. To estimate gestational age.
5. To confirm wellbeing of pregnancy.

Ultrasonography especially transvaginal sonography permits visualization of early pregnancy better than transabdominal sonography in early pregnancy. Transvaginal sonography permits an exquisite view of the gestational sac, yolk sac, amnion and early embryo. The gestational sac is the first definitive sonographic sign of early pregnancy. The gestational sac can be visualized by 4.5 menstrual weeks.[1] Yolk sac is the earliest embryonic landmark that can be recognized within gestational sac.

The presence of yolk sac virtually eliminates the possibility of ectopic pregnancy.[2] Cardiac activity is definitive sign of live pregnancy. It is seen by 40th menstrual day[3] and is always seen when embryo is 5 mm.[3-5] The menstrual dates are determined by various methods, as single method is not most accurate. Commonly used measurement is gestational sac size and embryonic size by crown rump length (CRL).

SECOND TRIMESTER (14-28 WEEKS)

Subjective Symptoms

Symptoms like nausea, vomiting and frequency of micturition usually disappear by this time, while amenorrhea continues.

The new symptoms that appear are as follows:
1. Progressive enlargement of lower abdomen
2. Quickening (Coming to life) indicates that mother has become aware of the existence of something, which is alive and moving within her. The *first* fetal movement felt by the mother is called quickening.

Summary: Signs of Early Pregnancy in First Trimester

1. *Breast changes:*
   - Engorgement of surface veins.
   - Pigmentation of primary areola.
2. *Pelvic organ changes:*
   - Blue or violet colored vagina and cervix (Chadwick's sign)—8th week
   - Pulsation of the vaginal and uterine arteries can be detected in the vaginal fornices (Osiander's sign)—8th week
   - Lips of cervix softened (Goodell's sign)—6th week
   - Irregularity in shape of the uterus (Piskack's sign)—8th week
   - Uterine contraction may be palpable (Palmer's sign)—4 to 8 weeks
   - The abdominal and vaginal fingers can be apposed below the body of the uterus (Hegar's sign)—8 to12 weeks

---

It appears around 18 to 20 weeks. Multiparous women appreciate earlier by about 2 weeks. Fetal movements continue to be present until the end of the pregnancy, and are important in the later months as an indication that the fetus is alive. Peristaltic movement of the intestine may sometimes be mistaken for fetal movements. The date of quickening, if definitely known from the patient, helps to cross-check the period of gestation and the probable expected date of delivery calculated based on the LMP.

General Examination

Skin Changes

Pigmentation over the cheeks and forehead in the form of dark brown patches, more noticeable in those who are fair skinned.

Breast Changes

Pigmentation is also seen on the breast. Secondary areola starts appearing at about 18 to 20 weeks seen more prominent in primigravidae. Montgomery's tubercles are prominent and extend to secondary areola. Colostrum becomes yellowish and thick.

Abdominal Examination

Pigmentation and striae is seen over the abdominal wall.

Inspection: A linear pigmented area stretching from the umbilicus to the symphysis pubis is of deeper color and is known as *linea nigra*. It starts appearing at 20 weeks of gestation.

Striae: Both pink and white striae may be visible to varying degree.

Palpation:
1. *Fundal height:* The uterus progressively increases in size. Duration of pregnancy can be roughly estimated based on the height of the uterus in relation to different levels on the abdomen. The fundus reaches the level of the umbilicus at about 22 to 24 weeks and just below the xiphisternum at the 36th week.
2. *Symphysiofundal height (SFH):* This should be measured with the woman in the dorsal supine position after passing urine. The upper border of the fundus is felt by the ulnar border of left hand and the point is marked. The distance between the upper border of symphysis pubis and marked point is measured using a measuring tape in centimeter. After 20 weeks the symphysiofundal height in centimeter correlates to number of weeks ± 2 cm upto 36 weeks. For example, at 24 weeks the SFH is 24 + 2 cm and at 36 weeks SFH is 36 + 3 cm (Figure 4.3).
3. *Braxton Hick contractions:* During pregnancy the uterus undergoes palpable but painless contraction at irregular intervals from the early stages of gestation. These contractions are referred to as Braxton-Hick contractions. It does not have any effect on dilatation of cervix. Nearing term, the contraction becomes more frequent with increase in intensity so as to produce some discomfort to the women. These are not however, positive signs of pregnancy, because similar contraction are sometime seen in women with hematometra and submucus fibroid. The detection of Braxton Hick contraction however, may be helpful in excluding the existence of abdominal pregnancy.
4. *Active fetal movement:* It can be felt by placing the hand over the uterus from 18 weeks onwards. When felt or seen it suggests evidence of pregnancy with a live fetus. The frequency and intensity varies and is stronger in last trimester.
5. *Palpation of fetal parts:* Fetal parts can be distinctly felt after 24 weeks of gestation. As pregnancy advances it is of great value not in detecting pregnancy but to ascertain the presentation and position of the fetus *in utero*.

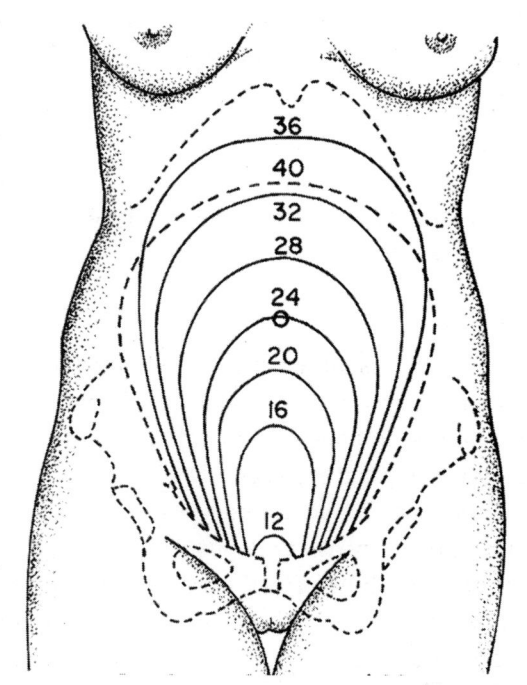

Figure 4.3: Level of fundus at different periods of gestation (weeks)

External ballotment: Ballotment of the fetal head is elicited with the patient in supine position by steadying the uterus with one hand applied to the side and gently pressing down the fetal head. The rebounding impact of the fetal head can be felt. It depends upon the amount of liquor amnii present in the uterine cavity. It is difficult to elicit in cases where abdominal wall is thick and when the liquor amnii is very much diminished in quantity (Figure 4.4).

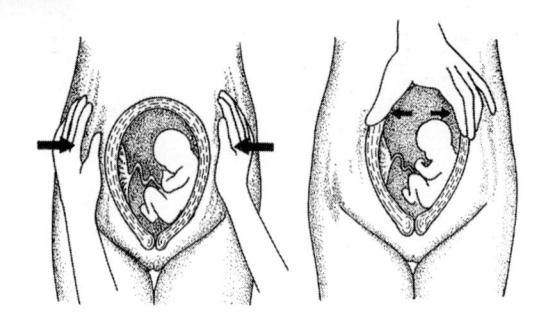

Figure 4.4: External ballotement

Auscultation: Fetal heart sound (FHS) is the most reliable and conclusive for the diagnosis of pregnancy. It can be heard around 18 to 20 weeks by stethoscope. The intensity of FHS varies with position of the fetus. The fetal heart rate is between 120 to 160 beats per minute.

Uterine souffle: This is a soft blowing sound best heard lower down at the sides of the uterus. This is due to increase blood flow through the distal dilated uterine vessel. This sound is synchronous with maternal pulse.

Vaginal Examination

Internal ballotement: This sign can be elicited between 16 and 18th week. To elicit this sign, patient is placed in the dorsal supine position. Two fingers are introduced into the vagina and with the tip of the fingers, a sharp tap is given upward through the fornix. The fetus is displaced upward and rebounds to its original position and falls back upon the examining fingers. This rebound phenomenon is ballotement. The test cannot be elicited in cases with scanty liquor amnii or when the fetus is transversely placed (Figure 4.5).

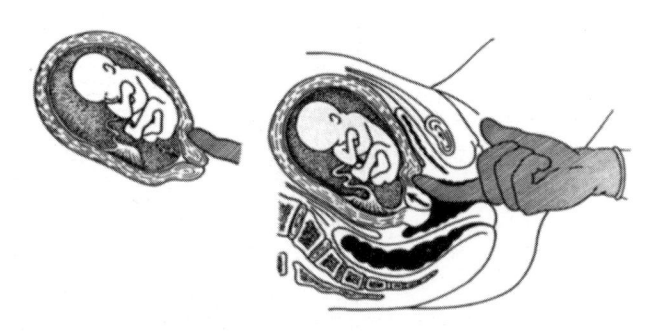

Figure 4.5: Internal ballotement

Investigations

Ultrasonography

The development of ultrasound has made it possible to measure the bones and soft tissue structure of the fetus. The optimal time to perform routine ultrasound in 2nd trimester is 18 to 22 weeks. At this time biparietal diameter, abdominal circumference and femur length measurements are taken. Examination at this time has the following advantages:

1. Accurate prediction of gestational age.
2. Allows diagnosis of multiple gestation.
3. Major structural anomalies can be recognized.
4. Placental localization.
5. Demonstration of viable healthy fetus increases maternal bonding.

Radiological Study

Radiological study is no longer in use. Evidence of fetal skeleton can be made out by 16 to 18 weeks, when seen in conclusive evidence of pregnancy. Realization of the hazards of radiation in pregnancy and the possibility of visualizing the fetus with ultrasound has restricted its use considerably.

THIRD TRIMESTER (29-40 WEEKS)

Subjective Symptoms

1. *Amenorrhea:* Persists.
2. *Enlargement of abdomen:* Uterus enlarges progressively to term when it fills almost the entire abdomen. This produces some maternal discomfort such as dyspnea.
3. *Frequency of micturition:* Reappears.
4. *Fetal movements:* They are more frequent and more pronounced.
5. *Lightening:* This occurs after 36 weeks, especially in primigravida. The falling forward of the uterus with the head sinking into the pelvis resulting in the so called lightening due to the relief of pressure exerted by the gravid uterus upon the diaphragm and therefore on the lungs and heart.

Objective Signs

1. *Cutaneous changes:* There is increased pigmentation and striae that become more prominent.
2. *Braxton-Hick contractions:* They are appreciated more frequently.
3. *Fetal movements:* They are more appreciable.
4. *Fundal height:* Duration of pregnancy can be roughly estimated noting the height of uterus in relation to the symphysis pubis.

    Signs of term pregnancy are full flanks with uterine height 4 cm below xiphisternum, and mature fetal head.
5. *Palpation of fetal parts:* It becomes much easier with progress of pregnancy. Fetal lie, presentation and position can be determined more clearly.
6. *Fetal heart sound:* It is best heard in an area that corresponds to the anterior shoulder of the fetus. Difficulty may arise to auscultate fetal heart sound in cases of obesity or hydramnios. In cases of intrauterine death fetal heart sound is not heard.

Investigation

Ultrasonography

Sonography not only confirms pregnancy but also permits evaluation of pregnancy being singleton or multiple, determining the fetal lie, presentation and visualization of cardiac pulsations. Ultrasonography has an important place in placental localization and to determine amount and distribution of amniotic fluid.

The fetus can be scanned for structural abnormalities and on the basis of several measurements a reasonably accurate estimate of the gestational maturity can be made.

DIFFERENTIAL DIAGNOSIS OF PREGNANCY

1. *Distended urinary bladder:* In cases of chronic retention of urine, the distended bladder may be mistaken for gravid uterus or as an ovarian cyst. Emptying the bladder before the examination solves the confusion.
2. *Leiomyoma of uterus:* Especially the intramural leiomyoma occasionally cause uniform enlargement of uterus. Absence of early symptoms and signs of pregnancy and negative immunological test should help toward the diagnosis. Ultrasound is very useful and shows absence of gestational sac.
3. *Cystic ovarian tumor:* The diagnostic signs and amenorrhea is usually absent. Absence of palpable Braxton Hick contractions, fetal parts, and fetal heart sound helps in the diagnosis. Ultrasound examination will reveal that there is no evidence of pregnancy.
4. *Pseudocyesis:* This is a psychological disorder, where the woman who has intense desire to become pregnant has the false belief that she is pregnant, although pregnancy does not exist. It is observed in women with long history of infertility or in women who is approaching menopause when her menstruation becomes scanty or ceased for a time.

    The woman believes her gradual enlargement of abdomen due to deposition of fat as that due to pregnancy and imagines that she feels fetal movements which may be intestinal movements. In

---

Summary of Diagnosis of Pregnancy

Subjective symptoms:
1. Amenorrhea of varying period
2. Nausea, vomiting (morning sickness)
3. Frequency of micturition
4. Breast changes
5. Skin changes
6. Quickening

Absolute signs:
1. Auscultation of fetal heart sound.
2. Palpation of fetal parts and perception of active fetal movements.
3. Ultrasonographic evidence of gestational sac and embryo in early pregnancy and later.

Probable signs:
1. Change in the size, shape, and consistency of uterus.
2. Softening of cervix.
3. Various signs described in early pregnancy.
4. Abdominal enlargement.
5. Braxton-Hick contraction.
6. External and internal ballotement.

some cases the condition may go on and eventually spurious labor may set in. Obstetrical examination reveals absence of positive signs of pregnancy. Ultrasound is useful in these cases.

REFERENCES

1. Fossum GT, Davajan V, Kletzky OA: Early detection of pregnancy with transvaginal US. *Fertil and Steril* **49**:788-91, 1988.
2. Nyberg DA, Mack LA, Harvey D, Wang K: Value of the yolk sac in evaluating early pregnancies. *J Ultrasound Med* **7**: 129-35, 1988.
3. Rempen A: Demonstration of viablilty in early pregnancy with vaginal sonography. *J Ultrasound Med* **7**:107, 1988.
4. Rempen A: Demonstration of viablilty in early pregnancy with vaginal sonography. *J Ultrasound Med* **9**: 711-16, 1988.
5. Timor-Tritsh IE, Farine D, Rasen MG: A close look at early embryonic development with the high frequency transvaginal transducer. *Am J Obstet Gynecol* **159**: 676-81, 1988.

5. Physiological Changes in Pregnancy

Wong Yat May

PART One

INTRODUCTION

Pregnancy is a unique stage where maternal adaptation occurs early to provide a favorable outcome for both the mother and fetus. These physiological changes occur at different rates throughout the whole body, which allow the pregnant woman to store additional energy in preparation for labor and delivery. The placenta is the initial place where these physiological changes occur. If the physiological changes were incomplete, it may lead to overt pathology in pregnancy. This chapter is aimed to provide the information on the relevant physiological changes that takes place during a normal pregnancy including the placenta.

PLACENTAL HORMONE SECRETION

The trophoblastic tissues of the placenta provide not only a pivotal role in regulating the fetal nutrition during pregnancy but also in the secretion of placental hormone to maintain the pregnancy. The numerous hormones that are produced by the placenta will be discussed here.

Human Chorionic Gonadotropin (hCG)

Human chorionic gonadotropin is produced by the syncytiotrophoblasts of the placenta. It has an α and β subunit. The α-hCG- is similar to the α subunit of luteinizing hormone (LH), follicular stimulating hormone (FSH) and thyroid stimulating hormone (TSH). hCG is primarily a luteinizing and luteotropic hormone with little FSH activity. It therefore, helps to maintain the corpus luteum in early pregnancy.[1]

Radioimmunoassay has been used to detect hCG in the serum. β-hCG is usually detectable in the maternal blood within 10 days of conception. The presence of its β subunit in the urine is the basis for home pregnancy test kits. Modern urine pregnancy test kit employs the ELISA (enzyme-linked immunoabsorbent assay) method to enhance its sensitivity. With ELISA, a much lower concentration of hCG (25-50 u/l) in the urine will be detectable. Hence, a positive urine pregnancy test will be evident as early as 8 to 10 days after fertilization.[2] The hCG rises rapidly in the fist trimester of pregnancy and peaks between the 8th to 10th weeks of gestation. This is then followed by a fall to a level, which is maintained for the rest of the pregnancy.

In a normal viable intrauterine pregnancy, the β-hCG level in the serum doubles every 48 hours. The peak of hCG in pregnancy persists for a longer period in multiple pregnancy and molar pregnancy.

Following termination of a pregnancy, the hCG level will disappear from the urine at a faster rate than from the serum. In the early stage of pregnancy, the function of the hCG is to maintain the corpus luteum, so that an adequate secretion of estrogen and progesterone can be maintained until the placenta has developed sufficiently to take over the production of these sex steroid hormones. These endocrine changes will provide a favorable environment for implantation and growth of the embryo.[3]

Human Placental Lactogen

Human placental lactogen (hPL) is a protein hormone secreted by the syncytiotrophoblast of the placenta. It is also sometimes known as human chorionic somatomammotropin (hCS) and chorionic growth hormone-prolactin (CGP). Its secretion follows that of the waning hCG level. It continues to rise until late pregnancy. hPL is lactogenic and essentially functions as a 'growth hormone' in pregnancy. Large quantities of hPL are found in the maternal blood, but very little reaches the fetal circulation. Hence, its effects are all on the mother's physiology. It promotes glucose conservation in the mother by mobilizing free fatty acids from the maternal stores. This lipolytic effect will reduce maternal glucose utilization by providing her with an alternative energy supply. The raised maternal blood glucose will then provide the fetus with an ample supply of glucose for its nutritional needs. hPL also acts to stimulate insulin secretion centrally and is partly responsible for the diabetogenic effects seen in pregnancy. The secretion of hPL parallels that of the placental size.[1]

Other Placental Hormones Production

Apart from hCG and hPL, there are other placental hormones that are produced and secreted. Pregnancy specific betaglycoprotein (SP-1) is a placental protein hormone produced by the syncytiotrophoblasts. It is secreted entirely into the maternal circulation and rises in parallel with hPL. Its exact function is unknown and its level has not been shown to correlate with the placental function. Estrogen is produced exclusively by the placenta during pregnancy. Its main function is at cellular level. In the cervix, estrogen reduces the adhesions between the connective tissue leading to softening of the cervix in pregnancy. It also aids in the growth of uterine muscle, increases the size of breast during pregnancy, increases the mobility of the nipple and causes ductal and alveolar development in the breast. Progesterone is produced and secreted initially by the corpus luteum and trophoblasts in early pregnancy. By the 35th day after fertilization, the placental syncytiotrophoblasts takes over the synthesis of this hormone, converting it from its precursor, cholesterol. It rises continuously throughout pregnancy like estrogen. Progesterone exerts its action mainly on the smooth muscle by reducing its excitability. The physiological actions of progesterone in pregnancy is reflected by a quiescent uterus antenatally, ureteric dilatation and reduced intestinal peristalsis.[4] It is also a hyperthermic agent.

A summary of the various hormones secretion in pregnancy and their functions is shown in Table 5.1.

Table 5.1: Summary of placental hormone secretion and their functions

	hCG	hPL
• **Site of production**	• Syncytiotrophoblasts	• Syncytiotrophoblasts
• **Pattern of secretion**	• Rise rapidly in 1st trimester. • Peaks at 8-10 weeks • Declines to a level and maintained at this for the rest of pregnancy.	• Peaks when hCG starts to fall. • Continues to rise throughout pregnancy.
• **Functions**	• Maintains corpus luteum	• Lactogenic • Act as maternal 'growth hormone'. • Conserves glucose in mother. • Stimulate insulin secretion

CARDIOVASCULAR SYSTEM

Plasma Volume

Plasma volume increases progressively toward 34 weeks of gestation before it starts to tail down. Its increase is notable from 10th week of pregnancy onward. The degree of increase is greater in multigravida than primigravida and in multiple pregnancies than singleton. It increases by almost 50 percent above non-pregnant value. At 34 weeks of pregnancy, the plasma volume in a healthy pregnancy is about 3800 ml. The plasma volume will start to decline by 200-300 ml from 34 weeks with a further drop noted at delivery, about 500-600 ml. It will return to the non-pregnant value by 6-8 weeks post-partum. The increase of this circulating volume is a healthy sign in pregnancy as it helps to accommodate the increased blood flow to the uterus and other organs. At the same time, this reduces the blood viscosity.[3]

Cardiac Output

Cardiac output rises by 1.5 L/minute within the first 10 weeks of pregnancy and reaches 6.5 L/minute by about 25th week of gestation. It is then maintained at this level until term. This represents a 30-50 percent increase during pregnancy. The increase in cardiac output is largely due to an increase in stroke volume as a consequence of the high circulating estrogen. In labor, cardiac output increases by 30 percent with each contraction. This increase is of a lesser extent when the patient is supine compared to lateral position. This is due to the interrupted blood flow from the uterus to the heart in a supine position because of compression of the inferior vena cava by the uterus. During each contraction, a rise in central venous pressure is noted which will account for the rise in cardiac output. This increase is even more noticeable during the pushing effort in the second stage of labor.[4]

Stroke Volume

Stroke volume increases by 10 percent during pregnancy due to the effect of circulating estrogen. During labor there is a further rise in stroke volume.

Pulse Rate

The pulse rate will increase by 15 beats/minute in pregnancy. Despite a rise in cardiac output and stroke volume during each contraction in labor, the pulse rate decreases at the height of a contraction although a small rise is seen at the beginning of a contraction.

Blood Pressure

The systolic blood pressure falls slightly during early pregnancy but rises again in late pregnancy. The diastolic blood pressure falls in first trimester of pregnancy and reaches its lowest level at 16 to 20 weeks of pregnancy. It rises again to reach its early pregnancy level by term. The level of rise during this period of time is about 15 mmHg. During supine position, a fall of blood pressure is noted as compared to one taken during sitting position. This is due the compression of the inferior vena cava and aorta at their bifurcation by the uterus when the patient is lying flat on her back. During a contraction in labor, a rise of central venous pressure will lead to an increase in arterial blood pressure by 10 to 20 mmHg. This increase is even more accentuated during pushing in the second stage of labor. In late pregnancy, the uterus may compress the aorta to a large extent and, thus, reduces the flow of blood to the right side of the heart. This in turn is compensated by an increase in systemic vascular resistance. If this compensatory mechanism is inadequate, the blood pressure will fall. Despite a fall in blood pressure, not many women develop supine hypotension as there are sufficient collateral venous return to the heart.[4]

Peripheral Resistance

At the beginning of a pregnancy, peripheral resistance is usually low but gradually increases thereafter. The low peripheral resistance is due to the circulating estrogen and progesterone. The progesterone acts as a muscle relaxant causing vasodilatation and hence a decrease in resistance.[5]

A summary of the cardiovascular changes in pregnancy is summarized in Table 5.2.

HEMATOLOGY

Red Cell Volume

Red cell mass increases in a linear fashion during pregnancy by about 20 to 30 percent with maximal effect seen in those taking iron supplements. The rise is more

Table 5.2: Cardiovascular changes in pregnancy

• Plasma volume	↑ progressively from 10 to 34 weeks gestation, then ↓
	↑ more in multigravida and multiple pregnancies
	Returned to non-pregnant value by 6-8 weeks post-partum
• Cardiac output	↑ from 10th week until 25th week, then maintained at this level until term
	~30-50% ↑ during pregnancy
	↑ with each uterine contraction
	↑ more in lateral than supine position
	↑ is due to estrogenic effect
• Stroke volume	10% ↑ in pregnancy
	↑ is due to estrogen
	↑ in labor
• Pulse rate	↑ by 15 beats per minute in pregnancy
	Small ↑ at beginning of uterine contraction
	↓ at the height of uterine contraction
• Blood pressure	Systolic/diastolic BP ↓ in 2nd trimester
	DBP is lowest at 16-20 weeks gestation
	BP ↓ in supine position compared to lateral
	BP ↑ during uterine contraction
• Peripheral resistance	Low in early pregnancy
	↓ due to vasodilatation from progestogenic effect

pronounced in multiple pregnancies as compared to singleton. This rise is due to an increase in the number and size of red cells, which aids the transport of oxygen and carbon dioxide. The increase in red cell volume and red cell production is regulated by an increase in demand for oxygen transport in pregnancy. As the total increase in red cell volume is less than that of the plasma volume, the concentration of red cells in the blood falls, hence physiological anemia in pregnancy is noted. These changes are still noticeable at 8 weeks post-partum but would have returned to normal by 4 to 6 months post-partum.[4]

Other Blood Constituents

The white cells count tends to increase slightly during pregnancy to about 10 to 15,000/ml. The platelet count generally tends to remain unchanged although there is a downward trend toward the end of pregnancy, hence the term gestational thrombocytopenia. Erythrocyte sedimentation rate (ESR) rises by fourfold in pregnancy, hence it is not accurate as a diagnostic marker in pregnancy. This rise is due to increased globulin and fibrinogen levels.[3]

Erythropoiesis

There is increased requirement for iron during pregnancy by both the mother and the fetus. In the mother, the increased iron requirement is to prepare for blood loss at delivery and lactation. Iron is constantly removed from its stores in the mother from liver, bone marrow and spleen. A falling serum ferritin level reflects this reduced storage of iron in pregnancy. The average iron concentration in the serum in late pregnancy is 35 percent below the non-pregnant level. Although this can be modified by iron supplements, it cannot be prevented. The iron binding capacity doubles in pregnancy.

Folic acid, which is readily available from fresh vegetables, liver and kidneys, tends to fall progressively toward term. Vitamin B_{12} level also tend to fall during pregnancy, with the level being lowest between 16 to 20 weeks gestation.[5] Table 5.3 summarizes the hematological changes in pregnancy.

Redistribution of Blood Flow in Pregnancy

The uterus receives the largest redistribution of blood flow during pregnancy. Before conception, the uterus receives its blood supply mainly from the uterine arteries. But during pregnancy, the ovarian arteries contribute significantly. During pregnancy, the uterine arteries dilate upto 1.5 times greater in diameter compared to that of a non-pregnant state. The spiral arteries that supply the placenta also dilate physiologically and can be 30 times larger than that of their prepregnancy diameter.[6] There

Table 5.3: Hematological changes in pregnancy

• Red cell volume	↑ in pregnancy
	2° to ↑ red cell mass
	↑ in red cell volume < plasma volume, hence red cells concentration ↓ ⇒ physiological anemia
• White cell count	↑ slightly in pregnancy
• Platelet count	⇔/↓ in pregnancy especially toward term
• ESR	↑ by 4 times in pregnancy
• Clotting factors	↑ fibrinogen, ↑ plasminogen
	↓ fibrinolytic activity

are two waves of trophoblastic invasion into the spiral arteries in pregnancy: at 10 weeks gestation and between 16 to 22 weeks gestation. This physiological invasion increases the capacity of spiral arteries and reduces/abolishes their response to vasoactive stimuli.[7,8] When these vessels fail to undergo these physiological changes, they will respond to the vasoactive stimuli and hence reduces its flow to the intervillous space. When this occurs, pre-eclampsia and intrauterine growth restriction will be seen clinically. The failure of this adaptation is also associated with a maternal serum uric acid of 300 umol/L or more, a biochemical abnormality that is used to monitor the severity of pre-eclampsia.[9] The uterine artery blood flow increases progressively in pregnancy; at 10 weeks gestation the flow is about 75 ml/min while at 34 to 40 weeks gestation, it is 500 to 600 ml/min. The vascular system of the placental bed is less well developed in the first pregnancies compared to subsequent pregnancies, hence the babies of subsequent pregnancies are 'larger' than the first.[4]

The venous system distends gradually in pregnancy. The mean of increase is about 50 percent. Hence, varicose veins and hemorrhoids are commoner in pregnancy. The increased pressure in the veins of the leg is due to a mechanical obstruction of the venous return by the pregnant uterus on the iliac veins and the inferior vena cava.[4]

The kidney receives increased blood flow during pregnancy and is about 400 ml/min above the non-pregnant value at 16 weeks and remains at this level until term.[2]

Blood flow through the skin and mucous membranes also increases in pregnancy, about 70 percent above the non-pregnant value by the 36th week of pregnancy. This increase in blood flow is associated with peripheral vasodilatation, hence the phenomena of 'feeling the heat', sweating easily and nasal congestion.[5]

A summary of the redistribution of blood flow is shown in Table 5.4.

RESPIRATORY SYSTEM

Physiological changes in maternal respiratory system facilitates an effective exchange of CO_2 between the fetus and mother. Mother's lungs are responsible for gas exchange whilst in the fetus the placenta is responsible. For an effective exchange of CO_2 from the fetus to the mother, the PCO_2 in the mother has to be higher than the fetus. Hence, resetting the maternal respiratory system is necessary to achieve this.

Table 5.4: Summary of distribution of blood flow in pregnancy

• Uterus	↑ in uterine artery blood flow
	Uterus receives largest redistribution of blood flow
• Venous system	Distends gradually in pregnancy
	↑ by 50%
	Varicose veins and hemorrhoids commoner in pregnancy
• Kidney	↑ in renal blood flow
• Skin/mucous membrane	↑ by 70% above non-pregnant value by 36th weeks
	Peripheral vasodilatation ⇒ 'Feeling the heat' as a symptom, sweating easily and nasal congestion noticed

The mechanical changes of the maternal respiratory system include flaring outwards of the lower ribs with the diaphragm rising 4 cm higher. The transverse diameter of the chest increases by 2 cm. Diaphragmatic movement is increased and costal breathing is reduced in pregnancy. Hence, the woman has to breathe in deeply. All these changes will rotate the heart forward and alter the electrocardiogram (ECG) signal.[4]

Tidal volume (volume of gas that is inspired and expired in each respiration) is increased by about 40 percent. The adaptation of the increase in tidal volume will allow a better mixing of gases and increased oxygen consumption, which rises by 20 percent. Inspiratory capacity rises by 5 percent, while the minute volume increases by 40 percent. Inspiratory capacity is a combination of inspiratory residual volume and tidal volume. Inspiratory residual volume is defined as the air inspired with maximal inspiratory effort in excess of tidal volume. Minute volume, the amount of air that is inspired per minute is increased by 40 percent.

The expiratory reserve volume decreases by 15 percent. Expiratory reserve volume is the volume of air that is expelled by an active expiratory effort after passive expiration. Residual volume similarly falls by 20 percent. Residual volume is the amount of air that is left in the lung after maximal expiratory effort. The fall in residual volume together with an increase in tidal volume causes more efficient gas mixing.

Vital capacity is the combination of inspiratory reserve volume, tidal volume and expiratory reserve volume.

Airway resistance decreases in pregnancy but oxygen consumption increases by about 15 percent in late pregnancy. This increase is compensated by an increase in oxygen carrying capacity in the blood. However, the increase in ventilation greatly exceeds that of oxygen consumption, hence the alveolar concentration of CO_2 falls. The fall of PCO_2 in pregnancy may be due to the effect of progesterone. In pregnancy, every 1 mmHg rise in PCO_2 increases the ventilation by 6.0/min, 4 times more than the non-pregnant state. Because of the increase in ventilation during pregnancy, the pregnant mother is often seen to be 'overbreathing' and may contribute to dyspnea in pregnancy.[4]

A summary of the respiratory changes in pregnancy is shown in Table 5.5.

RENAL SYSTEM

Increased frequency in micturition is common in pregnancy. Nocturia tends to occur later in pregnancy. Stress incontinence is not uncommon due to increased intra-abdominal pressure and relaxation of the bladder supports. Bladder tone decreases and its capacity increases progressively during pregnancy. However, there is generally no residual urine after micturation. Dilatation of the upper renal tract is also common; the right kidney and ureter more affected than the left because of dextrorotation of the uterus.[10] This dilatation may appear as early as 6 weeks and more marked in the multiparous. The renal dilatation is accompanied by a slowing of flow of urine down the ureter but no change in the ureteric

Table 5.5: Changes in respiratory system during pregnancy

• **Mechanical changes**	1. Flaring out of ribs
	2. Diaphragm is higher
	3. Transverse diameter of chest ↑
	4. ↑ Diaphragmatic movement
	5. Rotate heart forward ⇒ ECG changes
• **Increase**	• Tidal volume (by 40%)
	• Inspiratory capacity (by 5%)
	• Minute volume (by 40%)
	• Oxygen consumption
	• Ventilation ⇒ 'Overbreathing' in pregnancy ⇒ dyspnea
• **Decrease**	• Expiratory reserve volume (by 15%)
	• Residual volume (by 20%)
	• Airway resistance
• **No change**	• Respiratory rate
	• Vital capacity

Table 5.6: Physiological changes of the renal system in pregnancy

• **Increase**	Frequency of micturation
	Nocturia
	Stress incontinence
	Bladder capacity
	Dilatation of renal pelvis and ureters (right side more than left)
	↑ in kidney size and weight
	↑ in renal plasma flow
	↑ in GFR
• **Decrease**	Bladder tone
• **No change**	Residual urine ⇔ despite other changes within renal system

tone or contractions. As a result, the kidney is increased by 1 cm and their weight by 20 percent.[4]

Renal plasma flow increases from 1st trimester of pregnancy. By the 20th week of gestation, the flow has increased by 30 to 50 percent above non-pregnant value and remains at this level until 30 weeks of gestation. It will then start to decline gradually but still remains above non-pregnant value. The glomerular filtration rate (GFR) increases soon after conception, reaching 60 percent above non-pregnant value by 16th week of pregnancy and remains at that level from thereon until term. The rise in GFR may be due to a rise in cardiac output initially and later on, from a fall of resistance in the efferent glomerular arteriole. The reduction of plasma albumin in pregnancy also contributes to this rise in GFR. With a reduction in plasma albumin, the plasma oncotic pressure decreases hence GFR rises. The increase in GFR is associated with some physiological changes noted in pregnancy, namely proteinuria, glycosuria, hence the name a 'leaky kidney' is coined in pregnancy. Creatinine clearance also increases during pregnancy.[10,11] Table 5.6 shows a summary of the physiological changes in the renal system during pregnancy.

GASTROINTESTINAL SYSTEM

An increase in appetite is commonly seen during early pregnancy, which tends to decrease as the pregnancy progresses. Altered taste is not an uncommon complaint by the pregnant mother in early pregnancy. Craving for food is also commonly noted. Salivary secretion on the other hand remains within the normal range of the non-pregnant woman. Although there is no evidence to suggest a higher incidence of dental caries in pregnancy, spongy gums will be noticed due to gingival edema from fluid retention in pregnancy.[3]

In general, because of the effect of the progesterone, relaxation of the entire intestinal musculature is seen. Hence, heartburn and esophageal reflux is common in pregnancy because of the relaxation of the cardiac sphincter of the stomach. Gastric secretion is reduced and so is the motility of the stomach. Hence, the stomach emptying time is doubled in pregnancy. As a result, food will stay longer in the stomach, which potentially can be hazardous when the woman goes into labor as a risk of regurgitation during anesthesia may occur. In the large intestines, because of the delay in transit from lowered motility, reabsorption of water will occur, thus causing constipation.[12,13]

The liver is rarely palpable in pregnancy. The gallbladder empties more slowly in pregnancy although the constituent of the bile does not change. Cholestasis is a physiological phenomenon in pregnancy. There is stasis of bile with no change in the bile secretion. This could produce a generalized pruritus. Commonly, this condition is reproducible in subsequent pregnancies or when the woman is on the combined oral contraceptive pills or hormone replacement therapy. Albumin level in the plasma decreases in pregnancy but its total circulating amount is the same as in non-pregnant woman. Globulin level increases in pregnancy. Alkaline phosphatase level rises in pregnancy due to placental production of the heat stable enzyme.[4]

A summary of the alimentary system changes is noted in Table 5.7.

ENDOCRINE SYSTEMS

Hypothalamic-pituitary Axis

The pituitary gland enlarges in pregnancy. It increases in weight by 30 percent in the first pregnancy and 50

Table 5.7: Changes within gastrointestinal system during pregnancy

• **Increase**	• Appetite
	• Craving for food
	• Heartburn
	• Esophageal reflux
	• Stomach emptying time
	• Constipation
	• Alkaline phosphatase
	• Globulin
• **Decrease**	• Gastric secretion
	• Gastric motility
	• Large intestines motility
	• Gallbladder emptying
	• Plasma albumin
• **No change**	• Salivary secretion
	• Dental caries
	• Bile constituent and secretion

percent in subsequent pregnancies. This normal increase can produce headache. As the human chorionic gonadotropin rises, the follicular stimulating hormone (FSH) falls and remains low throughout pregnancy. The effect of pregnancy on luteinizing hormone (LH) is not known in pregnancy. However, there is blunted response of both FSH and LH to GnRH (gonadotropin-releasing hormone) in pregnancy. Initially, there is a progressive decrease in response of FSH to GnRH but eventually there will be no response, 3 weeks after ovulation. The LH response also disappears but not until some weeks after the loss of FSH response to GnRH.[14,15]

The level of TSH (thyroid-stimulating hormone) remains unchanged while the level of ACTH (adrenocorticotropic hormone) decreases. The number of prolactin secreting cells increases in pregnancy. Serum prolactin level doubles by term as compared to the non-pregnant level. Oxytocin and vasopressin levels remain low in pregnancy. The former will increase in its level during labor.

Adrenal Gland

Maternal adrenal gland does not enlarge during pregnancy but an increase in its secretion is noted. Plasma cortisol and corticosteroid increases during pregnancy, progressively from 12th weeks onwards. It can be 3-5 times higher than the non-pregnant level. Unbound cortisol does not change much during pregnancy as compared to the non-pregnant level. There is no change in the glucocorticoid receptor numbers during pregnancy.[16]

Thyroid Gland

The thyroid gland increases in size during pregnancy. A frank goiter may develop due to increased blood flow and hyperplasia of the follicular tissue. Clearance of iodide by the thyroid gland and kidney increases. Thyroid binding globulin (TBG) doubles during pregnancy. Free plasma triiodothyronine (T_3) and thyroxine (T_4) remain at the non-pregnant level whilst the bound fraction increases but the mother remains euthyroid.[17]

Parathyroid Gland

As the parathormone level increases during pregnancy, an increase in the calcium absorption by the mother is seen. However, neither calcitonin nor parathormone crosses from the mother to the fetus. At term, the parathormone level is higher in the mother but the calcitonin level is higher in the fetus, thus encouraging deposition of bone in the fetus.[4]

Pancreas

The pancreatic changes that occur during pregnancy are: (i) increase in the size of the Langerhans cells; (ii) increase in the number of β cells and (iii) increase in the number of receptor sites for insulin. Serum level of insulin rises during the second half of pregnancy and its response to glucose load is one of a greater increase than in the non-pregnant state. However, the blood sugar level does not fall as a result of this change. This resistance to insulin may be due to the diabetogenic hormones in pregnancy e.g. hPL, prolactin, etc. As pregnancy advances, the insulin resistance also increases. Glucagon level increases slightly during pregnancy. A glucose load suppresses glucagon further in pregnant compared to non-pregnant women.[18]

A summary of the endocrine changes in pregnancy is shown in Table 5.8.

CONCLUSION

Physiological maternal adaptation in pregnancy occurs early as this is necessary for implantation and healthy

Table 5.8: Endocrine changes in pregnancy

• **Pituitary gland**	↑ in size and weight ⇒ headache
	↑ in prolactin secreting cells ⇒ serum prolactin level ↑
	ACTH ↓
	↓ oxytocin until labor
	↓ vasopressin
	TSH ⇔
• **Thyroid gland**	↑ in size ⇒ frank goitre sometimes
	TBG ↑
	T_3/T_4 ⇔/↓
• **Adrenal gland**	⇔ in size
	↑ adrenal secretion
	↑ cortisol
	↑ corticosteroid
• **Parathyroid gland**	↑ parathormone
	↑ calcium absorption
• **Pancreas**	↑ size of Langerhans cells
	↑ number of β cells
	↑ number of insulin receptor sites
	↑ in insulin level
	↑ in insulin resistance

growth in early pregnancy. A thorough understanding of these changes in pregnancy is necessary for pathological processes to be assessed. The influence of age, parity, multiple pregnancy, race and other variables has to be understood and taken into account in order to appreciate the level of adaptation that occurs during pregnancy.

REFERENCES

1. Ganong WF: The gonads: Development and function of the reproductive system. In Ganong WF (Ed): *Review of Medical Physiology*. California: Lange Medical Publications, 12th edn, 342-74, 1985.
2. Chamberlain G: Diagnosis of pregnancy. In Turnbull A and Chamberlain G (Eds): *Obstetrics*, Edinburgh: Churchill Livingstone, 3rd edn, 219-23, 1994.
3. Llewellyn-Jones D: The physiology of pregnancy. In Llewellyn-Jones D (Ed): *Fundamentals of Obstetrics and Gynaecology*, Vol 1: Obstetrics, London: Faber and Faber Ltd, 4th edn, 41-53, 1986.
4. McFadyen IR: Maternal changes in normal pregnancy. In Turnbull A, Chamberlain G (Eds): *Obstetrics*, Edinburgh: Churchill Livingstone, 3rd edn, 151-71, 1994.
5. Stirrat GM: Physiological changes in pregnancy. In Stirrat GM (Ed): *Obstetrics*, Oxford: Blackwell Scientific Publications, 2nd edn, 7-22, 1986.
6. Bierniaz J, Yoshida T, Romero-Salinas G et al: Aortocaval compression by the uterus in late human pregnancy. IV circulatory homeostasis by preferential perfusion of the placenta. *American Journal of Obstetrics and Gynecology* **103**: 19-31, 1969.
7. Robertson WB, Brosens I, Dixon G: Uteroplacental vascular pathology. *European Journal of Obstetrics, Gynecology and Reproductive Biology* **5**: 47-65, 1975.
8. Zuspan FP, O'Shaughnessy RW, Vinsel J, Zuspan M: Adrenegic innervation of uteric vasculature in human term pregnancy. *American Journal of Obstetrics and Gynecology* **139**: 678-80, 1982.
9. McFayden IR, Price AB, Geirsson RT: The relation of birth weight to histological appearances in vessels of the placental bed. *British Journal of Obstetrics and Gynaecology* **93**: 476-81, 1986.
10. Dure-Smith P: *Radiology* **96**: 545-49, 1970.
11. Davison JM, Dunlop W: Renal hemodynamics and tubular function in normal human pregnancy. *Kidney International* **18**: 152-61, 1980.
12. Davison JS, Davison MC, Hay DM: Gastric emptying time in late pregnancy and labor. *Journal Obstetrics and Gynaecology of the British Commonwealth* **77**: 37-41, 1970.
13. Parry E, Shields R, Turnbull AC: The effect of pregnancy on the colonic absorption of sodium, potassium and water. *Journal of Obstetrics and Gynaecology of British Commonwealth* **77**: 616-19, 1970.
14. Jeppsson S, Rennevik G, Thorell JI: Pituitary gonadotropin secretion during the first weeks of pregnancy. *Acta Endocrinologica* **85**: 177-88, 1977.
15. Miyake A, Tanizawa O, Toshihiro A, Kurachi K: Pituitary responses in LH secretion to LHRH during pregnancy. *Obstetrics and Gynecology* **49**: 549-51, 1977.
16. Wintour EM, Coghlan JP, Oddie CJ, Scoggins BA, Walters WAW: A sequential study of adrenocorticoid level in human pregnancy. *Clinical Experience of Pharmacology and Physiology* **5**: 399-403, 1978.
17. Franklyn JA, Sheppard MC, Ramsden DB: Serum free thyroxine and free triiodothyronine concentration in pregnancy. *British Medical Journal* **287**: 394, 1983.
18. Puavilai G, Drogny EC, Domont LA, Bauma G: Insulin receptors and insulin resistance in human pregnancy: evidence for a post receptor defect in insulin action. *Journal of Clinical Endocrinological Metabolism* **54**: 247-53, 1982.

where it is transferred to the follicular fluid to be taken up by the grannulosa cells.

5. *Placental aromatase enzyme*: The enzyme is known as aromatase, the product of a CYP gene[16] and is a Flavoprotein.

   The principal cellular location of P-450 in placenta is syncytiotrophoblast. The main function of placental aromatase enzyme is to catalyse formation of estradiol 17-β from androstenedione.

6. *Estrogen secretion in different tissue location*: From 17-β hydroxysteroid dehydrogenase (17-β HSD) an isoenzyme in the tissue is responsible for secretion of estrogen. The androstenedione in tissues is converted to Estrone and Estradiol 17-β. This product has been found in extra uterine circulation as estrone whereas testosterone is converted into estradiol 17-β directly in all tissues by aromatisation. Metabolic clearance rate of estrogen precursor Dehydroepiandosterone Sulphate (DHEAS) increases 10/20 fold.[17] So near term the plasma level of DHEA becomes very low.

Contribution to Estrogen

Fetal adrenal cortex provides the principal source of estrogen. Anencephalics have small adrenal and as such these fetuses have very little estrogen. Further evidence is provided by fetal DHEA in maternal plasma, which is converted into estrogen in plasma of mother. Finally, it has now been established that the fetal DHEA is converted into estrogen.

1. *Estriol*: Large amounts of estriol are secreted from the syncytiotrophoblast.
2. *Estriol as index of fetal wellbeing*: In 1955 emphasis was placed on urinary estriol and truly it was found that in a large majority of cases low urinary estriol indicated either fetal distress or fetal death. But subsequent workers could not either reproduce or confirm these observations due to large variation of estriol secretion. Attempts to correlate serum estriol with fetal wellbeing also could not throw much light on the fetal status.
3. *Down syndrome*: There are different types of estriol circulating in maternal blood-free unconjugated estriol and conjugated estriol.

A rise in free unconjugated estriol indicates possibility of Down syndrome. This observation alongwith other two tests viz rise in hCG in midtrimester and low alpha-fetoprotein (triple test) raise the possibilities of Down syndrome.

Fetal Adrenal (Figure 6.3)

In early embryonic life the adrenal cortex is composed of only those cells which resemble fetal zone. The maternal ACTH does not cross the placenta and therefore it is obvious that the fetal pituitary secretion of ACTH takes place at the early weeks of pregnancy even in the absence of hypothalamicocorticotrophin releasing hormone, which is responsible for the fetal zone of adrenal cortex.

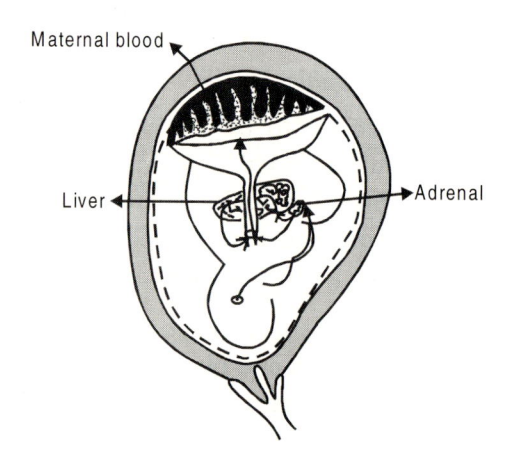

Figure 6.3: Fetal adrenal

The normal adrenal cortex continues to grow throughout the pregnancy. The adrenal gland becomes at least twenty-five times larger than those of adults. It is possible that in addition to the ACTH there must be some secretion of growth stimuli to the adrenal gland. It is also possible that the fetal adrenal gland by its large size provides most of the steroids necessary for the biosynthesis of other hormones like C-19 steroid so vitally necessary for the biosynthesis of estrogen.

Precursors of steroid biosynthesis in fetal adrenal gland— Most of the workers believe that progesterone and pregnenolone produced in the placenta are utilised for synthesis of cortisol and DHEA.

1. *Progesterone*: In the epochmaking classical experiment carried out by Dicsfaluzy, it was observed

that interruption of cord circulation led to rapid fall of estrogen but the level of progesterone continued for sometime till the placenta become nonfunctioning. In normal pregnancy there is a gradual rise of estradiol and estriol alongwith progesterone.

2. *Progesterone biosynthesis*: Cholesterol is initially converted into pregnenolone in mitochondria, a reaction catalysed by cytochrome P-450.

   In the second step of conversion the pregnenolone is converted into progesterone in microsome. This process is catalysed by 3, β hydroxysteroid dehydorgenase.

   In human, the placenta produces prodigious amount of progesterone.

3. *Source of cholesterol for placental biosynthesis*: It was found that maternal plasma cholesterol was the principal precursor of progesterone biosynthesis in pregnancy. This proves that the *de novo* synthesis of cholesterol in trophoblast is minimal.

4. *Progesterone synthesis and fetal wellbeing*: Fetal wellbeing is very closely related to the placental production of estrogen and progesterone. Experimentally it has been observed long ago, that following ligation of umbilical cord of fetus but placenta remaining intact, will result in very low maternal plasma level in estrogen but the progesterone decline does not take place similarly. It takes some time after fetal death that the placental production of protein hormones like hCG and progesterone come to a low level.

5. *Progesterone metabolism during pregnancy*: The clearance rate of progesterone in pregnant women increases near term thereby reducing the plasma level of progesterone and triggering the onset of parturition. Another interesting observation that merits mentioning is the conversion of progesterone 5-alpha to dihydroprogesterone, which resists the pressor effect on blood vessels in pregnancy.

   Another aspect of progesterone metabolism is that it is converted into very potent mineralocorticoid deoxy corticosteroid (DOCA). DOCA is increased strikingly in both maternal and fetal compartment.

6. *Transfer of steroids*: The steroids secreted from the syncytiotrophoblast enter the blood directly and this phenomenon does not need any receptor binding. The steroids must pass through the cytotrophoblast before reaching intervillous space.

ENDOCRINOLOGY OF LABOR

The exact mechanism of onset of labor is not clearly understood. However, it is a special characteristic of myometrium by which the myometrium is triggered to action producing effective contraction. The characteristics of these contractions are as follows:

A. One contraction tends to be triggered by the subsequent one.
B. It spreads in all directions in contrast to the skeletal muscle contraction, which acts only along its axis.
C. It produces gradual retraction and shortening of the muscle fibers.

All these special features of the myometrium are brought about by the influx of calcium into the muscle. The sequential events are as follows:-

a. Calcium binds to calmodulin calcium binding regulatory protein.
b. Calmodulin inturn binds to activate myosin light chain kinase.
c. Activation of calcium ion and increase of intracellular cytosolic calcium concentration.
d. Calcium promotes contraction.
e. cAMP and cGMP promote relaxation.

   How are these changes brought about:

1. *Progesterone withdrawal*: This was the assumption arising out of the concept that withdrawal of progesterone removes the relaxed state of myometrium. However, this has not been finally proved.

2. *Other mechanisms*: Increase of estrogen—It has been observed that there is a rise of estrogen which is synthesised in human pregnancy just before labor. The level of estrogen reaches incredible concentration and quantity.

   Factors leading to rise of estrogen are as follows:
   1. It has been shown that the estrogen is not formed from acetate or cholesterol or from C-21 steroid precursors like pregnenolone or progesterone.

2. In 1950, Ken Ryan found that human placental tissue effectively converts C-19 steroids to estrogen.
3. Liggins and colleagues identified the following events:
   a. Progesterone withdrawal.
   b. Corticotropin releasing hormone is transmitted from fetal hypothalamus via the hypophyseal portal circulation.
   c. This CRH reaches the fetal pituitary gland and produces increase of ACTH secretion followed by,
   d. Augmented increase of the fetal adrenal to the ACTH secretion.
   e. The augmented response converts C-19 steroids like androstenedione, the immediate precursor of estrogen.
   f. This androstenedione the immediate precursor of estrogen is synthesised in placenta by 17-alpha hydroxylation of 17-hydroxyprogesterone to DHEA and androstenedione.
   g. The androstenedione reaches the trophoblast where these C-19 steroid precursors are acted on by aromatase and estrogen is formed. Many observers have confirmed this.
   h. The other endocrine antecedents of parturition are a sharp drop in progesterone, rise of fetal cortisol and phenomenal rise of E_2.

Summarily all these changes finally point toward the steep rise of E_2 activated from fetal adrenal in response to the signal system from fetal hypothalamus for conversation of C-19 steroids into estrogens.

Other Experimental Evidences

Nitric Oxide Synthase Expression

The expression of ions (inducible nitric oxide synthase)/ is gradually reduced before or during labor.

The epithelial cells undergo a process of apoptosis or programmed cell death before start of labor. The process is associated with the degradation of extracellular matrix followed by the biomechanical changes resulting in rupture of fetal membrane and onset of labor.

CONCLUSION

The forgoing discussion illustrates the vital role of the fetoplacental unit for its wellbeing *in utero* and its rapid growth.

REFERENCES

1. Halban J: Die Inner Secretion Van Ovarium and Placenta Und Ihre Bedeutung Fur Die Function Der Michdrusen. *Arch Gyneco* **73**:345, 1905.
2&3. Cunningham Mac Donald Gant, Leven Gilstrap Hankins Clark: The Placental Hormone. Williams Obstertrics, 20th Edition, **6**: 125-26, 1997.
4&5. Cole La, Kardana A, Ying Fc, Birken S: The Biological and Clinical Significance of Nicks In Human Chorionic Gonadotropin and Its Free B Subunit. *Yale J Niol Med* **64**: 627, 1991.
6. Cunningham Mac Donald Gant, Leven Gilstrap Hankins Clark: *The Placental Hormone.* Williams Obstetrics, 20th Edition, **6**: 128, 1997.
7. Bradbury Jt, Brown We, Guay La, 1950. Maintenance of the Corpus Luteum and Physiologia Action of Progesterone. Recent Prog Horm Res, 5: 151.
8. Cunningham Mac Donald Gant Leven, Gilstrap Hankins Clark, 1997. *The Placental Hormone.* Williams Obstetrics, 20th Edition, 6: Pp-130.
9. Odagiri E, Sherrpill BJ, Mount CD, Nicholson WE, Orth DN: Human Placental Immunoreactive Corticotropin, Lipotropin and B Endorphin: Evidence for a Common Precursor. *Proc Natl Acad Sci USA,* **16**: 2027, 1979.
10. Bogic LV, Mandel M, Bryant Greenwood GD: Relaxin Gene Expression in Human Reproductive Tissues by in situ Hybridization. *J Clin Endocrinol Metab*, **80**: 130, 1995.
11. Patel N, Alsat E, Logout A, Barin F, Hennen G, Porquer D: Glucose Inhibits Human Placenta Gh Secretion *in vitro. J Clin Endocrinol Metab* **1743**: 199, 1980.
12&14. Siler-Khodr TM: Chorioni Peptides. In Mcnellis D, Challis JRG, Mac Donald PC, Nathamielsz PW, Robert JM (Eds). *The Onset of Labor: Cellular and Integrative Mechanism.* An Nichd Workshop. Ithaca, Perinatology Press, 213, 1988.
13. Petraglia F, Woodruff TK, Botticelli G, Botticelli A, Grenazzani AR, Mayo KE, Vale W: Gonadotropin – Releasing Hormone Inhibin and Activin in Human Placenta. Evidence for a Common Cellular Localization. *J Clin Endocrinol Metab* **74**: 1184, 1982.
15. Siler-Khodr TM, Khodr GS: Content of Luteinizing Hormone Releasing Factor in the Human Placenta. *Am J Obstet Gynecol* **130**: 216, 1978.
16. Cunningham Mac Donald Gant, Leven Gilstrap Hankins Clark: The Placental Hormone. Williams Obstetrics, 20th Edition, **6**: 136,1997.
17. Gant NF, Hutchinson HT, Siiteri PK, Mac Donald PC: Study of the Metabolic Clearance Rate of Dehydroisoandrosterone Sulfate in Pregnancy. *Am J Obstet Gynecol* **111**: 555, 1971.

7. Immunology of Pregnancy

A Padma Rao

INTRODUCTION

Edward Jenner performed effective immunization against smallpox more than 200 years ago. Nevertheless the discipline of immunology is hardly four decades old and that of pregnancy immunology is only two decades old and is now a mature discipline. Immune responses in the placenta and in the mother in normal pregnancy differ in many ways from the classical immune responses. The fetal allograft which is 50 percent foreign to the mother is not rejected. The mother not only develops immune tolerance to the fetus and placenta, but also provides the fetus means to achieve immunocompetence including passive immunity by transfer of maternal IgG. Many of the disorders of pregnancy may be caused by alteration in the various beneficial immunological responses of normal pregnancy. A brief account of basic immunology will be followed by the beneficial alterations in immunology in normal pregnancy and their aberration in abnormal pregnancy.

BASIC IMMUNOLOGY

Immunology is the study of the immune system which deals with the physiological responses by which the body destroys or neutralizes foreign matter both living and nonliving, thus protecting the body.

1. *Definition of antigen:* Any foreign molecule that can trigger a specific immune response against itself or the cell bearing it is termed 'antigen'. Most antigens are either proteins or very large polysaccharides.

    The immune system consists of several diverse elements that interact to counteract the antigens that are expressed by the invading pathogens. The most important heroes of the immune system are the Lymphocytes; the B lymphocytes and T lymphocytes. Other cells that orchestrate with the lymphocytes are the macrophages, other leucocytes and natural killer (NK) cells. Besides cells, innumerable agents also join in this process. They are complements and cytokines. The body is capable of 2 major types of immune responses to an invader, the production of antibodies (humoral) and cell mediated response. The aim of the immune system is to destroy the invader either by direct action or neutralise through an antibody and carry the memory of the invader so as to promptly attack when the invader reappears.

2. *T lymphocytes:* One of the heroes of immune system, the T cell lymphocyte are of 3 types. T helper cell (TH), cytotoxic T cell and suppressor T cell; of these T-Helper

cell is the commander-in-chief, because it regulates and controls the action of almost all the cells and if it fails the entire immune system collapses as happens in the disease-AIDS.

3. *B Lymphocytes:* They produce antibodies under orders from T-helper cells. B cells themselves do not produce antibodies—instead they instruct 'plasma cells' to do the job, but carry a copy of the antibody to be formed by the plasma cell.

4. *Macrophages:* They are the vigilant cells present in all the tissues and cell linings. They are the security officers. They patrol the body and attack, destroy and swallow the enemy when sighted. When they fail in destroying the enemy (antigen) completely, they present the antigen to TH cells for further action.

5. *Natural Killer (NK) cells:* These cells are produced in the bone marrow and are the oldest cells of the immune system. They do not manifest specificity for antigens. They kill directly virus infected and cancer cells.

6. *Complement:* These are protein molecules - nearly twenty in number; they are found in the blood and tissues. Complement act as a cascade, one leading to the next. They help the macrophages to travel from blood stream to the tissues, they help the macrophages in the process of phagocytosis, which is one of the functions of macrophages. Complement can attack the bacterial membrane through the formation of membrane attack complex (MAC).

7. *Cytokines:* These are another group of protein messengers secreted by a variety of cells. "Kine" derived from Greek word means "action"; cytokines thus activate the cells of the immune system. There are nearly 20 known cytokines which include interleukins, colony -stimulating factors, interferons and tumour necrosis factor. Different cytokines do different things. Some stimulate growth of cells, some inhibit growth, some stimulate inflammatory responses, while others inhibit inflammatory response of cells.

8. *Antibody:* Plasma cells produce thousands of antibody molecules per second before they die in a day or so. The primary function of antibody is to bind to antigen and bring about the inactivation or removal of the offending toxin, microbe, parasite or foreign substances from the body. There are five major classes of antibodies. The terms antibody and immunoglobulin are used synonymously. The most abundant (75% of total serum immunoglobulin) are the IgG antibodies, also commonly called gamma globulin. IgG is the only one of the immunoglobulin isotypes that crosses the placenta. IgG and IgM provide the bulk of specific immunity against bacteria and viruses in the extracellular fluid. IgM is the first immunoglobulin to appear in the immune response (primary immune response) and is the initial type of antibody made by neonates; IgM is an important component of immune complexes in autoimmune diseases. IgM is also a potent activator of complement. IgE antibodies mediate allergic responses and participate in defences against multicellular parasites. IgA antibodies secreted by plasma cells are taken up by the lining of the gastrointestinal, respiratory and genitourinary tracts and secreted on to the surface. IgA antibodies generally do not circulate but act locally in the linings; they are also secreted by the mammary glands and hence are the major antibodies in breast milk. The functions of IgD are still unclear.

Electron microscopic studies reveal that the immunoglobulin molecule has the shape of letter "**Y**". The stem of the **Y** is called Fc portion. The amino acid sequences of Fc portion are identical for all immunoglobulins of a single class. In contrast the amino acid sequences of the antigen binding sites vary from immunoglobulin to immunoglobulin in a given class.

9. *Immunoregulation:* The first step in immunoregulation is to spot the foreign antigen. This is done by macrophages, which patrol to spot any foreign molecule, which is either engulfed straight away (phagocytosis) or if unable to completely destroy, present it (antigen) to the helper T- cells for further orders to the various cells involved in the immune process. This takes us to the topic of antigen

presenting cells (APC). Macrophages, B cells and dendritic cells perform as APCs.

It is to be remembered that T cells do not produce antibodies, but receive antigens and interestingly these cells can recognise an antigen that is presented to it only if the antigen is complexed with a body protein called major histocompatibility complex (MHC). MHC are genetic markers and can be compared to "name tag" to the cell. The T cells can identify the antigen only when it has the "name tag". Two classes of MHC occur, class I and class II. Class I MHC are produced by all cells of the body. Additionally the B cell, dendritic cell and the macrophages express MHC class II molecules. The T-cell differentiate into a TH1 cells and TH2 cells. TH1 cell immune responses is one of destruction and that of TH2 cell is one of growth. Normally the TH1 and TH2 responses are kept in equal balance. But in pregnancy the TH2 response is preferred. (See later).

10. *Some wonderful revelations:* The process of lymphocyte development occurs in such a way that a single lymphocyte can recognize just one antigen. This is true of T cells and B cells. One consequence of this is that the number of cells which can recognize any particular pathogen is quite small. Hence the first thing that the immune system must do after contacting antigen is to expand the number of cells which can recognise it to react against it. Clones of cells which recognise the antigen are driven to divide and differentiate. This process occurs mainly in the lymphoid tissue and is described as clonal selection.

Because each individual has two chromosomes carrying the MHC genes the maternal chromosome and the paternal chromosome, there are usually six different versions of class I MHC molecules, and six different versions of class II molecules. Because the MHC is dependant on the genetic make-up of the individual, it is very unlikely that two unrelated people will have the same MHC molecules. Since each individual has different MHC molecules, the performance of everyone's immune system is different. This affects susceptibility to diseases where the immune system is involved.

Some Clarifications of Nomenclature

1. *MHC and HLA:* In humans MHC proteins are termed HLA (Human leukocyte antigen) because they were first discovered on leukocytes. Therefore MHC and HLA are used interchangeably, though it is correct to use the term MHC instead of the term HLA.
2. *Categorizing cells by the presence of certain proteins in their plasma membranes:* T helper cells have the protein CD4 and so may be referred to as CD4 cells. Cytotoxic T- cells and suppressor T cells have CD8, NK cells have CD 56 and so on.

SUMMARY OF IMMUNOREGULATION

1. The immune system consists of several diverse elements that interact to counteract pathogens and cope with the antigens they express.
2. Antigens are taken up by antigen presenting cells, which process the antigen and present it to the T-cells.
3. The T-cell may have differentiated into a TH1 cell, which releases cytokines that activate macrophages. The macrophages go on to remove the source of the antigen.
4. If, however the T-cell has differentiated into TH2 cell, it activates B-cells. These produce more antibody which binds with antigen, leading to its removal.
5. When the antigen is gone, the B-cells continue to generate antibodies. Without a target antigen, these antibodies feedback on to the B-cell and signal a shutdown in antibody production.
6. The effectiveness of these system depends to some extent on the genetic makeup of the host. Specifically, there are genes that determine how well antigen-presenting cells process antigen etc.
7. Even the relative population levels of *TH1 to TH2* are genetically determined. The ratio of one population to the other will govern how the immune system will respond to antigen, either preferring antibody production or macrophage activation.

8. Now an endocrine regulation of immune response is noted. The differentiation of TH cells to TH1 may be caused by low estrogen and high prolactin and the differentiation to TH2 cells may be caused by high estrogen and high progesterone.[2]

PREGNANCY IMMUNOLOGY

We discussed what happens to a foreign molecule on entering the body—it is destroyed. But the placenta and fetus are 50 percent foreign to the mother and yet it is not destroyed. Why? The story begins with the earliest phase of pregnancy, viz. implantation of the zygote.

1. *Pregnancy has two parts:* The trophoblast and the decidua. The trophoblast (the foreign tissue) has to gain entrance into the decidua (maternal tissue). Therefore the trophoblast signals and recruits the migration of a family of lymphocytes to the uterine decidua. These serve a variety of *growth supporting functions* and some of the recruited lymphocytes even suppress the activity of cytotoxic cells. The NK cells recruited by the trophoblast into the decidua behave differently from those found in peripheral blood. They resemble Large Granular Lymphocytes (LGL) and do not possess the cytotoxicity of NK cells. We may refer to this LGL cells in the decidua as decidual NK cells. The surprising fact is that the stromal cells in the decidua and the decidual NK cells produce cytokines that are essential for the trophoblast *growth, proliferation* and *differentiation* and this is exactly what is needed for the growth and maintenance of pregnancy.

2. When the trophoblast grows it produces the hormone progesterone which functions locally, through the help of decidual leukocytes to induce apoptosis (programmed cell death) of the cytotoxic NK cells. In pregnancies that fail, the cytotoxic NK cells are seen in abundance.

3. The trophoblast that has proliferated invades and deports itself into the maternal blood and antipaternal alloantibody is produced which returns and binds to the placenta. Here it has immunotrophic functions and *blocks* the immune response locally (blocking antibody). By this process placenta becomes a privileged tissue. By ten weeks the process is complete and not only the fetus parasitized to the mother-to-be, it has established a lasting immunologic truce with her, which imprints itself on her immune system and lasts a life time.

4. The trophoblasts express a unique variety of MHC antigen known as HLA-G antigen which causes immune suppression and production of growth promoting cytokines. This renders the placenta a privileged organ resistant to immune damage by the concerned cells.

5. The syncitiotrophoblast which is derived from the cytotrophoblast forms a membrane directly in contact with the maternal blood and all the immune factors contained in it. This membrane (syncitiotrophoblast) completely surrounds the fetus and functions as a biological dialysis membrane involved in two-way exchanges of all molecules entering or leaving the fetal circulation. It is interesting to note that the syncytiotrophoblast does *not* express any antigen and thus escapes immune recognition (a camouflage effect).

6. All the extravillous trophoblasts mentioned below also express HLA-G antigen. The extra villous trophoblasts are: (a) the anchoring cytotrophoblasts, (b) the cytotrophoblasts that migrated into the myometrium, (c) the endovascular trophoblasts that erode into and alter the structure of the maternal arterioles to render the vessel dilated and non-contractile, which phenomenon is necessary for protecting a normal pregnancy and is absent in those pregnancies with placental insufficiency. Thus in pre-eclampsia HLA-G antigen is decreased.

7. The trophoblast allows the passage of IgG antibodies to the fetus from the very earliest stage of conception. Thus the fetus is protected from most of the infections.

8. The TH1 response is suppressed (destruction avoided) and TH2 response is preferred (growth and proliferation of trophoblasts).

All points mentioned above have been scientifically explored with sophisticated methods. It is now possible to identify B and T lymphocytes and other cells. Can you believe that it is possible to follow one single cell in the blood stream and study its functions? In spite of the great advances made in the study of immunology, only some of postulates proferred some 35 years ago are answered; most of them are still puzzles. The postulates were:[4]

i. Fetal tissues are antigenitically deficient because of immunological immaturity.
ii. The uterus is an immunologically privileged site.
iii. The placenta is devoid of transplantation antigen and acts as an immunologically inert protective barrier between mother and fetus.
iv. The placenta is protected against immune attack by a local mechanical or hormonal barrier.
v. Maternal immune responses are nonspecifically diminished during pregnancy.
vi. The maternal immune response is specifically diminished during pregnancy by the process of immunological enhancement.
vii. The maternal immune response is suppressed by the fetus.

Much more research is needed to prove or disprove all the above postulates.

Aberrations in Pregnancy Immunology in Complicated Pregnancy

1. *Rejection of the early implantation embryo of assisted reproduction:* the lymphocytes in the decidua do not function as they do in normal pregnancy to cause growth of trophoblast, but destroy it. The decidua withers away.

2. *Recurrent spontaneous abortion (RSA) and pregnancy loss:*[5] The immunologic causes for pregnancy loss and implantation failure are the result of abnormalities in antibody responses. These responses fall into two categories: autoimmune and alloimmune.

i. *Autoimmune factors:* There are four different autoimmune problems that can cause RSA and pregnancy loss. A woman may have one or more of these underlying problems: antiphospholipid antibodies; antithyroid antibodies, antinuclear antibodies and lupus-like anticoagulant. Thirty percent of women with "unexplained" RSA will be test positive for an autoimmune problem.

- *Antiphospholipid Antibodies (APL antibodies):* In pregnancy phospholipids act like a sort of glue, holds the dividing cells together, and are necessary for growth of the placenta into the wall of the uterus. Phospholipids also filter nourishment from the mother's blood to the baby, and in turn, filter the baby's waste back through the placenta. APL (antibodies) can be IgG, IgA or IgM. The IgG APL antibodies cross the placenta, cause thrombosis, decrease prostacyclin production, cause damage to the placenta and to the fetus; thus causing pregnancy loss and pre-eclampsia at any period of pregnancy, early or late.

- *Antinuclear antibodies (ANA):* Antinuclear antibodies react against normal components of the cell nucleus. They can be present in a number of immunologic diseases, including systemic lupus erythematosus (SLE or Lupus) and in persons taking hydralazine and procainamide or isoniazid. In addition, ANA is present in some normal individuals or those who have collagen vascular diseases. The presence of ANA indicates there may be an underlying autoimmune process that affects the development of the placenta and can lead to early pregnancy loss.

- *Antithyroid antibodies:* Women with thyroid antibodies face double the risk of miscarriage as women without them. Increased levels of thyroglobulin and thyroid microsomal (thyroid peroxidase) autoantibodies show a relationship in an increased miscarriage rate, and as many as thirty percent of women experiencing RSA are positive for one or both antibodies. Chances of a loss in the first trimester of pregnancy increase to 20 percent, and there is also an increased risk of post-partum thyroid dysfunction. Therefore, antithyroid antibody, testing should be routine in women with a history of two or more losses or thyroid irregularities.

ii. *Alloimmune factors:* There are two possible reasons that women with alloimmune problems lose their pregnancies in miscarriage: Either her immune system does not recognize the pregnancy, or she develops an abnormal immunologic response to the pregnancy.

Successful pregnancy has been associated with the presence of circulating "blocking antibodies." These are antibodies that are formed by a woman's immune system when she is pregnant, and they "mask", or disguise the pregnancy so it is not recognised as "foreign".

Pregnancies that end with RSA have been associated with the absence of these blocking antibodies.

For some women who lack the blocking antibodies, immunization with their husband's white blood cells may be an effective treatment. However, a leukocyte antibody detection assay (LAD) should be performed prior to initiating this treatment.

Also IV immunoglobulin treatment may be effective for some women who lack blocking antibodies because the immunoglobulin, which comes from thousands of donors, appear to contain small amounts of antibodies to R80K, which is an antigen recently identified on the surface of syncytiotrophoblasts. The R80K antibodies is a kind of protein marker to which the blocking antibodies respond during a successful pregnancy.

Maternal-fetal HLA compatibility and fetal loss: The idea that maternal-fetal incompatibility with respect to MHC antigens is advantageous for successful human pregnancy was proposed in the 1960's, but not yet been fully accepted. It was thus proposed that HLA compatibility is a significant risk factor for fetal loss.[6]

3. *Pre-eclampsia:* HLA-G antigen expressed in the trophoblasts in normal pregnancies and which enhances maternal tolerance to the fetal allograft is greatly less in pre-eclampsia.

Additional evidence for alterations in immunity in the pathogenesis of pre-eclampsia includes; the disease is prominent in nulliparas followed by normal pregnancies, decreased prevalence after heterologous blood transfusions and long cohabitation before successful conception of all of which are evidences for the formation of some antibody protection for the paternal tissue. The pathological changes in the placental vasculature in pre-eclampsia resemble allograft rejection. Finally there are increased levels of inflammatory cytokines in the placenta and maternal circulation in pre-eclampsia as well as evidence of increased natural killer cells and neutrophil activation, all of them being evidence of decrease of the physiological maternal tolerance of the placenta and fetus.[7]

4. *Intrauterine growth restriction (IUGR):* This is associated with placental insufficiency. Deficient HLA-G antigen on intravascular trophoblast is a possibility.

5. *Blood group incompatibilities:*
   i. *Isoimmunization occurring with Rhesus antigen:* The fetal Rh positive RBC escape into maternal circulation, which contains Rh negative RBC. The Rh positive fetal cells are foreign to the mother. She therefore develops antibodies against the fetal cells. The antibodies are IgG antibodies. These IgG antibodies from the mother cross the placenta and cause hemolysis of fetal cells.
   ii. *ABO-incompatibility:* The antibodies of ABO system are nearly always of IgM type and hence do not cross the placenta which explains why the incidence of hemolytic disease in the newborn due to ABO incompatibility is much less than expected. Twenty-five percent of antibodies of ABO system however can be of IgG type and can cross the placenta and cause A-O isoimmune hemolysis.[8]

6. *Trophoblastic disease and tumors:*
   i. *Hydatidiform mole:* The karyotype of complete hydatidiform mole is XX (90%) and XY (10%).[9] All the 'X' are paternal in origin therefore it is completely mismatched with maternal host. The antigens expressed by the trophoblasts of molar pregnancy is believed to be similar to those expressed in normal pregnancy. The decidual NK cells (LGL) are also seen in molar pregnancy as in normal pregnancy. It is not clear why then the trophoblasts proliferate excessively and also penetrate into the myometrium and perforate the uterus. It is interesting to note that ABO compatible partners are protected from development of choriocarcinoma from postmolar pregnancy; group

A woman with group 'O' partner, show higher risk of development of choriocarcinoma.[10] How ABO antigens could influence postmolar trophoblast proliferation is immunologically obscure.

ii. *Choriocarcinoma:* Immunological cause of occurrence of choriocarcinoma is not understood. It may be associated with a small increase in HLA compatibility.

Synopsis of Pregnancy Immunology

Immune coexistence between mother and embryo is established very early in pregnancy. This involves alloimmune recognition, stimulation of TH2 response and suppression of TH1 cytotoxic response. Lack of immune recognition results in rejection of the embryo by autoimmune reactivity and activation of cytotoxic NK cells.[3]

REFERENCES

1. Arthur J Vander, James H Sherman, Dorothy S Luciano: Immunology Defences Against Foreign Matter, Human Physiology. 6th Edition, McGraw- Hill, Inc. New York, 700-37, 1994.
2. Gil Mor Dr. Assistant Professor, Department of Obstetrics and Gynaecology, Yale University School of Medicine, Slides on Immunology. Website:http://info.med.yale.edu/obgyn/reproimmuno/
3. Alan E Beer, Joanne YH, Kwak MD: Immunology of Normal Pregnancy. *Immunology and Allergy Clinics of North America* **18(2):** 249-70, 1998.
4. Fox H: Immunopathology of the placenta. *Pathology of the Placenta*, Saunders London, 327-33, 1978.
5. Carolyn B Coulam, Nancy P Hemenway: Immunology May Be Key to Pregnancy Loss: *I N C I I D Fact Sheet*. Website:: http://www.inciid.org/immune.html
6. Carole Ober: Immunogenetics'98. HLA and Pregnancy: The Paradox of the Fetal-Allograft. *American Journal of Human Genetics* **62:** 1-5, 1998.
7. Report of the National High Blood Pressure Education Program working Group on High- Blood Pressure in Pregnancy, National High Blood Pressure Education Program working Group on High Blood Pressure in Pregnancy. *American Journal of Obstetrics Gynaecology* **183:**S4, 2000.
8. Barbara J Stoll, Robert M Kliegman: Haemolytic disease of the Newborn. In Richard E Behrman, Robert M Kliegman, Hal B Jenson (Eds): *Nelson Text Book of Paediatrics*, 16th edition; Harcourt Asia PTE. Ltd. Printed in India at Thomas Press(I)Ltd. Noida 525.
9. Kajii T, Ohama K: Androgenic origin of hydatidiform mole. *Nature* **268:** 633-34, 1977.
10. Bagshawe KD, Rawlins G, Pike MC, Sylvia D Lawler: ABO Blood-groups in Trophoblastic Neoplasia. *The Lancet* 553-55, 1971.

8. Fetus, Placenta and Membranes

Anita Thomas
Pratap Kumar

PART One

Introduction

INTRODUCTION

Benirschke observed that the placenta is the most accurate record of the infant's prenatal experiences. Yet most physicians shy away from examining the placenta which will provide a wealth of information. The knowledge about the afterbirth can be traced far back in human history. The term placenta is derived from the Latin word for circular cake.

Interest in the placenta was derived from its role in nidation and in the transfer of nutrients from mother to fetus. Scientific interest in the placenta also evolved from its enormous diversity in function and from the varied metabolic, endocrine and immunological functions of the trophoblast.

The ensuing discussion deals with placental development, structure, circulation, functions and its clinical significance in practice. The amnion and umbilical cord is also discussed with special emphasis on amniotic fluid and its clinical relevance. Pertinent aspects of fetal anatomy are discussed with special emphasis on fetal circulation.

PLACENTA

The human placenta is a villous hemochorial structure, which plays a critical role in maternal fetal transfer, has a complex synthetic capacity and plays a role in the immunological acceptance of the fetal allograft. The placenta as expelled from the uterus appears to be complete in itself. However, this is only the fetal placenta and the maternal component comprising of the placental bed and uteroplacental vessels is also a part of the functioning unit of the placenta.

Development

The ovum is fertilised in the fallopian tube and enters the uterine cavity as a morula which rapidly sheds its surrounding zone pellucida and converts itself into a blastocyst (Figure 8.1).

The outer cell layer of the blastocyst then proliferates to form the primary trophoblastic cell mass from which the cells infiltrate between those of the endometrial lining: the latter degenerates and the trophoblast comes in direct contact with the endometrial stroma. This is completed by the 10th or 11th postovulatory day (Figure 8.2).

Fetus, Placenta and Membranes

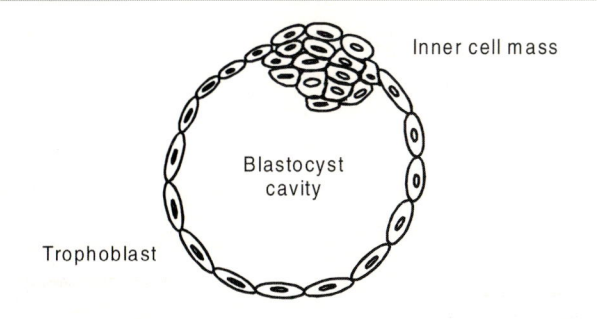

Figure 8.1: Blastocyst showing inner cell mass and trophoblast

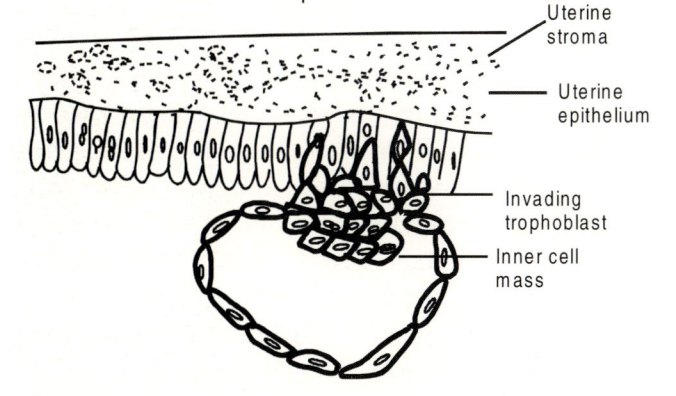

Figure 8.2: Trophoblast shown penetrating the uterine epithelium

In the 7-day zygote the trophoblast differentiates into two layers an inner layer of clear mononuclear cells the cytotrophoblasts with well-defined limiting membranes. The outer layers are formed by the fusion of the cytotrophoblasts and hence are multinucleated with no intercellular membrane though some remnants of such membrane can occasionally be found on electron microscopy.

Between 10th and the 13th postovulatory days a series of intercommunicating spaces or lacunae develop in the rapidly enlarging and dividing trophoblastic cell mass.

The lacunae become confluent and as the trophoblastic cells erode the maternal vessels, become filled with blood to form later the intervillous spaces. Between the lacunae spaces there are columns having a central core of cytotrophoblasts surrounded by syncitiotrophoblasts. These are not true villi but these form the framework from which the villi later develop. From these pillars branching sprouts appear. Those columns extend as far as the decidua and a mesenchymal core develops in them from the extraembryonic mesenchyme, which form the villous vessels. In due course these vessels establish continuity with those developing from the body stalk and inner chorionic mesenchyme (Figure 8.3).

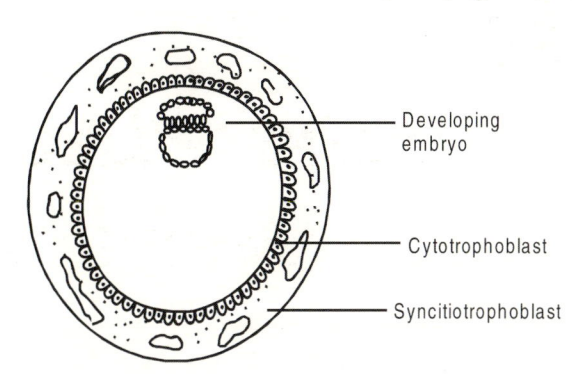

Figure 8.3: Differentiation into cyto and syncitiotrophoblasts

The distal part of the columns (toward the decidua) is not invaded by mesenchyme but only serves to anchor it to the basal plate. These cells proliferate and spread laterally separating the syncitiotrophoblast into two layers the definitive syncitium on the fetal aspect and the peripheral syncitium on the decidual side which eventually degenerates and is replaced by a fibrinoid material and is known as the Nitabuch's layer.

From the columns (primary villus stem) off shoots appear which are made up of syncitiotrophoblasts initially. Cytotrophoblasts appear later, which get finally invaded by a mesenchymal core. Hence, the primary villi grow and divide to form the secondary and tertiary villi. The placenta is a vascularised villous organ by the twenty-first day (Figure 8.4).

During the early weeks of gestation the cytotrophoblasts penetrate the peripheral syncitiotrophoblasts and spread into the underlying decidua even up to the myometrium where they fuse to form typical multinucleated giant cells the function of which is unknown. Groups of cytotrophoblasts also grow into the lumen of the spiral arteries extending as far as the decidual myometrial junction. These cells destroy the muscular and elastic layer of the vessels wall which finally get replaced by a fibrinoid material which is derived from the maternal blood and proteins secreted by the trophoblastic cells. This primary wave of invasion weakens

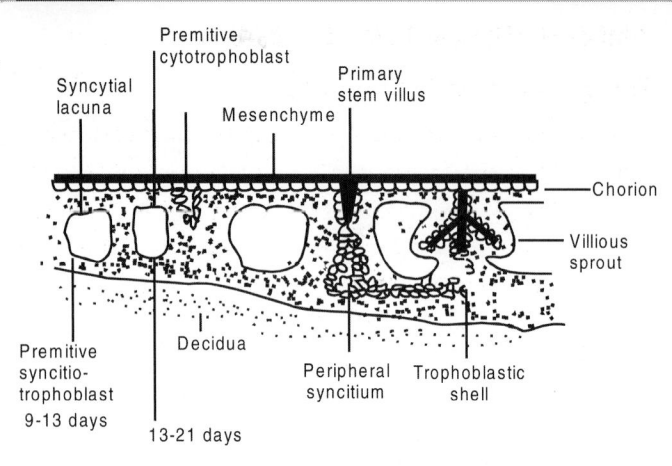

Figure 8.4: Development of placenta during the first 21 days

the spiral arteriolar wall, which dilates considerably and is an important factor in augmenting blood flow to the placenta.

During the fourth month there is a further proliferation of cytotrophoblasts and this second wave of invasion involves the myometrial portion of spiral arterioles extending up to their origin from the radial arteries.

The placental septa appear during the third month protruding into the intervillous spaces from the basal plate and divides the placenta into 15 to 20 lobes. These are simple folds of the basal plate and the lobes thus formed are not functional or structural subunits of the fetal placenta as the placenta works as one unit. The placental lobule is derived from a single secondary stem villous with its many tertiary villi just below the chrorial plate.

The definitive form of the placenta is achieved by the fourth month and continued growth may occur upto term due to continuous arborization and formation of fresh villi.

In the first trimester the villi are large and have a mantle of trophoblasts consisting of an inner layer of cytotrophoblasts and an outer layer of syncitiotrophoblasts, the stroma has small fetal vessels. During the second trimester the villi are smaller the mantle less regular and the cytotrophoblasts less numerous and the stroma has more collagen and fetal vessels become larger and moving toward the periphery of the villous. In the third trimester the villi are much smaller in diameter, the cytotrophoblasts irregular and thinned out. The fetal vessels are dilated and lie just below the thinned out trophoblasts. This brings the maternal and fetal circulation into close approximation providing conditions for optimal maternal-fetal transfer.

Structure

Full term placenta is discoid in shape with a diameter of about 15 to 25 cm and is 3 cm thick. It weighs about 500 gm and occupies one-third of the uterine wall. At birth it separates from the uterine wall at the Nitabuch's layer and is expelled approximately 30 min after the birth of the child. When viewed from the maternal side it has 15 to 20 cotyledons seen as slightly bulged areas separated by grooves formed by the decidual septa. The fetal surface is smooth and a number of arteries and veins are seen converging on the umbilical cord. The umbilical cord is usually eccentric and occasionally marginal. Rarely it inserts into the chorionic membrane outside the placenta, i.e. vilamentous insertion.

Circulation

Cotyledons receive blood through 80 to 100 special arterioles that enter the intervillous space through the basal plate at regular intervals. The lumen of the spiral artery being narrow pushes blood into the intervillous spaces and bathes the branches of the villous tree with oxygenated blood. As the pressure decreases blood flows back toward the decidua and enters the veins. The intervillous space contains about 150 ml of blood which is replenished 3 to 4 times/minutes. Exchange does not take place in all villi, only those in which fetal vessels are in intimate contact by possessing microvilli. The placental membrane, also called the placental barrier, separates the maternal and fetal blood. This initially consists of four layers: (a) endothelial lining of fetal vessels, (b) connective tissue of the villi, (c) the cytotrophoblasts and (d) the syncitiotrophoblasts. The layers get thinned out after the fourth month thus increasing exchange. As the maternal blood is separated from the fetal blood by a chorionic derivative the placentation in humans is said to be hemochorial in type.

Function

1. *Exchange of metabolic and gaseous products between maternal and fetal blood.* Exchange of O_2 and CO_2 occurs by simple diffusion.
2. *Glucose is transported by facilitated diffusion.*
3. *Transmission of maternal antibodies.* Antibodies are taken into the syncitiotrophoblasts by pinocytosis and subsequently transferred to fetal capillaries. In this manner the fetus can acquire passive immunity.
4. *Hormone production.* It produces several hormones like progesterone, estriol, and human chorionic gonadotropin. These hormones are produced by the syncitiotrophoblasts and excreted through maternal urine. Another hormone is the human placental lactogen that supports fetal growth by increasing maternal blood glucose, i.e. makes the mother diabetogenic.

Clinical Correlation

Most maternal hormones do not cross the placenta. Thyroxin crosses at a slow rate. Some synthetic progestins can cross at a rapid rate and cause masculinization of the female fetus.

Although the placental barrier is a protective mechanism several viruses can cross over like rubella, cytomegalovirus, coxsackie, variola, varicella, measles and poliomyelitis and can cause fetal infection, which in turn can result in fetal death or birth defects.

Drugs and drug metabolites too can traverse the placental barrier and may cause serious damage to the embryo.

In the rhesus incompatible fetuses the antibodies produced in the Rh –ve mother against the Rh +ve fetus in a previous pregnancy can cross over and cause hemolysis in subsequent pregnancies resulting in intrauterine death or hemolytic diseases of the newborn.

The Nitabuch's layer provides the plane of separation of the placenta. Absence of the Nitabuch's layer results in an adherent placenta.

The invasion of the spiral arterioles provides adequate supply of blood to the fetus. Absence of the secondary wave of invasion could cause vasospasm of the spiral arterioles, which is the primary event in pre-eclampsia.

AMNION AND UMBILICAL CORD

Development of Membranes

The morula becomes a blastocyst by formation of a central fluid filled cavity. This separates the primary trophoblastic cell mass from the inner cell mass which forms the embryo. This inner cell mass is eccentrically placed and then becomes a bilaminar disc. The layer facing the blastocyst cavity forms the primitive endoderm and that facing the cytotrophoblastic cells forms the primitive ectoderm. A slit like space appears between the cytotrophoblast and the primitive ectoderm by 12th postovulatory day and is the amniotic cavity. At the same time the endodermal cells on the other side migrate and line the blastocyst cavity to form the primitive yolk sac. Extraembryonic yolk sac then appears separating the yolk sac from the blastocyst wall. This mensenchyme also insinuates between the amniotic cavity and the trophoblasts (Figure 8.5).

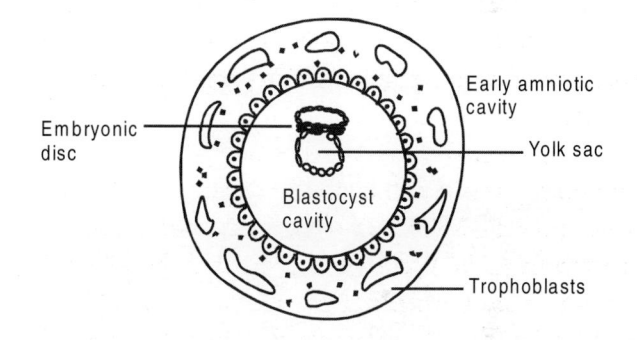

Figure 8.5: Early stage of formation of amniotic cavity

Small cystic spaces appear in the extraembryonic mesenchyme and fuse to form the extraembryonic coelom dividing the mesenchyme into two portions one apposed to the trophoblast the parietal extraembryonic mesenchyme and the other which covers the yolk sac the visceral extraembryonic coelom. This coelom also separates the amnion from the inner aspect of the chorion at all places except one portion, which forms the body stalk from which the umbilical cord is derived (Figure 8.6).

Subsequently, the amniotic cavity enlarges and surrounds the enlarging embryo and the part of the yolk sac, which gets incorporated into the embryo and forms the primitive gut. The gut communicates with the yolk

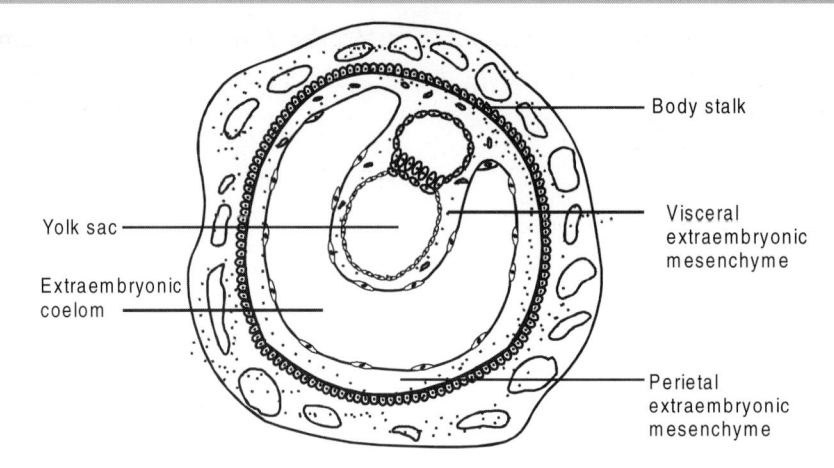

Figure 8.6: Relation between developing amniotic cavity, extraembryonic celom and primitive body stalk

sac through a channel, which elongates and thins out and forms the vitelline duct. The extraembryonic yolk sac becomes removed further away from the embryo to finally get incorporated into the body stalk. With further expansion the amniotic cavity enlarges and finally the mesenchyme covering the amnion fuses with the lining chorion to form the amniochorion (Figures 8.7 and 8.8).

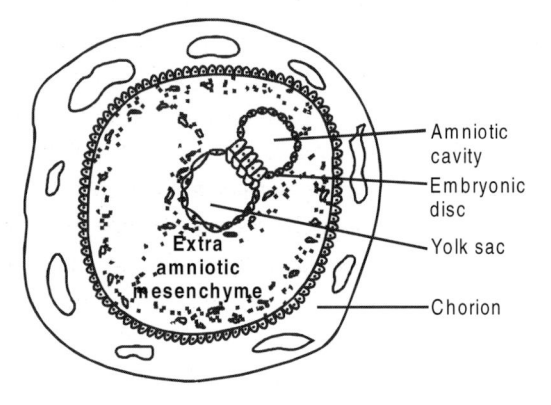

Figure 8.7: Relation between developing amniotic cavity and extraembryonic mesenchyme

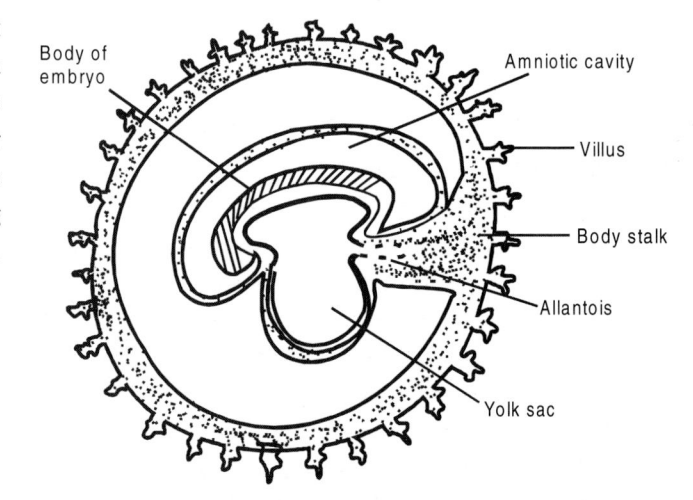

Figure 8.8: Relationship between expanding amniotic cavity and developing embryo

the fetus develops the ability to swallow, the fluid swallowed is digested and excreted. Additional contribution comes from the amniotic membrane secretions. At term there is an exchange of 500 ml every 24 hr.

Composition of the Amniotic Fluid

As a result of the mixed origin its composition is heterogeneous. Some cells and cellular debris are suspended in a clear solution, the osmolarity of which decreases as pregnancy progresses. The cells may be fetal squamous, amniotic cells and fibroblasts. Nitrogenous wastes are present like urea, creatinine and uric acid from the functioning kidney. Amino acids are in the same concentration as maternal plasma. Proteins

The amniotic fluid at 12 weeks is approximately 50 ml and increases to 150 ml at 16 weeks and to a maximum of 1000 ml at 36 weeks and falls again before term.

Formation of amniotic fluid: Initially the fluid is formed from the primitive cells of the amniotic vesicle. Later it is a transudate from the fetal skin and umbilical cord. In the second trimester as the skin becomes keratinised there is contribution from fetal urine and lung secretions. As

increase in concentration as pregnancy progresses and contains mainly albumin. Alfa fetoprotein is formed in early pregnancy but in concentrations ten times less than fetal blood. Lipids increase as pregnancy progresses, half of which is in the form of fatty acids. Lung secretions contribute phospholipids, lecithin and cholesterol. Carbohydrates are half of that found in maternal serum predominantly glucose. Inorganic salts are found in same concentrations as maternal plasma. Estrogens and progesterone with their metabolites are also found. Insulin levels increase toward term and are higher in diabetic pregnancies. Pigment from bilirubin and meconium may stain the amniotic fluid. Amniotic fluid pH is slightly acidic pH 7.0 as compared to maternal plasma.

Clinical Correlation

Amniocentesis where a small quantity of fluid is drawn for examination is done at 16 weeks.

- Fibroblast found in the amniotic fluid is used for karyotyping. In the presence of renal defects glial cells are found.
- Excess of liquor or polyhydramniosis is found in association with open neural tube defects when, the spinal fluid leaks out and is also observed in gut atresias.
- Oligohydramnios or decreased fluid occurs with renal agenesis and in cases of intrauterine growth restriction. Insulin levels in the amniotic fluid are higher in diabetic pregnancies.
- Amniotic fluid alpha fetoprotein is raised in open neural tube defects, abdominal wall defects but is abnormally low in Down syndrome.
- Bilirubin levels in the amniotic fluid decreases toward term but may be raised in cases of fetal hemolysis.
- Meconium may be present in late pregnancy and labor and is often taken as an indicator of fetal distress but correlates with biochemical incidence in only 20 percent of cases.
- Amniotic fluid has antibacterial properties because of its pH and it contains interferon and lysozyme.
- Preterm prelabor rupture of membranes and draining out of the amniotic fluid can cause lung hypoplasia and clubfoot.

- Occasionally tears in the amnion can result in amniotic bands that can encircle any part of the fetus particularly the limbs and rarely result in amputation.

FETUS

1. *Fetal growth and development*: Birthweight of a baby has profound influence on the survival and perinatal morbidity. As gestational age advances birthweight increases and charts are plotted for a particular population demonstrating the normal and abnormal range using centiles or standard deviations. Large for gestational age is usually taken as more than the 90th centile and small for gestational age as below the 10th centile. This can be determined antepartum by fetal measurement using ultrasound.

2. *Fetal circulation*: The fetal circulation is designed in such a way that a major part of the oxygenated blood coming from the placenta is diverted to the brain. Blood from the tertiary villi courses through a number of veins in the chorionic plate and eventually forms a single channel the umbilical vein. This vein enters through the umbilical cord traverses intra-abdominally to the liver dividing into two, the smaller one supplies the liver and the larger carries the major portion of the blood to the inferior vena cava. Vena caval blood flows into the right atrium then through the foramen ovale into the left atrium. Some mixing with much less oxygenated superior vena caval blood may occur in the right atrium. Superior vena caval blood is directed toward the right ventricle from where it enters the pulmonary artery but only 8 percent of the blood reaches the lung, the rest being diverted through the ductus arteriosus to the descending aorta. The left atrial blood mixes with the returning blood from the pulmonary veins and enters the left ventricle. Blood pumped into the root of the aorta supplies the brain through the carotid vessels and the lower part of the body though the descending aorta. Blood from the descending aorta is diverted through the two umbilical arteries arising from the internal iliac vessels to return to the placenta for oxygenation (Figure 8.9).

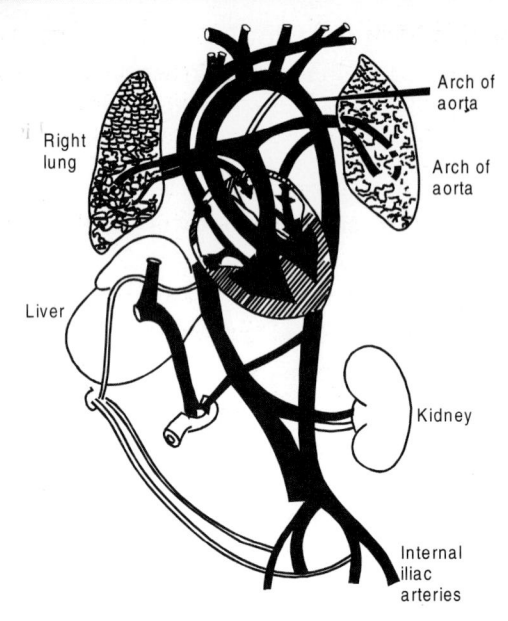

Figure 8.9: Fetal circulation

3. *Fetal blood*: Fetal hemoglobin first appears at 11 weeks of gestation and persists into neonatal life gradually being replaced by adult hemoglobin. It has increased affinity for oxygen, which allows larger amount of oxygen to be transported at lower partial pressures of oxygen. Despite the increase in the hemoglobin concentration the viscosity is not increased, as the red cells are more deformable and fibrinogen less concentrated.
4. *Immune system*: IgG is transported across the placenta from around 16 weeks of gestation conferring on the newborn a certain degree of protection. The fetus in response to an infection can produce IgM.
5. *Gastrointestinal tract*: Functional development is complete by 36 weeks. The gut contains amniotic fluid from which water is extracted and together with degenerated cells from the intestine forms meconium which gains its color from bile pigment.
6. *Respiratory system*: Lung development can be divided into four stages. In the first (5-17 weeks) pseudoglandular stage the bronchi and terminal bronchioles form. In the second (13-25 weeks) canalicular stage the bronchi and terminal bronchioles enlarge and respiratory bronchioles and alveolar ducts develop. By 24 weeks surfactant storage organelles appear within the type II penumocytes. During this period lungs become vascular. From 24 weeks till birth the alveolar ducts give rise to the terminal air sacs, the epithelium becomes thin approximates the blood supply. In the fourth (alveolar) stage from fetal life to 8 years mature alveoli develop and proliferate.

Lung fluid is essential for development by 'splinting' the air sacs. It is produced at the rate of 5 ml/kg body weight. This enters the pharynx through the trachea and is swallowed. Amniotic fluid is important for development probably by providing unrestricted breathing movements. Fetal breathing movements are seen 30 to 40 percent of the time in association with rapid eye movement sleep. It increases with increase in glucose level and in the evening.

Surfactant is formed in the lamellar bodies of the type II cells. It is a glycerophospholipid composed mainly of phosphatidylcholine (lecithin). There is a large increase in the production after 30 weeks. From 30 to 35 weeks' phosphatidylinositol increases and after 35 weeks the levels of phosphatidylinositol decreases while that of phosphatidlglycerol increases. It also contains glycoproteins known as apoproteins the most important of which is SPA. Surfactant reduces the surface tension and hence ensures that the terminal alveoli are kept open.

7. *Urinary system:* Function of the kidney is not vital during fetal life because the excretory function is mainly carried out through the placenta. Tubular reabsorption is low as indicated by the sodium content of fetal urine. At 30 weeks the fetus produces 10 ml/hr of urine which increases to 30 ml/hr later, contributing to the amniotic fluid.
8. *Clinical correlation*: The unique architecture of the fetal circulation allows the most oxygenated blood to be supplied to the heart, brain and liver accounting for the brain sparing effect in intrauterine growth retardation.

The transfer of IgG antibodies to the fetus can be disadvantage when IgG red cell D-antigen is transferred to the fetus. Anti Ro antibody in patients with connective tissue disorders can cause fetal heart block.

Oligohydramnios can result in lung hypoplasia particularly when it occurs early in gestation at the canalicular period. Corticosteroids given to the mother can act through fibroblast pneumocyte factor to stimulate the type II pneumocytes to produce surfactant in preterm babies prior to delivery. Fetal breathing movement decreases with narcotic analgesics and alcohol and also during labor. Indomethacin increases FBM. Indomethacin the prostaglandin inhibitor increases renal vascular resistance and decreases renal blood flow when given to patients for the treatment of preterm labor or polyhydramnios. It can also cause premature closure of the ductus arteriosus.

BIBLIOGRAPHY

1. Barker Graham, Bennett Philip; Embryology. In De Swiet Michael, Chamberlain Geoffrey (Eds): *Basic Sciences in Obstetrics and Gynaecology*. 2nd Ed Churchill Livingstone 27-52, 1992.
2. Benirschke K: The placenta: How to examine and what you can learn. *Contemporary Obstetrics and Gynaecology* **17**:117, 1981.
3. Sadler TW, Leland Jill, Redmond S, Sulik KK: Fetal membranes and placenta. In *Langmans Medical Embryology*. 7th ed. Williams and Witkins 101-21.
4. Sadler TW, Leland Jill, Redmond S, Sulik KK. Fetal circulation. In *Langmans Medical Embryology*. 7th ed. Williams and Witkins 224-28.

9.

Devendra Kanagalingam
Sabaratnam Arulkumaran

PART **One**

History and Examination of a Pregnant Mother

Introduction

Pregnancy, labor and delivery should be a normal physiological event. In the majority it is so but in a minority the pregnancy is complicated by pre-existing illness or obstetric conditions that may be acquired during the course of the pregnancy and labor. Patients coming to a hospital or a clinic have some illness for which they have come to seek a remedy. The pregnant mother with no illness attends the antenatal clinic, in order to ensure that she develops no complications that will jeopardize her pregnancy. We should consider the pregnant mother as a woman and not as a patient, unless there is a pathology which needs treatment during her pregnancy, labor or delivery. The pregnant mother, although healthy, may be anxious. Therefore, the clinics where the mothers are seen should be pleasant and give an atmosphere of calm and friendliness so that the mothers are not apprehensive to come to these clinics. Antenatal care is not a norm for many pregnant mothers in this world, but wherever the facilities are provided these should be appropriate, accessible and affordable. It is useful to follow a set pattern of taking an obstetric history and performing a clinical examination in every mother so that the important points that are relevant to the pregnancy outcome are not missed.

HISTORY

Obstetric History

The obstetric history should start with an introduction whereby the staff should introduce themselves and the purpose of the interview. The mother should be offered a comfortable seat in privacy to enable her to talk to the doctor or midwife without hindrance. The name, age, and social status should be established. It will be useful to find out how far the pregnancy has advanced and whether she has any concerns about this pregnancy. If she has any complaints then one should listen to the presenting symptoms of the particular problem. A detailed history of the presenting complaint should be taken. For example if there was bleeding one should establish when the bleeding started; whether it was precipitated by any particular event; whether there was associated pain; the quantity of bleeding and whether she is continuously bleeding. It is important to elicit past history of bleeding in the current pregnancy. If the complaint was abdominal pain one should establish the onset whether it was continuous or colicky in nature; the site; whether it is radiating; whether there are any associated symptoms and whether there are any relieving or aggravating factors. The chapters in the book relating to antepartum hemorrhage, pre-eclampsia, diabetes and other medical and obstetric conditions will give the details of the presenting symptoms pertaining to each of the conditions.

Past Obstetric and Gynecological History

The obstetric performance in the past may influence the current pregnancy outcome. The past reproductive history should be taken in a chronological order. The year in which each pregnancy occurred; the gestation at which the pregnancy ended; the mode of delivery; the condition of the baby, and birth weight, should be noted. If it was a miscarriage or premature delivery, possible reason and the details of the event may be of relevance to manage this pregnancy.

A gynecological history should follow the obstetric history as it may be of some relevance to the current pregnancy. A history of previous myomectomy may influence the way the labor and the delivery is managed. Other conditions that may be of relevance should be noted including the cervical smear history.

Past Medical and Surgical History

Past medical and surgical history may be of importance. A detailed history of pre-existing medical conditions including any medications she is currently taking should be noted. Some medical conditions might jeopardize the progress of pregnancy to term or might affect the fetus. The medication may have to be changed because to avoid teratogenic effect to the fetus. History of allergy especially to drugs (e.g. allergy to latex) needs to be noted. Inquire how the medical condition influenced the pregnancy and how the pregnancy influenced the medical condition in the past and current pregnancy. More often than not the condition may not cause any problems, but if there is any doubt then appropriate medical or surgical opinion should be sought.

Family History

Family history should include history of multiple pregnancy, diabetes, hypertension and congenital disorders. The history of consanguineous marriage is of importance. Appropriate counseling may be necessary if there is a risk to the mother or her unborn baby.

Social History

Whether the mother is supported, her financial status, and whether she is in need of financial support are important but delicate questions. The living conditions, the family members living with her at home and the history of diet, smoking, alcohol consumption and any drug abuse is of relevance. Eliciting such a history might be sensitive and one should use discretion in how the questions are worded so that the woman does not get offended, but at the same time is able to volunteer the information. This applies also to domestic violence for which some advice may be given depending on the situation.

It is always useful to end such a history with a systems enquiry going through the central nervous system followed by cardiovascular, respiratory, renal and gastrointestinal systems. This avoids one missing symptoms related to any of these systems.

History of Present Pregnancy

The gestation at which a woman is seen should be clearly established and this starts with enquiring about the last menstrual period. The gestation may be influenced depending on whether the cycles were regular or irregular, and the cycle length. History of previous hormonal contraception, the date of cessation of contraception and the number of spontaneous cycles prior to the conception is of importance. If the pregnancy started immediately after the contraception was terminated then it could be difficult to decide the gestation and where facilities exist, one should arrange for an ultrasound scan to establish the dates.

History of bleeding in early pregnancy is not that uncommon and a detailed history as to whether she had any bleeding and the dates that it occurred need to be noted. Any infection or medication taken during the pregnancy is of relevance and specific enquiries regarding this should be made. Based on the last menstrual period (LMP) and the regularity of the cycles, the expected date of delivery should be calculated. If the cycles were regular and were 28 days in length with no immediate past history of oral contraception or bleeding in early pregnancy then Nagele's rule can be applied. The conventional way of calculating the expected date of delivery is to add one year and subtract three months and add seven days to the last menstrual period. Alternatively, one could add nine months and seven calendar days to the last menstrual period. Based on this a calculation can be made as to the number of weeks the woman is pregnant. If an ultrasound was performed in early gestation one should check whether the date calculated by the ultrasound tallies with the gestation calculated based on the LMP according to Nagele's rule. The period of gestation may not correspond with the period of amenorrhea in those who have irregular cycles and who were on contraception and did not get regular cycles subsequent to cessation of taking the hormones. The ultrasound examination done during the first trimester is accurate and the difference in gestation calculated based on LMP may be within one week of the gestation estimated by the crown rump length.

First Trimester

It is useful to elicit the history in the first trimester as to whether the pregnancy was planned and whether the mother had preconception folic acid. The effect of folic acid is maximal if it was started preconceptionally, and it is useful for a pregnant mother to take folic acid at least during the first trimester. Whether the pregnancy was suspected based on symptoms, the date on which the pregnancy test was positive and results of early ultrasound examination should be noted. This will help to verify the gestation calculated based on the last menstrual period. In many centers the booking and the antenatal care is provided by the midwife or general practitioner. Shared antenatal care is popular and is provided by the family practitioner or midwife and the consultant team in the hospital. The type of care needed is determined by the history. Should the pregnancy be uncomplicated and the pregnancy progresses well then the care is provided by the midwife and/or the family practitioner. The surroundings where they provide the care is more friendly compared to a busy hospital set-up. If the mother develops complications like pre-eclampsia or antepartum hemorrhage she is best looked after by the consultant team. If it is a mild complication the visits can alternate between the family practitioner and the consultant team in the hospital.

In the first trimester a number of routine blood tests are carried out; hemoglobin and full blood count; blood group and the rhesus status; immune status for rubella, test for syphilis and hepatitis. In some centers mothers are tested for HIV. Additional tests may be needed to screen for thalassemia or sickle cell disease depending on the personal or family history.

Second Trimester

In the second trimester screening and diagnostic tests for fetal anomalies are undertaken. In centers where facilities are available serum screening by triple test is offered to select those at high risk of Down syndrome. In some centers screening for Down is done by a first trimester nuchal translucency scan. If the nuchal translucency scan or the triple test indicates a high risk of Down syndrome pre-natal diagnosis is offered which is done by amniocentesis at about 15-16 weeks gestation. Between 18-20 weeks by gestation detailed scanning is offered to identify the number of fetuses; biometry of the fetus; placental position and to identify any major fetal abnormalities. Should there be doubt about any abnormality especially that of the soft tissue like cardiac abnormality, then an additional scan is offered at about 21 weeks. This would permit the clinician to make a diagnosis of lethal anomalies and if necessary to offer a termination under 24 weeks gestation which is the legal limit to offer medical termination of pregnancy.

In those where a placental position is found in the lower pole an additional scan is arranged at about 34 weeks to exclude the possibility of low lying placenta. It is important in taking a history to see whether the woman has undergone any of these tests and to identify the test results in the records and to explain the findings. If there is any concern, further consultation with the appropriate medical personnel should be arranged. In certain situations an appointment with a social worker may need to be arranged.

In the second trimester it is the norm to request a woman to come for antenatal check-up every four weeks. During this time the mother's blood pressure is recorded followed by urine examination for albumin, sugar, ketones and nitrites. This is tested by using a dipstick which has color indicators that identifies abnormal amounts of these substances in urine. Ask for presence of fetal movements, especially the first time the mother felt them, which is known as quickening. This is usually around 20 weeks in the first pregnancy and it is felt at about 16 weeks in women who had a previous pregnancy beyond 20 weeks. If there were any admissions the outcome should be enquired in detail to rule out the possibility of the problem recurring or giving rise to complications later in pregnancy. During the second trimester visits uncover any complaints the mother has and explore whether she has any concerns. Pregnancy lasts for nine months and the mother could be anxious about unknown things for a long period. The opportunity should be taken in the clinics to reassure the mother if the pregnancy progresses without complications.

Third Trimester

In the third trimester enquiry about fetal movements should be followed by checking the blood pressure and urine examination. Attention is paid to the growth of the symphysis—fundal height. The symphysis—fundal height (SFH) after 20 weeks corresponds to the weeks of gestation plus or minus 2 cm up to 36 weeks. Subsequent to that the SFH is 36 plus or minus 3 cm and at 40 weeks it is plus or minus 4 cm. This is related to the reduction of amniotic fluid toward end of pregnancy and/or the descent of the head into the pelvis. SFH larger than dates may indicate the possibility of wrong dates, macrosomia, multiple pregnancy or fibroids. Polyhydramnios may be one of the causes and in such situations there is difficulty in palpating the fetal parts. Measuring the SFH is from the top most point of the fundus to the upper margin of the symphasis pubis. The top most point of the fundus could be on the right or the left of the maternal abdomen and there is no need for correction of the position of the uterus. The upper margin of the symphysis is identified by palpating from the suprapubic region above the hair margin and going downward in the midline to feel the bony prominence. The SFH identifies if the baby's growth is satisfactory.

Gestational diabetes and gestational hypertension tend to occur more commonly in the third trimester. These problems may have been identified and should be elicited in the history. The hemoglobin estimation is repeated at 28 weeks of gestation and if the mother is rhesus negative an antibody test is performed. It is important to find out whether these tests were performed and if so to check the results.

History of the Presenting Complaint

This relates to any complaints or complications that have arisen in this pregnancy at the time of presentation to the clinic. A history of vaginal bleeding, abdominal pain, symptoms related to elevated blood pressure like headache, reduced fetal movements; pruritus or rash on the abdomen are some of the presentations. Whatever the complaint a detailed history is important to direct examination and investigations. It is useful to know the opinion of the midwife or the doctor who saw her prior to that. Prior to examination it is useful to summarize the history in a succinct manner and present it to the woman so that the accuracy of the history can be determined. This will also indicate to the mother that you have taken some interest in identifying the key issues related to her pregnancy.

EXAMINATION

Examination of the Patient

General examination of the pregnant woman is like any other patient where one looks for general condition of the individual including pallor for anemia, inspection of the conjunctiva for jaundice, the peripheral pulse, blood pressure, cardiovascular and respiratory systems.

The difference with the pregnant woman is on the abdominal examination. Unlike a patient who has no other mass when healthy, the pregnant woman will have the uterus which distends the abdomen and displaces the gut to the sides and posteriorly. The retroperitoneal structures on the posterior abdominal wall would be difficult to palpate. Unless indicated, the liver, spleen and kidneys are not palpated in late pregnancy. This is because of the difficulty in reaching these organs, because of the distended uterus. The woman should be asked to lie on the couch comfortably, preferably in a semi-reclined position in order to avoid supine hypotension. At times the mother will feel uncomfortable and one should be able to detect that because she might go pale, start sweating and feel uncomfortable in which case it is best to ask her to lie on her side. The abdomen is exposed from the xiphisternum to the upper hair margin near the symphysis pubis. Therefore, care should be taken to have the examination in private. It is preferable to have a chaperone who could be a midwife or a nurse or nursing assistant even in the presence of her partner. Thyroid as well as breast examination are important. Allowance should be given for the physiological enlargement of the thyroid, and the breasts. There should be no lumps or any obvious abnormality that is found on inspection or palpation. The examination of the breasts need not be done on repeated visits, but it may be appropriate to have it done on the first or second visit to the antenatal clinic. The examination of the abdomen should consist of inspection, palpation, auscultation and at times percussion.

Inspection

On inspection the enlargement or distention of the abdomen should be noted, usually it will be pear shaped if it is singleton and it will be fairly globular distending the whole abdomen from the symphysis pubis to the top of the fundus and the flanks laterally in multiple pregnancy. The way the uterus presents itself may give a clue as to the lie of the fetus. From the umbilicus there might be a line of pigmentation going downward to the symphysis pubis and may also extend up to the xiphisternum at times and is know as linea nigra. It is not always present. Because of the stretching of the anterior abdominal wall due to the increased intra-abdominal pressure, the subcutaneous tissue gives way giving rise to 'stretch marks' known as 'striae gravidarum'. These are usually purplish in color but in a mother who has had a previous pregnancy they have a silvery pale discoloration and is known as 'striae albicans'. The umbilicus might be flush with the surface or may be everted. One should look for surgical scars especially transverse suprapubic scars due to previous cesarean section. This may be hidden below the hairline and one should look for it if it was mentioned in the history. The laparoscopic scars may not be easily visible as it is usually in the lower margin of the umbilicus. The scars have to be defined in terms of the surgery the women has had so that it will be more meaningful in describing the scar. The hair distribution is like an inverted triangle, but depending on the ethnicity it may differ. Prominent hair distribution on the abdomen might suggest a possibility of an android type of pelvis, especially if the woman is of muscular (stocky) build. There may be superficial veins on the abdomen which may have to be described. Toward the end of pregnancy it is easy to see the fetal movements and if one observes the fetal movements it is useful to mention that and to verify whether the mother felt the movement.

Palpation

The fundosymphyseal height should be measured in centimetres and has been described earlier. It is useful to locate the fundus and mark this point. Start the measurement from that point to the top of the symphysis pubis and call it fundosymphyseal height. The tape should be kept on the surface of the abdomen rather than dipping into the abdomen wall which might increase the number of centimetres in an obese mother. It is best to have the tape with the measurements on the under-surface while doing the measurements to avoid subjective errors in measurement of the fundalsymphysial height. The fundosymphyseal height approximately corresponds to the weeks of gestation + or −2 cm up to 36 weeks and + or −3 cm thereafter. Should there be a discrepancy beyond this deviation one should think about wrong dates. If that is verified to be correct then a small uterus may indicate intrauterine growth restriction or the possibility of oligohydramnios. A large uterus may indicate the possibility of multiple pregnancy, polyhydramnios, fibroids in the uterus or a large baby. This is an indication for an ultrasound examination to make sure the baby is of normal size. Clinical smallness should be verified by ultrasound measurement as the ultrasound might reveal that the size of the fetus is compatible with the gestation, i.e. ultrasonically normal size.

Lie and Presentation

Lie is the relationship of the longitudinal axis of the fetus to the longitudinal axis of the uterus. If the breech or the head is just above the symphysis pubis in the pelvis in the midline then it is likely to be a longitudinal lie, although the opposite pole might be deviated to one or the other side of the abdomen because of the tilt of the body of the uterus off the midline. Presentation is the lower most fetal part which overlies the pelvis. Usually it is the cephalic presentation and in a small number it might be the breech presentation. Very rarely, neither the head nor the breech might be presenting in which case the baby might be in the oblique or transverse lie. Lie and presentation is of little relevance before 28 weeks gestation and may be difficult to palpate. However, it would be easy after 28 weeks of gestation and one should identify the lie and presentation of the fetus. They are of greater importance at term especially in early labor.

Position and Station

The position is the relationship of the denominator of presenting part to the fixed points of the maternal pelvis. The fixed points of the maternal pelvis are the sacral promontory posteriorly and the symphysis pubis anteriorly. Posterolaterally are the sacroiliac joints and anterolaterally are the ileopectineal eminences. The most prominent and definable peripheral point of the presentation is called the denominator. The denominator for a vertex presentation is the occiput; the sacrum is for the breech and the mentum or the chin for the face presentation. If the occiput of the fetus is just against the sacral promontory it is defined as occipitoposterior and if it is just behind the symphysis pubis it is called occipitoanterior. If the occiput is facing the right ileopectineal eminence it is called right occipitoanterior and the opposite side would be left occipital anterior. Similarly, if the occiput is facing the sacroiliac joint it will be termed as sacroposterior and it may be on the right or left side. The breech presentation will be also defined according to the relationship of the sacrum of the fetus to the fixed points of the maternal pelvis.

The vertex is a diagonal area subtended by the anterior fontanelle anteriorly, the posterior fontanelle posteriorly and the two biparietal eminences. In a well flexed head it is the vertex that presents to the pelvis. The descent of the head into the pelvis can be defined abdominally as well as vaginally. Five fingers are needed to cover the head above the symphysis it is called five fifths and if only two fingers are needed to cover the head above the brim it is called two-fifths. With progress of the pregnancy toward term the head descends into the pelvis and when it is only two fifths palpable then it is termed 'engaged' which means the maximum diameter of the head has passed through the pelvic brim. Another way of defining the descent is by vaginal examination and is called the station of the presenting part and it refers to the leading part of the fetus in relation to the ischial spines. This can be assessed only by vaginal examination. In the vertex presentation one has to look at the descent of the bony part of the head rather than soft tissue swelling or the caput which might give a false impression of the descent. The female pelvis is suited to have the fetal head at term in a three-dimensional manner and hence if the head is only one-fifth palpable the leading part of the head should be at or below the ischial spines. Malpresentations and malpositions have different findings on palpation and have difficulties in labor and will be discussed in different chapters.

Attitude

The relationship of the fetal parts to each other is the attitude. The fetus usually presents in a flexed attitude whereby the knee joints and the hip joints are flexed as well as the shoulder and elbow joints. The head is also in a flexed position in relation to its trunk. When the head is well flexed the occiput (the prominence of the head on the side of the fetal spine) is at a lower level than the sinciput. It may not be easy to define the attitude on abdominal palpation if the abdomen is tense and if the woman is obese. This is of little significance antenatally, but is of significance if one is to deliver a breech with an extended head or when the labor is not progressing well in a vertex presentation when the head is deflexed.

Estimation of Fetal Weight

It is good practice to estimate the fetal weight after 28 weeks of gestation. This is clinically difficult, but some effort should be made in order to make sure the baby is not too small or too large for that gestation. An approximate weight estimation depending on the gestation and symphysis of fundal height is given in Table 9.1.

If fetal movements or uterine contractions are felt during the time of palpation this should be verified with the patient and mentioned in the notes. The amount of amniotic fluid is not always easy to determine but if the fetal parts can be palpated and if the head is ballottable then one should be able to guess whether there is a normal amount of amniotic fluid. If there is excessive amniotic fluid there might be difficulty in palpating the fetal parts. Excessive amniotic fluid is called polyhydramnios and it usually presents with abdominal discomfort. The abdomen might look shiny and striae gravidarum might be seen both in the upper and lower abdomen. This is more common with multiple pregnancy, but can present with singleton pregnancy, especially when there is diabetes in the mother, or when there is certain fetal anomaly. If fetal parts are difficult to palpate, the abdomen is tense and if fluid thrill can be elicited it is highly suggestive of polyhydramnios. The fluid thrill is not a definite indicator of polyhydramnios as it could be elicited even without polyhydramnios. An ultrasound examination would be useful to check whether there is any fetal anomaly and also to confirm polyhydramnios. On ultrasound examination a single vertical pool depth of more than 8 cm or an amniotic fluid index (a four quadrant analysis) of greater than 25 cm is considered to represent polyhydramnios. In the absence of fetal anomaly and multiple pregnancy check the blood sugar and if necessary proceed to a glucose tolerance test.

Auscultation

It is important to auscultate the fetal heart. This could be by using a Pinard stethoscope. But in current practice a Sonicaid which is a small device with a Doppler ultrasound facility is used so that not only the midwife or the doctor, but also the woman herself, her partner and the family can listen to the fetal heart sounds. The fetal heart sounds are best heard over the anterior shoulder of the fetus. Once the head is palpated, the shoulder should be palpated and it is demarcated by the groove which is neck between the head and the shoulders. This prominent part of the shoulder which can be palpated anteriorly on the anterior abdominal wall will be the place where one should place the fetal stethoscope in order to auscultate. The fetal heart sounds are transmitted to the anterior shoulder and could be heard easily. In an occipitoposterior position when the baby's back is lying against the maternal spine, the fetal heart can be auscultated in the midline between the umbilicus of the mother and the symphysis pubis as well as in the flanks where the anterior shoulder is felt. Usually, the anterior shoulder lies in the midpoint between the umbilicus and the anterior superior iliac spine. However, this is not a definitive point as the position of the umbilicus might vary as well as the anterior shoulder depending on the descent of the head. When using a fetal stethoscope a light pressure should be used so that it does not cause discomfort to

Table 9.1: Fetal weight on the basis of fundal height and BPD

Gestations	Symphysis of fundal height	Approximate biparietal diameter (weeks in gestation ÷ 4)	Approximate fetal weight in grams/kg
22 weeks	22 cm + or - 2 cm	5.5 cm	500 - 600 grams
28 weeks	28 cm + or - 2 cm	7 cm	1 - 1.2 kg
32 weeks	32 cm + or - 2 cm	8 cm	1.5 - 1.8 kg
34 weeks	34 cm + or - 2 cm	8.5 cm	2 - 2.4 kg
36 weeks	36 cm + or - 3 cm	9 cm	2.5 - 2.9 kg
38 weeks	38 cm + or - 3 cm	9.5 cm	3 - 3.5 kg
40 weeks	40 cm + or - 4 cm	9.5-10 cm	3.5 - 4 kg

the mother and the hand with which the stethoscope was placed should be removed so that it does not dampen the sounds which are conveyed. The fetal heart is a low pitched sound and the double click of the heart can be heard on auscultation. The normal fetal heart rate at term is between 110 and 160 beats per minute. Term is defined as a period between 37 and 42 weeks. A gestation below 37 weeks is considered pre-term and over 42 weeks is considered post-term.

Percussion

Percussion is rarely used in an obstetric examination. In early pregnancy one palpates for the liver or the spleen if indicated. Percussion might be of value to determine the lower margin of the liver or the spleen. Similarly, if there is difficulty in palpating the uterus in early pregnancy in an obese woman, percussion might help to delineate the upper margin of the uterine fundus. Eliciting fluid thrill is also an art of percussion, but as mentioned earlier it has limited value in obstetric practice.

Pelvic Examination

Pelvic examination is performed in an obstetric patient only when indicated. There are only a few occasions when such an examination is done in the antenatal period. If a cervical smear needs to be performed then a speculum examination is done. Women might present to the clinic with a history of vaginal bleeding or rupture of membranes before the onset of labor. After a detailed history, speculum examination may be important to confirm the bleeding or the leaking of amniotic fluid. In the case of leakage of amniotic fluid, if there is no fluid seen then the mother can be asked to cough or strain and close observation must be done to see whether there is any liquid coming through the cervical os. At times it is difficult to confirm even though she is definitely leaking fluid based on the history. Additional examinations may need to be performed such as Nitrazine color indicator test.

In the case of bleeding it is best to rule out the possibility of placenta previa by an ultrasound examination. If the woman is hemodynamically unstable because of the bleeding; the mother should be attended to first by resuscitation. The management of a woman with antepartum hemorrhage is discussed in detail in other chapters. The main purpose of speculum examination in antepartum hemorrhage is to rule out the possibility of local causes such as laceration, cervical polyp or very rarely a cervical cancer. At times a swab has to be taken from the cervix or from the upper vagina in order to find out whether there is any infection. To identify streptococcus a lower vaginal swab and a rectal swab is taken.

A digital examination is warranted in early pregnancy to confirm the size of the uterus and to elicit some of the signs discussed in the chapter that deals with diagnosis of pregnancy. A speculum and digital examination may need to be done if the woman presents with bleeding. In pregnancies at term a digital examination is performed in labor or prior to induction of labor to assess the condition of the cervix or the progress of cervical dilatation. This is discussed in the chapters related to spontaneous and induced labor. It is important to perform an abdominal examination whether it is in early or late pregnancy or in labor prior to vaginal examination. The combined findings will provide more information for clinical management.

10.

Suku Mathew George
Pratap Kumar

Miscarriage

INTRODUCTION

Syn: Abortion: Human reproduction is an inefficient process with high pregnancy losses occurring at every stage. Miscarriage and Abortion are interchangeably used to describe a pregnancy loss in the initial trimesters. However, most lay people attribute the term miscarriage to a spontaneous loss while abortion is reserved for an induced termination. In this discussion these terms have been used appropriately. Definition, incidence, etiopathology, classification and management issues are discussed.

DEFINITION

The WHO defines miscarriage (abortion) as expulsion or extraction of a fetus or an embryo weighing 500 gm or less from its mother's womb before 20 weeks of pregnancy. The criterion for viability of pregnancy varies from 24 weeks in United Kingdom to 28 weeks in most developing countries. including India.

INCIDENCE

The incidence of clinically evident miscarriage ranges from 10 to 15 percent of all pregnancies. However, when very early pregnancies, in the 14 days period following conception even before a woman misses her period, are considered the miscarriage rate will be between 45 to 55 percent. These so-called biochemical pregnancies, diagnosed only by the presence of βhCG in the serum of these women have been increasingly recognised due to the availability of assisted reproductive techniques. These early miscarriages may manifest as heavy periods and are of no clinical consequence except in infertile women.

PATHOLOGY

Hemorrhage into the decidua basalis and necrotic changes in the adjacent tissues is the hallmark of miscarriage. The ovum becomes detached partially or completely and begins to stimulate uterine contractions that result in painful expulsion. When the sac is opened fluid is seen to surround the crumpled fetus or in case of blighted ovum an empty sac is noted. Microscopically placental villi appear thick and edematous. Carneous mole is an ovum that is seen surrounded by a capsule of clotted blood with degenerating chorionic villi scattered through it. This type of appearance is associated with a miscarriage that occurs slowly allowing

PART One

Introduction

blood to collect between the decidua and chorion and to coagulate in layers. In larger fetuses there may be evidence of maceration.[1]

CLASSIFICATION

Miscarriage could be spontaneous or induced. The different types of spontaneous miscarriage are depicted in Table 10.1.

Table 10.1: Types of miscarriage

- Threatened miscarriage
- Inevitable miscarriage
- Incomplete miscarriage
- Complete miscarriage
- Missed (abortion) miscarriage
- Induced abortion
- Septic miscarriage
- Recurrent miscarriage

All of these are complicated by some form of vaginal bleeding and have characteristic physical findings (Figure 10.1).

Threatened Miscarriage

The term threatened miscarriage is used when vaginal bleeding within the first 28 weeks of gestation complicates a pregnancy. This is usually associated with dull aching lower abdominal pain. Vaginal examination done at the time will indicate a closed cervical os. Upto a third of these women will progress to inevitable miscarriage regardless of the treatment offered. The best predictor of a pregnancy that will continue to term is the presence of fetal cardiac activity on ultrasound. Over 90 percent of live intrauterine gestations with threatened miscarriage will progress to term (Figure 10.1A).

Inevitable Miscarriage

It is characterized by vaginal bleeding, cramping lower abdominal pain associated with an open cervical os and products of conception often palpable through the os, i.e. in the cervical canal (Figure 10.1B).

Incomplete Miscarriage

In this category of women, there is a history of passage of products of conception as fleshy masses in addition to vaginal bleeding and pain. Due to incomplete nature

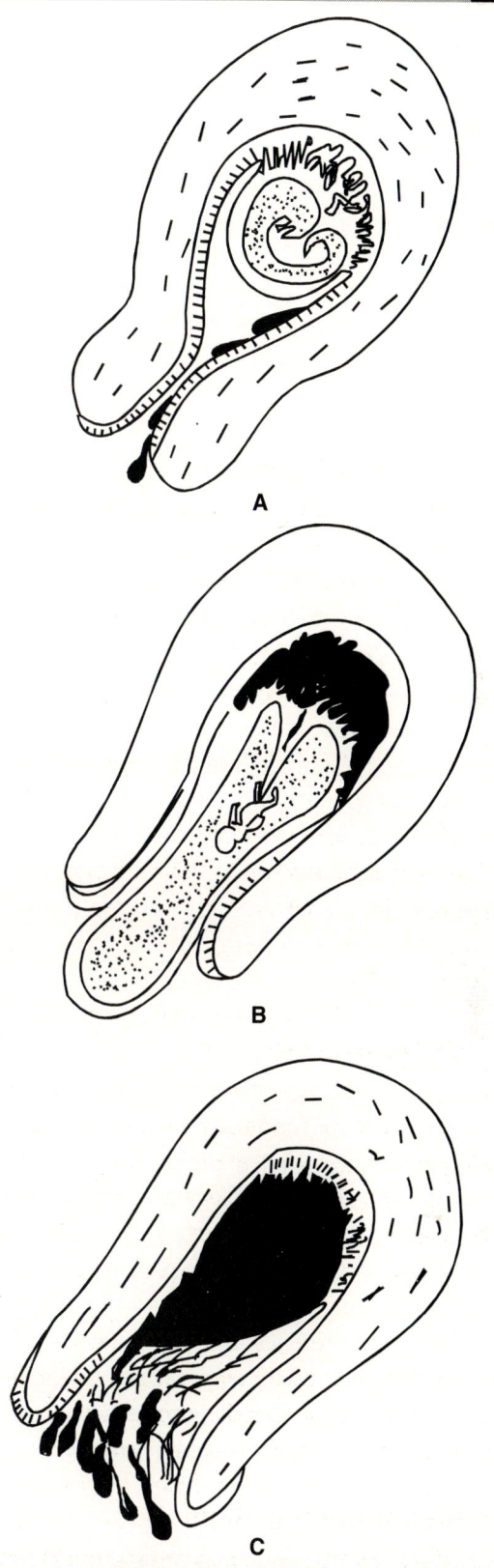

Figures 10.1A to C: Stages of miscarriage

of the miscarriage there is often considerable hemorrhage with symptoms of shock (Figure 10.1C).

Complete Miscarriage

This is characterized by a history of pain and passage of products followed by absence of pain and bleeding or minimal bleeding if present. The cervical os is closed at vaginal examination and the uterine size is less than the period of amenorrhea. With progress of time, the pregnancy test becomes negative and symptoms of pregnancy disappear.

Missed Miscarriage (Abortion)

This term is used when the fetus/embryo has died but is retained in the uterus for a period of time without symptoms of miscarriage. The uterus is less than the period of amenorrhea and the woman may have minimal vaginal bleeding often streaks of dark altered blood.

Based on the ultrasound findings missed miscarriage is classified as to be of two types: When an empty gestational sac is visualized with an absent embryonic pole it is termed as blighted ovum and when a gestational sac with an embryonic pole without cardiac activity is visualized it is termed early fetal demise. When unrecognized for a long duration of time it may lead to consumptive coagulopathy due to disseminated intravascular coagulation.

Recurrent Miscarriage

It is the term used when there have been more than three successive spontaneous miscarriages. It is a distressing uncommon clinical problem in reproduction. A definite cause can be established in only 50 percent of the cases, leaving the couple distraught and frustrated. Repeated spontaneous pregnancy losses are likely to be a chance phenomena in the majority of cases. In early miscarriages, there is usually a chromosomal abnormality of the conceptus while in late abortions the fetus is structurally normal with a maternal abnormality responsible for the miscarriage.[2]

Septic Miscarriage (Abortion)

Occasionally a spontaneous miscarriage or an induced abortion is complicated by infection either ascending from the lower genital tract or iatrogenically introduced while performing induced abortion. This can manifest as local genital tract infection or in severe cases as a systemic infection with sepsis.

ETIOLOGY OF MISCARRIAGE

Many etiological factors have been attributed, although only a few have been conclusively proven to be responsible for causing miscarriage.

Miscarriage can be due to fetal, maternal or paternal factors.

Fetal Factors

The most common cause of abortion is a maldeveloped embryo. This may range from complete absence of the fetus to major or minor anomalies. This is often caused by a defect in number of chromosomes (aneuploidy), an addition (trisomy), a deletion (monosomy) or a defect in one or many of the chromosomes. These abnormalities amount to over half of the miscarriages and they tend to increase with advancing maternal age. The miscarriages, which result from the implantation of these embryos, seem to be nature's way of preventing the birth of abnormal fetuses.

Maternal Factors

Systemic factors include (i) maternal medical disorders like diabetes, thyroid disorders and connective tissue disorders, (ii) infections with herpes virus, microorganisms like *Mycoplasma, Listeria monocytogenes, Ureaplasma urealyticum*. Other infective agents like rubella virus, *Toxoplasma gondii* is occasionally responsible. A non-specific infection with high pyrexia also may cause miscarriage. (iii) excessive maternal smoking and alcohol intake also have been incriminated. (iv) psychological factors like increased stress, sudden shock though attributed is rarely responsible.

Local factors (Luteal phase defect): Deficient amount of progesterone from the corpus luteum of the ovary upto 8 to 10 weeks of gestation may affect decidual development. However, evidence has shown that this factor is very uncommon and difficult to prove. Except in proved cases of luteal phase deficiency, routine administration of progestogens to pregnant women is not advisable.

Uterine abnormalities: The most common abnormality is cervical insufficiency. A competent cervix is essential for retaining pregnancy. In some women this sphincteric action of the cervix is deficient leading to characteristic midtrimester losses of live fetuses. The miscarriage process is usually painless and rapid with expulsion of a live fetus often with intact membranes.

Other uterine abnormalities that can cause miscarriage are defects in mullerian ducts with fusion defects like, bicornuate uterus, septate uterus and double uterus. Implantation over the relatively avascular septum can lead to abnormal decidual development and miscarriage. Most mullerian anomalies have associated cervical insufficiency. These can cause pregnancy losses in first and second trimesters. Hysteroscopy and laparoscopy in non-pregnant women can diagnose these abnormalities. Surgical correction of these defects can dramatically improve prognosis in women with recurrent miscarriage. Administration of diethylstilbestrol (DES) to a pregnant woman can result in characteristic uterine anomalies in their female offspring viz.: T-shaped uteri among others. These women can have recurrent miscarriages and are often benefited by treatment for cervical insufficiency. However, this is not a common occurrence in the developing world.

An acquired cause that can cause spontaneous miscarriage is the presence of submucous myomas that distorts uterine cavity. Removal of these myomas may result in term pregnancies. Other rare causes are acquired intrauterine adhesions due to overzealous uterine curettage in the post-abortal or puerperal period. These adhesions develop due to destruction of large area of endometrium leading to defective implantation. This when suspected can be diagnosed easily with hysteroscopy and treated by lysing these adhesions at the same sitting.[1]

Immunological factors: There is increasing evidence that abnormal immune function in the mother can lead to miscarriages. A successful pregnancy depends on a number of immunological factors that allows the retention of an antigenically foreign fetus in the mother without initiating a host versus graft rejection.

The presence of antiphospholipid antibodies, viz. lupus anticoagulant (LAC) and anticardiolipin antibodies (ACA) are recognized causes of recurrent miscarriage associated with thromboembolic episodes.

Other newly discovered abnormalities are the deficiencies of some factors essential for coagulation like protein C, protein S and antithrombin II. In all these abnormalities there is abnormal decidual development with abnormal capillary development and formation of microthrombi in the uteroplacental circulation. An increasing understanding of these factors will lead to newer modalities of treatment for women with unexplained recurrent miscarriage.

Paternal Factors

Presence of chromosomal abnormalities in either of the parent such as balanced translocations can result in spontaneous miscarriages, hence the importance of performing peripheral blood karyotyping of the couple with recurrent pregnancy losses.

CLINICAL FEATURES

Apart from symptoms of pregnancy all types of miscarriage have some amount of vaginal bleeding and pain of varying degree. The characteristic clinical features are summarized in Table 10.2.

MANAGEMENT

All patients with miscarriage require careful and sympathetic counseling. They should be reassured that the chance of a future successful pregnancy is over 80 percent. Baseline investigations such as hemoglobin and blood group and typing should be performed. Rhesus-negative women should receive anti-D immunoglobulin in doses ranging from 50 to 150 micrograms depending on the duration of pregnancy.

Threatened abortion is best managed by a pelvic ultrasound examination to determine whether a fetus is present and, if so, whether cardiac activity is observed. Over 90 percent of women with a live fetus will go on to deliver a baby at term. Management of these women consists of reassurance and emotional support.

Table 10.2: Types of miscarriage and their clinical features

Miscarriages	Uterine size	Symptoms	Cervix	USG
Threatened	Corresponding	Bleeding, Pain	Closed	Live fetus, Retrochoreal hemorrhage
Inevitable	Same or less	Bleeding, Pain	Open with palpable products	Absent cardiac activity, Retrochoreal hemorrhage
Incomplete	Smaller	Heavy bleeding, Signs of shock	Open	Retained products seen
Complete	Smaller	No bleeding	Closed	Empty cavity
Missed	Smaller	Absent or minimal bleeding	Closed	Empty gestational sac in blighted ovum or fetus without cardiac activity in early fetal demise

Hospitalization, bed rest or administration of progestogens has not been proven to be of benefit. A repeat ultrasound examination can be performed a week later to confirm a growing fetus and to reassure the family.

Inevitable Miscarriage

Women with inevitable miscarriage need hospitalization, analgesics for control of pain and a pelvic ultrasound examination. The uterine cavity needs to be evacuated with either suction evacuation or manually with ovum forceps. Administration of misoprostol vaginally in doses upto 400 mcg has been successfully used.

Incomplete Miscarriage

These women may have significant blood loss and signs of shock. Hence, they need to be admitted for prompt resuscitation and analgesics are given for pain. Hypovolemia when present is initially corrected with crystalloid and later with compatible cross matched blood. Broad-spectrum antibiotics are administered to prevent infection and once the patients condition is stabilised, the remaining products of conception is evacuated from the uterus. In some patients, there may be spontaneous passage of products, thus avoiding the need for surgical evacuation. If necessary, an ultrasound examination can be done to confirm an empty uterus.

Complete Miscarriage

These women require ultrasound examination to ensure an empty uterine cavity and also to rule out the possibility of an extrauterine pregnancy. If the diagnosis is uncertain and in women where no prior ultrasound is available serial β hCG estimation will aid in the diagnosis.

Missed (Abortion) Miscarriage

As mentioned earlier this is suggested by a uterus smaller than the period of amenorrhea. An ultrasound examination needs to be performed to confirm the diagnosis and to ascertain whether it is an anembryonic pregnancy with an empty gestational sac or whether it is early fetal demise. These patients can be managed conservatively to await spontaneous expulsion. However this would involve further maternal anxiety, pain of expulsion and in some cases development of serious complications such as disseminated intravascular coagulation and infection. Hence it is preferable to evacuate the products of conception either surgically or by medical methods. A combination of mifeprestone and misoprostol can be used successfully to evacuate the uterus with minimal intervention.

Septic Abortion (Miscarriage)

With the easy access of broad-spectrum antibiotics and better surgical facilities this condition is fortunately becoming rare, but when diagnosed require urgent hospitalization and prompt institution of parentral antibiotic therapy. Once infection is controlled careful evacuation of uterus is performed preferably under ultrasound guidance. In some cases severe sepsis may lead to renal failure and disseminated intravascular coagulation and even death. These patients are also at risk of chronic pelvic inflammatory disease and infertility.

Recurrent Miscarriage

Although by definition three consecutive pregnancy losses constitute recurrent miscarriage, investigation of the couple can be done after two miscarriages in the first trimester or after a single second trimester loss. Most of the etiological factors thought to be responsible for sporadic miscarriage have not been proven to cause recurrent miscarriages.

Royal College of Obstetricians and Gynecologists (RCOG) in England recommended that the investigation of recurrent miscarriage should include:
- Peripheral blood karyotyping in both partners, karyotyping of all fetal products,
- A pelvic ultrasound scan to assess ovarian morphology and the uterine cavity and
- Screening tests for antiphospholipid antibodies (both the lupus anticoagulant and anticardiolipin antibodies) performed on two separate occasions at least six weeks apart.

The place of all other investigations including a search for newly described thrombophilic defects is unproven and such tests should only be performed in the context of research studies. A clinical geneticist should see the couple with recurrent miscarriage who have undergone the above investigations and those with karyotypic abnormalities. Women with persistently positive tests for antiphospholipid antibodies are offered treatment with low dose aspirin together with low dose heparin during pregnancy (also the subject of on-going research).[3] Treatments of unproven benefit such as routine progesterone administration should be abandoned except in cases with proved luteal phase defect. Investigations such as glucose tolerance test, thyroid function and hysterosalpingogram need be individualized to patients.

Women with recurrent miscarriage and a double uterus (uterine septum) should undergo hysteroscopic evaluation and reparative surgery. If cervical insufficiency is diagnosed, cervical encirclage is done by placing a stitch at the level close to the internal os in early second trimester. This may be accomplished by putting a purse string suture with non-absorbable material at the cervicovaginal junction as described by McDonald. The suture can be inserted at the actual level of internal os after dissecting the bladder anteriorly off the cervix using merselene tape as described by Shirodkar. The latter method is preferred in women with a short cervix due to previous surgery. These operations are successful in treating cervical insufficiency when the patients are appropriately selected.

Couples with otherwise unexplained recurrent miscarriage should be counseled regarding the potential for successful pregnancy without treatment.

Induced Abortion

Deliberate termination of pregnancy before the viability of fetus is termed as induction of abortion. No other topic in obstetrics has generated such intense controversy and ethical debate over the rights of the unborn fetus continues to this day. Induction of abortion is protected by legislation in countries where it is permitted. In India it is governed by the provisions of the Medical Termination Act of 1971 which was revised in 1975. Under the provisions of the Act abortion can be induced upto the 20th gestational week if
  i. The continuation of pregnancy would involve serious risk to life or grave injury to the physical and mental health of the pregnant woman.
  ii. There is a substantial risk of the child being born with serious physical and mental abnormalities so as to be handicapped in life.
  iii. The pregnancy is caused by rape both in case of major and minor girl and in mentally imbalanced women.
  iv. The pregnancy resulted as the result of failure of contraception in any married couple.

According to the revised rule, a registered medical practitioner is qualified to perform medical termination of pregnancy (MTP) provided he has assisted at least 25 such procedures in an authorised training center and is certified or has undergone six months house surgeon training in obstetrics and gynecology or is a qualified obstetrician and gynecologist. Termination can be performed only in government hospitals or other institutions approved by it. Pregnancy can be terminated only by the written consent of the woman or her legal guardian in case of a minor or a mentally unsound person. Termination is permitted only upto 20 weeks of gestation and when it exceeds the 12th week opinion of two medical practitioners is required. The procedure has to be performed confidentially and has to be reported to the director of health services of the state in the prescribed form.

Preabortion Assessment

Individual patient counseling should be an integral part of termination of pregnancy because this is an emotionally difficult time for many women. It is also essential that a thorough physical assessment be performed. If there are any discrepancies in uterine size and gestational age, an ultrasound examination is essential. Baseline investigations such as hemoglobin, blood group and Rh typing should be performed prior to the procedure. Assessment prior to induced abortion may be viewed as an opportunity to ascertain each woman's cervical cytology history. Women who have not had a smear within the last year may be offered a smear taken at this time.[4] For minimising the risk of post-abortion infective morbidity antibiotic prophylaxis should be administered. Common regimens include, Ciprofloxacin 500 mg with 300 mg Tinidazole twice daily for 7 days or doxycycline 100 mg twice daily for 7 days, commencing post-abortion. Contraception should be discussed with the patient and appropriate method started at this time.

Methods of Termination

First Trimester Methods

- Suction curettage
- Dilatation and evacuation
- Mifeprestone 200-600 mg orally followed by misoprostol 400-600 mg orally
- Methotrexate 1.5 mg/square meter of body surface area intramuscularly followed by 400 mg of Misoprostol vaginally 1 week later.

Conventional suction termination should be avoided at gestations of less than 7 weeks due to high incidence of failure.[4] From 7 weeks onward, suction curettage is the method of choice till 12 weeks. Dilatation of the cervix can be either rapid dilatation by gradual insertion of metal dilators under anesthesia or paracervical block. It can also be slow dilatation achieved by introduction of hygroscopic agents such as laminaria tents or by the local application of prostaglandins.

Mifeprestone, a progesterone antagonist acts by competitive inhibition of the receptors in the endometrium and has a high efficacy of over 90 percent upto 9 weeks of gestation when used in conjunction with misoprostol. The drug is presently undergoing clinical trials and is awaiting approval by the Indian FDA. When used under 7 weeks it is given in doses of 200 mg followed by 400 mcg of misoprostol 48 hours later orally. Between 7 and 9 weeks misoprostol is administered intravaginally

Methods in the Second Trimester

- Dilatation and evacuation
- Extra-amniotic instillation of Ethacridine lactate, prostaglandins E2 and F2∝
- Intra-amniotic instillation of hypertonic (20%) saline, hypertonic urea, prostaglandins E2 and F2∝
- Intravaginal misoprostol/gemeprost
- Intramuscular administration of PGF2∝
- Combination of above methods

The disadvantage of the above methods is that woman has painful uterine contractions for hours and often have incomplete abortion with retention of the placenta necessitating its removal by instrumentation. The incidence of hemorrhage and infection is high. The use of hypertonic saline is associated with hypernatremia and disseminated intravascular coagulation. Hysterotomy, which involved laparotomy and removal of the fetus in second trimester through a uterine incision, has been abandoned due to the availability of better methods and the risk of uterine rupture in subsequent pregnancies.

Before she is discharged following abortion, future contraception should have been discussed with each patient and contraceptive supplies should have been offered if required. The chosen method of contraception should be initiated immediately following abortion. Sterilization can safely be performed at the time of induced abortion. It is safe and effective to insert an IUCD for contraceptive use immediately following induced abortion.

Complications

Complications are relatively more frequent in second trimester terminations. With the advent of effective agents such as prostaglandins terminations in mid trimester are becoming safe. Immediate complications include cervical tears and injury due to manipulation and perforation of the uterus. These can lead to hemorrhage and may warrant discontinuation of the procedure. Hemorrhage during the procedure can be minimized by using oxytocics such as intravenous oxytocin infusion or methyl ergometrine. Perforation of the uterine cavity can lead to serious consequences such as injury to bowel, bladder and rarely major blood vessels. If perforation of uterus is suspected the procedure should be stopped and resuscitative measures should be undertaken as appropriate. If bowel injury is suspected it is prudent to perform laparoscopy or laparotomy to confirm the diagnosis. Once the injury is repaired the remaining products can be evacuated under direct vision. Use of hypertonic saline can result in hypernatremia; convulsions and disseminated intravascular coagulation. Prostaglandins are relatively safe but can cause vomiting, diarrhea and occasionally cervico-uterine injuries. Genital tract infection of varying severity, including pelvic inflammatory disease, occurs in upto 10 percent of cases. The risk is reduced when prophylactic antibiotics are given or when lower genital tract infection has been excluded by bacteriological screening. Infection, if diagnosed, should be aggressively treated with broad-spectrum antibiotics.

Late complications include chronic pelvic inflammatory disease, infertility due to tubal block and uterine synechia formation giving rise to amenorrhea and infertility (Asherman's syndrome). Other complications include cervical insufficiency and uterine rupture in pregnancy. Failure to immunize the Rhesus-negative woman can lead to isoimmunization in future pregnancies.

SUMMARY

Miscarriage when occurs is unsuspected and devastating to the involved couple. The various types progress from an early threat of miscarriage to end in complete expulsion of the conceptus. Most miscarriages are sporadic and are nature's way of avoiding the birth of a malformed fetus. When recurrent, treatable causes should be looked for aggressively and remedial measures undertaken where possible. Increased understanding of the immunology of pregnancy promises the possibility of preventing some of these recurrent losses.

Induced abortion when indicated should be offered to women after adequate counseling which should include the available options. Contraceptive advice should be a part of this counseling. Complications can be minimized by choosing the appropriate method for the gestation and the use of prophylactic antibiotics.

REFERENCES

1. Cunningham FG, Mac Donald PC, Garri NF, Leveno KJ, et al: Abortions. In *Williams Obstetrics*. 20th edn, Appleton and Lange, Prentice Hall International inc. 579-606.
2. Scott JR: Recurrent miscarriage: Overview and recommendations. *Clinical Obstetrics and Gynecology* **37**:623, 1994.
3. RCOG Clinical Guideline development group. *Clinical Guideline in Recurrent Miscarriage*: RCOG Press, UK.
4. RCOG Clinical Guideline development group. *Clinical Guideline in Induced Abortion*: RCOG Press, UK.

11. Ectopic Pregnancy

Idora Mohamed

INTRODUCTION

Abnormal implantation of a blastocyst or a fertilized ovum outside the uterine cavity is termed as ectopic pregnancy. This condition is a major public health concern as there is a rise in its incidence worldwide. In the 19th century, the reported mortality from an ectopic pregnancy was 70 percent (Parry and Lea). In 1884, Lawrence Tait published the first cases of surgical management where a laparotomy was performed to remove a ruptured tube. Thankfully, after a century of rapid technological advances, the diagnosis and management of ectopic pregnancy has been dramatically improved.

INCIDENCE

In northern Europe between 1976 and 1993, the incidence increased from 11.2 to 18.8 per 1000 pregnancies. In the United States, admissions to hospital for ectopic pregnancy increased from 17,800 in 1970 to 88,400 in 1989. In 1992, it had increased to 10,8000 accounting for 2 percent of all pregnancies. These changes were greatest in women over 35 years of age. In the United Kingdom (UK) the incidence is 11.5 per 1000 pregnancies (around 11,000 cases per year). There have been four reported deaths in the UK confidential enquiries in the year 1994-1996. Increases in the incidence have been attributed to rising rates of pelvic inflammatory disease, mainly caused by *Chlamydia trachomatis*

PATHOPHYSIOLOGY

Why a fertilized ovum can implant in an apparently normal fallopian tube is still unknown. Normal transport of the ovum from the ovary to the uterine cavity takes 3 to 4 days. The fertilized ovum normally invades the uterine decidua on the sixth to seventh day after conception. Important factors that are involved in its transport include the tubal contractility, ovarian hormones and the cilial action within the tubes. Estrogens stimulate tubal contractility but progesterone decreases its activity. Progesterone has been shown to reduce local prostaglandin secretion and relaxes the isthmic portion of the tube. This may allow the fertilized egg to cross into the uterus.

The uterus will still undergo changes of early pregnancy. The isthmus and the cervix begin to enlarge and soften. The endometrium decidualizes. After fetal death it will degenerate and shed, explaining the irregular vaginal bleeding that is often seen. In the event where a uterine evacuation was performed and the curettage yields only decidual changes without trophoblastic tissue, an ectopic must be suspected.

Arias-Stella Reaction

The endometrial glands show marked secretory and proliferative activity, forming tall, vacuolated cells that have hypertrophic and hyperchromatic nuclei. This is not specific for ectopic pregnancies and the incidence varies from 3 to 100 percent. It can also be seen in normal pregnancy, abortions, chorioepithelioma, endometriosis and patients on long-term estrogens and progestogens.

SITES OF IMPLANTATION

Tubal

Almost all (97%) of extrauterine pregnancies occur in the fallopian tube. The sites in order of frequency are ampullary, isthmic, fimbrial and interstitial (Figure 11.1, Plate 1).

The trophoblast invades the epithelium of the tube, proliferating into the deeper muscular wall causing erosion into the maternal blood vessels causing a hematoma and tubal dilatation. This might explain the pain that patients complain of before other complications of an ectopic arises. As the trophoblast proliferates further, it will eventually lead to serosal rupture and hemoperitoneum. The trophoblast does not differ histologically from a normal intrauterine pregnancy, but the embryo in an ectopic is usually stunted or frequently absent.

A tubal abortion occurs when the conceptus passes through the fimbria into the abdominal cavity. This is more likely in cases with implantation around the fimbria and ampulla of the tube. If the implantation is in the isthmus, rupture is the more common outcome. If the site of implantation is on the mesosalpinx, rupture may occur into the broad ligament, causing a broad ligament hematoma. Implantation in the interstitial or the intramyometrial portion of the tube is also called a cornual pregnancy. As it is surrounded by the muscle fibers of the uterus, the rupture classically occurs later because of the increased distensibility of the tube. It would be more difficult to diagnose, causes more tissue damage and has a great potential to bleed heavily due to the rich blood supply from branches of the uterine and ovarian arteries.

Ovarian

Ovarian pregnancy is rare. The incidence is reported as being in between 1/2000 and 1/8500 deliveries. If the implantation was directly on the ovary it is a primary ovarian ectopic. To diagnose this, the tube on the involved side must be normal, the affected ovary is in its normal anatomic site with presence of the utero-ovarian ligament. More importantly, the gestational sac wall contains ovarian tissue on histologic examination.

A secondary ovarian ectopic is the result of a tubal abortion and its reimplantation on the ovary.

Abdominal Site

This again is rare with rates reported between 1/3400 and 1/8000 deliveries. It is usually secondary, as a result of a tubal abortion or rupture where the viable fetus is transferred into the peritoneal cavity. In a primary implantation, the pregnancy is surrounded with peritoneal tissue and the tubes and ovaries are normal.

If it is not diagnosed, the remaining fetus which usually is unable to survive is retained. Then there will be spontaneous resorption, suppuration or lithopedion formation. If the pregnancy continues, it may even proceed to the third trimester. The clinical features of an abdominal pregnancy may develop causing mainly gastrointestinal symptoms—nausea, vomiting, constipation, diarrhea and pain. Suspicion should be aroused when uterine contractions do not occur with oxytocin stimulation. The condition sometimes becomes apparent only at laparotomy where massive hemorrhage can occur. The maternal mortality as a result of this is estimated at 10 percent.

Cervical Site

The implantation here is below the internal cervical os with the trophoblastic tissue eroding into the endocervical mucosa and eventually into the fibrous substance of the cervical wall. Its frequency is between 1/10000 and 1/16000 deliveries.

The overdistended cervix will cause painless vaginal bleeding. The challenge is in its management. A balloon tamponade with Foley's catheter or "occlusion compression" suture of the cervix may help. At time a hysterectomy may become necessary as a result of uncontrollable bleeding from the placental implantation in the cervix that cannot contract well.

Other Sites

Other uncommon sites that have been reported include the vagina, intraligament and in a rudimentary horn.

A heterotopic pregnancy is an intrauterine pregnancy coexisting with an ectopic, which is usually tubal. The incidence quoted in the literature varies from 1/10,000 to 1/30000 deliveries but it is on the rise with the advent of *in vitro* fertilization and multiple embryo transfers.

ETIOLOGY AND RISK FACTORS

Logically, any mechanism that interferes and delays tubal transport will contribute to the cause of ectopic pregnancy. However, there will be a proportion of women with no identifiable causal or risk factors.

Tubal Damage

Most commonly, this is due to pelvic inflammatory disease or salpingitis. The risk is increased seven-fold in acute salpingitis. Gonococcal, tuberculosis and more commonly, chlamydia are known pathogens. With endosalpingitis, the tubal endothelium may be damaged causing adhesions and subsequent strictures or formation of sacs where the fertilized ovum could get trapped. The ciliary and peristaltic action will also be impaired.

Previous tubal surgery, either for sterilization or improvement of fertility and a history of previous ectopic pregnancy are other risk factors.

After sterilization, the chances of conceiving are very low. If there is a pregnancy, it has a higher probability of being an ectopic. In a large collaborative review in the United States, the 10-year cumulative probability of ectopic pregnancy after sterilization was 7.3 per 1000 procedures. This is most probably due to the formation of a tuboperitoneal fistula after destruction of the tube allowing migration of sperms through it to fertilize the ovum.

In those with a previous ectopic, the chances of getting another ectopic is as high as 10 percent, which is why early examination of these patients in the next pregnancy is important.

Intrauterine Contraceptive Devices (IUCD)

There is no proven direct relationship between the increased incidence of ectopic to IUCD use. In a meta-analysis of 16 studies, the incidence is not increased in current IUCD use, but is mildly elevated in those who had IUCDs inserted before. The reason for this is that the risk of pregnancy is low, but if pregnancy does occur, an ectopic is more likely.

Assisted Reproduction

The incidence of ectopic pregnancy after assisted reproductive techniques is increased by 2 to 3 times the background incidence. The incidence is reported to be 4 percent. The main risk factor is tubal infertility. In *in vitro* fertilization, the embryo could get deposited into the tube directly or by uterine contractions. However, in a diseased tube with impaired action, re-expulsion of the embryo would not occur. The high levels of estrogen and progesterone could also contribute as it affects the effective beating of the cilia and alters tubal transport.

PRESENTATION

Almost all ectopic pregnancies are diagnosed between 5 and 12 weeks' gestation. The most common symptoms are low abdominal, back or pelvic pain, which is usually unilateral, and vaginal bleeding. The pattern of the bleeding is usually—but not always—scanty, dark and intermittent, unlike the profuse bleeding that occurs in a miscarriage. The fact that a patient with regular menses is late for a single period or has irregular or abnormal bleeding should suggest potential pregnancy. If there is free blood in the peritoneal cavity, the diaphragmatic irritation will be transmitted as shoulder tip pain. When there is significant hemoperitoneum, the patient will have syncopal attacks or even come in a state of circulatory collapse. The presence of known risk factors can increase suspicion, but any sexually active woman presenting with abdominal pain and vaginal bleeding after an interval of amenorrhea has an ectopic until proven otherwise.

Initial examination should be the vital signs and a general examination to estimate signs of blood loss with hypovolemia. In cases of an unruptured ectopic, the patient complains of a localized pain to one iliac fossa. In significant hemoperitoneum, guarding, rebound tenderness and decreased bowel sounds may be present.

The vaginal examination will aid in making a more conclusive diagnosis. During speculum examination, the cervix should be closely examined for signs of a spontaneous abortion. Blood oozing out from the os, with presence of fetal and placental tissue, points to an inevitable abortion. In an ectopic, the cervical os is closed. On bimanual examination the uterus will be somewhat smaller than the expected date. A pathognomonic sign of an ectopic is a positive cervical excitation test. This is done by gentle motion of the cervix to both sides of the lateral fornix. There is frequently marked tenderness due to the stretching of the involved site. Sometimes the posterior fornix will be very tender as the heavier affected tube lies in the pouch of Douglas. The examination should be carried out as gently as possible to avoid rupture of an unruptured ectopic. Rupture will lead to severe intraperitoneal bleed and collapse. When there are obvious signs of hemoperitoneum, a digital vaginal examination is of little value and may enhance further intraperitoneal bleeding.

INVESTIGATION

The major advances that have helped in making an early diagnosis of extrauterine pregnancy are highly sensitive rapid assays for beta-human chorionic gonadotropin (β-hCG) levels, use of ultrasound to evaluate the pelvis and application of laparoscopy as a diagnostic and therapeutic tool.

β–hCG Measurement

The easiest assessment of pregnancy in any woman in the reproductive age group with abdominal pain and abnormal vaginal bleeding will be a urine pregnancy test. It is highly sensitive being able to positively identify a positive hCG threshold level of 50 IU/L.

In instances where expectant management is feasible or in very early pregnancy around 5 weeks where the gestational sac might not yet be visualized, the serial serum β-hCG monitoring becomes an essential tool. In a normal pregnancy, the serum concentrations increase exponentially, doubling every 2 to 3.5 days in the fourth to eighth week of gestation and reaches a peak around the 8th to 12th weeks (Figure 11.2). A two-day sampling interval is helpful. If the doubling is less than 85 percent or the level starts reaching a plateau or decreasing, it is most likely to be an ectopic pregnancy.

Ultrasound

Imaging with a transvaginal probe has improved visualization of the gestational sac in early pregnancy. At about 5 weeks a gestational sac can be seen in the uterine lumen. This sac is surrounded by two layers of decidua, the capsularis and the parietalis, giving an

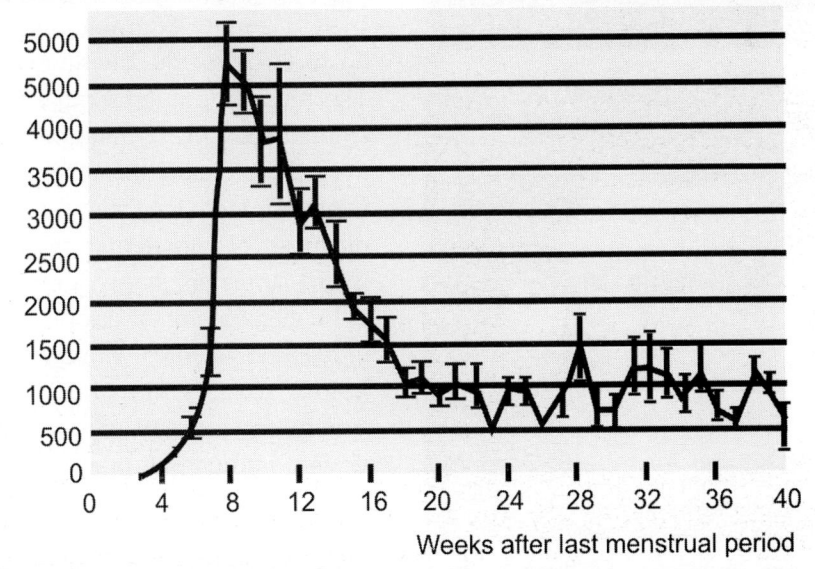

Figure 11.2: Levels of hCG in relation to gestational weeks in normal pregnancy

ultrasonographic appearance of a 'halo'. The presence made by these two concentric layers is strongly indicative of an intrauterine pregnancy and can be used to differentiate it from an ectopic pregnancy where there is only one decidual layer. In an intrauterine pregnancy, a fetal pole will be visualized at around the 6th to 7th weeks. By 9 weeks, the crude human features may be seen. After the death of an ectopic fetus, the central part of the decidua will undergo necrosis with some amount of fluid. This can be mistaken for an intrauterine sac and is termed a pseudogestational sac.

Other ultrasound findings include fluid in the pelvis which would indicate a collection of blood from either a leaking or ruptured ectopic and presence of dilated tube with the gestational sac within. Sometimes, this would appear as a complex mass in the adnexe or free fluid in the pouch of Douglas (Figures 11.3 and 11.4).

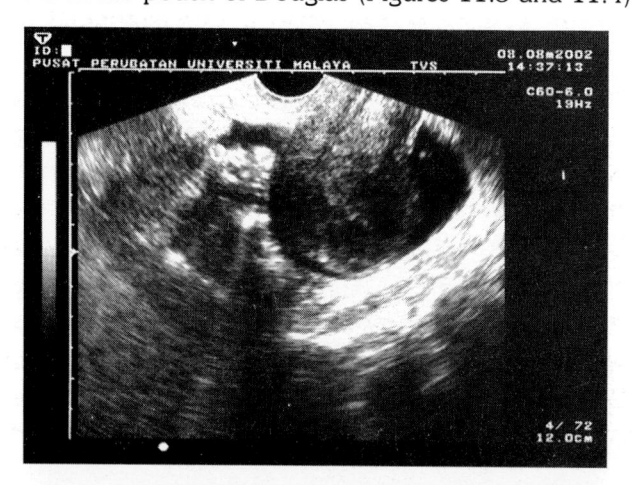

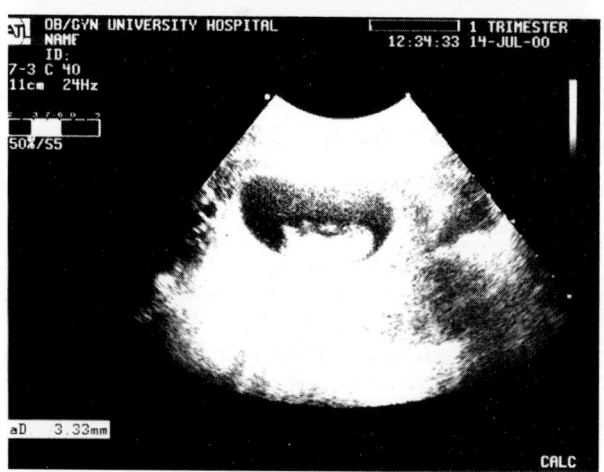

Figures 11.3A and B: Ultrasound picture of complex mass in adnexae

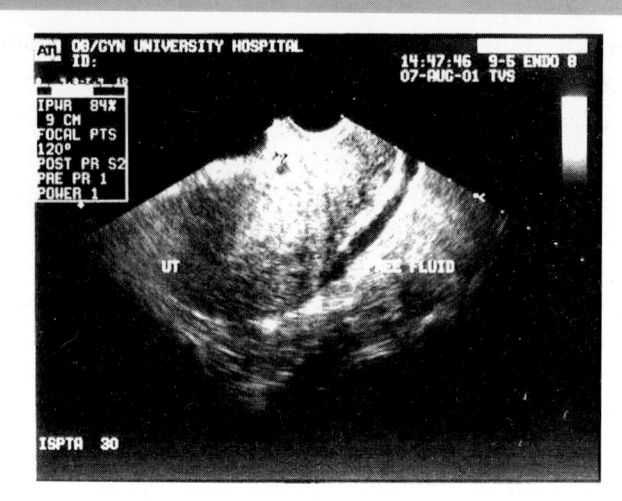

Figure 11.4: Free fluid in pouch of Douglas

Discriminatory Zone

This was proposed by Kadar et al where the hCG levels are correlated to the ultrasound features of an early intrauterine pregnancy. This is especially important in women with irregular vaginal bleeding in early pregnancy where the exact age of gestation is not known. An intrauterine sac seen when the hCG concentration was above the discriminatory zone almost always predicted an intrauterine pregnancy. When no sac is present above this level, an ectopic pregnancy must be considered. The recent recommended level is 1500 IU/L in the presence of a mass or fluid in the pouch of Douglas, but in the absence of these, a higher concentration of 2000 IU/L is advised.

Ultrasound examination done in a patient with an hCG below the discriminatory zone is not useful. The sensitivity in detecting an intrauterine pregnancy, spontaneous miscarriage or ectopic pregnancy when the hCG is below this level is 30 to 40 percent. The positive predictive value of ultrasound in making a diagnosis of intrauterine pregnancy is 80 percent and in an ectopic pregnancy is 60 percent. This means that if the diagnosis of an ectopic is made just based on the ultrasound features without considering the discriminatory zone, 4 out of 10 women would undergo surgical intervention unnecessarily and jeopardizing a desired intrauterine pregnancy.

Laparoscopy

Once the diagnosis has been established, a diagnostic laparoscopy is performed for the definitive diagnosis and

7. National CSSM progra – Complications during antenatal, intranata and postnatal period, Ministry of Health and Family Welfare, Govt. of India, 89, 1992.
8. Thaddeus S, Maine D: Too far to walk: maternal mortality in context. *Soc Sci Med* **38**:1091-110, 1994.
9. Essential Obstetric functions at first referral level: Report of a Technical Working Group. Geneva: WHO, 8-11, 1986.
10. Making Pregnancy Safer—A health Sector Strategy for Reducing Maternal and Perinatal Morbidity and Mortality. WHO, Geneva. 2000.

13. Antenatal Care

Onnig Tamizian
Sabaratnam Arulkumaran

PART TWO: Feto-maternal Medicine

AIMS OF ANTENATAL CARE

- Provision of education, reassurance and support to the pregnant woman and her partner
- Advice on minor problems and symptoms encountered in pregnancy
- Assessment of maternal and fetal risk factors prior to and at the onset of pregnancy and as they develop throughout pregnancy
- Provision of prenatal screening and management of abnormalities detected
- Determination of timing and mode of delivery where complications arise.

Effective antenatal care needs to focus on what should be achieved at each key stage of the pregnancy. Antenatal care needs to be provided as part of a broadly agreed and implemented program but 'fine tuned' to the individual requirements of the mother and fetus as assessed at booking and as these requirements evolve during the course of the pregnancy. The current emphasis is provision of as much of the antenatal care as possible in the community and the primary care team setting and this is partly in response to what the women would prefer themselves.

Routine antenatal care is provided by means of antenatal visits to the community midwife, GP or hospital specialist at regular intervals. The majority of the antenatal care visits are however with the community midwife. In general, these visits are at 4 weekly intervals to 28 weeks, two weekly intervals to 36 weeks and weekly thereafter until delivery. Clearly the timing, frequency as well as the lead professional for these visits is altered according to the presence or evolution of any problems during the pregnancy.

PRECONCEPTION COUNSELING

In an ideal world antenatal care would commence at the preconception stage where health education (general advice about nutrition, lifestyle, avoidance of teratogens, folic acid supplementation, etc) and risk assessment can be focused toward a planned pregnancy. Preconception counseling is of much greater importance in two main groups of women.

1. Ones with underlying medical conditions that may be affected by or may influence the outcome of a pregnancy. Examples of such conditions include diabetes, various endocrinopathies, hemostatic or thrombotic problems and cardiac disease. Patients following organ transplantation (kidney, liver, heart and lungs) are also now contributing to the ranks of these patients along with survivors of childhood malignancies. A multidisciplinary approach to optimize/stabilize the underlying condition and planning care

during the antenatal period is a key component to optimizing pregnancy outcome.

2. Ones where there are identifiable factors that would suggest the couple are at a high risk of fetal anomaly. Such identifiable factors may include a previous child affected by a single gene disorder or syndromic disorder, a family history of a genetic disorder or history of parental chromosomal abnormality.

Counseling is a major part of prenatal diagnosis. The majority of parents to be, do not perceive themselves at risk and 95 percent of abnormalities do occur unexpectedly, in pregnancies not considered at risk.

GENERAL ADVICE ABOUT LIFESTYLE

Pregnancy can be both an exciting and worrying time for the mother and her partner. Part of the role of the health care professionals (usually fulfilled by the community midwife and general practitioner) caring for the mother is the provision of information about everyday activities that may or may not be affected by or have an effect on the pregnancy.

1. *Alcohol:* Pregnant women are advised to limit alcohol consumption and a consumption of under 20 gm/week (2 units) appears to be generally safe. Heavy alcohol consumption (greater than 12 units or 120 gm/day) is associated with development of fetal alcohol syndrome. The syndrome is characterized by growth retardation, neurological and structural defects (facial, cardiac, joints). A lesser degree of alcohol consumption but still greater than 8 units/day may also be associated with fetal alcohol syndrome as well as other associated features such as increased risk of miscarriage and reduced head circumference.

2. *Smoking:* It should be strongly discouraged in pregnancy. The target should be cessation of smoking, but if not possible, then cutting down to as few as possible is advisable. Smokers (especially those smoking > 20/day) have a slightly higher incidence of miscarriage, a slightly higher perinatal death rate (20% increase in 20/day smokers, and 35% increase if > 20/day) and babies of smokers are 150 to 300 gm lighter than babies of non-smokers. Furthermore, smoking is associated with a three-fold increase in risk of cleft palate. Smoking during pregnancy, however, does not affect long-term mental or motor development. The mechanisms involved include interference of carbon monoxide with oxygen transfer, shifting the oxygen dissociation curve to the left in both maternal and fetal hemoglobin and reduced intervillous blood flow. Appropriate advice and support should be provided for women who wish to try stopping smoking, with optimum benefits achieved if smoking is stopped prior to conception.

3. *Sex during pregnancy:* Patient inhibition to ask and failure to address the issue by health professionals has resulted in considerable misconceptions. In general with an uncomplicated pregnancy, there are no contraindications to coitus or other form of sexual enjoyment in pregnancy including cunnilingus and masturbation. There is no evidence that these have a damaging influence on the fetus or risk inducing premature labor. With advancing gestation certain coital positions may be physically awkward. There may be a decline in some women in sexual desire and activity in early pregnancy and toward the end of pregnancy. Coitus may best be avoided with premature rupture of membranes and where there have been recurrent episodes of APH and in the presence of a placenta previa major.

4. *Exercise:* Exercise in pregnancy should be encouraged, though with advancing gestation physical constraints may limit sporting activities. Exercise can improve cardiovascular function, lower blood pressure and improve self-esteem and confidence. Swimming is often helpful throughout pregnancy especially with advancing gestation as it is essentially a non-weight bearing exercise. It is advisable however to avoid hyperthermia, dehydration and exhaustion.

5. *Diet:* Dietary extremes are associated with risks in pregnancy. Obesity is associated with gestational diabetes, hypertension and monitoring difficulties. Malnutrition is associated with maternal anemia and fetal growth restriction, while deficiency of certain vitamins predispose to congenital abnormalities; folic

acid deficiency is linked to the risk of neural tube defects (NTDs). A balanced diet rich in fresh fruit and vegetable is recommended. It is prudent to avoid unpasturized milk and cheeses and pates. Pregnant women should avoid eating liver due to its high vitamin A content. Vegans should have Iron and vitamin supplementation and ethnic groups lacking sunlight are advised to have extravitamin D.

6. *Work:* A job provides satisfaction, self esteem and confidence, along with financial peace of mind. Women can continue working in pregnancy as long as they wish and as long as they and their baby remain well. Avoidance of exposure to hazardous chemicals, smokey environments, excessive lifting and exercise and at least an 8-hour rest at night is recommended.

First Trimester

Antenatal care in the first trimester starts with a visit to the GP after a missed period and confirmation of pregnancy. This visit is followed by a booking visit with the community midwife. It also provides an ideal opportunity for the woman to discuss any anxieties she may have. During this visit routine blood tests are performed—FBC, blood grouping and antibody screen, rubella, syphilis, hepatitis B and HIV serology and hemoglobin electrophoresis if appropriate. Urine is tested for glucose and protein and a midstream specimen is sent for culture and sensitivity to detect asymptomatic bacteriuria. The hospital booking visit may be any time between 12 and 20 weeks and varies from hospital to hospital but there is an increasing tendency for earlier referral especially in older women who may wish screening tests for chromosomal abnormalities in the first trimester. Many hospitals offer a first trimester ultrasound scan for pregnancy dating and measurement of nuchal translucency at the 10 to 14 weeks stage. Nuchal translucency measurements may be combined with serum markers such β-hCG and PAPP-a as a sensitive screening test for trisomy 21. Toward the end of the first trimester (11-12 weeks) is the time when prenatal diagnostic testing such as chorionic villus sampling may be performed in selected groups of patients. The purpose of the booking visit is to obtain a comprehensive history, establish gestational age and identify any maternal or fetal risk factors. Details are obtained on medical, family, social and previous obstetric history and a general physical examination performed. The estimated date of confinement is also confirmed or amended after the initial dating scan. A variety of screening tests are routinely performed in pregnancy.

Hematological Investigations

These include hemoglobin estimation and a complete blood picture if indicated. Blood group determination and antibody screen is also performed to identify rhesus negative women who will need prophylaxis against rhesus isoimmunization.

Full blood count: This is the most commonly performed hematological investigation in pregnancy. Pregnancy is associated with a physiological dilutional anemia due to a greater increase in plasma volume than red cell mass and therefore the lower limit for a 'normal' Hb is 10.5 g/dl in pregnancy as opposed to 11.5 g/dl in the non-pregnant female. Many women enter pregnancy with a low iron reserve and therefore if anemia is detected in pregnancy it should be appropriately investigated by assessment of ferritin, total iron binding capacity (TIBC), serum and red cell folate and serum B_{12} levels based on the blood picture. The most common cause of anemia in pregnancy is iron deficiency anemia. FBC estimation is performed 4-8 weekly in the second half of pregnancy and a low hemoglobin on admission in labor is an indication for sending a specimen to the lab for 'group and save' in case of intrapartum or postpartum bleeding.

Blood grouping and screening for antibodies: Blood grouping at booking, enables the determination women who are rhesus negative and therefore may be at risk of rhesus isoimmunization. The incidence of rhesus disease has dramatically fallen over the last thirty years following the introduction of anti-D administration. Despite screening at 28 and 34 weeks or after any potential sensitizing event and administration of prophylactic anti-D at these times, a small number of RhD negative women still develop anti-D antibodies because of small silent hemorrhages predominantly in the third trimester or because of failure of timely administration of anti D immunoglobulin. Screening for red cell antibodies should be repeated in all women in early pregnancy in subsequent pregnancies, even if rhesus positive, as there may be other clinically significant antibodies as a consequence of previous pregnancy or blood transfusion. An antibody screen is performed to detect the presence of antibodies that may put the baby at risk of hemolytic disease or result in difficulties with cross-matching blood for the mother if required at any stage of pregnancy, labor or postnatally. If antibodies are detected, the titer is determined and subsequent samples taken for further estimations at appropriate time interval.

Screening for hemoglobinopathies: These tests are not performed routinely in all patients. Hemoglobin electrophoresis should be performed in women of ethnic or racial origins in whom the incidence of hemoglobinopathies is high. These include women of Cypriot, Eastern Mediteranean, Middle Eastern, Indian and Southeast Asian origin where the incidence of thalassaemia is greatest and women of African or Afro-Carribean origin who are at risk of sickle cell disease. If a patient herself is affected then consideration should be given to testing her partner, as this will have implication on counseling and prenatal testing. Persistent anemia is also an indication for hemoglobin electrophoresis in any woman irrespective of racial origin.

Microbiological Investigations

These include serum screening for evidence of immunity to rubella, as well evidence of infection or immunity to hepatitis B, and evidence of infection with HIV.

Rubella: Rubella infection suffered by the mother, especially in early pregnancy can have devastating consequences for the fetus. In an attempt to reduce the incidence of congenital rubella defects, vaccination has been undertaken since the 1970s. Despite the policy of vaccination, present data show that around 2 percent of primigravida and 1 percent of multigravida are nonimmune to rubella in the UK and it is recommended that these women receive postpartum rubella vaccination. Vaccination in pregnancy is not recommended but there have been no reports of adverse outcome where this has been performed inadvertently in pregnancy.

HIV: HIV infection in the mother has implications for the mother, the developing fetus and health care professionals involved in the mother's care. The current recommendations from the government in the UK are for universal screening for HIV for all antennal bookings. This has come about by difficulties in effectively targeting affected women even in areas of high prevalence. There is now clear evidence that the vertical transmission from mother to fetus can be significantly reduced (by two-thirds) by treatment of the mother with antiretrovirals in pregnancy and labor and the infant for 6 weeks postnatally. Furthermore the risk of transmission can also be reduced by delivery by cesarean section and avoidance of breastfeeding. It should also be borne in mind that HIV testing performed as part of routine antenatal screening is not used by insurance companies as a marker of high risk. However, even in the presence of infection, the HIV antibody test may be negative during the incubation period, thus in high risk situations a repeat test three months after exposure is recommended.

Hepatitis B: Screening for hepatitis B aims to determine whether the patient has ever been exposed to the virus, and whether is immune to the virus or whether she is a potential risk of transmitting the infection to the neonate, her partner and to health care professionals. A combined course of active and passive immunization can then be undertaken in the neonate at risk after birth. The importance of preventing hepatitis B infection in the neonate is that while in the adult patient the virus is cleared within 6 months in 90 percent of infected individuals, in neonates 90 percent become chronic carriers with the risk of post infective hepatic cirrhosis and hepatocellular carcinoma

Syphillis: Screening for syphilis is also routinely performed with around 250 cases detected annually in the UK. The rationale for screening for syphilis lies in the fact that early treatment of the disease can prevent congenital syphilis in the neonate. Treatment confers benefits to mother too, by preventing development of cardiovascular and neurological complications of the advanced stages of the disease.

Screening for Urinary Tract Infection

A urine specimen is sent at the booking visit, for culture to detect and treat asymptomatic bacteriuria. The rationale being that some cases asymptomatic bacteriuria and a lower urinary tract infection may lead to complications such as pyelonephritis and predispose to preterm labor.

Miscellaneous Tests

Other blood tests may be performed on an individual basis. Thus, if there is a history of thyroid disease, thyroid function tests may be required. In patients with hypertension or renal complications or diabetes, baseline urea, creatinine and electrolytes would be advisable. Long-term diabetic control is monitored by means of serum HbA1c estimation. Where epilepsy is poorly controlled despite adequate doses of anticonvulsants it may be useful to assess serum levels prior to further dose increases or as a means of confirming compliance. Patients with a family or personal history of coagulation disorders may need screening for bleeding disorders or thrombophilia and checking of coagulation factor levels.

Second Trimester

Early in the second trimester, around 16 weeks, serum screening tests are performed for assessment of risk of open neural tube defect and Down syndrome. Prenatal diagnostic testing in the form of amniocentesis may be performed around 16 weeks and a detailed ultrasound scan to assess fetal anatomy is usually performed at 19 to 20 week stage by which time the results of serum screening should have been available and reviewed. Where cardiac anomalies are suspected, a further ultrasound may be required at 22 to 24 week stage. Toward the end of the second trimester of pregnancy the patient is seen 4 weekly and at each visit BP, urinalysis, fundal height is checked as well as maternal wellbeing and fetal activity enquired about. Any concerns or queries the mother has are discussed or addressed such as giving up work and maternity leave.

Screening for NTD

It is important at this stage to make the distinction between the double/triple test and the role of maternal serum alpha fetoprotein (MSAFP) alone which is used as a screening tool for open neural tube defect. Anencephaly and open spina bifida each have an incidence of 1 per 1000. AFP is produced first by the yolk sac and subsequently by the fetal liver and enters the amniotic fluid by fetal urination and its level continues to rise till 30 to 32 weeks after which it declines. During the period of screening (15-20 weeks gestation) the levels of AFP rise at around 15 percent per week. In cases of open neural tube defects, AFP leaks into the maternal serum leading to raised MSAFP levels. A level greater than 2.2 multiples of the median (MoM) is considered elevated (multiple of median is calculated by dividing an individual MSAFP by the median for the gestational week). A raised MSAFP in addition to open NTD may be a result of abdominal wall defects, congenital nephrosis, upper fetal bowel obstruction, placental or umbilical cord tumors, sacrococcygeal teratoma, multiple pregnancy, gestation more advanced than thought, bleeding in early pregnancy amongst other causes. Management of elevated MSAFP includes confirmation of gestation and exclusion of multiple pregnancy along with high resolution ultrasound to exclude an anatomical cause. A knowledge of elevated MSAFP in the absence of fetal structural malformation should trigger a modification of prenatal care to provide enhanced fetal or maternal surveillance as it is a marker for adverse perinatal outcome such as risks of fetal death, IUGR, early and late pregnancy bleeding and preterm delivery while there are conflicting reports whether it may be a marker for subsequent development of pre-eclampsia.

Triple/Double Test

This test refers to the estimation of serum AFP, beta hCG and unconjugated estriol in the maternal blood at around 16 weeks gestation (triple test) or more commonly the use of alpha fetoprotein (AFP) and βhCG alone (double test) as a screening test for trisomy 21. Down syndrome is the most common cause of congenital mental retardation with a birth prevalence of 1 in 700 and has great clinical and societal significance in terms of severity and compatibility with life. Studies have shown that MSAFP levels in pregnancies affected by Down syndrome are 25 percent lower than in women with chromosomally normal fetuses and this is independent of age. Similarly, the levels of another hormone produced by the fetoplacental unit, unconjugated estriol (MSuE3) are also 27 percent lower in pregnancies affected by Down syndrome. The most effective marker to date, however, appears to be the placental specific product hCG with levels being twice as normal in pregnancies affected by Down syndrome or other chromosomal abnormalities. While MSAFP and MSuE3 rise between 14 and 21 weeks, hCG levels drop. More recently a combination of serum biochemical markers (β hCG and PAPP-1) have been combined with nuchal translucency measurements to screen for Down syndrome at the end of the first trimester.

Screening for Gestational Diabetes Mellitus

There appears to be no consensus as to who, when, how or even whether to screen for gestational diabetes mellitus (GDM). Universal biochemical screening has been suggested or universal screening limited to those over 25 has also been suggested. Screening all pregnant women at 28 weeks gestation would identify those with impaired glucose tolerance or diabetes with a sensitivity of 78 percent and specificity of 90 percent. The majority of units decide on who to screen on the basis of clinical risk factors including previous GDM, family history of diabetes (first degree relative with diabetes), previous macrosomic baby, previous unexplained stillbirth, obesity (BMI > 26), glycosuria on more than 1 occasion, polyhydramnios and large for gestational age infant in current pregnancy. This policy of selective screening would identify 50 percent of women with GDM. The timing of testing is also controversial as the later in pregnancy it is performed, the higher the detection rate since glucose tolerance progressively deteriorates. On the other hand, the earlier in pregnancy GDM is diagnosed and hyperglycemia treated, the greater the likelihood to have an influence on outcome.

Third Trimester

Monthly visits to the community midwife continue in the third trimester. FBC is checked and antibody screen is repeated at 28 and 34 weeks in rhesus negative women who are given anti-D prophylaxis at these times. In addition to BP, urinalysis, fundal height and maternal wellbeing and fetal activity from 36 weeks onwards fetal presentation is also assessed and if not cephalic referral to the hospital antenatal clinic organized for appropriate investigations and counseling. During the third trimester the mother and her partner need to be prepared for what to expect regarding onset and process of labor and delivery. The final routine antenatal visit often is in hospital and timed between 40 and 41 weeks where discussion takes place regarding induction of labor after 41 weeks. If the women wish to avoid induction after discussion of the rationale for induction and the risks involved in prolongation of pregnancy, then a plan of increased surveillance with CTG and ultrasound assessment of liquor volume can be individualized.

Antenatal care has undergone significant transformation over time to make it both more streamlined and responsive to women's needs. The major changes have been to concentrate care at the primary care team level, so that fewer hospital visits are the norm for the uncomplicated pregnancy.

14. Hyperemesis Gravidarum

Duru Shah
Sukhpreet Patel

INTRODUCTION

The gastrointestinal tract is commonly affected by the physiologic changes that occur during pregnancy. Nausea and vomiting during pregnancy (NVP) is a common experience, affecting 50 to 90 percent of all women.[1-4] Its association with pregnancy was documented on papyrus dating as far back as 2000 BC.

Although in most women NVP is usually limited to the first trimester, in 20 percent of the pregnant women symptoms continue throughout pregnancy.

Hyperemesis gravidarum is the most severe manifestation of the spectrum of NVP. Historically known as "pernicious vomiting of pregnancy", it is characterized by intractable nausea and vomiting, so severe as to cause dehydration, electrolyte and metabolic disturbances and nutritional deficiency necessitating hospitalization.

This chapter describes the epidemiology, pathogenesis, diagnosis, clinical features, and management of hyperemesis gravidarum.

EPIDEMIOLOGY

Hyperemesis gravidarum has an incidence of 0.3 to 2 percent of all deliveries.[3] Nausea and vomiting of pregnancy is more common in westernized countries, especially in urban as compared to rural areas. Various demographic factors have been hypothesized as contributing factors to NVP. These include occupational status,[5] maternal age, vomiting in prior pregnancy,[5] parity,[3] history of infertility,[5] interpregnancy interval,[7] corpus luteum in right ovary,[8] and prior intolerance to oral contraceptives.[2]

PATHOGENESIS

The pathogenesis of NVP is an enigma. In the 19th century, several theories were postulated, including toxemia, reflex (due to displacement or abnormalities of female reproductive organs), and neuroticism. Current theories include a combination of different perspectives.

A. *Metabolic and Endocrine Factors.*
1. hCG: One popular theory was that NVP was related to trophoblastic activity and gonadotropin production. This was possibly secondary to elevated serum hCG levels. Factors in favor of this theory are:
   a. A higher incidence of NVP in patients with multiple and molar pregnancies, in whom hCG levels are higher than normal pregnancies.

b. Women with NVP have higher serum hCG levels as compared with those who are asymptomatic.[9]
2. *Estrogen:* The etiologic role for estrogens is supported by the observation that women who have intolerance to OC pills because of side effects have a higher incidence of NVP.[2]
3. *Progesterone:* Either alone or in combination with estrogen, progesterone is believed to be important in NVP. Progesterone decreases smooth muscle activity, potentially prolonging gastric emptying and precipitating nausea and vomiting. Progesterone levels peak during the 1st trimester of pregnancy just when the incidence of nausea and vomiting peaks.

B. *Upper Gastrointestinal Dysmotility:*
During pregnancy esophageal, gastric and small bowel motility are impaired as a result of smooth muscle relaxation fostered by increased levels of female sex hormones. This dysmotility could contribute to NVP.
1. *Esophagus:* Hormonal changes are postulated to alter lower esophageal sphincter (LES) function causing an incompetent sphincter. This alteration may contribute not only to heartburn, but also to NVP. LES pressures are abnormally low during all 3 trimesters, with a nadir reached at 36 weeks gestation accompanied by heartburn.[10]
2. *Stomach:* A delay in gastric emptying during pregnancy may be important in NVP. Progesterone, a smooth muscle relaxant, inhibits gastric emptying in early pregnancy when levels are highly elevated. In late pregnancy, the large gravid uterus contributes to the manifestations of upper gastrointestinal symptoms by mechanically compressing the stomach.
3. *Small bowel:* Alterations in gastrointestinal transit time especially in the small bowel, have also been implicated in NVP.

C. *Psychological factors:* Previously, about 50 percent of obstetricians believed that NVP was psychologically based. This syndrome was attributed to a subconscious attempt to reject an unwanted pregnancy; symptoms ceased in early pregnancy when fetal movement began owing to the inability to deny further the fetus's existence.[11] It has been observed that women with nausea and vomiting during the first trimester of pregnancy had more unplanned or undesired pregnancies.[12] Also, when psychosocial factors are taken into account in the search for a cause, the results of treatment of hyperemesis gravidarum are more successful and persist over a longer time.[7]

D. *Infection:* Newer data now indicates that 90 percent of women with hyperemesis gravidarum are infected with *Helicobacter pylori*. Chronic infection of *Helicobacter pylori* has been suggested as one of the important factors in the pathogenesis of hyperemesis gravidarum by Hayahawa et al.[13] In a review of literature done by Eliakim et al it was observed that *Helicobacter pylori* infection functions as a contributing factor to hyperemesis gravidarum.[14]

E. *Hyperthyroidism:* In normal pregnancy, when hCG levels are highest at 10 to 12 weeks gestation, there is suppression of serum TSH. When serum hCG exceeds about 200 IU/ml, hyperthyroidism is likely to be found.[15]

F. *Liver dysfunction:* The increased hormonal load during pregnancy, compounded by the slow hepatic adaptation to this load, is also believed to cause hypermesis. The liver is a major site for steroid hormone inactivation. Serum transaminase levels are elevated in 15 to 25 percent of hospitalized women with hyperemesis. Not all patients with hyperemesis gravidarum however, develop abnormal serum levels of liver enzymes.

G. *Altered lipid metabolism:* The frequent alterations in serum lipids and lipoproteins in pregnant women are speculated to be related to altered hepatic estrogen metabolism during pregnancy. These alterations support the belief that an increased sensitivity of the liver to an altered hormonal milieu contributed to hyperemesis gravidarum.[2]

H. *Immunological:* Immune parameters regarding IgG, IgM, C3, C4 and lymphocyte count were significantly higher in patients with hyperemesis gravidarum than in controls in a study done by Leylek et al.[16] They concluded that immunological activity in pregnancy may have an effect or role on the stimulatory mechanism of hCG in hyperemesis patients.

DIAGNOSIS AND CLINICAL FEATURES

NVP occurs within weeks of missing the period, symptoms usually peak between 10 and 16 weeks of gestation and definitely disappear by week 20. Patients usually present with signs of dehydration, ketosis, and electrolyte and acid-base disturbances. These include sunken eyes, loss of skin elasticity, dry tongue with ketotic odor of breath, tachycardia, hypotension. Weight loss (more than 5% of body weight) may occur. In severe cases icterus may develop. When the diagnosis of hyperemesis gravidarum is made, the associated conditions of multiple gestation and molar pregnancy should be excluded (Tables 14.1 and 14.2).

Table 14.1: Symptoms of hyperemesis gravidarum

1. Excessive vomiting
2. Epigastric pain
3. Giddiness
4. Oliguria
5. Symptoms of complications
   a. Wernicke's encephalopathy: restlessness, insomnia, convulsions or coma.
   b. Korsakoff's psychosis: mental confusion with loss of memory of recent events.
   c. Peripheral neuritis.
   d. Ophthalmic complications: blurring of vision, diplopia, blindness.

Table 14.2: Signs of hyperemesis gravidarum

On General examination:
1. Anxious appearance
2. Weight loss > 5 percent of total body weight
3. Sunken eyes
4. Loss of skin elasticity
5. Dry tongue with ketotic odor of breath
6. Tachycardia
7. Hypotension
8. Fever
9. Icterus (in severe cases)

Per vaginum examination:
1. Confirmation of pregnancy
2. Determination of size of uterus: larger than weeks of gestation in twins and molar pregnancy

Vomiting beyond the 20th week of gestation is uncommon and should prompt a search for other causes. The differential diagnosis for NVP includes
1. Peptic ulcer disease.
2. Gastroenteritis.
3. Appendicitis.
4. Severe gastroesophageal reflux.
5. Cholelithiasis and cholecystitis.
6. Nephrolithiasis and pyelonephritis.
7. Hepatitis.
8. Pancreatitis.
9. Gastric carcinoma (rare).

OUTCOME OF PREGNANCY

Various studies suggest that NVP is a favorable prognostic indicator, with decreased risk of miscarriage,[1,5] stillbirth,[2] fetal mortality,[2-4] preterm delivery,[2,6] low birth weight,[2,6] and perinatal mortality.[1]

No increased risk of malformations has been reported in children born to symptomatic mothers.[3]

NVP was first recognized as a potential cause of death from starvation in the 18th century. Today, hyperemesis gravidarum rarely causes death. It was a significant cause of maternal death before 1940, because of the lack of understanding about the associated fluid, electrolyte and metabolic disturbances.

PATHOLOGY

The changes in various organs are the generalized manifestations of starvation and severe malnutrition.

1. *Liver:* There is centrilobular fatty infiltration of the liver without necrosis.
2. *Kidneys:* Occasionally, there may be fatty change in the cells of the first convolute tubule, related to acidosis.
3. *Brain:* Small hemorrhages may be seen in the hypothalamic region giving the manifestation of Wernicke's encephalopathy.

Other Changes

1. *Metabolic changes*: Starvation leads to depletion of glycogen store in patients with hyperemesis gravidarum, thus mobilizing fat stores which produces ketone bodies. These ketone bodies are excreted through the kidneys and respiratory tract. Therefore, ketone bodies in urine and ketotic odor of breath are common findings in severe cases (Figure 14.1).
2. *Biochemical*: Electrolyte disturbances due to dehydration, such as, hyponatremia, hypokalemia and hypochloremia may be seen. In severe cases

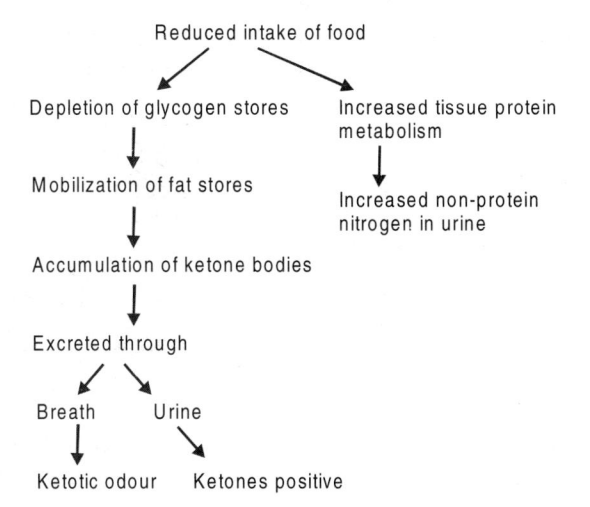

Figure 14.1: Flow chart showing metabolic changes in hyperemesis gravidarum

hepatic dysfunction can lead to elevated blood urea nitrogen and uric acid. Prolonged starvation may produce hypoglycemia, hypovitaminosis and hypoproteinemia (Figure 14.2).
3. *Hematological*: Hemoconcentration is a result of dehydration. Mild leucocytosis with eosinophilia may be seen in a few patients.

INVESTIGATIONS

Laboratory findings usually show evidence of dehydration with increased urine specific gravity and ketonuria and increased serum blood urea nitrogen, creatinine, and hematocrit levels. Electrolyte disturbances are commonly found, including alterations in serum sodium, potassium levels and pH. Hypokalemia can produce ECG changes if severe. Elevation of liver enzymes and total bilirubin may also occur (Table 14.3).

Table 14.3: Investigations in hyperemesis gravidarum

1. Hematological
   a. Serum electrolytes
   b. BUN
   c. Hematocrit
   d. Liver function tests
2. Urine Analysis
   a. Reduced volume
   b. Dark color
   c. High specific gravity
   d. Acidic pH
   e. Presence of ketones
   f. Diminished or absent chlorides
3. Hormonal
4. Diminished TSH
   a. Elevated free T3
5. ECG—changes of hypokalemia
6. Fundoscopy—retinal hemorrhages and detachment.

Complications

These include jaundice due to hepatic dysfunction, stress ulcers due to excessive vomiting, pancreatitis, and renal failure. Neurological complications are a result of vitamin deficiency, and can occur in the form of Wernicke's encephalopathy, Korsakoff's psychosis and peripheral neuritis. Ophthalmic complications include retinal hemorrhages and retinal detachment (Table 14.4).

Table 14.4: Complications of hyperemesis gravidarum

1. Jaundice
2. Stress ulcers in stomach
3. Neurological complications
   a. Wernicke's encephalopathy
   b. Peripheral neuritis
   c. Korsakoff's psychosis
4. Ophthalmic complications

MANAGEMENT

Simple Nausea and Vomiting of Pregnancy

Mild to moderate NVP during the first trimester is usually tolerated by most patients with conservative management. These measures include reassurance that these symptoms are common and almost self limited. Frequent (every 2 to 3 hours) small meals, rich in carbohydrates (for example, biscuits, toast) and low in fats effectively reduce symptoms. Food and odors that

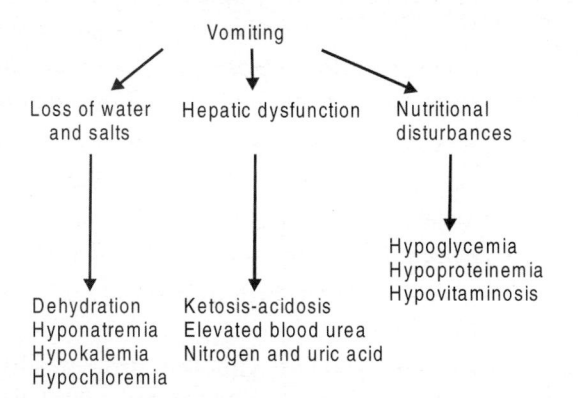

Figure 14.2: Flow chart showing biochemical changes in hyperemesis gravidarum

precipitate symptoms should be avoided. Iron tablets, if taken should be withheld, since it may contribute to nausea and vomiting (Table 14.5).

Table 14.5: Initial steps in treatment of simple nausea and vomiting of pregnancy

1. Reassurance
   - Physiological.
   - Transient nature.
   - Overall good prognosis.
2. Dietary modifications
   - Avoid emetogenic foods and odors.
   - Frequent small meals.
   - Low protein and low fat diet.
   - High, easily digestible carbohydrate diet.
   - Avoid iron supplements.
3. Exclude other causes.
4. Trial of medications.
   - Discuss benefits and risks.
5. Alternative therapies and/ or psychotherapy.

Hyperemesis Gravidarum

Hospitalization

Hospitalization is essential in severe cases for monitoring vital parameters such as temperature, pulse, respiration, blood pressure and fluid intake and output. Investigations which are essential for management of this condition can be repeated as required after hospitalization. These especially include urine examination for ketones and estimation of serum electrolytes.

Intravenous Hydration

The mainstay of therapy for hyperemesis gravidarum includes correction of hypovolemia and electrolyte disturbances with intravenous fluids. Nothing should be given by mouth until dehydration in corrected. Afterwards, small, frequent feeds, gradually advancing from liquids to solids can be attempted as tolerated.

Intravenous hydration accomplished with dextrose and dextrose saline also helps in correcting ketosis. Approximately 2-3 liters of fluid is required to correct hypovolemia in extreme cases of hyperemesis gravidarum. Intravenous potassium supplementation may be required in a few patients, but should be done with adequate monitoring.

Parental vitamins should be administered when hyperemesis gravidarum is prolonged, particularly because thiamine deficiency manifesting as Wernicke's encephalopathy has occurred in severe cases.

Total parental nutrition has also been used in extreme cases (Table 14.6).

Table 14.6: Therapy for hyperemesis gravidarum

1. Diagnosed by severe nausea and vomiting accompanied by
   - Dehydration
   - Metabolic/electrolyte disturbance
   - Weight loss > 5 percent total body weight
2. In addition to evaluation and therapy outlined for nausea and vomiting alone, the following should be considered:
   - Hospitalization
   - Intravenous hydration
   - Correction of electrolyte/metabolic disturbances
   - Antiemetics
   - Nutritional support
   - Alternative therapy
   - Therapeutic abortion—if all therapeutic measures fail; only when maternal life is threatened.

Pharmacologic Agents

A. *Antihistamines and Anticholinergics*:
   1. Meclizine
      - *Pregnancy category B*: Epidemiological studies in pregnant women, do not indicate that meclizine increases the risk of abnormalities when administered during pregnancy.
      - *Adverse reactions*: Drowsiness, dry mouth and on rare occasions blurred visions.
      - *Dosage*: 25 mg every 6 hours as required.
   2. Diphenhydramine and Dimenhydrinate:
      - *Pregnancy category B:* Reproduction studies on animals revealed no evidence of harm to the fetus. There are, however, no adequate and well controlled studies in pregnant women. Both were widely used in pregnancy before 1970 until an association with cleft lip and palate was reported. Dimenhydrinate stimulates the uterus in later stages of pregnancy.
      - *Dosage*: 25 mg 3 to 4 times daily
   3. Scopolamine
      - *Pregnancy category C*: Scopolamine was observed to produce frequent chromosomal aberrations and sister chromated exchanges. Animals treated with this drug produced malformations including deformed limbs and trunks.

B. *Antiemetics and antinauseants:*
   Phenothiazines—Chlorpromazine and Prochlorperazine
   - *Pregnancy category C*: The use of phenothiazines in pregnancy reveals conflicting data regarding teratogenicity. Phenothiazines cross the placenta and are eliminated from fetal and neonatal tissues more slowly than in adults; therefore, potential toxicity can occur. Both structural malformations and neonatal extrapyramidal effects are reported.
   - *Dosage*: Prochlorperazine—25 mg every 8 hours orally, intramuscularly, or rectally as needed.

C. *Promotility Agents:*
   Metoclopramide
   - *Pregnancy Category B*: There are no adequate and well-controlled studies in pregnant women.
   - *Dosage*: 10 mg orally upto four times a day Continuous subcutaneous metoclopramide has been used on an outpatient basis in women with Hyperemesis gravidarum with good results.

D. *Other Agents:*
   1. *Doxylamine:*
      - *Pregnancy category B*: The unsubstantiated beliefs that doxylamine is unsafe during pregnancy has been refuted in many studies.[17]
      - *Dosage*: 10 to 12.5 mg orally one or 2 times a days (with pyridoxine 25 to 50 mg).
   2. *Corticosteroids:*
      - *Pregnancy category C*: 40 mg prednisolone daily in 2 divided oral doses was found to be beneficial in severe hyperemesis gravidarum. The rationale is that steroids are beneficial in treating chemotherapy induced emesis and may help in other conditions in which vomiting is thought to have a central origin.
   3. *Ondansetron*
      - *Pregnancy category C*: The literature is limited with regards to the use of ondansetron during pregnancy. Therefore, ondansetron cannot be recommended for treatment of hyperemesis gravidarum because larger trials are needed to ascertain the long-term fetal effects (Tables 14.7 and 14.8).

Table 14.7: FDA classification of drugs used in nausea and vomiting of pregnancy

Generic names	FDA classes
Pyridoxine	A
Doxylamine	B
Cyclizine	B
Meclizine	B
Dimenhydrinate	B
Diphenhydramine	B
Metoclopramide	B
Scopolamine	C
Promethazine	C
Prochlorperazine	C
Chlorpromazine	C
Cisapride	C
Droperidol	C
Ondansetron	C
Corticosteroids	C

Table 14.8: Definition of food and drug administration (FDA) classification

FDA classification	Definition
Category A	Well controlled studies in humans show no fetal risk
Category B	Animal studies show no risk, but human studies inadequate Or Animal studies show some risk, but not supported by human studies
Category C	Animal studies show risk, but human studies are inadequate or lacking Or No studies in humans or animals
Category D	Definite fetal abnormalities in human studies, but potential benefits may outweigh the risks.
Category X	Contraindicated in pregnancy, fetal abnormalities in animals or humans, risks outweigh benefits.

E. *Alternative treatments*

Alternative nonpharmacologic treatments should be considered if conventional treatments fail or if the patient does not wish to incur the risks associated with pharmacotherapy.

1. *Acupressure:* Acupressure on the point PC6 above the wrist on the palmar side has been found to prevent some types of nausea and vomiting. Studies have shown a significant decrease in nausea, vomiting and retching during pregnancy.[18]
2. *Psychotherapy:* In a study by Leeners and colleagues, they found that when psychosocial factors were taken into account in the search for a cause, the

results of treatment were more successful and persisted over a long time.[7]

3. *Pyridoxine (Vitamin B₆):*
   - Pregnancy category A:
   - *Dosage:* 12.5 to 25.0 mg every 8 hours, or pyridoxine, 25 to 50 mg orally 2 to 4 times day in combination with doxylamine, 10.0 to 12.5 mg orally one to two times a day, is effective in controlling hyperemesis gravidarum in a large proportion of women.

4. *Ginger:* Powdered root of ginger in the dose of 1gm daily has been found to reduce symptoms in women with hyperemesis gravidarum.

5. *Sensory afferent stimulation:* Transcutaneous nerve stimulation (TENS) is under investigation for the treatment of hyperemesis gravidarum.

6. *Medical hypnosis:* It has been suggested that medical hypnosis should be considered as an adjunctive treatment option for women with hyperemesis gravidarum.[19]

Termination of Pregnancy

Therapeutic abortion is a rare and last resort, to be used only when maternal life is threatened.

REFERENCES

1. Brandes JM: First trimester nausea and vomiting as related to outcome of pregnancy. *Obstetrics and Gynecology* **30**:427, 1967.
2. Jarnfely-Samsioe A, Samsioe G, Velinder G: Nausea and vomiting in pregnancy: A contribution to its epidemiology. *Gynecol Obstet Invest* **16**:221, 1983.
3. Klebanoff MA, Koslowe PA, Kaslow R *et al*: Epidemiology of vomiting in early pregnancy. *Obstetrics and Gynecology* **66**: 612, 1985.
4. Tierson FD, Olsen CL, Hook EB: Nausea and vomiting of pregnancy and association with pregnancy outcome. *American Journal of Obstetrics and Gynecology* **155**:1017, 1986.
5. Weigel MM, Weigel RM: The association of reproductive history, demographic factors, and alcohol and tobacco consumption with the risk of developing nausea and vomiting in early pregnancy. *American Journal of Epidemiology* **127**:562, 1988.
6. Medalie JH: Relationships between nausea and /or vomiting in early pregnancy and abortion. *Lancet* **2**:117, 1957.
7. Leeners B, Sauer I, Rath W: Nausea and vomiting in early pregnancy/hyperemesis gravidarum. Current status of psychosomatic factors. *Z Geburtshilfe Neonatol* **204(4):** 128-34, 2000.
8. Samsioe G, Crona N, Enk L *et al*: Does position and size of the corpus luteum have any effect on nausea of pregnancy? *Acta Obstetrics and Gynecology Scandinavia* **65**:427, 1986.
9. Masson GM, Anthony F, Chau E: Serum chorionic gonadotropin (hCG), schwangerschaftsprotein 1 (SPI), progesterone and estradiol levels in patients with nausea and vomiting in early pregnancy. *British Journal of Obstetrics and Gynecology* **92**:211, 1985.
10. Van Thiel DH, Gavaler JS, Stremple: Lower esophageal pressure in women using sequential oral contraceptives. *Gastroenterology* **71**:232, 1976.
11. Semmens JP: Female sexuality and life situations: An etiologic psycho-socio-sexual profile of weight gain and nausea and vomiting in pregnancy. *Obstetrics and Gynecology* **38**:355, 1971.
12. Fitzgerald CM: Nausea and vomiting in pregnancy. *British Journal of Medical Psychology* **57**:159, 1984.
13. Hayakawa S, Nakajima N, Karasaki-Suzuki M, Yoshinaga H, Arakawa Y, Satoh K, Yamamoto T: Frequent presence of Helicobacter pylori genome in the saliva of patients with hyperemesis gravidarum. *American Journal of Perinatology* **17(5):**243-47, 2000.
14. Eliakim R, Abulafia O, Sherer DM: Hyperemesis gravidarum: A current review. *American Journal of Perinatology* **17(4):** 207-18, 2000.
15. Hershman JM: Human chorionic gonadotropin and the thyroid: Hyperemesis gravidarum and trophoblastic tumors. *Thyroid* **9(7):**653-57, 1999.
16. Leylek OA, Toyaksi M, Erselcan T, Dokmetas S: Immunologic and biochemical factors in hyperemesis gravidarum with or without hyperthyroxinemia. *Gynecology and Obstetrics Invest* **47(4):**229, 1999.
17. Bishai R, Mazzotta P, Atanackovic G, Levichek Z, Pole M, Magee LA, Koren G: Critical appraisal of drug therapy for nausea and vomiting of pregnancy: II. Efficacy and safety of diclectin (doxylamine-B6). *Canadian Journal Clinical Pharmacology*; **7(3):**138-43, 2000.
18. Carlsson CP, Axemo P, Bodin A, Cartensen H, Ehrenroth B, Madegardlind I, Navander C: Manual acupuncture reduces hyperemesis gravidarum: A placebo-controlled, randomized, single-blind, crossover-study. *J Pain Symptom Manage* **20(4):**273-79, 2000.
19. Simon EP, Schwartz J: Medical hypnosis for hyperemesis gravidarum. *Birth* **26(4):**248-54, 1999.

15.

Onnig Tamizian
Sabaratnam Arulkumaran

Minor Disorders of Pregnancy

The anatomical and physiological changes in pregnancy are associated with what are perceived by many women as minor disorders or 'nuisance' problems of pregnancy. The majority of women will put up with these as normal 'part and parcel' of pregnancy, not wishing to appear to be making a fuss. Professionals involved in the care of pregnant women have a role to offer advice and reassurance regarding the nature of these symptoms. The majority of theses complaints are trivial in medical terms but may be the cause of considerable discomfort and distress to many pregnant woman.

NAUSEA AND VOMITING

Nausea and vomiting are very common problems of early pregnancy and can result in the first trimester being viewed as a miserable time. Up to three quarters of women experience nausea and in up to half vomiting occurs. Vomiting may start as early as 6 weeks gestation and usually settles by 13-14 weeks. The precise etiology is unknown but it may be a response to rising estrogen and/or very high hCG levels as it is more common in multiple pregnancy or with a molar pregnancy. Psychological factors may also have a role through their direct action on the emetic center in the midbrain. Symptoms tend to recur in a quarter of women in a subsequent pregnancy.

In the majority of women symptoms can be controlled by dietary advice. Small, frequent meals each day consisting of non-fatty, dry and high calorie foods is recommended with adequate fluid intake between but not with meals. If the vomiting is precipitated by reflux then the use of alginates or antacids may help. In the majority of women the nausea is mild and the vomiting occasional and dietary measures are often adequate. About 10 percent of pregnant women suffer moderate nausea and vomiting, affecting the woman's daily activities, making her feel miserable and at risk of dehydration. There is reluctance from patients to take medication in pregnancy but these patients may benefit from an antiemetic agent such prochloperazine, cyclizie or metoclopramide. In a small minority of women, there is continuous nausea with frequent vomiting with an inability to keep food or fluids down (hyperemesis gravidarum). This group of patients are at serious risk of dehydration and ketosis and need hospital admission for intravenous fluids and antiemetics in order to break the cycle of vomiting—dehydration—ketosis—vomiting. It is essential to exclude other causes

PART TWO

Feto-maternal Medicine

of nausea or vomiting such a UTI, deranged liver or thyroid functions, multiple pregnancy or a molar pregnancy. Provided there is no underlying cause treatment is conservative and usually the vomiting settles. In extremely rare cases parenteral feeding may become necessary if the problem persists for prolonged period of time and adequate nutrition cannot be achieved in any other way.

HEARTBURN

Heartburn is a common problem in pregnancy mediated by relaxation of the physiological sphincters of the stomach due to elevated progesterone levels. The resulting reflux of the acid gastric contents and bile irritates the lower esophagus and may also contribute to nausea and vomiting. The problem is aggravated by smoking and wearing tight clothing. Simple measures such as small frequent meals, avoiding bending soon after eating, sleeping more propped up and cessation of smoking may all help. Pharmacological treatment includes the use of alginates and or antacids such as Maalox (aluminium and magnesium hydroxide) 10 ml three times daily 20 to 30 minutes after meals and at bed time or Gaviscon (sodium alginate, sodium bicarbonate, calcium carbonate) 10 ml three times daily 20 to 30 minutes after meals and prior to bed time. In intractable cases a H_2 antagonist preparation such as ranitidine may safely be used in pregnancy.

BACKACHE

Backache is common in pregnancy and may arise *de novo* or exacerbate pre-existing back problems. The shift of a woman's center of gravity, from its prepregnancy position, where it passes through the knees, to gravid situation where it now moves forward and is in front of the knees, is the principal contributory factor. During pregnancy, in order to maintain stability on her feet, each woman subconsciously has to alter her posture to account for the presence of the gravid uterus. The alteration in the posture is an increase in the lumbar lordosis. The hormonal milleiu of pregnancy (progesterone and relaxin in particular) lead to relaxation of ligaments and joints, which in combination with the exaggerated lumbar lordosis put pressure on the nerve roots producing pain. Simple measures include advice regarding avoidance of high heels, analgesia, bed rest and a firm mattress (can be achieved by placing boards beneath the mattress). In some cases the use of a pregnancy brace girdle may help.

CARPAL TUNNEL SYNDROME

Carpal tunnel syndrome refers to the tingling sensation experienced in the distribution of the median nerve in the hand and in some cases radiating up the forearm. The pregnant patient may present complaining of being unable to use her hand in the morning because her fingers feel stiff and she has a tendency to drop things but symptoms improve during the course of the evening. In the first instance the patient will need to be reassured that there is no underlying sinister pathology involved and that it will improve after the pregnancy is over. The underlying pathophysiology is due to compression of the median nerve secondary to edema underlying the flexor retinaculum. Referral to the physiotherapist or surgical appliances will provide the patient with splints that keep the wrist(s) in dorsiflexion and thus relieving pressure on the median nerve.

CONSTIPATION

Constipation is one of the most common problems encountered in pregnancy and it is due to the smooth muscle relaxant effect of progesterone. The resulting reduced gut motility is also aggravated in late pregnancy by the pressure from the enlarged uterus and from iron supplementation. The usual management strategy is to advise a fiber diet with fresh fruit and vegetables and increased intake of water. In cases where laxatives are deemed necessary, it is preferable to opt for agents that effectively add bulk to the stool and therefore increase peristalsis. Bulking agents are not absorbed from the GI tract so are safe to use in pregnancy. Agents that are often used include lactulose (15 ml twice daily) and Ispaghula husk (one sachet twice daily). Where stool softeners are required senokot is the ideal choice.

URINARY PROBLEMS

Urinary frequency is encountered from early on in pregnancy secondary to hyperdynamic circulation and supranormal urine production by the kidneys. As pregnancy advances the enlarging uterus and the presenting part may also directly irritate the trigone. Occasionally a retroverted uterus may fail to become spontaneously anteverted, and if remains retroverted after the 14th week may become incarcerated in the pouch of Douglas. This leads progressively to frequency and dysuria and eventually to urinary retention and overflow incontinence. Once the bladder has been decompressed by catheterization the uterus often anteverts spontaneously or can be anteverted by vaginal examination and manipulation.

In the latter half of pregnancy up to half of all women suffer some degree of incontinence (often minor) and patients may need reassurance that this is the case and will resolve in the puerperium. It is however important always to exclude urinary tract infections with any urinary symptoms.

PUBIC SYMPHYSIS DIASTASIS/PELVIC OSTEOARTHROPATHY

Progesterone can result in relaxation of the pubic symphysis joint and the surrounding ligaments as the pregnancy progresses. To some extent this is a physiological response to help increase the pelvic diameters and ease the passage of the fetus through the birth canal. However, occasionally this adaptation may become excessive resulting in significant separation of the pubic bones.

VARICOSITIES

The main contributory factor for the development of varicosities is a degree of pelvic venous obstruction due to pelvic pressure exerted by the growing uterus. Varicosities may arise *de novo* or may represent exacerbation of pre-existing ones and become worse with advancing pregnancy. Varicosities may affect the legs, vulva, abdominal wall and also present as hemorrhoids. Treatment during pregnancy is conservative.

Hemorrhoids can be troublesome and aggravated by pregnancy associated constipation. Conservative management includes prevention and treatment of constipation along with topical application of local anesthetics and provision of adequate analgesia. Very rarely surgical intervention may be required. The patient must be aware that they are slow to resolve and may persist for several months after pregnancy.

Varicose veins in the legs can be disfiguring and painful. Conservative methods include keeping the legs elevated whenever possible. Other measures include the use of surgical support stockings which are not comfortable at the best of time but less so in hot weather. If support stockings are to be used these should be put on while the patient is still horizontal before getting out of bed while the veins are relatively collapsed.

Abdominal wall varicosities, eventhough unsightly, rarely cause problems. Occasionally a varicocele of the round ligament may present as a groin swelling mistaken for an inguinal hernia but in view of the uterine enlargement this would be highly unlikely. Such varicosities settle after delivery.

Vulval varicosities often cause alarm in the patient so reassurance may be required. Usually they are confined to the vulva but may involve the perineum and extend around the introitus and this being the case if an episiotomy is required it should be directed away from them. Vulval varicosities disappear slowly after delivery.

Pregnancy is an exciting but also a worrying time for the patient. The biochemical, physiological and hormonal changes manifest themselves with a variety of symptoms. Patients need advice and reassurance that these changes are all part and parcel of pregnancy and benign in nature and will gradually resolve after pregnancy.

16. Basic Ultrasonography in Pregnancy

Jamiyah Hassan
Sofiah Sulaiman

INTRODUCTION

The first ultrasonic device for obstetrical use has been introduced into daily medical practice for more than half a century ago. In recent years the advances in ultrasound and computer technology have enabled the industry to produce more sophisticated scanning machines and today, diagnostic ultrasound is part of the daily medical practice. Ultrasound is a useful diagnostic tool in obstetrics. The ultrasound waves, as used today appear to be safe to the developing fetus.

Ultrasound technology uses sound waves to create images by 'bouncing' sound waves off tissues. The ultrasound waves used are of a very high frequency which is undetectable to the human ears. The common frequency used is usually between 3.5 and 7.0 megahertz. These sound waves are emitted intermittently through a transducer that is placed on the maternal skin and the transmission is enhanced by placing gel on the maternal skin at the point of contact with the transducer. The ultrasound pulse is then transmitted through one's body and is then reflected back to the receiving transducer by the various structures under study. The amount of ultrasound waves that is reflected back is dependent on the density of the tissue. The velocity of the sound waves varies from 331 to 4080 meters per second. Today due to the advances of the ultrasound machines the images are seen as realtime. During the last decade, the usage of ultrasound in obstetrics has increased due to realtime imaging, Doppler and color imaging.

SAFETY OF ULTRASONOGRAPHY

The issue of safety of ultrasound has been debated for many years especially to the developing fetus. Very high frequency ultrasound waves have been shown to produce heat and cause cavitations in cells. However diagnostic ultrasound in its current form has been shown to be completely safe for the fetus. Despite these reassurances scientists are still conducting studies on the safety of ultrasound. However, it is recommended that the usage of ultrasound in medical practice be not abused even though it is considered as safe. It is prudent to limit the usage where there are indications.

METHODS

There are two approaches in obstetric sonography. They can be performed transabdominally or transvaginally. Transabdominal mode is popular during the second trimester. If it is used in the first trimester a full bladder is usually needed to act as a "window" for better visualization.

Transvaginal approach is used most commonly during the first trimester of pregnancy. This approach allows the transducer to be closer to the structures under study and so allow a higher frequency beam to be transmitted. This will in turn provide more accurate images and the structures can be seen one week earlier than if the transabdominal approach is used. For a transvaginal approach a full bladder is not needed.

INDICATIONS FOR ULTRASOUND EXAMINATION IN OBSTETRICS

There are various indications for ultrasonography in obstetrics. The question of routine ultrasound versus ultrasound with indicated use has always been debated. Even though various studies on routine ultrasound has not shown a clear benefit other than incurring more cost, most couples will relate much better with the pregnancy if the fetus is seen on the screen.

Assessment of Early Pregnancy

Using the transvaginal approach the gestational sac can be visualized as early as four and a half weeks of gestation and the yolk sac at about five weeks (Figures 16.1, Plate 1 and 16.2).

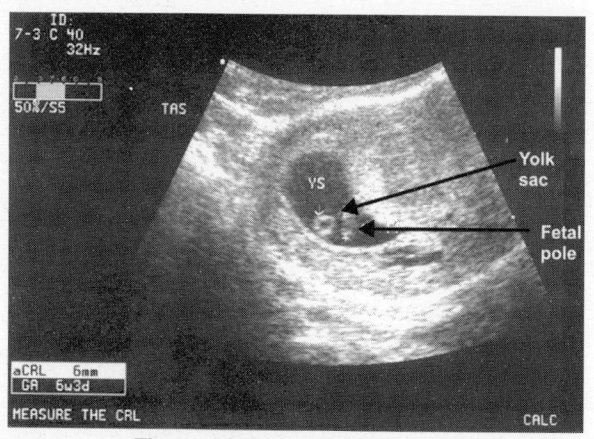

Figure 16.2: Early pregnancy

Complications of Early Pregnancy

Vaginal bleeding is the most common complication of early pregnancy. The causes of vaginal bleeding in early pregnancy include threatened, incomplete, complete and missed miscarriages. The diagnosis can be confirmed with the aid of the ultrasound examination.

In threatened miscarriage the fetal heart must be visualized on ultrasound and clinical examination should not reveal evidence of cervical dilatation. Fetal heart motion is usually clearly seen at 7 weeks using the transabdominal approach and a week earlier using the transvaginal approach. If this is observed, the probability of a continued pregnancy is greater than 97 percent. In missed abortion fetal poles which may not be appropriate to the gestational age is seen without the evidence of heartbeat. In blighted ovum the typical picture would be of a large gestational sac with no evidence of fetal poles. Ultrasonography is also useful in the early diagnosis of ectopic pregnancies (Figure 16.3). Definitive diagnosis can be made if the fetal heart is clearly visualized outside the uterine cavity. However, in some cases of ectopic pregnancy, where a pseudo-gestational sac is seen in the uterine cavity, a definitive diagnosis can be difficult. Ultrasound is also useful in the diagnosis of molar pregnancies (Figure 16.4) where the typical picture of cystic spaces within the uterine cavity or the "snowstorm appearance" is seen.

Determination of Dates

Determination of the maturity of the pregnancy is very important especially when the menstrual date is unclear. Gestational age can be determined with good accuracy using the ultrasound especially in the first trimester. The common parameters use in the first trimester include gestational sac diameter and crown-rump length. In later gestational age biparietal diameter, head circumference, abdominal circumference and intercerebellar diameters are used to determine the gestational age.

The following measurements are usually made:

Crown-rump Length (Figure 16.5)

Crown-rump length (CRL) measurement can be made between 7 and 13 weeks and this gives a very accurate estimation of the gestational age. The error of dating

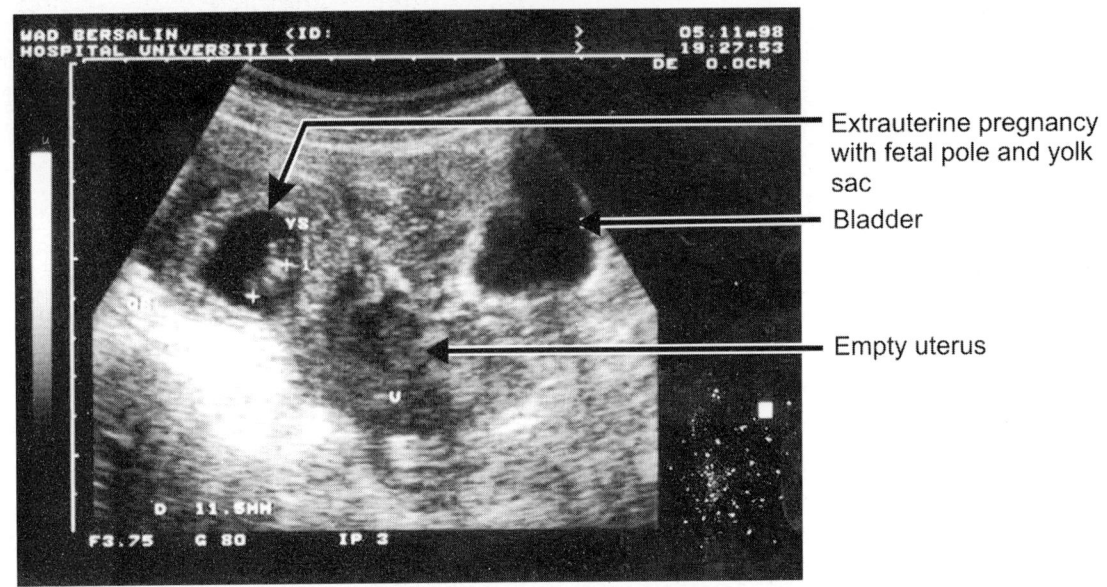

Figure 16.3: Ectopic pregnancy
- Extrauterine pregnancy with fetal pole and yolk sac
- Bladder
- Empty uterus

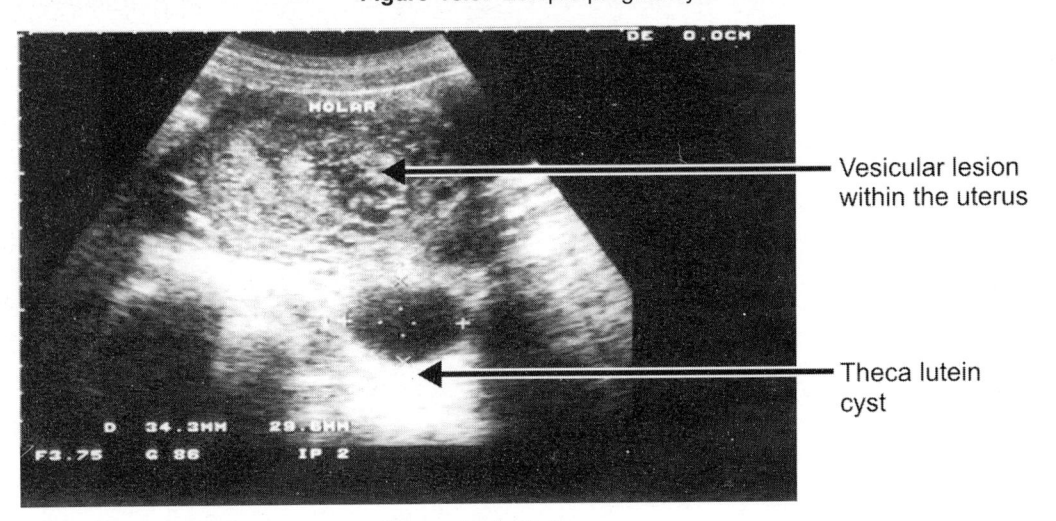

Figure 16.4: Molar pregnancy
- Vesicular lesion within the uterus
- Theca lutein cyst

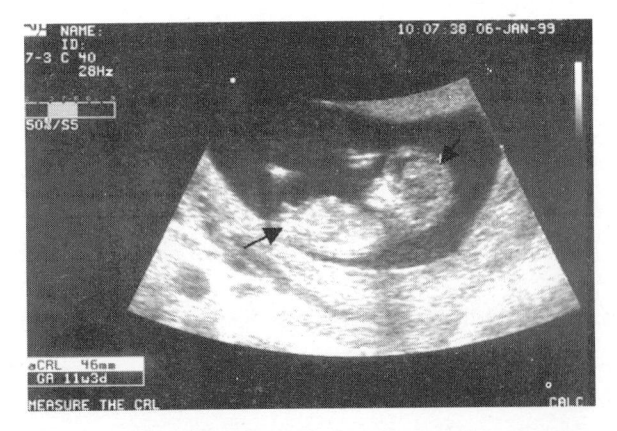

Figure 16.5: Crown-rump length

using the CRL as a parameter can be within 3-4 days of the last menstrual period. However, between 10 and 12 weeks of gestation when the fetal spine starts to move, care should be taken to ensure that the fetus is not hypo- or hyper-flexed as this will increase the error slightly.

Biparietal Diameter (Figure 16.6)

Biparietal diameter (BPD) is taken at the transverse plane between the two parietal eminences. This is usually measured from the 15th week onward. The error of dating using this measurement from the 15 to

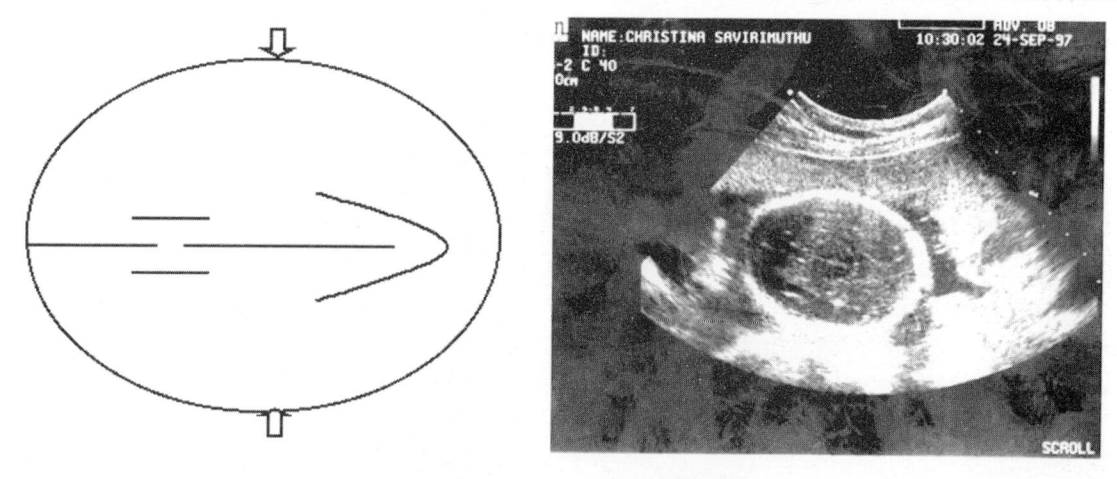

BASIC ULTRASONOGRAPHY IN PREGNANCY

Figure 16.6: Biparietal diameter

24 weeks is about 7 to 10 days. In the third trimester the error increases to 2 to 3 weeks. In dolichocephaly this measurement can grossly underestimate maturity and other measurements like the head circumference which does not change with head shape should be used to determine the gestational age.

Femur Length (FL) (Figure 16.7)

Femur length (FL) is measured in the longitudinal section without including the epiphyses. It is useful as a parameter for dating especially in the third trimester.

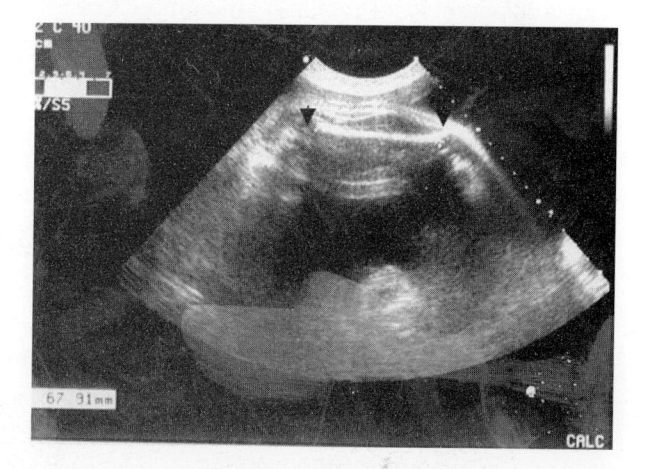

Abdominal Circumference (Figure 16.8)

Abdominal circumference (AC) is one of the most difficult measurements as it is operator dependent. In growth restricted fetuses the abdominal circumference is usually affected and thus this is not useful to date a pregnancy.

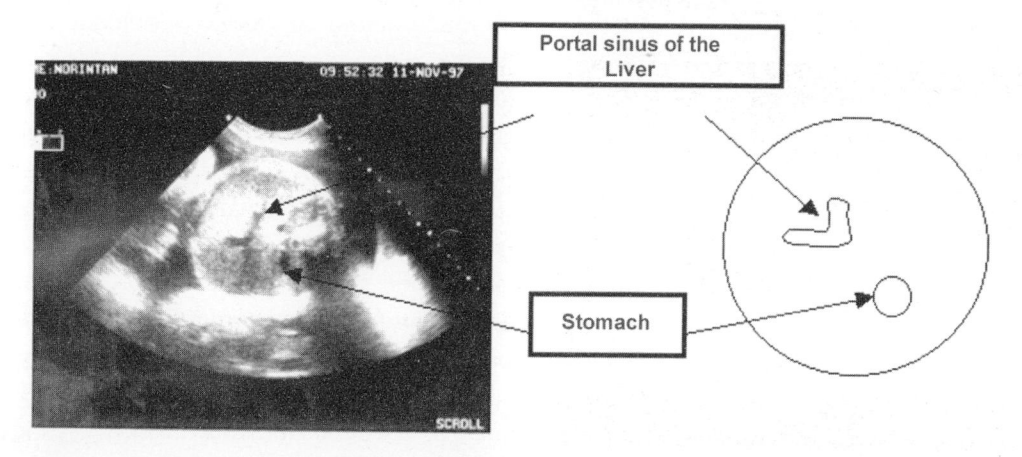

Figure 16.7: Femur length

Figure 16.8: Abdominal circumference: The plane of measurement should include the structures shown

Intercerebellar Diameter

This is a useful diameter to date a pregnancy especially before 24 weeks as it corresponds millimeter to millimeter to the gestational age in weeks.

Placental Localization

Ultrasonography is an important tool in the diagnosis of placenta previa, and other placental abnormalities. With the help of color Doppler other complications like vasa previa and placenta accreata can be diagnosed.

Multiple Pregnancies

Determination of chorionicity has become an important part of management of multiple pregnancy. This can be performed reliabily using ultrasound at 11 to 14 weeks gestation. In multiple pregnancy, ultrasonography is also valuable in determining the number of fetuses (Figure 16.9), gestational age and fetal malformations. In the latter part of pregnancy ultrasound can be used to monitor the growth of the fetuses and the development of complications like intrauterine growth restrictions, twin to twin transfusion and *in utero* demise.

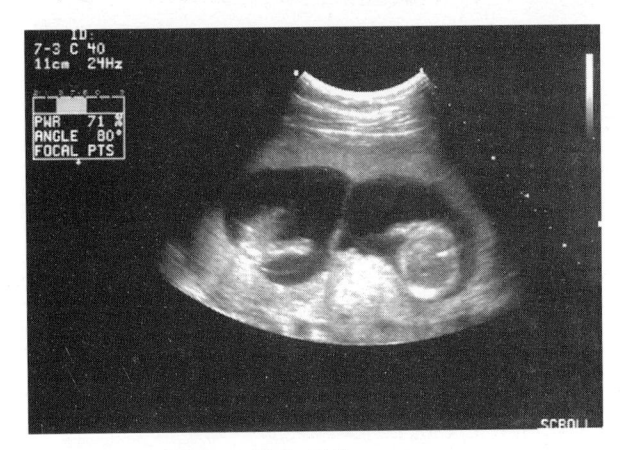

Figure 16.9: Twin pregnancy

Assessment of Amniotic Fluid

Excessive or decreased amount of liquor (amniotic fluid) can be identified by ultrasound. In both these situations, careful ultrasound examination should be made to exclude intrauterine growth retardation and congenital malformation in the fetus such as intestinal atresia, hydrops fetalis (Figures 16.10 and 16.11) or renal dysplasia with polyhydramnios in the absence of fetal abnormality screening for maternal diabetes is recommended.

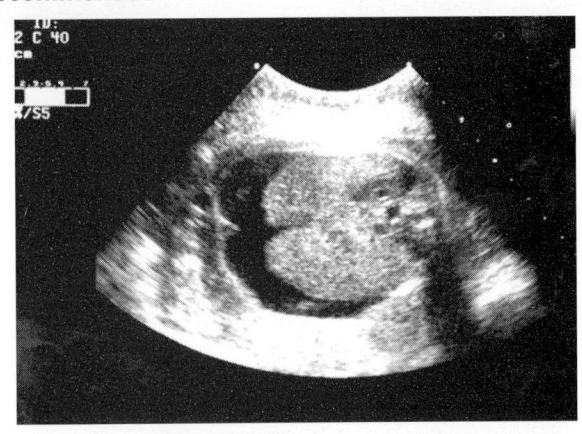

Figure 16.10: Fetal ascites

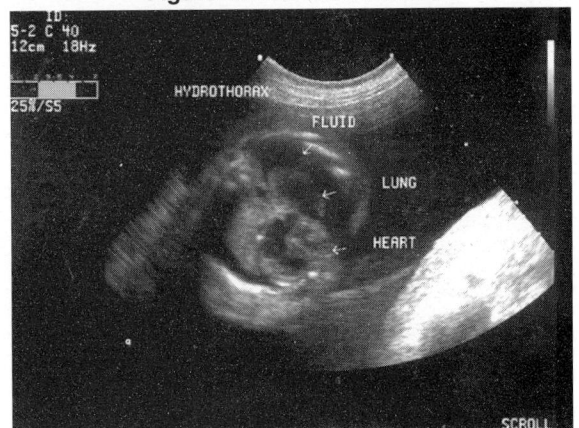

Figure 16.11: Fetal hydrothorax

Fetal Malformation

Structural abnormalities in the fetus can be reliably diagnosed by an ultrasound scan, and these can usually be made before 20 weeks. Systematic examination of the major systems is performed and structural anomalies like anencephaly, myelomeningocele, spina bifida (Figure 16.12), ventriculomegaly (Figure 16.13), gastrochisis (Figure 16.14), cyst in the umbilical cord (Figure 16.15), duodenal atresia and many others can be diagnosed. With more modern equipments, minor conditions such as cleft lips/palate and the more complicated assessment like the cardiac anomalies can be performed. Ultrasound can also be used to look for soft ultrasound markers for chromosomal abnormalities such as the fetal nuchal translucency (Figure 16.16), mild renal pyelectasis, sandal gap for condition like Down

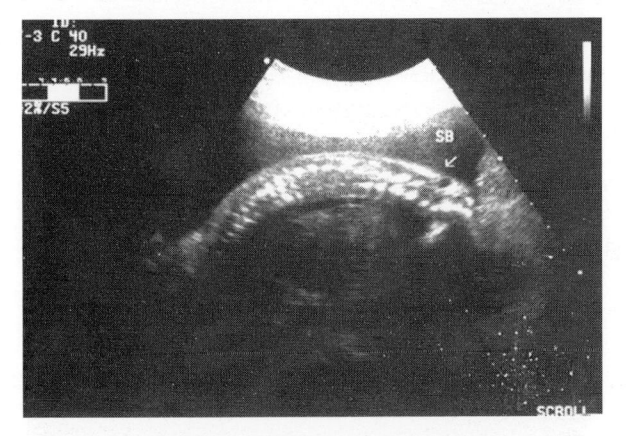

Figure 16.12: Spina bifida

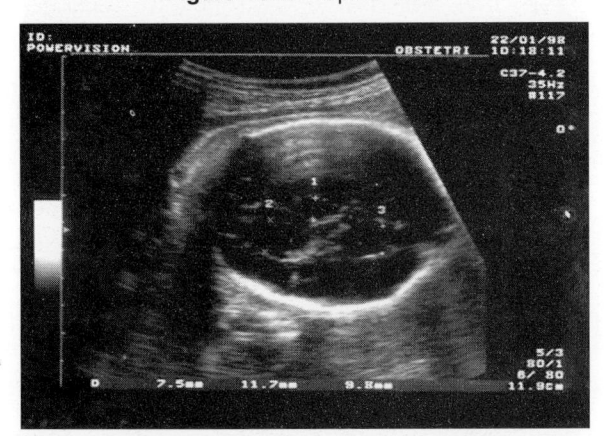

Figure 16.13: Fetal ventriculomegaly

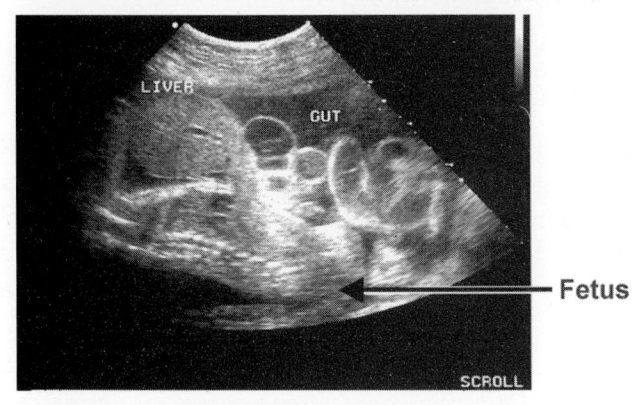

Figure 16.14: Gastrochisis

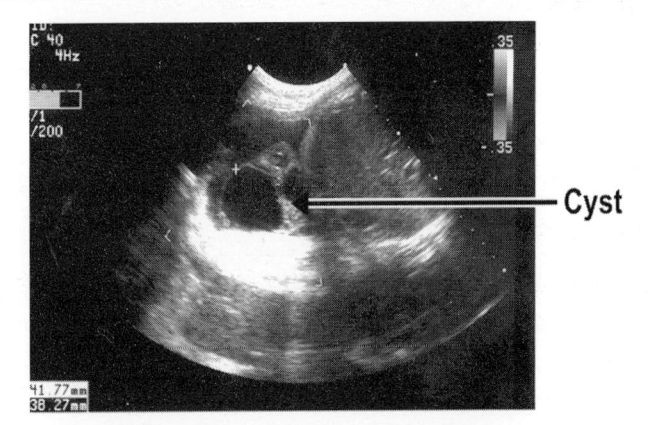

Figure 16.15: Cyst in the umbilical cord

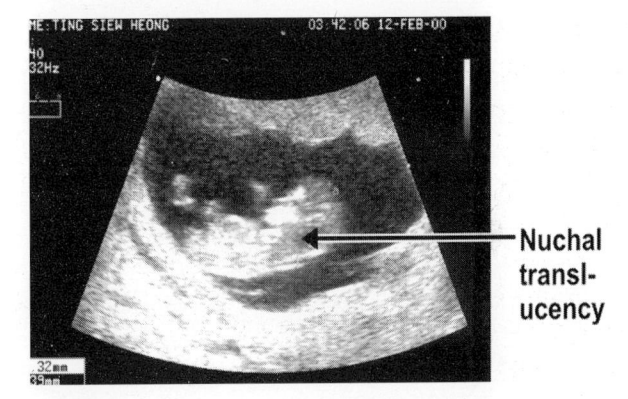

Figure 16.16: Nuchal translucency—soft marker for trisomy 21

Other Areas

Ultrasonography is of great value in other obstetric conditions such as:
a. Confirmation of intrauterine death.
b. Confirmation of fetal presentation in uncertain cases.
c. Evaluating fetal movements, tone and breathing in the biophysical profile.
d. Diagnosis of uterine and pelvic abnormalities during pregnancy, e.g. fibromyomata and ovarian cyst.

THE SCHEDULE

There is no hard and fast rule as to the number of scans a woman should have during her pregnancy. Ideally a scan is booked at less than twelve weeks (first trimester) to confirm pregnancy, exclude ectopic or molar pregnancies, confirm cardiac pulsation and measure the crown-rump length for dating.

syndrome. Ultrasound is also used for diagnostic procedures such as amniocentesis, chorionic villus sampling, percutaneous umbilical blood sampling and in fetal therapy.

A second scan is performed at 18 to 24 weeks to look for congenital malformations and to verify dates and growth. The placental position is also determined during this time.

A third scan may sometimes be done at around 34 weeks to evaluate fetal size and assess fetal growth. The total number of scan will vary depending on whether a previous scan has detected certain abnormalities that require follow-up assessment.

In a normal uncomplicated pregnancy a scan in the first trimester and a more detailed scan between 18 and 24 weeks gestation will suffice.

DOPPLER ULTRASOUND

The development in fetal Doppler ultrasound technology has enabled its application in obstetrics in the area of assessing and monitoring the fetal wellbeing.

Blood flow characteristics in the fetal blood vessels can be assessed with Doppler flow velocity waveforms. The blood vessels that are commonly used are the umbilical artery (Figures 16.17 and 16.18, Plate 2), the middle cerebral arteries and the uterine arcuate arteries.

Color Doppler is particularly important in the diagnosis and assessment of congenital heart abnormalities. Power Doppler uses amplitude information from Doppler signals rather than flow velocity information to visualize slow flow in smaller blood vessels.

BIBLIOGRAPHY

1. Bucher HC, Schmidt JG: Does routine ultrasound scanning improve outcome in pregnancy? Meta-analysis of various outcome measures. *BMJ* **307:** 13–17, 1993.
2. Duck FA, Starritt HC, ter Haar GR, Lunt MJ: Surface heating of diagnostic ultrasound transducers. *Br J Rad 62* 1005–13, 1989.
3. Evans DH, McDicken WN, Skidmore R, Woodcock JP: *Doppler Ultrasound: Physics, Instrumentation and Clinical Applications.* Wiley, Chichester, 1989.
4. Neilson JP. Ultrasound for fetal assessment in early pregnancy. Cochrane Review. The Cochrane Library Issue. Oxford Update Software, 1999.
5. Smith NC, Hau C: A six year study of the antenatal detection of fetal abnormality in six Scottish health boards. *Br J Obstet Gynecol* **106:** 206–12, 1999.
6. The value of ultrasound in pregnancy. RCOG Guidelines No 4, 1994.
7. Ultrasound Screening for Fetal Abnormalities. *Report of the RCOG Working Party*, RCOG, London, 1997.

17. Prenatal Diagnosis

Teresa WP Chow

PART TWO — Feto-maternal Medicine

INTRODUCTION

In recent years, the scope of prenatal diagnosis has expanded greatly with the development of screening tests like maternal serum biochemical screening[1] and fetal nuchal translucency.[2] Most women in the developed countries are offered some form of prenatal screening in pregnancy that may subsequently lead to a specific diagnostic test. However, some prenatal screening and diagnostic tests may not be freely available in some developing countries. Nevertheless, it is vital that each pregnant woman should always be counseled on the risks and benefits of prenatal screening and diagnostic tests so that informed choice may be made as a woman's approach to prenatal diagnosis is a personal one.

This chapter provides an outline of prenatal screening followed by an overall coverage of common indications for prenatal diagnosis and the associated risks and benefits.

PRENATAL SCREENING

Prenatal screening is becoming close to being a routine part of antenatal care. The main aim of prenatal screening is to identify "high risk" pregnancy. To date, there are few prenatal treatment modalities available for specific disorder and the general common goal of screening at present is to reduce the number of babies with disabilities born through "therapeutic abortions".

There is a definite distinction between prenatal screening and prenatal diagnosis. The former is generally non-invasive whilst the latter usually entails invasive procedure that carries a risk of fetal loss. Any prenatal screening test should meet the standard criteria for a screening test (Table 17.1). Only a few fetal conditions are sufficiently common for screening to be worthwhile. These include Down syndrome and neural tube defects, and in selected populations, conditions like the hemoglobinopathies.

The initial screening usually begins at the clinic when the woman presents for her first antenatal care. However, this may even begin as early as preconceptual where preconceptional counseling clinics are available. It is vital that a detailed assessment is carried out (Table 17.2). It is also imperative to bear in mind that there are ethnic differences in the prevalence of certain inherited disorders and the specific screening and diagnostic test has to be tailored accordingly. In addition, prescreening counseling is of paramount importance with respect to the individual's personal view and the associated risks of possible prenatal diagnostic tests.

Table 17.1: Criteria for screening

- Non-invasive and safe
- Easily available
- Simple
- Accurate
- Inexpensive
- Offered to all pregnant women
- Performed for specific disorders with relatively high prevalence with consideration of ethnic, racial and geographic background (for example, α and β-thalassemia in South-East Asians; sickle-cell disease in Africans; Tay-Sachs disease in Ashkenazi Jews; cystic fibrosis in Caucasians)
- Availability of prenatal diagnostic test
- Availability of treatment or management solution for identified affected cases

Table 17.2. Assessment and prenatal screening for prenatal diagnosis

History (as part of prenatal screening)	Prenatal screening test	Prenatal diagnostic test
• Maternal age (increase risk of fetal chromosomal anomalies with advanced age) • Ethnicity (increase prevalence of certain genetic disorder in certain ethnic group, e.g. thalassemia in South-East Asians) • Previous pregnancy outcome (e.g. previous Rhesus isoimmunization or fetal Barts hydrops, previous child with chromosomal abnormalities) • Family history and partner's history of certain genetic disorder (e.g. thalassemia, cystic fibrosis, hemophilia) • Medical history and drug history (e.g. association of fetal structural anomalies with diabetes mellitus and use of anti-epileptic drugs) • Occupational history (e.g. nursery workers and contacts with CMV/ parvovirus infected children)	• Fetal nuchal translucency • Maternal serum screening for neural tube defect and Down syndrome • Maternal full blood indices / electrophoresis (thalassemia) • Sickledex test (sickle cell disease) • Maternal blood group/rhesus antibodies • Maternal serum virology (CMV/ toxoplasmosis/ rubella/parvovirus); serology for syphilis • Ultrasound scan (fetal anatomy)	• CVS: fetal karyotype; DNA analysis for specific genetic disorder (e.g. α and β-thalassemia, cystic fibrosis) • Amniocentesis: fetal karyotype; PCR technique for diagnosis of fetal CMV/ toxoplasma infection • Fetal blood sampling: fetal karyotype; fetal hemoglobin and blood group (e.g. Rhesus disease); DNA analysis for certain genetic disorder (e.g. thalassemia, cystic fibrosis) • Comprehensive ultrasound scan (e.g. neural tube defect/ skeletal anomalies)

CVS=chorionic villus sampling; CMV= cytomegalovirus; PCR= polymerase chain reaction; DNA=deoxyribonucleic acid

Whilst routine antenatal hemoglobin estimation, screening for blood group and antibodies, syphilis infection and rubella antibodies are universally practised, fetal nuchal translucency and maternal serum screening for Down syndrome and fetal neural tube defects are not (Table 17.3).

The congenital abnormalities rate is 2 percent with major defects occurring in approximately 1 percent of live births. These anomalies may be structural, chromosomal, genetical or secondary to *in utero* viral infection (Table 17.4) but neural tube defects (NTDs) and Down syndrome are the most common major malformations and congenital mental handicap respectively. Therefore, prenatal screening programs for this structural and chromosomal abnormality were introduced.

Second Trimester Biochemical Screening

Maternal serum α-fetoprotein (AFP) screening for fetal open NTDs was developed in 1970s in Great Britain. This is performed at 15 to 20 weeks of gestation. Elevated AFP levels are associated with fetal open NTDs, anterior abdominal wall defects and other anomalies. The finding of lower maternal serum AFP levels in Down pregnancies led to the introduction of biochemical screening for Down syndrome in the late 1980s because although advanced maternal age is associated with Down pregnancies, 80 percent of Down pregnancies occur in women under the age of 35. The test includes maternal serum AFP, human β-chorionic gonadotropin (β-hCG) and unconjugated oestriol (uE$_3$) assay. β-hCG tends to be higher and uE$_3$ tends to be lower in Down

Table 17.3: Common routine prenatal screening tests

Screening tests	Purpose of tests	Available treatment modalities
Full blood count Blood indices Hemoglobin electrophoresis*	• Screen for anemia • Hemoglobinopathy screen	• Treatment of anemia • Expert management to avoid complications (e.g. sickling crisis) prenatal diagnosis/ therapeutic abortion/ counseling
Blood group and rhesus (Rh) antibody screening	• Screen for Rh status prevent isoimmunization	• Appropriate prophylaxis in Rh negative cases • Prenatal diagnosis/fetal blood transfusion in affected cases
Hepatitis B* screen/ HIV mothers	• Identify positive mothers	• Appropriate prophylaxis to prevent transmission to baby
Syphilis serology	• Identify positive mothers	• Effective treatment of seropositive women, sexual partner(s) and infant
Rubella status	• Identify seronegative mothers	• Immunization to seronegative mothers postdelivery
Urinalysis	• Screen for asymptomatic bacteriuria	• Treat positive cases to reduce incidence of acute urinary tract infections and hence preterm deliveries
• Ultrasound (US) • Serum screening /NT (not universal)	• US: early dating/ identify multiple fetuses • Screen for structural anomalies/ Down	• US: avoid induction for post-term • Prenatal diagnosis/ therapeutic abortion/ counseling

* Only in selected populations

Table 17.4. Classification of common congenital abnormalities[3]

Congenital abnormality	Common Examples	Incidence per 1000 birth
Structural	Neural tube defects (Incidence trend has been reported to decrease with the introduction of periconceptual folic acid)	Varies with geographic areas:- 0.38 in the Netherlands; 0.5 in the States; 2-3 in the UK; 1.8 in China; 3.9 in Northern India.
	Congenital heart defects	Overall: 3 - 8
Chromosomal	Down syndrome (Trisomy 21) Turner's syndrome (45 XO) Trisomy 13 (Patau syndrome) Trisomy 18 (Edward's syndrome)	1.3 0.3 0.2 – 0.03 0.3 – 0.08
Genetic	Alpha-thalassemia Beta-thalassemia Sickle cell disease Cystic fibrosis (CF)	Prevalence determined by ethnic and geographic factors:- *Carrier frequency* of α-thalassemia: Chinese 1/15 -1/30; β-thalassemia: Asians 1/10-1/30; Sickle cell trait: Afro-Caribbeans 1/10, West Africans up to 1/4; CF: 1/3300
Whites		
Congenital infection	Cytomegalovirus, toxoplasmosis, rubella, varicella, parvovirus; syphilis	CMV: 5- 22; toxoplasma: 0.1-1 Prevalence varies with geographic areas.

pregnancies. Using this "triple screen" or its modifications (AFP and hCG) between 15th and 20th week of gestation combined with maternal age and ultrasonically corrected gestational age to calculate the risk of Down syndrome is more precise than using maternal age alone. Approximately 60 percent of chromosomal abnormal infants can be detected with this test but with the disadvantage of 5 percent false-positive rate.[1] In other words, one in 20 women less than 35 years will be classified as high risk. Inhibin A is relatively new and it may be used in future as an additional marker to increase the detection rate.

Screening Ultrasound for Fetal Structural Abnormalities

Routine anomaly scanning at between 18 and 20 weeks of gestation is often carried out in the developed countries as screening for fetal structural abnormalities. However, this is not a routine practice in places with constraints of resources and expertise. Although anomalies are an important cause of perinatal mortality, the eventual outcome is not significantly affected by the diagnosis of lethal fetal anomaly. The value of routine screening ultrasound for anomaly thus remains controversial[4] but routine ultrasound scan in early pregnancy has been shown by meta-analysis of randomised controlled trials to be of value as it results in the reduction of induction of labor for "post-term pregnancies" as well as early detection of early multiple pregnancies.[5] The risks of false-positive findings of uncertain significance on routine anomaly ultrasonography and hence possible unnecessary anxiety generated on women should be considered when anomaly ultrasound screening is offered as a routine. This should also be weighed against the availability of prenatal diagnostic tests and policies on termination of pregnancy in a country.

Fetal Nuchal Translucency

Observation of a strong association between abnormal accumulation of fluid behind the fetal neck and chromosomal abnormalities led to the introduction of new method of screening by fetal nuchal translucency (NT) in the first trimester.[2] This is a screening ultrasound that involves sonographic measurement of a translucent space on the fetal neck between 10th and 14th week of gestation. The advantage of this early screening is that termination of pregnancy if opted for may be carried out in the first trimester (Table 17.5).

An increase in nuchal translucency (NT) measurement based on fetal crown-rump length measurement has been shown to be associated with fetuses with major chromosomal abnormalities and sex chromosomal abnormalities. The individual's risk for Down syndrome can be predicted based on information on maternal age, gestation and NT measurement.

This screening method has been shown to identify about 80 percent of fetuses with Down syndrome for a false-positive rate of 5 percent.[2] However, it is operator-dependent and a high quality ultrasound machine is required. The role of routine NT screen in a low risk population is yet to be clarified.

Table 17.5: Screening for Down syndrome

	Maternal age only	Maternal 2nd trimester serum biochemical screening	Fetal nuchal translucency (NT)	Fetal NT + Maternal 1st trimester serum screening
Method	History	Blood test	Ultrasound scan	Ultrasound scan and blood test
Timing of test	Any time	15–20 weeks gestation	10–14 weeks gestation	10-14 weeks gestation
Detection rate	25%	About 60%	About 80%	About 90%
False-positive rate	5%-10%	5%	5%	5%
Advantages	• Simple, cheap	• Relatively cheap	• Early test • Screen for all aneuploidy/cardiac anomalies	• Early test
Disadvantages	• Poor sensitivity	• Laboratory dependent • Requires dating scan • Affected by other factors e.g. diabetes, ethnicity • Specific for Down	• Operator-dependant • Requires high-quality scan machine	• Operator-dependent • Requires high-quality machine • Requires standardisation of assay kits

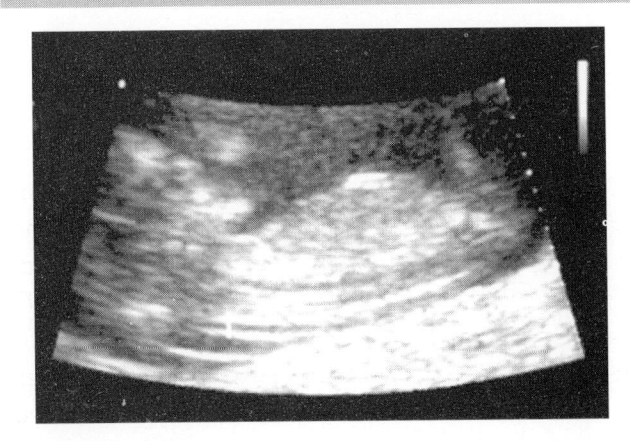

Figure 17.1: First trimester normal fetal NT measurement

First trimester biochemical screening
Maternal serum free human β-chorionic gonadotropin (β-hCG) and serum pregnancy-associated plasma protein A (PAPP-A) increases and decreases respectively in trisomy 21 pregnancies. The combination of maternal serum β-hCG and PAPP-A with maternal age alone provides a detection rate for trisomy 21 pregnancies of 67 percent for a 5 percent false-positive rate.[6]

Studies have shown that by combining fetal NT measurement (Figure 17.1) with these two biochemical markers and maternal age, the detection rate improves to 89 percent at a 5 percent false-positive rate.[6] However, until the availability of robust assay kits that meet international standards, first trimester biochemical screening is only currently carried out on research basis. There is insufficient evidence at present to recommend routine first trimester screening for Down syndrome by biochemical markers and fetal NT measurement.

PRENATAL DIAGNOSTIC TESTS

Diagnostic tests are carried out on pregnancies that have been identified as "high-risk" from a screening test. Except for comprehensive sonographic structural examination of the fetus, these prenatal diagnostic tests are usually invasive and carry a small risk of fetal loss. All women who are rhesus negative should be given anti-D immunoglobulin prophylaxis after any invasive procedure.

Diagnostic Ultrasound

The development of high-resolution ultrasound machine is the main catalyst for advance of prenatal diagnosis. A fairly large proportion of fetal structural abnormalities can be identified by ultrasound scan with NTDs being the common examples. In addition, many cases of fetal anomalies associated with major chromosomal abnormality or a syndrome may be detected. The advent of 3-D ultrasound further improves diagnosis of some fetal abnormalities like cleft lip and palate and skeletal anomalies. However, its value is yet to be evaluated.

Amniocentesis

Amniocentesis was in fact established well before the general availability of ultrasound. It is generally carried out at or after 15th week of gestation whereby a fine bore needle is passed through the maternal abdomen under ultrasound guidance into the amniotic cavity to remove a small amount of amniotic fluid (Figure 17.2) containing fetal fibroblasts for culture for fetal chromosomal analysis for which result is available 2 to 3 weeks later. With the new interphase fluorescent *in situ* hybridization (FISH) technique using chromosome-specific probes on uncultured amniocytes, rapid and accurate results can be obtained.

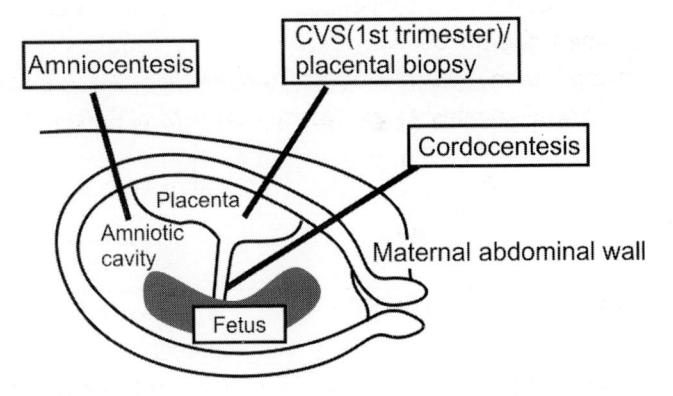

Figure 17.2: A schematic diagram showing the common prenatal diagnostic tests

In addition to fetal karyotyping, the fetal cells in the amniotic fluid can also be used for enzyme analysis in metabolic disorders and DNA (deoxyribonucleic acid) analysis for single gene defects. However, amniocentesis for DNA analysis has now generally been superseded by early trimester chorionic villus sampling. The supernatant of the fluid has also been used for assay of AFP and acetylcholinesterase for fetal NTD and

Table 17.6: Some common investigations from prenatal diagnostic procedures

CVS	Amniocentesis	Fetal blood sampling
Cells • Chromosomal analysis /FISH (Direct preparations: results within 48 hours; Cultured preparations: results in 1–2 weeks) • DNA analysis for single gene defects (e.g. thalassemia) and fetal infections (e.g. CMV and toxoplasma)	Cells • Chromosomal analysis (Cultured preparations: results in 2-3 weeks; FISH technique: rapid results but only for specific selected probes like trisomy 13, 21 and 18) • DNA analysis for single gene defects (e.g. thalassemia) • PCR technique on detection of viral or protozoa – specific nucleic acid in amniotic fluid in the diagnosis of fetal infections	Cells – usually in cases of late presentation • Chromosomal analysis/ FISH Direct from white blood cell: results with 48 hours) • DNA analysis for single gene defects (e.g. thalassemia) and fetal infections • Enzyme analysis in inborn metabolic disorders (rarely done) • Blood group, hemoglobin and haematocrit in the investigation of Rhesus disease • Platelets assessment in the assessment of allo-immune thrombocytopaenia (a condition due to maternal sensitization to fetal platelet antigens)
	Supernatant • Bilirubin assessment in rhesus disease) • Surface active Phospholipids for lung maturity (rarely used now)	Serum • Viral or parasitic antibodies in cases of suspected infection like toxoplasmosis and CMV infection – low diagnostic sensitivity. Now replaced by PCR on amniotic fluid.

bilirubin level in cases of rhesus hemolytic disease in the third trimester as well as surface active phospholipids level for fetal lung maturity assessment. In addition, fetal infections like toxoplasmosis and cytomegalovirus infection can now be detected by the use of polymerase chain reaction (PCR) technique on the amniotic fluid (Table 17.6).

Amniocentesis is associated with a miscarriage rate of 0.5 percent to 1percent. Amniocentesis before 15 weeks is not recommended due to the association of higher miscarriage rate and neonatal talipes and respiratory disorders.

Chorionic Villus Sampling

The introduction of chorionic villus sampling (CVS) has enabled early prenatal diagnosis in the first trimester. The test is carried out at 10 weeks or after under ultrasound guidance whereby small amount of chorionic (placental) tissue is obtained for fetal karyotyping or DNA analysis for specific genetic defect (Figure 17.2). Rapid karyotyping from the direct preparation allows the fetal karyotype result to be available within 48 hours although interpretation can be difficult with confined placental mosaicism which has an occurrence rate of 1 to 2 percent. This is a phenomenon whereby the placenta and fetus has differing karyotypes and it is more often encountered with direct preparation than with CVS culture and amniocentesis. The procedure related miscarriage risk is about 1 percent.[7] Transabdominal technique is generally associated with lower risk of miscarriage as compared with the transcervical route.

Cordocentesis or Fetal Blood Sampling

Cordocentesis involves percutaneous cord blood sampling with a fine needle under ultrasound guidance (Figure 17.2). The umbilical vein at the placental cord insertion is the common target but other site for sampling may include the fetal intrahepatic umbilical vein. This procedure is usually performed at or after 20 weeks' gestation. The procedure-related fetal loss rate varies with the fetal condition with an overall fetal loss rate of about 1 percent in a normal fetus.

The indications for fetal blood sampling are becoming rare with the introduction of CVS but it allows rapid fetal karyotyping in cases of late presentation. Another indication for such procedure is the assessment of rhesus isoimmunization whereby *in utero* fetal transfusion may be carried out at the same time.

Fetoscopy

The introduction of small fiberoptic scopes into the amniotic cavity under ultrasound guidance allows direct visualization of the fetal external features for diagnosis of some congenital fetal skin diseases and some multiple malformation syndromes. This is now rarely performed with the advent of high-quality ultrasound imaging and 3-dimensional ultrasound technology.

Fetal Tissue Biopsies

Tissue biopsy is also rarely performed especially now with the advent of molecular technology whereby DNA analysis can usually replace for instance the need of liver and muscle biopsy in the diagnosis of rare enzyme deficiencies[8,9] and Duchenne muscular dystrophy[10] respectively. Fetal skin biopsy may be performed for the prenatal diagnosis of some congenital skin conditions[11] but as many of the responsible genes have been identified, PCR-based DNA analysis has superseded the need for skin biopsy.

COMMON FETAL ABNORMALITIES

Structural Malformations

Neural Tube Defects

Neural tube defects (NTDs) have been the most common major fetal structural malformations in most countries. However, the incidence has been reported to decrease with the introduction of periconceptual folic acid. The etiology is multifactorial with variable geographical preponderance.

NTDs include anencephaly, encephalocele and spina bifida. Anencephaly or absence of the cranial vault is lethal whilst the prognosis of encephalocele (skull defect usually involves the occipital bone) is determined by the severity of the defect. Spina bifida commonly affects the caudal end and the level of defect determines the severity of clinical presentations which range from paralysis of the lower legs to urinary and fecal incontinence. It may be associated with hydrocephalus and mental retardation. The risk of recurrence is about 5 to 10 percent when a parent or previous sibling has had NTD. Women on antiepileptic treatment or women with poorly controlled diabetes mellitus are also at risk of pregnancies with NTDs.

Women who were screened positive on mid-trimester serum α-fetoprotein screening would in the past be referred for amniocentesis whereby acetylcholinesterase assay from the amniotic fluid would be carried out to diagnose open NTDs. However, the advent of high-resolution ultrasound imaging has since superseded the place of amniocentesis for diagnosis. Anencephaly and encephaloceles can be detected by first trimester transabdominal or transvaginal ultrasound scan. Spina bifida, on other hand, may not be detected in the first trimester, but is diagnosed in the routine 18 to 20 weeks anomaly scan. 3D ultrasound may have a role in the diagnosis but 2D ultrasound provides more than 95 percent sensitivity in the detection of NTDs. The typical ultrasound features of spinal bifida include "lemon" shape of the fetal skull and/or "banana" shaped cerebellum.

Congenital Heart Defects (CHDs)

Cardiac abnormalities are the most common congenital abnormalities, representing about 10 percent of all congenital malformations, with ventricular septal defect being the most common CHDs. About 50 percent of these cardiac defects are major whilst the remaining 50 percent are asymptomatic. CHDs are responsible for more than half the deaths from lethal malformations of childhood. The etiology is mainly multifactorial and at least 90 percent of fetuses with CHD are from pregnancies without any risk factor although some are associated with chromosomal anomalies like Down syndrome. Pregnant women with poorly controlled diabetes mellitus or a family history of CHD are at increased risk of having babies with cardiac defects. Other predisposing factors to CHD include drugs like lithium and viral infection like rubella.

Ultrasound scan is the mainstay of diagnosis of CHD. The best time to perform fetal heart examination or fetal echocardiography is at 18 to 20 weeks' gestation. However, the sensitivity of prenatal detection of CHDs varies with the operator's skill and quality of the ultrasound scan machine. It has been shown that the detection rate of major cardiac defects is only 26 percent when using the four-chamber view alone.[12] Sensitivity can be raised up to 61 percent by additionally examining the outflow tracts, but this is highly dependent on the expertise of the sonographer.[12] Recently, increased fetal NT measurement at 10 to 14 weeks of gestation has been shown to be associated with chromosomally normal fetuses with major defects of the heart and great arteries.[13] Hence, the clinical implication is that fetuses with increased NT measurement should be referred for a fetal echocardiography performed by a specialist.

Chromosomal Abnormalities

Chromosomal abnormalities can be broadly be classified into aneuploidies and sex chromosomal abnormalities. The former implies abnormal numbers of chromosomes with trisomies being the most common. Most of the trisomies occur due to non-dysjunction in meiosis whereby paired members of chromosomes fail to separate from one another. This occurs more frequently with advanced maternal age. Rarely, trisomies may also arise from unbalanced translocations, in which part of one chromosome breaks off and attaches to another chromosome or mosaicism.

Most of the trisomies result in miscarriage in the first trimester except for trisomies 13 (Patau syndrome), 18 (Edward's syndrome) and 21 (Down syndrome).

Down Syndrome (Trisomy 21)

Down syndrome is the most common chromosomal anomaly at birth. Whilst trisomies 13 and 18 are generally associated with severe major structural abnormalities that can be diagnosed on routine anomaly scan and are incompatible with life, Down syndrome may not present with any structural anomalies on routine antenatal anomaly scan. The characteristic features of a Down individual include mental retardation, typical flat facies with protruding tongue, slanting of the eyelids with small skinfolds at the inner corner of the eyes, depressed nasal bridge and decreased muscle tone. Congenital heart defects also occur in about 40 percent of these individuals and they are at increased risk of childhood leukemia.

Fragile X Syndrome

This sex chromosomal anomaly is the second leading cause of mental retardation after Down syndrome, affecting about 1 in 1000 males and 1 in 2000 females. Approximately 2 to 6 percent of males and 2 to 4 percent of females with unexplained mental retardation carry the full fragile X mutation. The underlying pathology of this syndrome is caused by a mutation in the fragile X mental retardation (FMR)1 gene,[14] which is located on the long arm of the X chromosome. Individuals with fragile X syndrome have distinct behavioral and physical features, including mild-to-profound mental retardation, delayed language development, attention deficit-hyperactivity disorder, poor eye contact, short attention span, hand flapping and biting, and features of autism. Male subjects with the disorder typically have macro-orchidism in addition to a long face with prominent ears and jaw and hyperextensible joints.

Although the fragile X mutation gene is transmitted by a female, fragile X inheritance does not conform to the usual rules governing X-linked traits as there are asymptomatic transmitting males and a proportion of females who inherit the gene are also affected. Prenatal diagnosis has been developed using polymerase chain reaction technique for DNA analysis on chorionic villus and amniotic fluid cell samples.

Genetic Disorders (Table 17.7)

Hemoglobinopathies

Hemoglobinopathies are among the most common genetic disorders worldwide. These disorders are typically inherited as autosomal recessive disorders from parents who are healthy carriers. The most common disorders are the sickle cell disorders and the thalassemias.

Table 17.7: Examples of genetic disorders that can be diagnosed prenatally

Disorder	Inheritance
Thalassemia (α and β)	Autosomal recessive
Cystic fibrosis	Autosomal recessive
Hemophilia A	X-linked recessive
Sickle cell anemia	Autosomal recessive
Fragile X syndrome	X-linked
Congenital adrenal hyperplasia	Autosomal recessive
Duchenne type muscular dystrophy	X-linked recessive
Myotonic dystrophy	Autosomal dominant
Spinal muscular atrophy	Autosomal recessive
Familial retinoblastoma	Autosomal dominant

Thalassemia

Thalassemia is a common genetic blood disorder whereby defect in the synthesis of the globin chains results in red cells being formed with abnormal hemoglobin (Hb) content. The hemoglobin molecule consists of four globin chains, each of which is associated with a heme complex. There are basically three normal hemoglobins in man, HbA ($\alpha_2 \beta_2$), HbA$_2$ ($\alpha_2 \delta_2$) and HbF ($\alpha_2 \gamma_2$). The synthesis of the globin chains—alpha (α), beta (β), delta (δ) and gamma (γ) are under separate control. Normal adult Hb has more than 95 percent of HbA. The synthesis of α chain and β chain are under the control of four genes (two from each parent) and two genes (one from each parent) respectively.

There are two main groups of thalassemia, α- and β-thalassemias, depending on whether the defect occurs in α or β globin chain synthesis.

α-thalassemia is common in South-East Asians, especially among the Chinese. α^+-thalassemia (one defective genes on chromosome 16) and α^0-thalassemia (two defective genes) are the two carrier states of α-thalassemia (Figure 17.3). HbH is a form of α-thalassemia in which there is only one functional α gene. α-thalassemia major or HbBarts (γ_4) in which there are no functional α genes present, is incompatible with life and fetuses with this defect usually develop hydrops *in utero*.

Normal adult Hb
(4 functional genes):-
> 95% HbA
HbA2 1.5-3.5%
HbF <1%

$\alpha+$- that trait (1 defective gene)

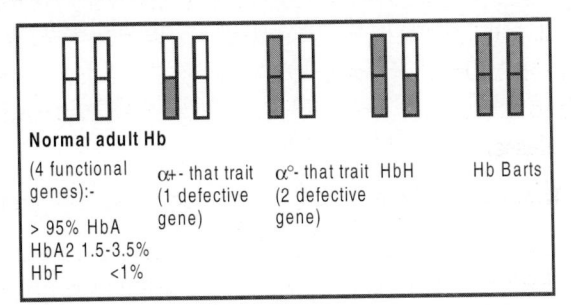

α°- that trait (2 defective gene)

HbH

Hb Barts

Figure 17.3: Types of α-thalassemia based on genotype and hemoglobin pattern

β-thalassemia, unlike α-thalassemia, rarely arises from the complete loss of a β globin gene. The β globin gene is present, but produces little β globin protein with varied degree of suppression. In some cases, the affected gene makes essentially no β globin protein (β^0-thalassemia). In other cases, the production of β chain protein is just lower than normal (β^+-thalassemia). The severity of β thalassemia depends in part on the type of β-thalassemic genes that a person has inherited. β-thalassemia is common in the Mediterranean, Middle Eastern, Indian and South East Asian. Over 160 different β thalassemia mutations have been identified and usually a given ethnic group possesses specific mutations. If both parents are β-thalassemia carriers (β-thalassemia minor), as in other autosomal recessive disorders, the offspring has a 25 percent chance of acquiring β-thalassemia major whereby the child would be anemic requiring regular transfusion and also would run the risk of the complications of iron overload.

Routine full blood count with red blood indices is a useful screening test for thalassemia. Both α- and β-thalassemia carriers may not have low hemoglobin count but will usually present with significantly or mildly decreased mean corpuscular volume (MCV) and mean corpuscular hemoglobin (MCH). The screening and management of women with thalassemia in pregnancy is summarized in Figure 17.4.

Sickle cell disorder

Sickle cell disorder is a hemoglobin variant of the β globin chain whereby one amino acid is replaced by another. Hemoglobin carries oxygen to the various organs of the body. In sickle cell anemia (homozygous HbSS) the hemoglobin assumes a sickle shape following the release of oxygen. This abnormal shape causes the cells to clump together making their passage through smaller blood vessels difficult called sickling resulting in sickle cell crisis. Symptoms of the condition are rarely apparent before the age of 6 months.

Sickle cell trait is not to be confused with sickle cell anemia. It occurs when a person inherits the usual hemoglobin from one parent and sickle hemoglobin from the other (HbAS). The trait itself rarely causes health problems, though it may occasionally cause blood to appear in the urine and special attention is required when having an operation or needing an anesthetic. This disorder is commonly seen in the African-Caribbean or Mediterranean.

Sickle cell carriers can be detected with solubility testing, on peripheral smear, and on hemoglobin

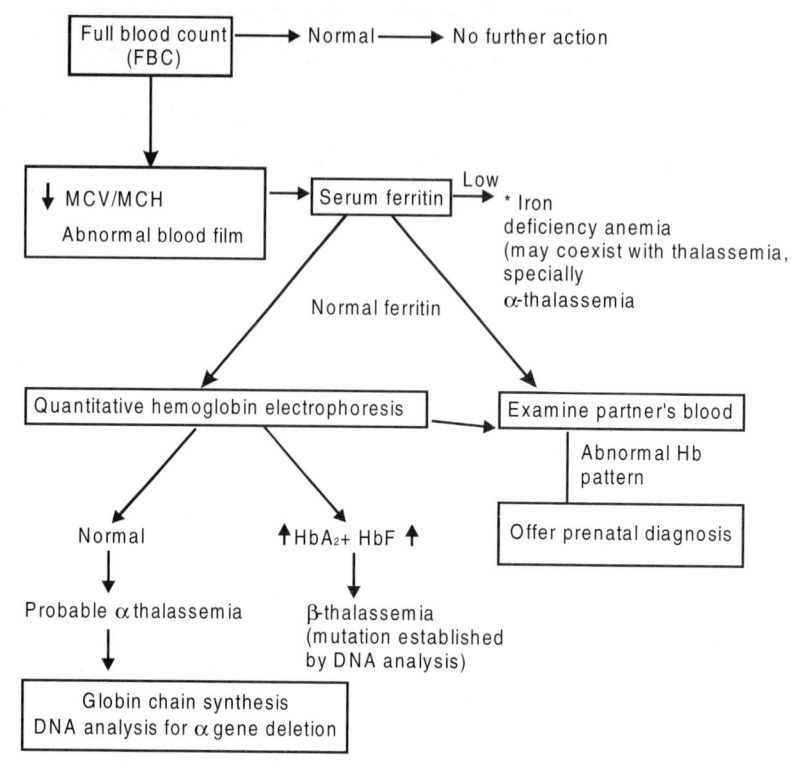

Figure 17.4: Flow chart showing summry on screening and management of thalassemia in pregnancy

electrophoresis. Prenatal diagnosis is now possible by DNA analysis.

Cystic Fibrosis (CF)

Cystic fibrosis is the most common lethal genetic disease of childhood in Caucasians. Manifestations of this disease relate not only to the disruption of exocrine function of the pancreas but also to intestinal glands, biliary tree, bronchial glands (resulting in chronic bronchopulmonary infection with emphysema) and sweat glands (resulting in high sweat electrolyte with depletion in a hot environment). Despite advances in treatment, there is no cure for CF. Majority of CF related deaths are a result of pulmonary complications. CF has great phenotypic variations with multiple, different mutations. The responsible gene, the CF transmembrane conductance regulator (CFTR), has been mapped to chromosome 7 and more than 600 mutations and DNA sequence variations have been identified in the CFTR gene. However, the Delta F508 mutation is found in about 70 percent of CF.

Prenatal diagnosis is offered to couples who are carriers or who had a previously affected child.

Congenital Viral and Parasitic Infections

Primary maternal viral and parasitic infection is generally uncommon but fetal infection with rubella, cytomegalovirus (CMV), toxoplasmosis, varicella and parvovirus as a result can have potentially serious effects on the fetus (Table 17.8). Antenatal presentations may vary from confirmed maternal viral infection on serological test or incidental detection of abnormalities like hydrops or ventriculomegaly on ultrasound (Table 17.8).

With the introduction of rubella immunization program, CMV has become the most common congenital viral infection worldwide. Congenital CMV infection occurs in about 1 percent of all live births in developed countries and in an even higher rate in developing countries. Generally, the highest risk for symptomatic fetal infection with fetal damage is among infants born to mothers who have had primary infection during early pregnancy. Transmission risk to

Table 17.8: Characteristics of the common congenital infections

Infective agent	Maternal infection and risk of fetal infection	Features congenital infection
Rubella	• Fetal infection in 1st trimester: highest risk of fetal damage	• Cataracts, hearing loss, mental retardation; heart defects • IUGR, hepatomegaly, thrombocytopenia
CMV	• <26 weeks: greatest risk of severe fetal infection • 90% of infected fetus are asymptomatic at birth but 10-15% will develop sequelae later in life	• Microcephaly, ventriculomegaly, cerebral calcification; hydrops • Heart defects; IUGR, hepatomeagly, thrombocytopenia • Mental retardation, cerebral palsy, hearing loss
Varicella	• ≤ 20 weeks: risk of fetal damage is greatest (2%) [15]	• Scarring with a dermatomal distribution; eye defects • Hypoplasia of bone/ muscle of limb; neurologic abnormalities
Toxoplasmosis	• 24-30 weeks: transmission risk to fetus highest • 1st trimester fetal infection: highest risk of fetal damage	• As for congenital CMV infection
Parvovirus	• First half of pregnancy: 10% excess fetal loss; 3% with hydrops fetalis; 90% healthy child	• Aplastic anemia; fetal hydrops; fetal demise (rare)

fetus is also generally highest in early pregnancy with the exception of toxoplasmosis where transmission risk to fetus is highest when women contract the parasite early in their third trimester of pregnancy although clinical fetal damage is highest if fetal infection occurs in the 1st trimester (Table 17.8).

The only definitive prevention of congenital viral or parasitic infections is the prevention of infection in the mother, best obtained by vaccination like in the case of rubella vaccination. There are no vaccines available against most of the perinatally transmitted viruses except for rubella. The development of CMV vaccine is underway but the effectiveness and safety is yet to be established. There is no therapy for established viral infection in the fetus, with the exception of symptomatic treatment by *in utero* transfusion for parvovirus B19 anemia. Antepartum screening for toxoplasma infection as carried out in countries with high prevalence of Toxoplasmosis, like France and Austria, allows consideration of antepartum chemoprophylaxis to reduce the severity of congenital toxoplasmosis. The effectiveness of antenatal antiparasitic treatment in women with presumed toxoplasmosis in the reduction of the congenital transmission of *Toxoplasma gondii* is undetermined[16] but antenatal treatment has been shown to significantly reduce the severity of congenital toxoplasmosis.[17]

Infections which occur early *in utero*, such as rubella, CMV, and varicella are amenable to prenatal diagnosis by PCR technique assay on amniotic fluid or even fetal body cavity and fetal blood and hence overcoming the drawbacks of serology and culture (parvovirus cannot be cultured). However, fetal prognosis is difficult to establish in cases of confirmed infections. In addition, these diagnostic facilities may not be freely available.

FUTURE DEVELOPMENT

3-Dimensional Ultrasound

In additional to 3-Dimensional ultrasound imaging,[18] realtime 3D has also been developed whereby dynamic 3D fetal echocardiography can be performed. Although there may be advantages in using the 3D technique, its diagnostic significance had not been evaluated.

Magnetic Resonance Imaging (MRI)

Fetal MRI[18] has been used to differentiate intracerebral lesions and fetal chest malformations as well as estimation of fetal organ volume. As with 3D ultrasound, the clinical value has not been determined.

Multicolor FISH

This new FISH technique employs the application of combinatorial labeling to enable simultaneous detection of all 24 human chromosomes in individual cells. Multicolor FISH is capable of not only identifying the gene-expressing segments of chromosomes of marker chromosomes but also translocations, insertions, and cryptic chromosome abnormalities (i.e. chromosome rearrangements) not visible using light microscopy.[19]

Comparative Genome Hybridization (CGH)

This is a new robust FISH method that enables the comprehensive analysis of the gain or loss of chromosome material. CGH has been successfully applied in the genomic analysis of products of conception after spontaneous miscarriage or following surgical evacuation because it does not require fetal tissues to be viable and it can be applied to DNA from archival clinical materials.[19]. CGH analysis has also been shown to be effective in detecting confined mosaicism in all placental tissues. Another advantage of CGH over the conventional FISH technique is that it does not require DNA probes or any prior indication of the chromosome or region of interest.

Fetal DNA in Maternal Circulation

Successful FISH testing of nucleated fetal red blood cells for determination and prenatal noninvasive diagnosis of chromosomal disorders has been reported.[19] The potential applications of fetal DNA in maternal plasma include the investigation of sex-linked disorders and fetal rhesus D status determination.

Recently cell-free fetal DNA has been found to be present in much higher fractional concentrations than fetal nucleated cells in maternal plasma. This opens up a new field of investigation and provides a potentially easily accessible source of fetal genetic material for prenatal diagnosis. The existence of circulating cell-free fetal DNA in maternal plasma provides a new source of fetal genetic material for noninvasive prenatal diagnosis.

Preimplantation Genetic Diagnosis (PGD)[20]

It is a new tool for genetically investigating embryos prior to implantation. PGD involves *in vitro* fertilization or intracytoplasmic sperm injection followed by removal of one or two cells from an embryo at the eight-cell stage. DNA is amplified by polymerase chain reaction and analysed for abnormalities by one of several techniques, one of the most common of which is fluorescence *in situ* hybridization. It is used to diagnose single gene defects, such as cystic fibrosis and thalassemia, and also for diagnosis of chromosome disorders. PGD has also been used for evaluation of couples who have recurrent *in vitro* fertilization failure or habitual spontaneous abortion.

In contrast to traditional methods of prenatal diagnosis, couples undergoing PGD minimise the risk to face the difficult decision whether or not to terminate a pregnancy.

IMPORTANT TERMS

Cytogenetic Analysis or Karyotyping

Amniocytes, chorionic villus cells or circulating blood lymphocytes obtained from the amniotic fluid, placenta or fetal blood respectively by invasive prenatal diagnostic procedures are cultured in the laboratory until enough cells in mitosis are available for chromosomal analysis. Mitosis is then arrested at metaphase when each chromosome has replicated into two chromatids attached at the centromere. The cells, which are spread onto slides, are then stained. Chromosomes from single cells are usually photographed and their images are then cut out and pasted onto a piece of paper, forming a karyotype. Computer imaging can now be used to produce visual display of the karyotype. With chorionic villus samples that are rich in cells in mitosis, a "direct" analysis in 24 to 48 hours is feasible which is adequate to exclude abnormal numbers of chromosomes or aneuploidy. However, this is not adequate for the detection of chromosomal aberrations such as deletion or inversions.

Mosaicism

This occurs when a person has more than one type of chromosomal make-up. In Down syndrome, for instance, mosaicism means that some cells of the body have trisomy 21, and some have the typical number of chromosomes. In addition, whilst mosaicism can occur in just one cell line (e.g. some blood cells have trisomy 21 and the rest do not), it can also occur across cell lines (e.g. skin cells may have trisomy 21 while other cell lines do not).

DNA (Deoxyribonucleic Acid) Analysis

Analysis with the use of DNA specific probe for the diagnosis of conditions like fragile X syndrome, sickle cell disease, thalassemia can now be carried out. Chorionic villus samples are especially rich in fetal DNA material.

Polymerase Chain Reaction (PCR)

This is a technique in molecular biology whereby a small fragment of DNA can be rapidly cloned or duplicated to produce multiple DNA copies. PCR can be used to identify individuals from minute amounts of tissue or blood to diagnose genetic diseases.

The supplies necessary for carrying out PCR are available in a kit form. It is important to emphasize that PCR is not flawless. The use of PCR requires great care. The main concern is contamination. PCR is so sensitive that it is possible to accidentally multiply minute amounts of contaminating DNA.

FISH (Fluorescent *in situ* Hybridization)

FISH is rapidly becoming an integral part of prenatal diagnostic programs. This technique employs a variety of chromosome-specific and single-gene specific DNA probes with fluorescent tags to identify the organization of genes and to look for deletions, rearrangements and duplications of the chromosomes. Rapid (within 6 to 8 hours) accurate diagnosis of some major chromosomal abnormalities is now possible using commercially available DNA probes specific for chromosome 13, 18, 21, X and Y on direct chorionic villus samples, amniotic fluid and fetal blood. However, in the presence of maternal cell contamination misdiagnosis is a possibility.

REFERENCES

1. Howe DT, Gornall R, Welleslay D, Boyle T, Barber J: Six-year survey of screening for Down syndrome by maternal age and mid trimester ultrasound scans. *British Medical Journal* **320(7235)**: 606-10, 2000.
2. Pandya PP, Snijders RJ, Johnson SP, De Lourdes Brizot, Nicolaides KH: Screening for fetal trisomies by maternal age and fetal nuchal translucency thickness at 10 to 14 weeks of gestation. *British Journal of Obstetrics and Gynecology* **102(12)**: 957-62, 1996.
3. Tolmie JL: Chromosome disorders. In: Whittle MJ, Connor JM (Eds): *Prenatal Diagnosis in Obstetric Practice*. 2nd edn, Blackwell Science Ltd, Oxford, 34- 57, 1995.
4. Smith-Bindman R, Hosmer W, Feldstein VA, Deeks JJ, Goldberg JD: Second-trimester ultrasound to detect fetuses with Down syndrome: A meta-analysis. *The Journal of the American Medical Association* **285(8)**: 1044-55, 2001.
5. Neilson JP: Routine ultrasonography in early pregnancy. In: Neilson JP, Keirse MJNC, Crowther C, Hofmyer J, Hodnett C (Eds): *Pregnancy and Childbirth Module of the Cochrane Database of Systemic Reviews*. The Cochrane Collaboration. (Disk and CD-Rom) Issue 3, Oxford, 1996.
6. Spencer K, Souter V, Tul N, Snijders R and Nicolaides KH: A screening program for Trisomy 21 at 10 to 14 weeks using fetal nuchal translucency, maternal serum free beta-human chorionic gonadotropin and pregnancy-associated plasma protein–A. *Ultrasound in Obstetrics and Gynecology* **13(4)**: 231-37, 1999.
7. MRC Working Party on the Evaluation of Chorionic Villus Sampling. Medical Research Council European trial of chorion villus sampling. *Lancet* 1491-99, 1991.
8. Lam CW, Sin SY, Lau ET, Lam YY, Poon P, Tong SF: Prenatal diagnosis of glycogen storage disease type 1b using denaturing high performance liquid chromatography. *Prenatal Diagnosis* **20(9)**: 765-68, 2000.
9. Marie S, Flipsen JW, Duran M, Poll-The BT, Beemer FA, Bosschaart AN, Vincent MF and Van den Berghe G: Prenatal diagnosis in adenylosuccinate lyase deficiency. *Prenatal Diagnosis* **20(1)**: 33-36, 2000.
10. Nevo Y, Shomrat R, Yaron Y, Orr-Urtreger A, Harel S, Legum C: Fetal muscle biopsy as a diagnostic tool in Duchenne muscular dystrophy. *Prenatal Diagnosis* **19(10)**: 921-26, 1999.
11. Schimizu H, Suzumori K: Prenatal diagnosis as a test for genodermatoses: its past, present and future. *Journal of Dermatology Science* **19(1)**:1-8, 1999.
12. Tulzer G: Fetal cardiology. *Current Opinion in Pediatrics* **12(5)**:492-96, 2000.
13. Hyett J, Perdu M, Sharland G, Snijders R, Nicolaides KH: Using fetal nuchal translucency to screen for major congenital cardiac defects at 10-14 weeks of gestation: Population based cohort study. *British Medical Journal* **318(7176)**: 81–85, 1999.
14. de Vries Bert B A, Halley DJJ, Oostra BA, Niermeijer, MF: The fragile X syndrome. *Journal of Medical Genetics* **35(7)**:579-89, 1998.
15. Pastuszak AL, Levy M, Schick B, Zuber C, Feldkamp M, Gladstone J, Bar-Levy F, Jackson E,. Donnenfeld A, Meschino W, Koren G: Outcome after maternal varicella infection in the first 20 weeks of pregnancy. *New England Journal of Medicine* **330(13)**:901-05, 1994.
16. Wallon M, Liou C, Garner P et al: Congenital toxoplasmosis: Systematic review of evidence of efficacy of treatment in pregnancy. *BMJ* **318**: 1511–14, 1999.
17. Foulon W, Villena I, Stray-Pedersen B et al: Treatment of toxoplasmosis during pregnancy: A multicenter study of impact on fetal transmission and children's sequelae at age 1 year. *Am J Obstet Gynecol* **180**: 410–15, 1999.
18. Ogle RF and Rodeck CH: Novel fetal imaging techniques. *Current Opinion in Obstetrics and Gynecology* **10(2)**: 109-15, 1998.
19. Pergament E: The application of fluorescence *in situ* hybridization to prenatal diagnosis. *Current Opinion in Obstetrics and Gynecology* **12(2)**:73-76, 2000.
20. Hanson C, Jakobsson AH, Sjogren A, Lundin K, Nilsson L, Wahlstrom J, Hardarson T, Stevic J, Darnfors C, Janson PO, Wikland M, Hamberger L: Preimplantation genetic diagnosis (PGD): The Gothenburg experience. *Acta Obstetricia et Gynecologica Scandinavica* **80(4)**:331-36, 2001.

18.
Anemia in Pregnancy

Shripad Hebbar

PART TWO — Feto-maternal Medicine

INTRODUCTION

Anemia in pregnancy is a major health problem in developing countries. More than two-thirds of pregnant women in India are anemic and most of the times it is due to deficiency of iron and folic acid. Study of anemia in pregnancy is important because it is directly or indirectly responsible for maternal deaths (20-30%)[1,2] and it is associated with high perinatal loss. Anemic patients have poor tolerance for potential blood loss during delivery and are poor subjects for surgery. For this purpose, screening for anemia is routine in all antenatal clinics.

According to WHO (1975), the pregnancy anemia is defined as hemoglobin level below 11 gm/dl as this cannot be explained by physiological hemodilution that occurs in pregnancy. If this cut off value is considered 40 to 80 percent of pregnant women in India and neighboring countries are anemic.[3] It has been observed that the pregnant women in India do well when Hb per cent is above 10 gm/dl and levels below this value may be accepted to consider them as anemic. For the purpose of management, anemia in pregnancy is arbitrarily classified as mild (8.7 to 10 gm/dl), moderate (6.6 to 8.6 gm/dl) and severe (6.5 gm/dl and below).[4]

PHYSIOLOGICAL CONSIDERATIONS

There is striking increase of blood volume during pregnancy. This rise starts at about 8 weeks of gestation and reaches its maximum at 32 to 36 weeks—a mean value of 85 mL/kg.[5] There is disproportionate rise in plasma volume (50%), compared to red cell volume (30%) resulting in physiological hemodilution. This results in fall in Hb percent by 2 gm/dl in later half of pregnancy.

The erythropoiesis is accelerated during pregnancy resulting in increased number of circulating RBCs. The bone marrow is hyperplastic. There is a gradual rise in red cell volume reaching 20 to 30 percent above non-pregnant values at term.

IRON DYNAMICS IN PREGNANCY

Iron is an essential constituent of the body, being necessary for formation of hemoglobin and for oxidative processes of living tissues. The body contains about 4 gm of iron most of which is present as hemoglobin (70%).[6]

Good dietary sources of heme iron are animal products such as meat; non-heme iron is found in fresh leafy vegetables, lentils, legumes and beans. Iron is poorly absorbed by mouth and administration with food may further impair the absorption. Compounds containing calcium and magnesium, including antacids, mineral supplements, bicarbonates, carbonates, oxalates, phytates, or phosphates may impair the absorption of iron by forming insoluble complexes. Some agents such as ascorbic acid and citric acid may actually increase the absorption of iron.

Iron is absorbed mainly in the duodenum and jejunum. The absorption is aided by the acid secretion of the stomach and is more readily affected when the iron is in ferrous state or it is a part of heme complex. Absorption is also increased in conditions of iron deficiency or in the fasting state but decreased if the body stores are overloaded. The usual diet contains 15 to 20 mg of iron.[6] Only about 5 to 15 percent of this, is normally absorbed. Following absorption, the majority of the iron is bound to transferrin and is transported to the bone marrow, where it is incorporated into hemoglobin (70%); the reminder is contained in the storage forms: ferritin or hemosiderin or as myoglobin (29%), with smaller amounts occurring in the heme containing enzymes or in plasma bound to transferrin (0.2%)[7]. The majority of iron released after destruction of RBC is reused (Table 18.1).

Table 18.1: Distribution of iron

Location	Form	Distribution(%)
1. Hemoglobin iron		• 70
2. Tissue iron		• 29
• Storage iron	• Hemosiderin	
	• Ferritin	
• Essential iron	• Myoglobin	
	• Enzymes	
	• Cytochromes	
	• Peroxidases	
	• Catalases	
3. Plasma transport iron	• Transferrin	• 0.19

Apart from hemorrhage, iron is mainly lost from the body in the feces, urine, from skin and sweat, but the total loss is very small. Iron is also lost in small amount in the breast milk and in menstrual blood. This loss is replaced by the absorption of about 1 to 1.5 mg of iron daily (Figure 18.1).[6]

In pregnancy the demand for iron is increased to meet mainly the needs of expanded red cell mass (450 to 500 mg) and, to a lesser extent, the requirements

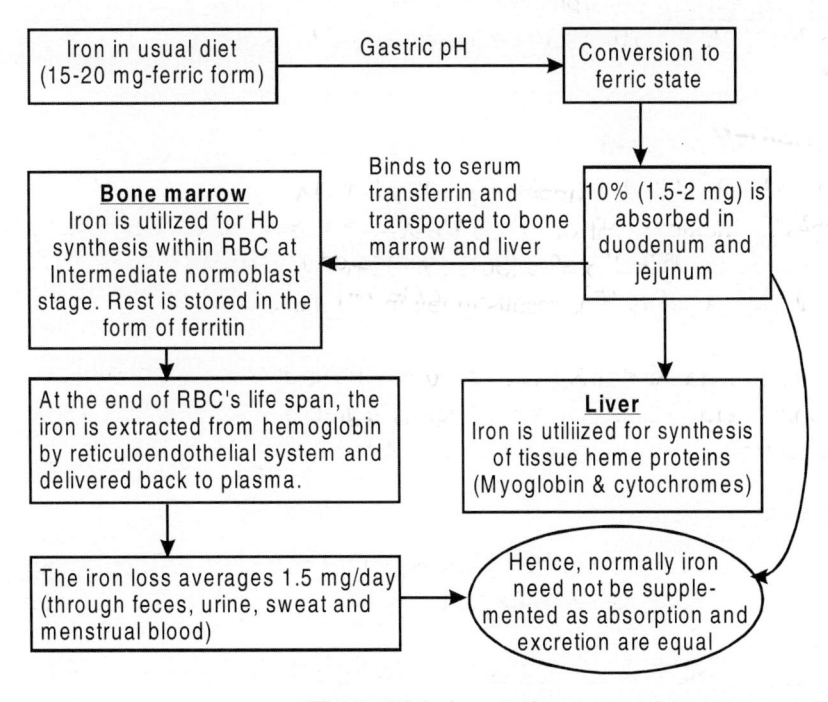

Figure 18.1: Iron cycle

of the developing fetus and placenta (400 mg). In addition, variable amount of iron is lost following delivery of placenta (100 ml of blood loss is equivalent to 50 mg of iron). However, due to pregnancy, iron loss through menstruation is suspended. In total, the iron requirement is around 950 to 1100 mg during pregnancy (Table 18.2). The fetus derives its iron from the maternal serum by active transport across the placenta predominantly in the later half of gestation. Hence, the requirement of iron rises from 2.8 mg in non-pregnant state to 6.6 mg/day especially in third trimester of pregnancy. This can be met only by additional supplementation of iron.[7]

Table 18.2: Iron requirements in pregnancy

Required for	mg
• Red cell expansion	450-500
• Fetus and placenta	400
• Blood loss at delivery	100-200
• External iron loss (in sweat, urine and feces)	300
Total requirement	950-1100
Iron saved due to amenorrhea	300
Net requirement	950-1100

CLASSIFICATION OF ANEMIA IN PREGNANCY

Anemia in pregnancy can be due to the followings:
1. Lack of production of blood (hemopoietic)
   a. Iron deficiency
   b. Folic acid deficiency
   c. Protein deficiency
   d. Combined deficiency
2. Blood loss (hemorrhagic)
   a. Bleeding during pregnancy
   b. Hookworm infestation
3. Increased breakdown of RBCs (hemolytic)
   a. Malaria
   b. Sickle cell disease
   c. Hemoglobinopathies
4. Decreased production (very rare)
   a. Aplastic anemia
   b. Myelosuppression

As such iron and folic acid deficiency are very common and hence will be discussed in detail.

Iron Deficiency Anemia in Pregnancy

Causes of Increased Prevalence

- Poor intake
  - Diet deficient in iron containing foods
  - Vomiting in pregnancy
- Poor absorption
  - Presence of phosphates, phytates
  - Increased pH of gastric juice (achlorhydria)
  - Ferric ions in the gut instead of ferrous form
  - Lack of vitamin C
- Increased utilization
  - Demands of pregnancy more if multiple pregnancy
- Excessive iron loss
  - Repeated pregnancies, especially at short intervals
  - Menorrhagia prior to pregnancy
  - Hookworm infestation
  - Chronic malaria

In addition, chronic infections and intestinal malabsorption also contribute to development of anemia. Presence of asymptomatic bacteriuria may also impair erythropoiesis during pregnancy.

Another problem posed by anemia in pregnancy in tropics is its polymorphism. Pregnancy tends to interfere with maternal erythropoiesis by competing for the available raw materials such as folic acid, vit B_{12} and proteins apart from iron.

Clinical Features

The symptoms are of gradual onset. They include fatigue, lassitude, anorexia, and breathlessness on exertion, dizziness, headache, insomnia, palpitation and dyspepsia. On examination, there is varying degree of pallor of skin and mucous membranes, tachycardia and swelling of legs, glossitis and stomatitis. In chronic cases, koilonychia may be present. A soft systolic murmur in mitral area and crepitations at the base of the lungs may be present.

Maternal and Fetal Consequences

There is evidence indicating that pregnancy induced hypertension, abruptio placenta[8] and puerperal venous thrombosis occur more frequently in patients with iron deficiency or megaloblastic anemia. Maternal risks are also increased because of inability to withstand hemorrhage, susceptibility to infection and development of heart failure if anemia is severe. Studies have shown that stillbirths and preterm labor[9,10] are more common in anemic mothers. Though the neonate will not be anemic at birth if there is little or no reserve iron, anemia develops rapidly in neonatal period. There is a close relationship between maternal hemoglobin levels and the birth weight of infants. There is also a higher incidence of small for date infants.[11]

Diagnosis

Iron deficiency anemia *per se* is diagnosed by (Table 18.3):

a. Appearance of microcytic-hypochromic erythrocytes in peripheral smear.
b. Low serum iron (less than 60 μg/dl) accompanied by a high total iron binding capacity (over 300 μg/dl) or transferrin saturation of only 15 percent or less.
c. Lack of stainable iron in an otherwise normal bone marrow.
d. Low serum ferritin (less than 12 μg/L)
e. Response to iron therapy

Table 18.3: Normal blood values in pregnancy

Contents	Ranges
Hemoglobin (Hb)	>11 g/dl
Hematocrit (Hct/PCV)	32-36%
Mean corpuscular volume (PCV)	85 ± 9 μm³
Mean corpuscular hemoglobin (MCH)	28 ± 3 pg
Mean corpuscular hemoglobin concentration (MCHC)	33 ± 3 g/dl
Serum iron	75 μg/dl
Total iron binding capacity (TIBC)	300-400 μg/dl
Saturation percentage (serum iron/TIBC)	16-60%
Serum folate	6-12 μg/L
RBC folate	165-760 μg/L
Serum B$_{12}$	190-950 μg/L

Appropriate investigations should be undertaken to detect the cause. Stool examination should be carried out to detect worm infestation and to rule out occult blood loss. Routine examination of urine is essential and culture and sensitivity should be obtained in cases of suspected urinary tract infection. Appropriate investigations should be carried out to diagnose malaria, pulmonary tuberculosis and kala azar in endemic areas.

Prognosis

If detected early and appropriate treatment is instituted, both maternal and fetal prognosis is good. However, if patient present with severe anemia with congestive cardiac failure and left uncared for, maternal mortality may result. As stated earlier, anemia either directly or indirectly contributes to 20 to 30 percent of maternal deaths in third world countries.

Prevention

Every woman needs iron supplementation during pregnancy. Govt of India has evolved National Anemia Prophylaxis Programme which is operational since 1972 and it is aimed at distribution of iron tablets containing 60 mg of elemental iron and 500 μg of folic acid daily during last 100 days of pregnancy. Patient should be educated regarding role of balanced diet rich in iron and folates. Adequate measures should be undertaken to eradicate dysentery, malaria, bleeding piles, urinary tract infection and of course, hookworm and other worm infestations. Every effort should be made to detect anemia at the earliest. Hemoglobin estimation should be carried out at least four times in pregnancy; at first antenatal visit, about 24 to 26 weeks' gestation, between 32nd and 34th weeks (period of maximum hemodilution) and finally before term.[12]

Treatment

The mainstay of treatment includes
1. Oral iron therapy
2. Parenteral iron therapy
3. Blood transfusion

The main aim of therapy is to achieve hemoglobin of at least 10 gm/dl at term. It is important to remember that in the first week following iron therapy, there is no rise in hemoglobin; only a reticulocytosis[6] is observed. Hemoglobin starts rising only from the second week onward by 1 gm/dl/week. If the desired hemoglobin rise is unlikely to be achieved by term, like those who present in late pregnancy with moderate to severe anemia, blood transfusion must be considered.

Oral iron therapy

The preferred route of administration of iron is oral, usually as ferrous salts (ferrous sulfate, ferrous gluconate, ferrous fumarate etc). One tablet will provide approximately 60 mg of elemental iron and it should be administered three times daily. The response to this dosage is fast, and is evidenced by significant increase in reticulocyte count within 5 to 10 days of initiation of therapy. There is significant rise in hemoglobin concentration by 0.1 to 0.2 gm/dl/day starting from the second week of treatment. Hemoglobin rises by 2 gm/dl over a period of 3 to 4 weeks.[6]

However, there are certain disadvantages with oral iron therapy. The absorption may be affected by several factors mentioned earlier and hemoglobin may not rise as expected. Hence, oral iron therapy should be reserved for those cases of mild to moderate anemia remote from term.

Another problem with oral iron therapy is gastrointestinal intolerance in about 10 percent of cases. The most common side effects are nausea, vomiting, constipation, abdominal cramping and diarrhea. Since these side effects are dose related, the treatment of choice is to reduce the dose to tolerable limits. Another useful maneuver is to give iron pill with meals rather than after meals. Although this decreases the amount of iron that is absorbed and prolongs the time necessary to achieve normalization of hemotological indices, it is frequently the only way to continue treatment.

Oral iron therapy is generally continued until hemoglobin concentration reach normal values, which may take some weeks and then for a further 3 months or more to restore body iron stores. Parenteral iron therapy should be considered in those cases who cannot tolerate oral iron therapy or when the compliance is not good.

Parenteral iron therapy

Two compounds are available for use:
1. Iron dextran (Imferon).
2. Iron sorbitol (Jectofer).

Of the two, iron dextran is more widely used. Commercially available preparation contains 100 mg of elemental iron in 2 ml ampoule. It can be given both intravenously and intramuscularly.

The total dosage is calculated according to the hemoglobin concentration and body weight of the patient; allowance is also made for additional iron to replenish iron stores. Dosages can be calculated from one of the following formulae:[13]

[(Normal Hb - Patient's Hb) × Weight(kg) × 2.21] + 1000 = Milligrams of iron needed.

For example, the iron required by a pregnant woman with a hemoglobin concentration of 7 gm/dl and a weight of 50 kg is:

[(14-7) × 50 × 2.21] + 1000 = approx 1775 mg.

Another simpler formula easier to remember is to give 250 mg of elemental iron for each gram of hemoglobin below normal. In the hypothetical case just mentioned the calculation is:

250 mg × 7 = 1750 mg.

The preferred site for intramuscular injection is upper and outer quadrant of the buttock deep into the gluteal muscle. After intramuscular injection iron dextran is absorbed preliminarily through lymphatic systems, about 60 percent is absorbed after 3 days and upto 90 percent after 1 to 3 weeks.[6] The reticuloendothelial cells gradually separate iron from iron dextran complex. Absorption of drug inadvertently deposited in subcutaneous tissue may take months or even year. Seepage of drug along the needle tract into subcutaneous tissue also causes ugly staining of the skin and painful subcutaneous inflammation. This could be avoided by:[14]

- Ensuring that the needle surface does not have any iron dextran solution
- Using the Z technique (i.e. the subcutaneous tissue is drawn to one side before the needle is inserted) so that the needle tract is zigzag and
- Injecting 1.0 ml of saline after the iron solution is injected

After initial test dose of 1 ml, the injections are given daily or on alternate days in doses of 2 ml intramuscularly till the total dose is reached. However, 10 to 15 percent of women develop fever, myalgia or arthralgia and 1 to 2 percent have arthritis, 7 to 15 days after initiation of IM iron therapy.[15] These respond readily to commonly used analgesics; but once the symptoms develop, the majority of women refuse to take the remaining doses of IM iron. In these cases intravenous iron therapy may be considered. However, these days intravenous iron therapy is becoming obsolete.

The main advantage of intravenous therapy is the certainty of its administration to correct the hemoglobin deficit and to fix up the store iron. It eliminates repeated and painful intramuscular injections and the treatment is completed in a day, at the maximum two and patient is discharged much earlier from the hospital.

Severe anaphylactoid reactions may occur after administration of iron dextran and fatalities have been reported. Hence, intravenous iron should be given only in those institutions where all facilities for emergency resuscitation are readily available. Some patients may develop peripheral vascular flushing, tachycardia, hypotension and syncope. *Thrombophlebitis* may occur at the site of injection, although the incidence is reduced by administering iron dextran in sodium chloride 0.9 percent rather than glucose 5 percent.

In total dose infusion, the iron requirement is calculated as outlined earlier. It is mixed with 500 ml of 0.9 percent sodium chloride. The initial rate for 0.5 ml test dose should not exceed 5 drops per minute and if this is well tolerated the rate of infusion may be increased gradually to 45 to 60 drops per minute. Patient should be closely observed for adverse reactions.

Iron sorbitol (Jectofer) injection is less painful. It should not be administered intravenously. Single intramuscular dose should not exceed 100 mg. There may be severe systemic reactions with cardiac complications, which may be fatal, such as complete atrio-ventricular block, ventricular tachycardia, or ventricular fibrillation. A transient metallic taste or loss of taste sensation may occur.

Place of blood transfusion

All patients with severe anemia (Hemoglobin less than 6 gm/dl)[4] should be hospitalized for blood transfusion, especially when they present in later weeks of pregnancy. Those who fail to respond to iron, folic acid and vit B_{12} therapy and those who need surgery are also candidates for blood transfusion. Not only there is dramatic response in oxygen carrying capacity of the blood; erythropoiesis too, is stimulated. Patient should be closely observed for transfusion reactions and signs of circulatory overload. As a routine diuretic (frusemide 20 mg) should be administered intramuscularly prior to blood transfusion to produce negative fluid balance. Packed cell or exchange transfusion must be considered when cardiac failure is present.

Management during Labor

Patient should be confined to bed with a position comfortable to her. Adequate amount of cross-matched fresh blood should be available on demand. Maternal oxygenation helps to reduce fetal hypoxia. Strict asepsis should be maintained to prevent puerperal sepsis. Delay in second stage of labor should be curtailed by prophylactic forceps. Prophylactic administration of methyl ergometrine 0.2 mg helps in minimizing blood loss. However, it is contraindicated if congestive cardiac failure is present. If there is a tendency for postpartum hemorrhage and patient is likely to go into shock methyl ergometrine should not be withheld. Administration of prostaglandin PGF2α (Prostodin) 250 μg may be considered, if administration of methergin is feared or if contraindications to methyl ergometrine are present.

Management of Puerperium

Patient should be closely observed for development of infection, congestive cardiac failure and puerperal venous thrombosis. Blood transfusion in puerperium is considered only if there is severe anemia. Patient should be discharged with appropriate contraceptive advice and hematinics.

Megaloblastic Anemia

Megaloblastic anemia is the second most common cause of nutritional anemias seen in tropics; contributing to 3 to 4 percent of all anemias seen during pregnancy. Incidence is more common in multiparae (5 times than non-pregnant) and in multiple gestation (8 times more common).[16] Though folic acid and vit B_{12} deficiency cause same clinical picture, the deficiency of former is more prevalent. Vit B_{12} has longer storage life and as such its deficiency is rare. It occurs usually after 40 years of age and by that time woman would have completed her family. Even if it occurs earlier, infertility is more common.

Pathophysiology

Folic acid has important role in synthesis of thymidine portion of DNA. Deficiency[17] causes defective DNA synthesis within RBCs. The RNA synthesis proceeds normally leading to increase in cytoplasm compared to the nucleus. There is impaired growth and maturation of erythrocytes, granulocytes and megakaryocytes. The net effect is ineffective erythropoiesis.

Etiology

As such there is increased demand for folic acid during pregnancy. Non-pregnant requirements of 180 μg/day is increased to 400 μg/day.[18] The requirement is further increased in multiple pregnancy, infection and chronic blood loss. The drugs like phenytoin and sulfasalazine also inhibit folate absorption. Folate is heat labile and rapidly destroyed by extensive cooking. When combined deficiency of iron coexists, administration of iron alone results in hyperplastic bone marrow, which leads to increased folate demand and if extra folic acid is not supplemented there is exacerbation of megaloblastic anemia.

Clinical Features

In addition to signs and symptoms of iron deficiency anemia mentioned earlier, patient may present with hemorrhagic patches under the skin and conjunctiva and hepatosplenomegaly. There is increased incidence of pregnancy-induced hypertension, abruptio placenta and fetal malformations.[19,20]

Diagnosis

Macrocytosis as evidenced by raised MCV (>100 μm^3) is one of the hallmarks of folic acid deficiency. Peripheral smear shows macrocytic-normochromic erythrocytes, some of which may exhibit Howell-Jolly bodies (which are residual nuclear inclusion bodies within RBCs). Changes are clearly demonstrated in buffy coat preparation, which shows hypersegmented neutrophils (5 or more lobes), giant polymorphs and megaloblasts. There may be leucopenia and thrombocytopenia. Serum folates are below 3 μg/dl and red cell folate levels are below 80 μg/L. Bone marrow shows megaloblastic changes.[14]

Management

Prophylaxis with 500 μg of folic acid is indicated in all pregnant women. Most of available prenatal multi-vitamin preparations contain 1 mg of folic acid.

Once megaloblastic hematopoiesis is established, daily administration of folic acid 5 mg orally will lead to rapid recovery, as evidenced by reticulocytosis within a week. The treatment should be continued in postpartum period. Parenteral administration is indicated in women with malabsorption syndrome. Ascorbic acid (Vit C) 500 mg given orally once a day, enhances the action of folic acid by converting it into folinic acid. If there is vit B$_{12}$ deficiency, 250 μg of cynacobalamin is administered[13] parenterally every week, as oral preparations of vit B$_{12}$ have unreliable absorption.

Severely anemic patients, especially nearing term need blood transfusion along with daily administration of folic acid 1 mg and vit B$_{12}$ 100 μg for a week.

Both folate and vitamin B$_{12}$ deficiencies may mask an iron deficiency. Red cell synthesis is inhibited during vitamin deficiency, available iron is underused, and increased saturation of transferrin occurs. As soon as therapy with folate or B$_{12}$ is initiated, red cell synthesis starts again, use of iron is maximal, and iron deficiency becomes apparent. Hence, it is important to supplement iron along with folate and B$_{12}$.

Dimorphic Anemia

Dimorphic type of anemia is more prevalent in low socioeconomic groups of tropics. Poor dietic sources, faulty dietic habits and intestinal malabsorption are main culprits. There is deficiency of iron, folic acid and proteins. Peripheral smear shows features of both iron and folate deficiency as mentioned earlier. Bone marrow is predominantly macrocytic. The treatment consists of supplementation of all precursors.

SUMMARY

1. Anemia in pregnancy is a major health problem in developing countries. It is directly or indirectly responsible for 20 to 30 percent of all maternal deaths.

```
                Ascertain type of anemia
                and severity of anemia
                         │
     ┌───────────────────┼───────────────────┐
     ▼                   ▼                   ▼
┌─────────────────┐ ┌─────────────────┐ ┌─────────────────┐
│Iron deficiency  │ │Megaloblastic    │ │Dimorphic anemia │
│anemia           │ │anemia           │ │                 │
└─────────────────┘ └─────────────────┘ └─────────────────┘
     │                   │                   │
     ▼                   ▼                   ▼
┌─────────────────┐ ┌─────────────┐   ┌─────────────────┐
│Determine whether│ │Folic acid   │   │Give iron, folic │
│normal Hb% can be│ │and vit B_12 │   │acid and vit B_12│
│reached by term  │ │             │   │                 │
└─────────────────┘ └─────────────┘   └─────────────────┘
```

┌─────────────────────────┐   ┌─────────────────────────────┐
│Pregnancy remote from term│   │Pregnancy nearing term or   │
│   │   │severe anemia (Hb%<6 gm/dl) │
└─────────────────────────┘   └─────────────────────────────┘
         │   │
         ▼   ▼
┌─────────────────────────────┐   ┌─────────────────────────┐
│Start oral iron therapy. If │   │Consider blood transfusion│
│there is GI intolerence or   │   │   │
│compliance is doubtful,   │   └─────────────────────────┘
│advise parenteral iron therapy│
└─────────────────────────────┘

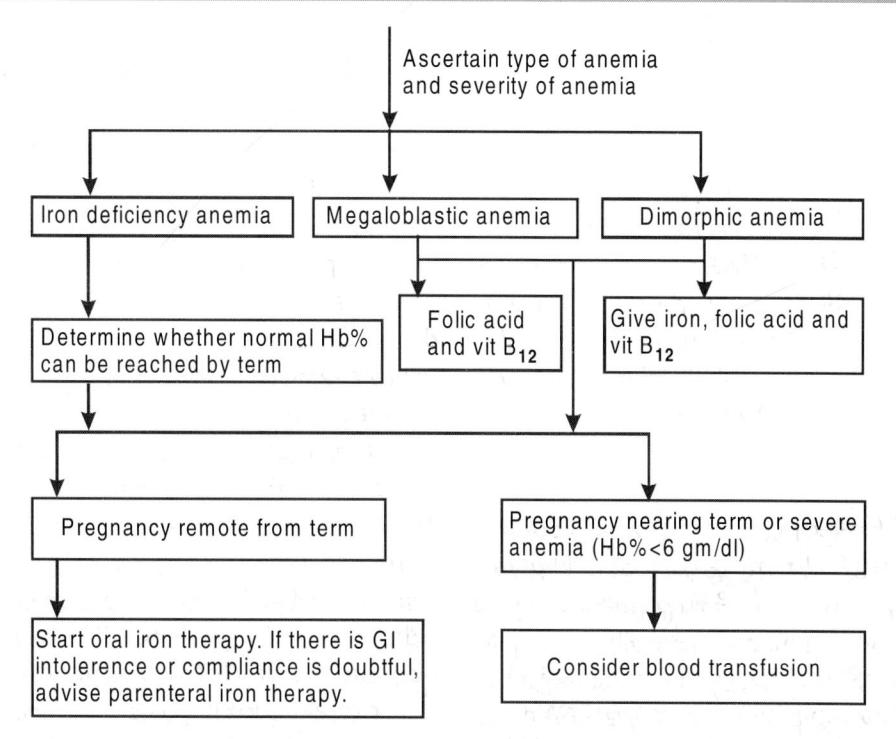

Figure 18.2: Schematic representation of management of anemia in pregnancy

2. Though there is absolute rise in total RBC volume in pregnancy, the hematocrit falls as there is physiological hemodilution due to disproportionate rise in plasma volume. As such anemia is said to exist when Hb percent is less than 10 gm/dl as it cannot be explained by state of physiological hydremia.

3. In pregnancy, there is extra-need for iron by about 1000 mg which cannot be supplemented by diet alone. This can be met only by additional supplementation of iron in antenatal period.

4. Iron and folate deficiency are the most common cause for anemia in pregnancy. Most of the times, the deficiency is pre-existent and becomes revealed during pregnancy.

5. There is increased incidence of PIH, abruptio placenta, preterm labor and puerperal venous thrombosis when pregnancy is complicated by anemia. There is also increased incidence of small for date infants.

6. The main aim of therapy is to raise the hemoglobin to at least 10 gm/dl by term. This can be achieved by oral iron therapy if pregnancy is remote from term. If patient cannot tolerate oral route, parenteral administration of suitable iron salt should be considered. Severe anemia (Hb%<6 gm/dl) needs blood transfusion especially nearing term.

7. Every effort should be made to minimize the blood loss during third stage of labor. Patient should be closely monitored for development of infection, congestive cardiac failure and venous thrombosis in puerperium.

8. Most of the times, megaloblastic anemia responds to oral folic acid therapy. Some patient may need vit B_{12} in addition. It is important to remember that there may be deficiency iron and proteins in addition and as such it is imperative to correct all deficits.

REFERENCES

1. Viteri FE: The consequences of iron deficiency and anemia in pregnancy. *Adv Exp Med Biol* **352**:127, 1994.
2. Rao BK: Maternal mortality in India: A collaborative study. *J Obst Gyn India* **3**:859, 1980.
3. Sood SK, Madan N, Rusia U, Sharma S: Nutritional anemia in pregnancy and its health implications with special reference to India. *Ann of Nat Acad of Med Sci* **25**:41-50, 1989.
4. Pinto Y: The obstetrical behaviour of the pregnant anemic woman. *J Obstet Gynecol of India* **21**:154-59, 1971.

5. Longo LD: Maternal blood volume and cardiac output during pregnancy. *Am J Physiol* **245:** R720-R729, 1983.
6. *Martindale The complete drug reference,* Edited by Kathleen Parfitt, Pharmacological Press, 32nd Edition, 1346-48, 1999.
7. *Basic Sciences in Obstetrics and Gynecology,* 2nd Edition, Edited by Michael de Sweit, Churchill Livingstone, 203, 1992.
8. Hibbard BM: The role of folic acid in pregnancy with particular reference to anemia, abruption and abortion. *Br J Obstet Gynecol* **27:**155, 1964.
9. Scholl TO, Hediger ML, Fischer RL, Shearer JW: Anemia vs Iron deficiency: increased risk of preterm delivery in a prospective study. *Am J Clin Nutr* **55:**985-88, 1992.
10. Prema K, Neelakumari S, Ramalakshmi BA: Anemia and adverse obstetric outcome. *Nutrition Reports International* **23:** 637-43, 1981.
11. Goodfrey KM, Reman CWG, Barker DJP, Osmond C: The effect of maternal anemia and iron deficiency on the ratio of fetal weight to placental weight. *Br J Obstet Gynecol* **98:**886, 1991.
12. Ian Donald: *Practical Obstetrical Problems,* PG Publishing Pte. Ltd, 5th Edition, 198-221, 1989.
13. Fernando Arias: *Practical Guide to High Risk Pregnancy and Delivery,* 2nd Edition, Mosby Year Book, 1993.
14. Prema Ramachandran: Anemia in pregnancy. In Ratnam SS *et al* (eds): *Obstetrics and Gynecology for Postgraduates.* Orient Longman Limited, **1:**49, 1992.
15. Stein ML, Gunston KD, May RM *et al*: Iron Dextran in the treatment of Iron Deficiency Anemia of Pregnancy: Haematological response and incidence of side effects. *S Afr Med J* **79:** 195-96, 1991.
16. Rothman D: Folic acid in pregnancy. *Am J Obstet Gynecol* 108-49, 1970.
17. Hoffbrand AV, Jackson BF: Correction of DNA synthesis defect in vit B_{12} deficiency by tetrahydrofolate; evidence in favor of methyl-folate trap hypothesis as a cause of megaloblastic anemia in vit B_{12} deficiency. *Br J Obstet Gynecol* **83:**643, 1993.
18. National Academy of Sciences, National Research Council, Food and Nutrition Board: *Recommended daily allowances* 10th Edition, Washington DC, 1989.
19. Center of Disease Control: Recommendations for the use of folic acid to reduce the number of spina bifida and other neural tube defects. *MMWR* **41:**1, 1992.
20. Pritchard JA, Whalley PJ, Scott DE *et al*: The influence of maternal folate on intrauterine life. *Am J Obstet Gynecol* **105:** 388-89, 1969.

19. Diabetes in Pregnancy

Lavanya Rai

INTRODUCTION

Diabetes in pregnancy may be gestational (90%) or pregestational (10%) when it antedates pregnancy. Pregnancy is a diabetogenic state due to impaired insulin sensitivity. Pregnancy worsens diabetes, while poorly controlled diabetes results in fetal, neonatal and maternal complications. Fetal hyperinsulinemia occurring as a result of maternal hyperglycemia is responsible for all the perinatal complications. As gestational diabetes is asymptomatic, glucose challenge test is done for screening while glucose tolerance test is used in diagnosis. Insulin therapy is required in 15 percent of gestational diabetics and in all pregestational diabetics during pregnancy. Oral hypoglycemic drugs are not used during pregnancy. Diet and exercise also play a significant role in controlling blood sugar. Preconception counseling improves the outcome of pregnancy in pregestational diabetic women. Gestational diabetes recurs in subsequent pregnancies and increases the risk of Type 2 diabetes in later life.

Diabetes mellitus (DM) is a common medical disorder encountered in pregnancy. In certain populations such as Asians, particularly Indians the prevalence of diabetes is high.[1,2] Obesity and advanced maternal age are other risk factors for diabetes. Perinatal mortality and morbidity are high in untreated diabetic pregnancies. However, this has decreased considerably with screening, antepartum fetal surveillance and insulin therapy.

Diabetes in pregnancy is of 2 types:

1. **Gestational diabetes** (GDM): This is defined as glucose intolerance of variable severity with onset or first identified during the present pregnancy.[3] Gestational diabetes constitutes 90 percent of diabetes in pregnancy.[2]

    Gestational diabetes generally occurs in the latter half of pregnancy. Therefore it has no effect on organogenesis and does not cause congenital defects. It generally disappears after delivery as the hormonal levels revert back to normal. If it fails to disappear it suggests that there may be overt diabetes which may have antedated or begun concomitantly with the pregnancy.

2. **Pregestational diabetes:** It is pregnancy in a known or overt diabetic. This may be either type1 (Insulin dependent diabetes mellitus) or type 2 (Noninsulin dependent diabetes mellitus). Type 1 occurs in a younger age group and end organ complications are likely to be more in these patients. They are prone for ketosis. Hence they tend to have increased maternal and obstetric risks. Type 2 is rare during pregnancy. It may be seen in obese or women above 35 years of age.

PREGNANCY AS A DIABETOGENIC STATE

Pregnancy alters the carbohydrate metabolism in such a way that more glucose is made available to the fetus. Figure 19.1 summarizes the changes in carbohydrate metabolism during pregnancy. The physiological changes which occur during pregnancy result in a higher postprandial glucose level with a slight decrease in fasting glucose concentration. Elevated placental hormones such as estrogens, progesterone, prolactin and human placental lactogen (hPL) act as insulin antagonists. They oppose the action of insulin, making it less effective. This causes a state of insulin resistance. Thus there is a progressive decline in insulin sensitivity. This is further aggravated by increased body weight and caloric intake during pregnancy. hPL affects protein, fat and carbohydrate metabolism. It promotes lipolysis and the available free fatty acids (FFA) are used for the mother's own metabolism, to ensure the availability of adequate glucose for the fetus. As a result the glucose level increases to meet the fetal needs. Elevated FFAs also increase insulin resistance. Plasma cortisol also rises during pregnancy and this adds to the " contrainsulin" effect of other hormones. In response to this, the maternal pancreas increases the production of insulin to keep the carbohydrate metabolism stable. Thus, there is an increase in the insulin level but it is ineffective, because there is a peripheral resistance to its action.

Gestational diabetes develops when the pancreas, despite the production of insulin, cannot overcome the effect of these counter-regulatory hormones. Established diabetes becomes worse during pregnancy. Insulin requirement increases in these patients and control of blood sugar becomes difficult.

SCREENING FOR DIABETES

Gestational diabetes is asymptomatic and hence the need for screening. However, there is no consensus regarding the method or type of screening tests. Two methods of screening that are in practice today are:
1. Universal screening
2. Selective screening

All pregnant women are screened in the universal screening protocol while selective screening is done only in the presence of risk factors for gestational diabetes. These risk factors are depicted in Table 19.1.

Table 19.1: Risk factors for gestational diabetes

Historical factors	Clinical factors in the present pregnancy
• Age >30 years	Hydramnios
• Previous GDM	Congenital fetal anomalies
• Family history of DM	Pre-eclampsia
• Bad obstetric history	Obesity > 90 kg
• H/O Macrosomia	Recurrent UTI
• Prev Fetal anomalies	Recurrent Moniliasis multiple pregnancy

* UTI—Urinary tract infection

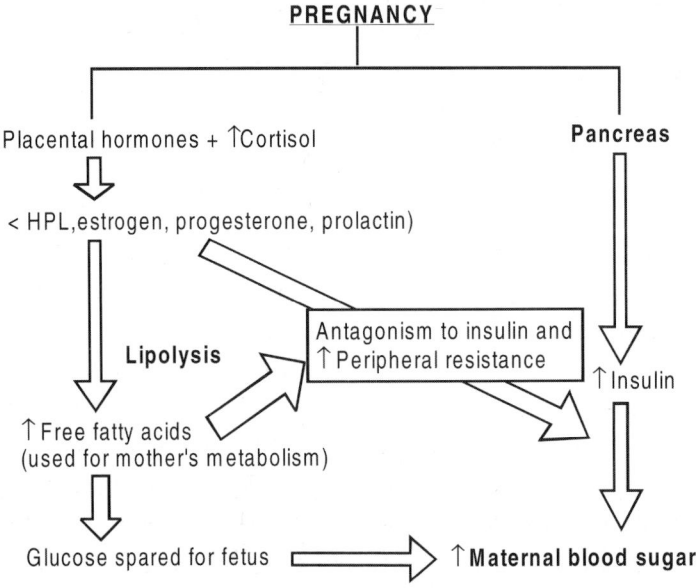

Figure 19.1: Changes in carbohydrate metabolism during pregnancy

If selective screening is adopted majority of gestational diabetes can be missed because the risk factors are present in only 30 percent of those who develop glucose intolerance during pregnancy.[4] At the same time universal screening in populations with a low prevalence (0.5-1%) is not cost effective. Therefore, it is better to do universal screening in populations with a high prevalence (> 5%) while selective screening can be used in areas with a low prevalence.[5] As Asians are a risk group for diabetes many hospitals in India practice universal screening.

The very concept of screening for GDM and its cost effectiveness has been challenged in recent years.[6] However screening is advisable till better evidence becomes available as detecting GDM identifies women at risk for future type 2 DM besides decreasing the perinatal morbidity and mortality for the index pregnancy.

Screening Test

Glucose challenge test (GCT) is commonly used in screening for gestational diabetes. No special preparation is necessary for this test. Fifty grams of oral glucose is given between 24 to 28 weeks of gestation irrespective of the time or the meal and blood glucose is determined 1 hour later. A plasma value of $\geq$ 7.8 mmol (140 mg/dl) is considered significant to perform the confirmatory diagnostic test. Though this test is generally done in the second trimester, a high risk patient can be tested during the booking visit. GCT has a high sensitivity (79%) and specificity (83%) compared to other screening tests, such as random or postprandial glucose estimations.[7,8] Moreover GCT has been extensively evaluated compared to other screening tests. Screen negative patients should ideally have a subsequent testing around 34 weeks. Repeat screening may become positive as insulin resistance becomes more marked with advancing pregnancy.

There is no role for urine glucose screening, because glycosuria is frequently seen as a result of lowered renal threshold during pregnancy. However, persistent glycosuria should be considered as an indication to rule out diabetes.

Diagnostic Test

Oral glucose tolerance test (OGTT) is performed for the diagnosis of gestational diabetes. It may be done using the WHO (World Health Organization) or NDDG (National Diabetes Data group) guidelines, recommended by American College of Obstetricians and Gynecologists.[9,10]

We use the 100 gm 3 hr OGTT proposed by NDDG.[10] After an overnight fast, with unrestricted diet for the preceding 3 days, the fasting blood sugar is determined. Then 100 gm of oral glucose is given, followed by glucose estimations at the end 1, 2 and 3 hr. The upper limit of normal are depicted in Table 19.2. Diagnosis of gestational diabetes is made when any two values are abnormal. Opinion is divided as to which glucose threshold values to use for diagnosis of GDM. Recently after the 4th International Workshop—Conference on GDM, the American Diabetes Association (ADA) has adopted more stringent criteria for diagnosis.[11] The values recommended by ADA are fasting $\geq$ 5.3 mmol/l (95 mg/dl); 1 hour $\geq$ 10 mmol/l (180 mg/dl); 2 hours $\geq$ 8.6 mmol/l (155 mg/dl) and 3 hour $\geq$ 7.8 mmol/l (140 mg/dl).

Table 19.2: Normal values of glucose tolerance tests

OGTT	Oral glucose (gms)	Fasting	1-hour	2-hour	3-hour
NDDG[10]	100	5.8 (105)	10.6 (190)	9.2 (165)	8.1 (145)
WHO[9]	75	<6 (108)		<8 (144)	

Venous plasma values in mmol/l, (mg/dl)

It has been found that even women with one abnormal value are at risk for fetal macrosomia. Generally 15 percent of pregnant women have a positive glucose challenge test and of these only 15 percent have abnormal 3 hr GTT.[12]

The WHO recommends the 2 hour 75 gm OGTT.[9] This test is more simple as only 2 samples are taken. The normal values are shown in Table 19.2. The diagnosis of DM is made when the plasma glucose concentrations exceed 8 mmol/l (144 mg/dl) in the fasting state and or the 2 hr value is ≥ 11 mmol/l (200 mg/dl). The values in between indicate impaired glucose tolerance which should be treated as GDM during pregnancy.[8]

In women who have normal OGTT in the presence of risk factors (Table 19.1) a repeat test may be advised at 32 to 34 weeks. It is also advisable in patients with one abnormal value during the initial test.

In many centers OGTT is directly performed as a one step approach in the presence of risk factors while the traditional two step approach with GCT followed by OGTT is carried out in a low risk population.[11,13] We follow this protocol where OGTT is performed for an abnormal GCT or in the presence of risk factors.

COMPLICATIONS

Maternal, fetal and neonatal complications are seen in untreated or poorly controlled pregestational and gestational diabetes. These are listed in Table 19.3. The complications are a direct result of hyperglycemia in the first trimester and the resulting fetal hyperinsulinemia in the second and third trimester.

Maternal Complications

Maternal complications are 2 to 4 folds higher in a diabetic pregnancy. Macrosomia results in higher incidence of operative delivery, prolonged labor and shoulder dystocia.

The prognosis in a poorly controlled pregestational diabetic is worse because of additional maternal and fetal complications compared to a gestational diabetic.

In a pregestational diabetic, blood sugar control is difficult because of the insulin resistance that accompanies gestation. Diabetic vasculopathy as indicated by retinopathy, neuropathy and nephropathy, develop in long-standing overt diabetes. There is no evidence to show that pregnancy exacerbates diabetic vasculopathy but established proliferative retinopathy and nephropathy may deteriorate. IUGR is seen when there is vascular disease because of uteroplacental insufficiency. Ketosis is likely to occur when pregnancy is complicated by hyperemesis, use of B mimetics, steroids and in the presence of infections.[12] Ketosis in pregnancy occurs more frequently and at a lower level of plasma glucose levels than in the non-pregnant state. Postpartum thyroiditis is a specific problem of type 1 pregestational diabetes after delivery.

Fetal and Neonatal Complications

Fetal anomalies and abortions are seen in pregestational diabetes when euglycemia is not maintained during periconceptional period. The incidence of congenital anomalies is about 4-fold higher than in normal

Table 19.3: Complications of diabetes in pregnancy

Maternal	Fetal	Neonatal
• Pre-eclampsia • Pyelonephritis • Polyhydramnios • Preterm labour • Operative delivery • Monilial vaginitis	• Macrosomia • Sudden IUD* • Shoulder dystocia	• Hypoglycemia • Hyaline membrane disease • Hypomagnesemia • Hyperbilirubenemia • Hypocalcemia • Hypertrophic cardiomyopathy • Hyperviscosity syndrome • Transient tachypnea • Birth injuries • Birth asphyxia
Pregestational • Difficult sugar control • Ketosis • Hypoglycemic attacks • Diabetic vasculopathy → IUGR** • Postpartum thyroiditis	• Congenital anomalies • Abortions	*Late Effects* • Obesity in adulthood • Type 2 diabetes

*IUD—intrauterine death, **IUGR—intrauterine growth restriction

pregnancy. These anomalies are believed to be due to the aberrant fuel mixture transferred to the fetus in poorly controlled diabetic women during organogenesis. The early growth delay shown by ultrasound and raised glycosylated hemoglobin (HbA1c >10%) at the end of the first trimester serve as indicators of congenital anomalies.[4,10] Neural tube defects, cardiac and renal anomalies occur with increased frequency in diabetic pregnancies. Caudal regression syndrome, a rare anomaly is characteristic of diabetic pregnancy. Early abortions are also increased in these women. Perinatal mortality is 4 percent in pregestational diabetes and 1 percent in gestational diabetes.[13] An infant of a diabetic mother (IDM) has a plethoric appearance due to polycythemia. Gestational diabetics have macrosomic babies while pregestational diabetics may have a macrosomic or an IUGR baby in the presence of vasculopathy.

The perinatal complications of IDMs is explained by Pederson's maternal hyperglycemia—fetal hyperinsulinism hypothesis as depicted in Figure 19.2.[14]

The fetus receives a continuous supply of nutrition from the mother but the placenta blocks the transfer of maternal insulin. The abundant supply of amino acids, glucose and free fatty acids not only stimulate fetal growth but also cause pancreatic beta cell hyperplasia resulting in fetal hyperinsulinemia. Insulin acts like a fetal growth factor resulting in a macrosomic baby. It favors fat deposition in insulin-dependent areas in the fetal trunk. The head size remains normal. This asymmetrical macrosomic baby therefore has a higher chance of shoulder dystocia during labor because there is a disproportionate increase in trunk size compared to the head. Sudden fetal death may occur due to hyperglycemia induced hypoxia and acidosis or hypoglycemia.

RDS is an important cause of neonatal death due to hyaline membrane disease. Surfactant production is impaired due to hyperinsulinemia, hyperglycemia and prematurity. Neonatal hypoglycemia is diagnosed when plasma glucose levels are below 2 mmol/l (40 mg/dl). The baby may be lethargic or have convulsions. Neonatal

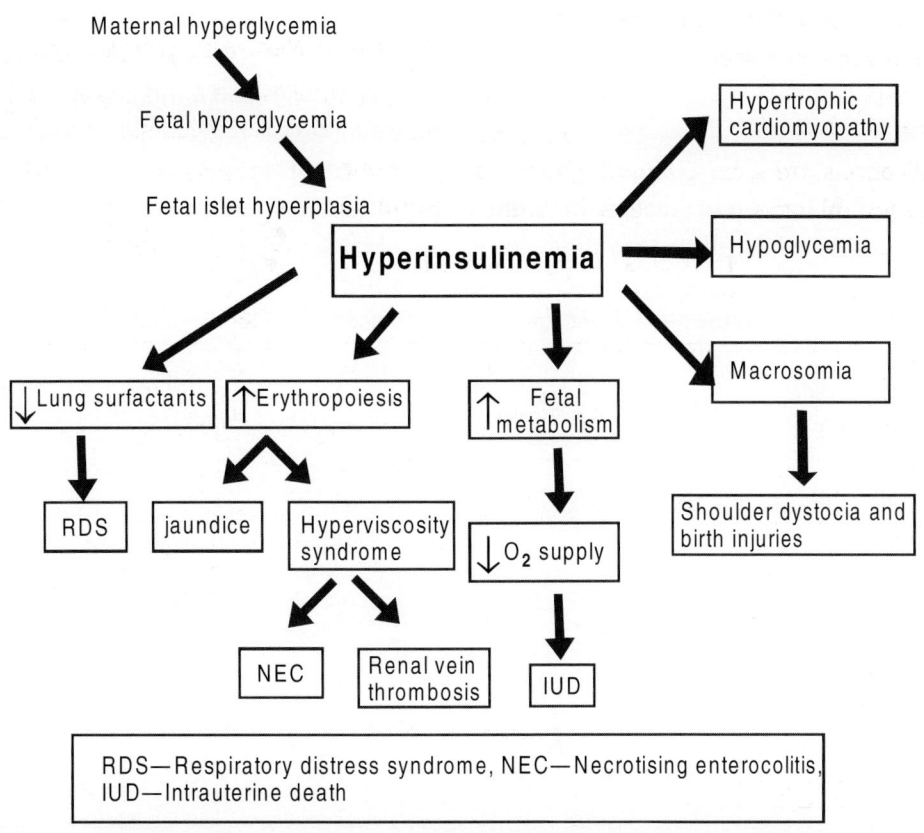

RDS—Respiratory distress syndrome, NEC—Necrotising enterocolitis, IUD—Intrauterine death

Figure 19.2: Pathogenesis of fetal and neonatal effects of GDM

gluconeogenesis is suppressed and the maternal nutrients are no longer available while the pancreas continues to secrete insulin. Low electrolytes are due to renal loss and decreased parathyroid hormone secretion in these babies. Prematurity and birth asphyxia further aggravate the neonatal complications in IDM.

Thus prevention of fetal hyperinsulinemia by proper control of maternal hyperglycemia will prevent all perinatal complications.

MANAGEMENT

Team care is ideal for the management of a diabetic pregnancy. Best results are obtained when the patients are seen in special diabetic clinics. The team consists of a physician, nutritionist, neonatologist besides the obstetrician and midwife. The diabetic lady is the most important member of the team because she has to actively participate in her own care.

Objectives

- A good glycemic control
- Antepartum fetal surveillance
- Delivery at the appropriate time
- Optimal neonatal support

Antepartum

A good glycemic control in the periconceptional period reduces the chance of fetal anomalies in a pregestational diabetic. The risk of perinatal complications are low when control is good during the latter half of pregnancy.

Antenatal visits may have to be more frequent compared to a low risk pregnant woman. Admission or care in day assessment units may be required for stabilization of blood sugar, adjustment of the insulin dose and to manage any complications if they arise. Investigations required for the management of diabetes in pregnancy are shown in Table 19.4.

Antenatal visits should be every 2 weeks until 32 to 34 weeks and weekly thereafter. Routine monitoring of blood pressure, weight gain, fetal movements, proteinuria and fetal growth are made at these visits. Pregestational diabetics are better managed in hospital or day assessment unit from 34 weeks onward, especially if there is difficulty in blood sugar control.

INVESTIGATIONS (Table 19.4)

1. *Blood sugar monitoring:* Weekly assessment is required. The aim is to keep fasting < 6 mmol/L (108 mg/dl)) and 2 hr postprandial < 7 mmol/L (126 mg/dl).[1] This is best achieved by evaluating the fasting and postprandial (2 hour) values around the main meals (post-breakfast, lunch and supper-sugar profile). This is useful in deciding on whether to start insulin or in adjusting the dosage of insulin. Home glucose monitoring is popular in developed countries

Table 19.4: Investigations of diabetes mellitus in pregnancy

Maternal	Fetal
• Blood sugar profile	• MSAFP – 16-20 wk
• Urine Microscopy ⎫ Booking,	• USG – Booking, 18-20 wk
• Urine C/S ⎭ 28, 32 and 36 wk	• 3rd trimester- serial scans for growth and amniotic fluid
	• Echocardiography-22 wk
	• NST and or Biophysical profile from 32 wk
Pregestational	• Umbilical artery Doppler
• Proteinuria ⎫ Every visit	
• Ketonuria ⎭	
• HbA1c ⎫	
• Fundoscopy ⎬ Every trimester	
• Renal function tests ⎭	

MSAFP—Matenal serum alpha-fetoprotein, C/S—culture and sensitivity, NST—nonstress test, HbA1c—Glycosylated hemoglobin

and this ensures better patient participation and control.
2. *Urine microscopy and culture with sensitivity (C/S)* is done to screen for asymptomatic bacteriuria.
   Pregestational diabetic requires evaluation and surveillance for nephropathy, retinopathy and ketosis during pregnancy.
3. *HbA1c:* It must be done in the first trimester or as and when the patient reports. This gives retrospective assessment of diabetic control regardless of the day to day fluctuations of glucose. Hemoglobin combines with glucose to form glycosylated Hb and this indicates the blood glucose values during the preceding 8 to 12 weeks. A high HbA1c at the end of first trimester indicates that the sugar control was suboptimal during the period of organogenesis.
4. *Maternal serum alpha-fetoprotein* (MSAFP) estimation is done between 16 and 20 weeks to screen for neural tube defects. However, while interpreting the values one should bear in mind that the values are low in diabetic pregnancies.
5. *Ultrasound:* It is indicated in the first trimester for accurate dating of the pregnancy. An early growth lag in a pregestational diabetic is an indicator of fetal malformations or early abortion.[4]
   IInd trimester—detailed anomaly scan is performed at 18-20 weeks
   Fetal echocardiography to rule out cardiac anomalies is done around 22-24 weeks.
   IIIrd trimester—serial scan is done to monitor for macrosomia and hydramnios.
   In those at high risk with poorly controlled diabetes or poor obstetric history, twice weekly NST and biophysical profiles are done to monitor fetal wellbeing. In the others, the tests can be tailored according to the needs. Mother's perception of fetal movements also plays an important role in monitoring the fetus.
6. *Doppler of umbilical artery* to study the fetoplacental flow may be done in cases with diabetic vasculopathy where IUGR is likely to occur.

TREATMENT

Good management of diabetes involves diet therapy, judicious use of exercise, a well monitored insulin therapy and fetal surveillance. Figure 19.3 shows the management protocol for gestational diabetes. Once GDM is diagnosed with abnormal GTT, treatment is started based on sugar profile consisting of fasting and postprandial results. If they are normal, diet therapy is sufficient. When the abnormal profile is not controlled with diet, insulin is added. Majority of the GDM women can be controlled with diet alone. Only 15 percent require insulin therapy.[14,15]

1. *Diet therapy*: This is prescribed for all patients with diabetes. Diet is now called the medical nutrition therapy.[11] The total calories advised is 24-30 kcal/kg of the present body weight. In the obese diabetic 24 kcal is advised while a lean individual can take 30 kcal/kg. The calories should be distributed between 3 meals and 3 snacks. Bed time snack prevents fasting ketosis. Dietary control decreases postprandial hyperglycemia and it also improves the action of insulin. Gestational diabetics are initially managed with diet alone. They should be seen at 1-2 weekly intervals. Fasting and postprandial sugars are measured to ensure that glucose levels are normal. Diet is planned with the help of a nutritionist. Blood glucose levels, appetite and weight gain can be used to formulate a meal plan which can be adjusted through pregnancy. A high fiber, low fat diet is beneficial.
2. *Exercise:* Light exercise helps by lowering free fatty acids and increasing blood flow to insulin sensitive tissue. Contracting muscles help stimulate glucose transport thereby decreasing the blood sugar. Thus daily exercise can decrease insulin requirement. Exercise is better done after meals. Exercise involving the muscle of the upper part of the body is sufficient. It is safe and effective.
3. *Insulin regimes*: Oral hypoglycemic drugs are generally not recommended during pregnancy as they cross the placental barrier and cause fetal hypoglycemia. Insulin is indicated in all overt diabetics and gestational diabetics with fasting or postprandial hyperglycemia. The insulin regimes vary with the clinician's preference. The popular regimes use a mixture of short acting (soluble) and medium acting insulin (NPH or Lente). It is given

20-30 minutes before the main morning and evening meals. Two-third of the total dose (2/3 NPH + 1/3 soluble) may be given in the morning and the remaining one-third of the total dose (½ NPH+ ½ soluble) can be given in the evening.[2,15] Human insulin is preferred.

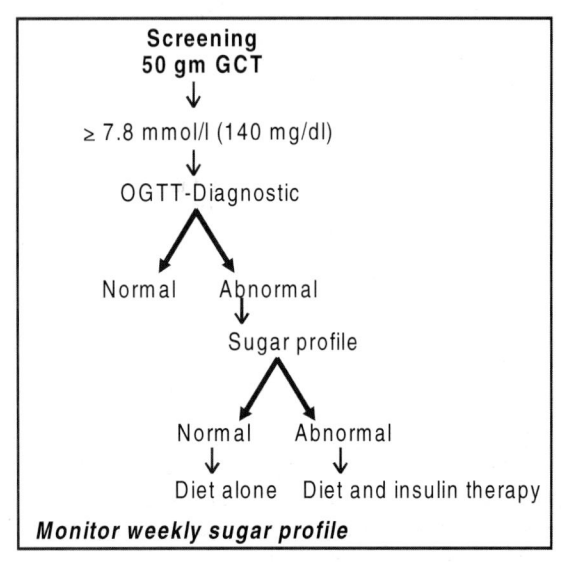

Figure 19.3: Management protocol of gestational diabetes

```
          Screening
          50 gm GCT
              ↓
      ≥ 7.8 mmol/l (140 mg/dl)
              ↓
         OGTT-Diagnostic
           ↙      ↘
        Normal   Abnormal
                    ↓
                Sugar profile
                 ↙      ↘
              Normal   Abnormal
                ↓        ↓
            Diet alone  Diet and insulin therapy

       Monitor weekly sugar profile
```

4. *Obstetric management:* The decision to deliver should be based on the degree of diabetes, nature of control, superimposed risk factors and fetal wellbeing. Pregnancy is not allowed to go beyond due dates even in well controlled diabetics.

   There are high chances of a cesarean section in a diabetic mother due to pregnancy complications or macrosomia. A cesarean section is not indicated for diabetes alone. It is important to maintain euglycemia during labor to minimize the risk of neonatal hypoglycemia. Continuous fetal heart rate monitoring is ideal. Partogram should be maintained. Epidural analgesia is helpful. Pain relief in labor prevents hyperglycemia that may result due to catecholamine release during uterine contractions.[13]

   In the event of an elective cesarean section or induction:
   - Skip the morning dose of insulin
   - Start an IV line with 5 percent dextrose and 5 units of insulin
   - Insulin may be given at the rate of 1.0 u/hr
   - Keep monitoring blood glucose hourly and maintain it between 4 to 6 mmol/l (72-108 mg/dl)

   Insulin can be given separately using a syringe pump. The dose of insulin may be adjusted depending on the blood sugar.

5. *Neonatal care:* The baby requires neonatal intensive unit or special care as blood glucose levels require close monitoring during the first 48 hr. Early breastfeeding is advocated to prevent hypoglycemia. Hematocrit levels should be checked at 1 and 24 hr. Early cord clamping during delivery prevents neonatal polycythemia.

6. *Postpartum care:* The insulin dose decreases drastically after delivery. A pregestational diabetic can be commenced on her prepregnancy regime. Breast feeding should be encouraged.

   GDM women on insulin can stop insulin after delivery. They should be monitored with blood glucose levels for 48 hours. A 2 hour 75 gm OGTT is indicated for GDM women at 6 weeks postpartum. Even if it is normal, gestational diabetes tends to recur in the subsequent pregnancy. These women have a 30 to 50 percent chance of developing DM within the next 15 to 20 years.[10,13] It will be worthwhile to encourage these women to continue the diet and exercise regimen adopted during pregnancy.

7. *Contraception:* Barriers and low dose pills can be used for contraception. As the estrogen content of these pills is low, glucose control is not a problem particularly with low dose triphasic pills. Depot preparations of injectable progesterone can be used. IUCD is not favored in pregestational diabetes. It can be used in gestational diabetics as it generally disappears after delivery. Pregestational diabetic women should have their children in early reproductive years as vascular complications are likely to increase with age.

8. *Prepregnancy counseling:* This plays an important role for pregestational diabetes. To prevent early pregnancy loss and congenital anomalies, medical care should begin before conception. A complete

assessment of the diabetic status and associated complications is done to find out if she is fit to go through pregnancy. HbA1c should be evaluated to indicate a good control before conception. The aim is to keep it below 8 percent. It would be advisable to do a fundoscopy and renal function tests to rule out diabetic vasculopathy. Folate supplementation given for 3 months prior to conception may reduce the incidence of neural tube defects.

Evaluation of thyroid function is also recommended in type 1 diabetes as hypothyroidism is frequently encountered in these women.[2] Those on oral hypoglycemic agents should be switched to insulin therapy preferably before conception.

CONCLUSION

Stevan Gabbe proposed the rule of 15 for GDM:[15]
- 15 percent of patients with positive GCT will have GDM
- 15 percent of GDM women will require insulin
- 15 percent of GDM will have macrosomia
- 15 percent of GDM will have impaired GTT after delivery

A good outcome is generally achieved in GDM women with adequate glucose control either with diet alone or with insulin therapy and careful fetal surveillance. Maternal and fetal prognosis today for women with well controlled pregestational diabetes is also satisfactory.

REFERENCES

1. J N Oats, NA Beischer: Gestational Diabetes. In John Studd (Ed): *Progress in Obstetrics and Gynecology* **6**:101-07, 1987.
2. Margarita De Veciana, M Elizabeth Mason: Endocrine disorders: Diabetes. In ArthurT Evans, KR Niswander (Ed), *Manual of Obstetrics*, 6th edn, Baltimore, Lippincott Williams and Wilkins, 127-48, 2000.
3. Third International Workshop Conference on gestational diabetes mellitus, Chicago, 1990, Summary and recommendations. *Diabetes* **40(suppl 2)**:197-201, 1991.
4. Gillmer MDG: Diabetes in Pregnancy, In: Weatherall DJ, Ledingham JGG, Warrell DA (Eds) *Oxford Textbook Of Medicine*, 3rd edn, Vol 2, Oxford, Oxford Medical Publications **2**: 1752-58, 1996.
5. Jacquiline de AC Soares, Anne Dornhorst, Richard W Beard: The case for screening for gestational diabetes. *British Medical Journal* **315**:737-39, 1997.
6. Jarrett RJ: Should we screen for gestational diabetes? *British Medical Journal* **315**: 736-37, 1997.
7. O' Sullivan JB, MahanCM, Charles D, Dandrow RV: Screening criteria for high risk gestational diabetic patients. *American Journal of Obst and Gynecology* **116**:895-900, 1973.
8. Michael Maresh, Richard Beard. In Michael De Swiet (Ed); *Medical Disorders in Obstetric Practice*, 3rd edn, Oxford: Blackwell Science Ltd, 423-58, 1995.
9. World Health Organization Expert Committee on Diabetes Mellitus; Technical report series no **646**:8, 1980.
10. ACOG technical Bulletin—Diabetes and Pregnancy –200- Dec 1994. *International Journal of Gynecology and Obstetrics* **48**: 331-39, 1995.
11. American Diabetes Association: Gestational Diabetes Mellitus – Clinical Practice recommendations 2000. *Diabetes Care* **23(Suppl 1)**: S77-S79, 2000.
12. Cunningham, Mac Donald, Gant, Leveno et al (Eds): Diabetes. In: *Williams Obstetrics*, 20th edn, International, Appleton and lange, 1203-21, 1997.
13. NA Beischer, EV Mackay, PB Colditz (Eds): The Endocrine System - Diabetes Mellitus. In Obstetrics and the New born- an illustrated text book , 3rd edn, London, WB Saunders, 324-38, 1997.
14. Cloherty John P, John P Cloherty and Ann R Stark (Eds): Diabetes Mellitus. In: *Manual of Neonatal Care,* 4th edn, Philadelphia, Lippincott- Raven, 11-20, 1997.
15. Steven G Gabbe, John T Queenan, John C Hobbins (Eds). Diabetes Mellitus. In: *Protocols for High Risk Pregnancies*, 3rd edn, Cambridge, Blackwell Science 253-63, 1996.

20.
Tropical Diseases in Pregnancy

NN Roy Chowdhury

PART TWO — Feto-maternal Medicine

INTRODUCTION

Multiple tropical diseases—viral, parasitic and water-borne pose special problems during pregnancy—three of them will be discussed here.

Chickenpox is uncommon in pregnancy, because 90 percent of the population are immune due to previous infection 1-2 percent babies may develop birth defects if it occurs between 8 to 20 weeks gestation; termination in these is justified. Pneumonia occurs in 10 to 15 percent mothers and may be fulminant. Viral hepatitis and malaria during pregnancy cause large number of maternal and perinatal deaths globally.

Viral hepatitis, the most common cause of jaundice in pregnancy carries a higher mortality in developing countries, causing 11 percent of maternal deaths in India especially due to hepatic failure and PPH. Hepatitis E is the most common cause of epidemics, intrauterine deaths and prematurity, which is associated with high perinatal loss.

Pregnant women are more susceptible to malaria, especially primigravidae and carry a higher mortality. Maternal complications include cerebral malaria, pulmonary edema, renal failure, anemia and hypoglycemia. Fetal problems include abortion, preterm labor, IUGR, IUFD and congenital malaria. Drug-resistant falciparum malaria is dangerous.

TROPICAL DISEASES

Climate has diverse effects on human behavior, nutrition spread of infection, and on health in general. In hot and dry or wet tropical climate, water-borne diseases like cholera and hepatitis are quite common. Malaria and gastrointestinal diseases increase during the rainy season. Giardiasis and trichomoniasis may cause morbidity among healthy individuals in large numbers. The importance of environmental factors in tropical infectious diseases affecting pregnant women is well established. With improvement of laboratory techniques and the discovery of new pathogenic viruses it is becoming more and more evident that many viral diseases may be transmitted to the offspring by the infected mother, who may or may not present evidence of disease herself. Obstetricians and pediatricians aided by the virologist are now able to diagnose many pathological conditions in the fetus and newborn infants, hitherto overlooked or not understood. In the consideration of fetal congenital abnormality, placental permeability is of the greatest importance. The transfer of substances from mother to the fetus has been shown to be a complex process.

In the less advanced countries, especially in the tropics, multiple disease entities are common due to parasitism, malnutrition, and diarrheal diseases. Chronic infections also damage important organs such as liver, and kidneys. Migration to urban slums increases the risk of gastrointestinal disease and tuberculosis.

Maternal infection with certain viruses during pregnancy may result in three separate effects on newborn child: (i) miscarriage, (ii) intrauterine fetal death, (iii) a teratogenic effect insufficient to kill the fetus. The rate of fetal loss appears to be directly related to the severity of the disease in the mother. Similarly miscarriage and preterm labor may be related to maternal toxicity with or without associated viral disease of the fetus. In these cases, infection may become apparent after an interval following birth.

Maternal viral infections causing congenital anomalies may be: (i) rubella, (ii) measles, (iii) varicella or chickenpox. Vaccinia or smallpox has been completely eradicated by vaccination during the last 3 decades, (iv) Poliomyelitis – number of cases has been considerably reduced by extensive use of oral polio vaccine.

Considering the damaging effects on pregnant women and their offsprings, three tropical diseases have been highlighted in this chapter.
1. Malaria.
2. Acute viral hepatitis causing jaundice.
3. Varicella or chickenpox.

Malaria in Pregnancy

Many experts believe that the true extent of malaria problem has been greatly underestimated. Each year 2.5 million people die of malaria most of whom are children. In pregnancy cerebral and other severe malaria has got a maternal mortality twice that among non-pregnant patients in Malayasia.[1] In the third trimester, it is ten times more in Thailand. Malaria is the most common cause of maternal mortality in Thailand.[2] Perinatal mortality is also very high—4 times more than the non-malaria sufferers due to stillbirth, prematurity and intrauterine growth restriction. Large-scale epidemics of malaria are becoming more frequent. Resistance to currently available anti-malarial drugs is a major problem across the tropical world. Over the last 10 years, the epidemiology of malaria has changed radically. Malaria should be recognized as a global priority in health care, more so when it occurs in pregnancy.

Incidence

Each year approximately 2.5 million die of malaria, many of whom are children. According to the latest WHO estimates, 40 percent of the population of the world live in areas where malaria is endemic. Around 300 million people are infected with malaria at any one time and a third of them will develop clinical disease. 80 percent of all malaria occurs in sub–Saharan Africa. In contrast, India has 8 percent of malaria cases, while the remaining 12 percent are spread over other countries across the world.

Why is the Incidence of Malaria Suddenly going up?

Many experts believe that the true extent of malaria problem had been greatly underestimated and the real figures are now estimated. There is a growing consensus that the problem of malaria is increasing rather than diminishing across the world.

Some of the reasons suggested for increase in the incidence of malaria in India are:
1. *Increased disease severity:* The number of hospital admissions due to malaria has increased greatly compared with the number due to other causes as more fatal cases are coming up.
2. Rural communities suffer more from malaria. For every death from malaria in the urban hospitals, 25 occur in villages.
3. *Changing epidemiology:* The normal pattern of malaria infection is changing. Large scale epidemics of malaria, where the number of cases increased dramatically for no apparent reason, now occur in India and the world.
4. *Drug resistance:* The development of drug resistance has intensified the problem. The emergence of resistance to chloroquine by *P. falciparum* was first documented in the late 1950s. Resistance to more

Table 21.1: Agents producing infection in pregnancy

A. *Bacteria*
- Group B streptococcal (GBS)
- *Mycobacterium (tuberculosis or leprae)*
- *Coliforms (E. coli)*
- *Salmonella typhi*
- *Shigella*
- *Gardnerella vaginalis*
- Bacteria monocytogenus

B. *Virus*
- Hepatitis B virus
- Human immunodeficiency virus
- Rubella
- Cytomegalovirus (CMV)
- Varicella-zoster
- Rubeola
- Parvovirus B-19

C. *Protozoa*
- *Plasmodium*
- *Toxoplasma gondii*
- *Trichomonas vaginalis*

D. *Fungi*
- *Candida albicans*
- *Trichophyton rubrum*
- *Actinomycosis*
- Others: *Cryptococcus, histoplasma,* coccidiodomycosis, etc.

E. Sexually Transmitted Infections
- HIV,
- Human papilloma virus (HPV),
- Syphilis,
- Gonorrhea,
- Chlamydia,
- Lymphogranuloma venerum,
- Granuloma inguinale,
- Chancroid.

TORCH—infection is the acronym used to refer to a group of infections wherein some of the organisms act as teratogens and affect the fetus severely. These TORCH infections include toxoplasmosis, rubella, cytomegalovirus and herpes simplex virus. In the group of other infections, syphilis is the most important, along with lysteriosis and parvovirus.

Diagnosis

A colony count of more than 100,000 units per ml of midstream voided sample of urine is diagnostic of UTI. The presence of pyuria suggests infection but is not diagnostic of UTI. A bedside Triphenyl tetra-zolium chloride test wherein the adding of affected urinary sample to this colorless solution changes its color to red is useful for the diagnosis of asymptomatic bacteriuria.

Management

Both symptomatic and asymptomatic bacteriuria should be properly treated. Women with recurrent UTI must be investigated for any structural abnormality or stone in the urinary tract. All patients should have urine analysis as an initial screening test at first antenatal check-up and urinary culture if it reveals pyuria, bacteriuria or nitrites. A clean catch midstream sample of urine collected in a sterile container after cleaning the introitus should be used for both these tests.

Treatment

The treatment of choice for asymptomatic bacteriuria is controversial as is the duration of treatment. The primary goal is to prevent pyelonephritis. Few patients without catheters who have asymptomatic bacteriuria develop serious complications and therefore routine antimicrobial therapy is not justified with only two exceptions: before urologic surgery and during pregnancy.[1] β-lactum antibiotics and cephalosporins have no known fetal risks and can be safely used at any time during pregnancy. For acute cystitis antibiotics are given for 7 of 14 days. Urinary tract prophylaxis should be considered in all pregnancies with urologic complications viz. ileal conduits, ureteral re-implantation, renal transplants and recurrent UTI. Long-term chemoprophylaxis should be suggested in patients with recurrent UTI or following acute pyelonephritis during pregnancy.[2]

Any UTI during labor or delivery, demands aggressive parenteral therapy followed by oral antibiotics during postpartum period. Cases catheterized during labor where possible should have their urine cultured and treated as each catheterization carries with it a risk of subsequent UTI.

Intra-amniotic Infections

Intra-amniotic infection (IAI) is an acute clinical infection of the amniotic fluid and intrauterine contents during pregnancy. It occurs in 1 to 2 percent of all deliveries, clinical presentation being fever, leucocytosis and/or uterine tenderness. Histologic chorioamnionitis is a different entity that is diagnosed histologically and may not be accompanied by clinical infection (Tables 21.2 and 21.3).

Pathologic Organisms

In the majority, the infection is polymicrobial involving both facultative and anaerobic microorganisms.

Table 21.2: Risk factors for intra-amniotic infection

- Prolonged rupture of membranes
- Internal fetal monitoring
- Frequent vaginal examinations during labor
- Coexistence of bacterial vaginosis

Table 21.3: Routes of intra-amniotic infection

- Ascending infection from lower genital tract following rupture of membranes
- Transplacental hematogenous spread secondary to maternal bacteremia
- Iatrogenic due to amniocentesis, cordocentesis, etc.

Escherichia coli and group B *Streptococcus* are the most common organisms and account for 60 percent of maternal or neonatal bacteremia.

Maternal and Fetal Effects

There is a 3 to 4-fold rise in perinatal mortality among low birth weight neonates born to women with IAI, but not in term neonates. RDS, intraventricular hemorrhage and clinical neonatal sepsis are also more common. There is no increase in perinatal mortality or neonatal sepsis among term neonates. Congenital pneumonia, however, is quite common and may prove fatal. Maternal bacteremia occurs in 2 to 6 percent of IAI cases with increased risk of dysfunctional labor, Cesarean delivery and puerperal sepsis.[3]

Diagnosis

Most constant feature is maternal fever. Leucocytosis, maternal or fetal tachycardia, uterine tenderness and foul smell of the amniotic fluid are other manifestations that may or may not be present. Amniotic fluid analysis will be helpful in women in preterm labor with intact membranes and suspected infection (Table 21.4).

Table 21.4: Investigations for diagnosis of IAI

- CRP measurement in maternal serum
- Amniotic fluid analysis for leucocytes and bacteria
- Amniotic fluid culture
- Measurement of amniotic fluid glucose concentration
- Detection of amniotic fluid esterase
- Detection of bacterial organic acids by gas-liquid chromatography
- USG for biophysical profile

Management

Treatment with antibiotics and delivery is the definitive treatment. In the majority, a broad-spectrum, parenteral, single agent therapy is required. Combination antimicrobial therapy should be given to more severe cases. Treatment should begin as soon as the diagnosis of IAI is made. Delivery should be accomplished vaginally if possible, as cesarean section increases the risk of maternal morbidity. CS should be considered if vaginal delivery is not imminent after a 12 hours interval from diagnosis of IAI. Postnatally, IV antibiotics should be continued for 2 days more and then replaced by oral antibiotics that should be continued for further 5 days.

Tuberculosis

Human tuberculosis is a bacterial infection caused by *Mycobacterium tuberculosis* and rarely by *Mycobacterium bovis*. The bacillus is carried on droplet nuclei expelled when people with pulmonary tuberculosis cough, sneeze or spit. *M. bovis* is transmitted through ingestion of contaminated milk (Table 21.5).

Table 21.5: Criteria for diagnosis of congenital tuberculosis

- A proven bacteriologic diagnosis
- A primary complex in the infant or fetal liver
- Manifestation of disease during the first few days of life
- Exclusion of the possibility of extrauterine infection

Congenital tuberculosis may develop when the mother develops active tuberculosis in pregnancy with bacteremia. It is believed to be a rare entity, but perhaps one that is increasing in frequency in this age of HIV infection and immunosuppression. Congenital tuberculosis may result from hematogenous spread through the placenta, into the umbilical vein, and subsequently pass into the fetus. This passage prompts formation of liver or lung granulomatous lesions.

Alternatively, placental or genital infection (endometritis) may contaminate amniotic fluid. Aspiration of contaminated fluid may result in a primary pulmonary infection. Ingestion of infected amniotic fluid may cause the development of gastrointestinal disease.

Although all routes of infection appear to occur with equal frequency, accurate determination of the site of infection requires a surgical biopsy of the appropriate organ. Despite the potential for transmission *in utero*, a newborn infant is probably at greater risk of acquiring tuberculosis postpartum than congenitally especially if born to a mother whose sputum contains acid-fast bacilli and whose condition remains undiagnosed and untreated.

Diagnosis

Tuberculin skin test (Montoux test) should be used for screening as it is safe during pregnancy and is reliable. A reaction of 10 mm or more after 48 to 72 hours of intradermal injection of 0.1 ml (5 units) of purified protein derivative (PPD) of tuberculin is considered positive. PPD positive women should be further investigated by chest X-ray and sputum examination.

Treatment

First line antituberculous drugs that can be used during pregnancy are isoniazid, rifampicin, pyrazinamide and ethambutol. Streptomycin is contraindicated as it has toxic effect on fetus. Second line of antitubercular drugs including para-amino-salicylic acid, ethionamide, cycloserine, kanamycin and capreomycin are not recommended for use during pregnancy. Since isoniazid can have central nervous system toxicity, pyridoxine (vit B_6) should be given concurrently. Routine use of pyrazinamide in pregnancy is not recommended because the risk of teratogenicity is undetermined. The standard recommended treatment for pregnant women with TB is a minimum of nine months of therapy with isoniazid, rifampicin and ethambutol. Pyrazinamide should be used only in cases with drug resistance to isoniazid or if indicated on susceptibility testing.

Breastfeeding is not contraindicated during the course of treatment or after the patient has become non-infectious. All babies born to TB patients should receive BCG vaccine and a course of prophylactic INH.

STDs

Sexually transmitted infections are caused by a wide variety of bacteria, viruses and protozoa. In pregnancy, such infections may cause chorioamnionitis, preterm labor, fetal infections, stillbirth or neonatal infection. STDs are more common in young age, low socioeconomic status and in primigravidae.

Syphilis

Syphilis is a chronic systemic infectious disease caused by a spirochete *Treponema pallidum*. In women, syphilis is almost always acquired by sexual contact. Multivariate analysis showed that women with live-born infants who had less than secondary level education, who did not watch television during the week before delivery (this was used as an indicator of socioeconomic status), who had a previous history of syphilis, or who had more than one partner during the pregnancy were at increased risk of syphilis.[4] The organism can cross the placenta to infect the fetus at any stage of pregnancy, resulting in congenital disease or stillbirth.

- *Maternal risks:* About one-third of untreated cases develop tertiary syphilis with involvement of cardiovascular, central nervous and musculoskeletal system, the manifestations being aortic aneurysm, tabes dorsalis, paresis, optic atrophy and gummas. There is a high risk of reactivation of maternal syphilis in the third trimester even if the mother does not show any symptoms. In this case further serological tests in the prenatal care and careful examination of the newborn must be initiated.[5]
- *Fetal risks:* If mother remains untreated the incidence of symptomatic congenital syphilis in neonates is 50 percent in primary and secondary, 40 percent in early latent and 10 percent in late latent phase of tertiary syphilis. The incidence of preterm birth and stillbirth significantly increases. Most of the infants with congenital syphilis look healthy at birth. A few have vascular bullous eruptions, usually on palms and soles. From 4 days to 3 weeks of life, symptoms may develop which include meningeal signs, lacrimation, nasal discharge, sore throat and generalised arthralgia.

Diagnosis

Demonstration of *T. pallidium* from infected lesion by dark-field microscopy of direct smear or by culture. An article by Obisesan et al[6] showed that if syphilis screening is done for all antenatal mothers, it is not cost-effective. If VDRL test is to be continued, efforts must be made to reintroduce TPHA-test, which is more specific-specificity. Because a lot of time and money is needed, the cost-effectiveness of this additional step is questioned at times (Table 21.6).

Table 21.6: Screening tests for syphilis

Screening Tests
- Rapid plasma reagin (RPR)
- Venereal disease research laboratory test (VDRL test)

Specific Tests
- Fluorescent treponemal antibody absorption (FTA-ASBS), microhemagglutination assay (MHA) and *Treponema pallidum* immobilization (TPI) tests are specific antitreponemal antibody tests and should be used to confirm all positive screening test

Management

Syphilis should be identified and treated before pregnancy. If the diagnosis is made during pregnancy, the aim of treatment is to cure the disease in the mother and to prevent congenital syphilis in the fetus or neonate. Benzathene penicillin G is the drug of choice that cures the maternal infection and prevents the congenital infection in 98 percent of cases.

After treatment, quantitative RPR or VDRL titers should be followed closely until negative or stable at a low titer of < 1:4. The quantitative titer declines 4-fold by the third or fourth month after treatment. Sexual partner should also be treated. Breastfeeding is not contraindicated.

Gonorrhea

Gonorrhea is a sexually transmitted disease caused by *Neisseria gonorrhoeae*—a gram-negative diplococcus. In most pregnant women, the infection remains asymptomatic and confined to cervix. Disseminated gonococcal infection (DGI) is more frequent in pregnant than in non-pregnant women. Acute salpingitis secondary to gonococcal infection may occur during first trimester but is rare after the twelfth week of gestation. Gonococcal cervicitis may lead to prelabor rupture of membranes, preterm delivery, chorioamnionitis and endometritis. Gonococcal ophthalmia neonatorum develops in 40 percent of newborn of infected mothers (Table 21.7).[3]

Table 21.7: Diagnosis of gonorrhea

- Microscopic exam of smear to demonstrate gram-negative diplococci within leucocytes.
- Culture in Thayer-Martin medium
- Immunoassay
- DNA detection assay

Treatment

During pregnancy the disease should be treated with cefixime 400 mg orally in a single dose or ceftriaxone 125 mg IM in a single dose or spectinomycin 2 g IM in a single dose. The single dose treatment should be followed by erythromycin base 500 mg orally 4 times daily for 7 days. Ocular prophylaxis and specific treatment should be provided to the infant after delivery.

Chlamydia Trachomatis Infection

Chlamydia trachomatis infection is one of the most prevalent sexually transmitted infections. During pregnancy, there is increased risk of preterm delivery, prelabor rupture of membranes and low birth weight delivery. Higher perinatal death rate and late onset postpartum endometritis have also been reported. Very few studies describe risk factors for chlamydial infection in pregnant women.[7]

In cases with *Chlamydia* cervicitis, colonization with *C trachomatis* occurs in approximately 50 to 60 percent of neonates, if delivered vaginally. 20 to 50 percent of infected infants will develop conjunctivitis within the first two weeks of life and 11 to 18 percent will develop pneumonia in the first 4 months of life.

Diagnosis

It can be made by culture in a susceptible tissue cell line. It is, however, costly and not widely available. Nonculture testing techniques appear to perform well in pregnant women, although studies are limited.[7] Other diagnostic tests are: Polymerase chain reaction, ligand chain reaction and serology.

Management

A wide range of antibiotics are effective against *C. trachomatis*: For pregnant women, azithromycin or erythromycin base in the same dose or amoxycillin 500 mg × 3 time daily for 7 days (98% cure) or clindamycin 450 mg × 4 times daily for 14 days can be given. Sexual contacts should also be treated. Erythromycin estolate should be avoided, as it may be associated with hepatotoxicity during pregnancy. If necessary stearate base should be used.

Postnatal
Ocular prophylaxis at birth with 0.5 percent erythromycin ocular ointment or 1 percent tetracycline reduces the incidence or neonatal inclusion conjunctivitis. Neonates/infants developing conjunctivitis or pneumonia are treated with oral erythromycin for 2 weeks.

Human Papilloma Virus Infection

HPV infection is the most prevalent sexually transmitted disease and the virus is the causative agent of condylomata acuminata (genital warts), juvenile laryngeal papillomatosis and many cases of cervical intraepithelial neoplasia and cervical cancer.

Genital warts may enlarge rapidly during pregnancy and may cause mechanical obstruction to labor. Perinatal exposure may result in the development of juvenile laryngeal papillomatosis, although the risk is small (about 1 in 400).[3]

Diagnosis
Most cases of HPV infection are subclinical. Pap smear may reveal evidence of infection in 10 to 30 percent of cases. White or pink verrucous friable growths may be present. Koilocytosis on Pap smear is an indication for colposcopy. Newer methods of diagnosis utilizing DNA technology are very sensitive and specific but are used only for research.

Treatment
It depends on the size, location and number of identified lesions. All visible lesions are treated. Cryotherapy with liquid nitrogen is a reasonable first line treatment modality. Recurrences are common due to subclinical and multifocal nature of HPV infection. A non-pregnant patient can be treated with podophylline, 5-fluorouracil and intradermal injection of interferon. These drugs can causes fetal toxicity so are not used during pregnancy. During pregnancy, topical application of 80 percent trichloroacetic acid (TCA) is effective for small lesions. Single application has a cure rate of only 20 to 30 percent, so weekly applications are required until the lesions disappear.[4] Laser vaporization is reserved for large, multiple or lesions refractory to TCA application or cryotherapy.

Cesarean section may be necessary for genital warts if patient presents with large obstructive lesions during pregnancy. Most lesions regress to some extent after delivery. Large lesions may get secondarily infected during postnatal period.

Vaginitis

Bacterial Vaginosis (BV)
It is the most frequent vaginal infection occurring in about 20 percent of pregnant women. It occurs due to altered vaginal microbial milieu. BV has been associated with preterm labor or delivery, amniotic fluid infection, chorioamnionitis and postpartum endometritis. About 6 percent of preterm deliveries may be attributable to bacterial vaginosis.[3]

Clinical features
About 50 percent of BV cases are asymptomatic. Thin watery non-pruritic discharge with a fishy odour is the most common symptom (Table 21.8).

Table 21.8: Criteria for the clinical diagnosis of BV

- The presence of a thin, homogenous discharge which adheres to the vaginal wall and a vaginal pH of > 4.5
- The release of a fishy odor on alkalization with 10% potassium hydroxide
- Clue cells on a saline wet mount

Management
Metronidazole is highly effective with a cure rate of 90 percent. The recommended dose is oral 250 mg × 3 or 500 mg × 2 for 7 days or a single dose of 2 gm. Alternatively, clindamycin 300 mg orally × 2 × 7 day can be given. These drugs should be given after the beginning of 2nd term. Since, nitromidazoles cross the placenta, there is some concern about their safe use during pregnancy. Intravaginal metronidazole and clindamycin cream are comparable to systemic therapy and can be safely used during pregnancy. The risk of preterm labor is not reduced with topical therapy.

Candidial vaginitis (CV)

Candida are saprophytic fungi present in vagina of 25 to 40 percent of asymptomatic women. 80-90 percent of candidial vaginitis is caused by *C. albicans* and the remaining by *C. glabrata* and others. *Candida* account for symptomatic vaginitis in 45 percent of pregnant patients. Alteration in the vaginal micro-flora, glycogen availability and depressed maternal cellular immunity all contribute to higher risk in pregnancy.

Diagnosis
The infection presents as vulval and vaginal pruritus, external dysuria and non-malodorous flocculent discharge. On examination there is erythematous vulval rash and a characteristic white cheesy discharge that adheres to the vaginal walls. Vaginal pH is usually less than 4.5. Typical mycelial forms and pseudohyphae are demonstrable in most cases on microscopic examination of material suspended in 10 percent potassium hydroxide.

Management
Topical application of antifungal agents is effective in nearly all patients. Imidazoles are the mainstay of treatment. These are broad-spectrum antifungal agents and include miconazole, clotrimazole tretraconazole and butaconazole. One-day, 3-day and 7-day courses can be used.

Trichomoniasis

Trichomoniasis is caused by *Trichomonas vaginalis*, an anaerobic protozoon, transmitted sexually.

Diagnosis
Motile trichomonads can be easily identified on microscopic examination of saline wet mount by their pear shape, flagella and rapid jerking motility. *Trichomonas* culture can be performed on Diamond's medium and is very sensitive and specific. All women with trichomoniasis should have a culture taken for *Neisseria gonorrhoeae* because of the frequency of co-infection.

Management
During first trimester, intravaginal 100 mg clotrimazole suppositories should be given daily for 14 days, which provides relief in 50 percent cases. After first trimester, a single 2 gm oral dose of metronidazole should be given.

Toxoplasmosis

Toxoplasmosis is caused by *Toxoplasma gondii*, an intracellular protozoon parasite. Cat is the definitive host that passes oocysts in its stool. Primary infection in an individual stimulates the immune system with formation of antibodies. The immunity is usually life-long preventing re-infections. Primary infection during pregnancy carriers with it the risk of fetal damage due to transplacental transmission of the organism. The incidence and severity of fetal damage is related to the gestational age at which infection occurs. The rate is lower in the first trimester but the effects are severe, manifested as miscarriage, stillbirth or severe neonatal disease. With increasing gestational age, the rate of fetal infection rises but the severity diminishes. Overall, 70 percent of infected fetuses are born without obvious damage, 10 percent suffer from only chorioretinitis, intracerebral calcifications, mental retardation and other evidence of parenchyma brain damage.[3] Primary infection acquired more than 6 months before conception does not affect the fetus that within 6 months carries a small risk (Table 21.9).

Table 21.9: Diagnosis

- Demonstration of *T. gondii* in blood and tissues.

Serological tests:
- IgM antibodies appear as early as 5 days after the infection, reach a maximum in 2 to 3 weeks and then decline over weeks and months to gradually disappear.
- IgG antibodies appear 1-2 weeks after the infection, reach a maximum in 6-8 weeks, maintain a plateau for months or years and then gradually decline but persist at low titers for life.
- Seroconversion or a 4-fold rise in IgG estimated at interval of 3 to 4 weeks indicates active disease.
- A positive IgG with negative IgM denotes chronic infection acquired months or years earlier.
- Chronicity is confirmed by similar titer in repeat test 3 weeks later.

Management
If the woman's pre-pregnant IgG titer is known to be stable, she is immunized with almost no risk to the fetus unless she is immunocompromised. Once a primary maternal infection is identified, Spiramycin should be

started immediately in a dose of 300 mg per day in two divided doses for 3 weeks followed by 2 weeks interval until delivery. The drug effectively reduces maternofetal transmission but does not alter the pathology of fetal infection. In cases with demonstrable fetal infection, 3 weeks of spiramycin alternated with 3 weeks of pyrimethamine sulfonamide combination till delivery has been found to give good results. Weekly blood count is mandatory with this regime as there is risk of bone marrow depression and the treatment should be discontinued until blood count is normal. Folinic acid 10 to 20 mg/d must also be given with this combination to prevent hematological effects. Termination of pregnancy should be recommended only if there is strong evidence of fetal infection.

Rubella Infection

Rubella infection is also called German measles. A 58 nm RNA virus belonging to the family Gaviridae causes it. The infection is acquired by respiratory droplets. The most frequent clinical finding in adults is a fine macular rash that starts on the face after an incubation period of 14 to 21 days and spreads to trunk and extremities within 1 to 2 days. Prodromal symptoms, e.g. fever, malaise, headache conjunctivitis may occur before rashes. The infectious period lasts from 7 days before to 5 days after the appearance of rash. There may be associated arthritis and cervical lymphadenopathy. After primary infection, the individual develops almost permanent immunity that can also be induced by vaccination. Reinfection rarely occurs.

If a pregnant woman gets primary infection with rubella and develops viremia, there is high risk of fetus getting affected due to transplacental transmission of viruses. Rubella is a potent teratogen. The fetal risk is highest (almost 80%) during first trimester and then gradually diminishes through the second trimester. Congenital defects involving almost every organ have been reported. 1/3rd of infected, but asymptomatic infants may develop encephalitis and type I diabetes in 2nd or 3rd decade of life. Infants born with congenital rubella may shed the virus for many months and thus can infect other susceptible persons.

Diagnosis

The diagnosis is based on detection of rubella-specific antibodies. Rubella specific Ig-M antibodies appear within one week after the onset of rash, remain positive for a few weeks and become virtually undetectable by 8th or 9th week. Rubella-specific IgG antibodies demonstrated by seroconversion in paired acute and convalescent specimens is indicative of acute infection. It can also be diagnosed by isolation of virus from the blood or throat. Rubella specific IgG antibodies remain present for the whole life after natural infection or vaccination.

Management

Prevention of maternal infection is the best therapy to avoid congenital rubella. Vaccination to all children at the age of 15 months as well as to all susceptible (seronegative) adults is the only effective strategy. Vaccination should not be given to pregnant women and during 3 months before conception.

If pregnant woman gets primary infection, counseling based on the gestational age is important. Termination should be considered for the first and early second trimester pregnancies.

Herpes Simplex Virus (HSV) Infection

HSV is a DNA virus of the herpes family. In human, two types of HSV_1 or HSV_2. Primary orolabial herpes is mainly a disease of childhood, acquired through close contact. Nearly all of such lesions are asymptomatic, in others florid vesiculo-ulcerating lesions occur in oropharynx and lips about a week after exposure. Adenopathy and viremia may persist for a week and viral shedding may continue for 6 weeks. Thereafter antibodies production limits the disease process but the virus remains dormant and occasional flaring up occurs with stress, fever or sunburn. During recurrence, viral shedding lasts upto a week.

During pregnancy, primary infection may stimulate preterm labor if associated with fever and systemic illness. Due to relative immunosuppression in pregnancy, dissemination of HSV may lead to death from hepatitis, encephalitis and general viral dissemination. Primary infection early in pregnancy may cause miscarriage. Severe neonatal morbidity including chorioretinitis, meningitis, encephalitis, mental retardation, seizures and death can result from intrapartum infection especially if mother is suffering from acute primary infection. The rate of neonatal disease is from 0.01 to 0.04 percent.[3]

Neonatal herpes affects about 1 in 15,000 newborns and the prognosis for disseminated disease with encephalitis is poor. Antiviral prophylaxis only partly prevents neonatal herpes infection, because it is not applicable to patients with no known clinical history but may excrete the virus (Table 21.10).[8]

Table 21.10: Diagnosis of HSV

- Presence of multinucleated giant cells in smears from freshly ulcerated vesicles
- Seroconversion in paired sample, first taken as early as possible after the appearance of rash and the second taken 10 to 15 days later. Since, the previously infected patient is at risk for recurrent disease, static levels of IgG are of no clinical significance
- Presence of HSV specific IgM antibodies confirms the diagnosis
- Tissue culture is the gold standard for diagnosis

Management

Only symptomatic treatment is required for recurrent HSV infection. Prophylactic use of acyclovir should be avoided during pregnancy. Acyclovir ointment can be used. Primary infection during pregnancy is an indication for hospitalization and close monitoring. Preterm labor, if it starts, should be appropriately treated. If liver enzymes are raised or there is abnormal neurologic testing, acyclovir should be given to prevent serious morbidity. The oral dose of acyclovir is 200 mg five times daily for 7 to 10 days or until clinical resolution. Intravenous acyclovir is given at 5 mg/kg dose every 8 hours for the same duration.

During labor, the perineum, vagina and cervix should be closely examined for the presence of any lesion if there is history of genital herpes. Cesarean delivery is indicated if lesions are present.

Cytomegalovirus Infection

Cytomegalovirus is a DNA virus of the herpes virus group. Most individuals get infected from it at some time in their life. The normal adult infected with CMV for the first time remains asymptomatic or can develop a syndrome of fever, malaise, lymphocytosis and lymphadenopathy.

About 2 percent of pregnant women develop primary CMV infection and 1 percent gets reactivation of latent infection. About 1/3 of these mothers may transmit the infection of the fetus/neonate at the time of delivery or *in utero*, perinatal transmission being the most common. Pregnant women shed the virus from their cervix more readily than non-pregnant and the rate of shedding increases with increasing gestational age. Virus excreted in breast milk or from other infected neonates in nursery can also infect the neonate. Infected children shed the virus in urine and respiratory tract for a long time.

About 5 to 10 percent of infected newborn are clinically symptomatic at birth with classic TORCH syndrome, i.e. hepatosplenomegaly, hyperbilirubinemia, petechiae, thrombocytopenia and growth retardation. Mortality may be as high as 20 to 30 percent with 90 percent of survivors suffering from late complications. Of the asymptomatic infected neonates, 5 to 15 percent develop some abnormality attributable to CMV within 2 years. CMV is the most common cause of sensorineural hearing loss. About 90 percent of infected infants are asymptomatic at birth and 85 to 95 percent of them develop normally, only 5 to 15 percent can develop sequelae of CMV infection. Various abnormalities attributable to CMV infection are hepatomegaly, seizures, splenomegaly, jaundice, learning disabilities, thrombocytopenia, chorioretinitis, petechiae, optic atrophy, hemolytic anemia, intracranial calcification, intrauterine growth restriction, long bone radiolucencies, mental retardation, microcephaly, dental abnormalities, ventriculomegaly, cerebral atrophy, pneumonitis, etc.[3]

Diagnosis

- Viral culture from cervix, vagina, urine, nasopharynx and blood is the most specific diagnostic test for maternal infection
- Detection of CMV-DNA sequences by *in situ* hybridization and polymerase chain reaction.
- CMV specific antibodies: Seroconversion or a significant rise in IgG titer on examination of paired

specimen suggests infection. CMV-specific IgM antibodies are usually present at 4 to 8 months after primary infection. They can increase periodically and can persist for years at low titer. Reactivation of latent CMV infection during pregnancy may not be accompanied by either an increase or reappearance of IgM antibodies.

Presence of fetal anomalies on ultrasound, e.g. cranial calcification, microcephaly, ventriculomegaly, hydrops or fetal death may point toward the possibility of CMV infection.

Treatment

Since vast majority of acute infections in normal immunocompetent individuals remain asymptomatic and in the rest mild, the treatment is only palliative. Currently, eradication of the virus is beyond the capacity of modern medicine. In immunocompromised patients, the antiviral drug gancyclovir provides temporary relief from severe effects. CMV vaccine is under the process of development. No effective fetal therapy is yet available.

IMMUNIZATION IN PREGNANCY

Infections in pregnancy can have far-reaching consequences. Prevention is desirable. It is, therefore, desirable to have a good knowledge of immunization. Pregnant mothers are at an equal risk of contracting any infection as her non-pregnant counterpart, if not more. Also, in pregnancy there are situations where extra-protection is desirable. In pregnancy, the immunization demanding situations are:

- Grave risk to mother and fetus due to infection.
- Exposure of the mother or other family members to the diseases in pregnancy.
- Epidemic
- Voluntary prophylaxis.

Different types of vaccines available include attenuated live vaccines, inactivated vaccines, immunoglobulins, and new technology-based vaccines. The therapeutic vaccines include tetanus, gas gangrene, diphtheria, antisnake venom, botulism and others. Inactivated vaccines are generally safe in pregnancy. Vaccines against bacterial infections are usually of these types.

Attenuated live vaccines: They give active immunity. However, the small near theoretical risk of transferring infection remains. But the benefits should be weighed against the risk involved. They are thus best avoided in first 12 weeks and last month of pregnancy. Common vaccines used for prophylaxis in pregnancy are tetanus toxoid, cholera and typhoid during epidemics.

Two most influential vaccines that have affected positively are: (i) Tetanus and (ii) anti-D vaccine. These two have given a spectacular result in their respective areas of protection.

Tetanus toxoid: The schedule currently recommended is:

- In first pregnancy two doses, four to six weeks apart.
- In next pregnancy, if it is within two years one booster dose is enough.
- If more than two years have passed before the next pregnancy, two doses are recommended.

Undoubtedly, tetanus toxoid has changed the face of maternal and neonatal tetanus. Amidst, a fear of increased ABO in compatibility due to tetanus toxoid was expressed. However, the risk is reduced with more pure preparations. Also, the benefits far outweigh the risks in favor of administration.

Hepatitis B: Hepatitis B vaccine is recommended for pregnant woman coming in contact with affected person or endemic areas. Recombinant hepatitis B surface antigen is to be given in 3 doses of 1 ml IM (20 µg). First and second dose is to be given one-month apart and third six months after. Prophylactic gamma globulin (16.5% 0.04 ml/kg) is also recommended for administration for exposure to HAV infections. HBIg and HB vaccine are administered for HBV exposure. These have a significant protective effect.

Antirabies vaccine is recommended even in pregnancy as benefits outweigh the risks and so should be given.

CONCLUSION

The concept of maternal immunization to prevent infectious diseases during a period of increased vulnerability in the infant is supported by historical

Table 21.11: Summary of recommendations of immunization during pregnancy

Live virus vaccine:
- Measles: Contraindicated
- Mumps: Contraindicated
- Polio: Not routine
- Yellow Fever: On travel

Inactive virus vaccine:
- Influenza: Voluntary
- Rabies: Same as non-pregnant.
- Hepatitis B: At high risk and –ve for B antigen

Inactivated vacterial vaccines:
- Pneumococcal pneumonia: same as non-pregnant
- Typhoid: Travel
- Plague: Selective vaccination of exposed persons.

Hyper-immunoglobulin:
- Hepatitis B: Postexposure prophylaxis along with HB vaccine initially and then vaccine alone at 1 and 6 months.
- Rabies: Postexposure prophylaxis
- Tetanus: Postexposure prophylaxis

experience and carefully conducted studies of various viral and bacterial vaccines. Candidate vaccines should be minimally reactogenic, immunogenic, and safe. Health education and access to immunization should be a priority if maternal immunization is to succeed as a disease prevention strategy. The potential effect on the incidence of disease in the newborn and young infant can only increase as more candidate vaccines that could be administered during pregnancy become available. In the future, common infections and other, more dreaded diseases, such as herpes simplex virus infection, cytomegalovirus, and human immunodeficiency virus infection, could be prevented with this intervention. Further research on the safety and efficacy of maternal immunization must continue if the occurrence of serious infectious diseases in neonates and young infants is to be reduced (Table 21.11).

REFERENCES

1. Nassar NT: Management of urinary tract infections. *Journal Medical Liban* **48(4):** 278-82, 2000.
2. Krcmery S, Hromec J, Demesova D: Treatment of lower urinary tract infection in pregnancy. *International Journal of Antimicrobial Agents* **17(4):**279-82, 2001.
3. Roy S: Approach to management of infections in pregnancy an overview. In Desai P, Patel P (Eds): *Medical Disorders in Pregnancy.* 1st edition, New Delhi: Jaypee, 172-90, 2000
4. Southwick KL, Southwick KL, Blanco S, Santander A, Estenssoro M, Torrico F, Seoane G, Brade W, Fears M, Lewis J, Pope V, Guarner J, Levine WC: Maternal and Cogenital syphilis in Bolivia, 1996: Prevalence and risk factors. *Bulletin of World Health Organization* **79(1):**33-42, 2001.
5. Vieker S, Siefert S, Lemke J, Pust B: Congenital syphilis after reactivation of "healed" maternal primary infection: Kliniks Padiatrik, **212(6):** 336-39, 2000.
6. Obisesan KA, Ahmed Y: Routine antenatal syphilis screening—a case against. *African Journal of Medical Sciences* **28(3-4):** 185-87, 1999.
7. Nelson HD, Helfand M: Screening for chlamydial infection. *Fetal Diagnosis and Therapy* **16(3):**187-92, 2001.
8. Braig S, Luton D, Sibony O, Edlinger C, Boissinot C, Blot P, Oury JF: Acyclovir prophylaxis in late pregnancy prevents recurrent genital herpes and viral shedding. *European Journal of Obstetrics and Gynecology and Reproductive Biology* **96(1):**55-58, 2001.

22.
Antepartum Hemorrhage

Eugene Leong Weng Kong

INTRODUCTION

Antepartum hemorrhage is an age old obstetric problem with high maternal mortality if not managed well. Perinatal mortality is also concomitantly high in untrained hands. Proper diagnosis is crucial as each form of antepartum hemorrhage requires its specific management. Prematurity is an issue, but with proper neonatal support prognosis is better than before. The advent of high resolution grey scale ultrasound has revolutionized the field of diagnosis in the arena of antepartum hemorrhage.

DEFINITION

Any bleeding from the genital tract after the 22nd week of pregnancy. It complicates 2 to 5 percent of all pregnancies.[1]

ETIOLOGY

Antepartum hemorrhage (APH) can be due to placenta previa, abruptio placentae, local causes or indeterminate antepartum hemorrhage. There are other less common causes of APH, for example, vasa previa, bleeding from a succenturiate lobe, a friable carcinoma of the cervix, velamentous insertion of the umbilical cord, uterine rupture, scar dehiscence, vaginal tear, postcoital bleed, medical causes (for example, Factor 8 deficiency) and vulvovaginal varicosities.

Placenta previa was found in 514 women out of 93,384 deliveries in a 22-year analysis, an incidence of 0.6 percent.[2] In a recent paper,[3] of a total of 32,162 deliveries the incidence of placenta previa was (n=117) 0.36 percents, abruptio placentae (n=232) 0.72 percent, antepartum hemorrhage from the lower genital tract (n=25) 0.07 percent and indeterminate antepartum hemorrhage (n=718) 2.23 percent.

The Confidential Enquiries into Maternal Deaths in the United Kingdom 1991-1993 reported 15 deaths directly due to antepartum and postpartum hemorrhage (mortality rate of 6.4 per million maternities), four due to placenta previa, three due to placental abruption and eight due to postpartum hemorrhage. Care was considered substandard in eleven cases (73 %). The number of direct deaths from antepartum hemorrhage, which had risen sharply in 1988-90, had fallen slightly but was still higher than in 1985-87.[4]

Antepartum Hemorrhage

In any patient presenting with per vaginal bleeding it is important to initiate adequate resuscitative measures. Needless to say an adequate history, physical examination and a gentle speculum examination are important.

Placenta Previa

Placenta that is situated wholly or partially within the lower segment at or after 28 weeks of gestation. There is ambiguity as to whether a diagnosis of placenta previa can be made at 22 weeks of gestation, as it has been traditionally believed that the lower segment forms and is identifiable from then on. Hence, before this period, a diagnosis of a low lying placenta is usually made. Its incidence is quoted to be in the region of 0.36 to 0.6 percent.[2]

Placenta previa is associated with a high maternal mortality in the unattended and in the poorly managed patient. There is a decreasing trend in the maternal mortality rate due to better transfusion services, better anesthetic support, increased availability of ultrasound expertise and a better understanding of its pathology. With increasing rates of cesarean section the incidence of placenta previa with accreta in subsequent pregnancies will increase[2] and may increase morbidity and mortality.

Fetal morbidity and mortality is also reduced with the use of dexamethasone, better neonatal care and conservative management.

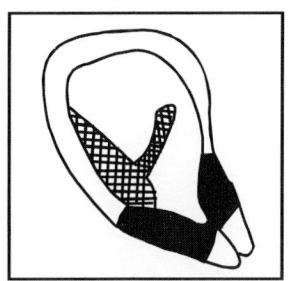

Figure 22.1A: Placenta previa type 1: Placenta just encroaching onto lower segment (darkened)

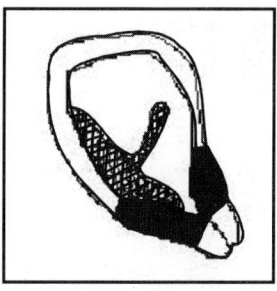

Figure 22.1B: Placenta previa type 2: Placenta extends to internal os

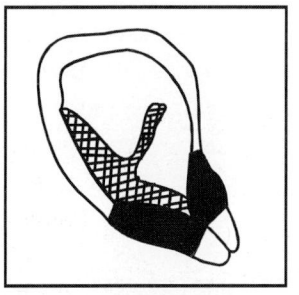

Figure 22.1C: Placenta previa type 3: Placenta covers internal os asymmetrically over the lower segment (darkened)

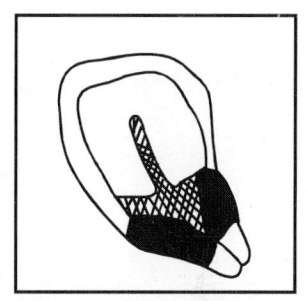

Figure 22.1D: Placenta previa type 4: Placenta covers os symmetrically overlying the lower segment (darkened)

Classification (Figures 22.1A to D)

- Type 1: Low lying placenta positioned close to the os (within 5 cm)
- Type 2: Marginal placenta previa located at the margin of the os
- Type 3: Partial placenta previa partially covering the internal os
- Type 4: Total placenta previa completely covering the os

Etiology and Associated Factors

- Implantation of the blastocyst at a site low in the uterine cavity gives rise to this condition.
- *Parity:* Placenta previa is more common in multiparous women
- *Maternal age:* Risk is 2 to 3 times higher in women over 35 years[5]
- *Uterine scars:* Scars from previous surgical procedures, for example myomectomy, submucous fibroids, TCRE (transcervical resection of the endometrium)
- *Smoking:* Associated with an increased incidence of placenta previa
- *Previous dilatation and curettage:* Prior damaged endometrium/myometrium is a risk factor for a lower implantation site
- *Previous placenta previa:* Associated with a recurrence rate of 4 to 8 percent

Complications Associated with Placenta Previa

- Massive antepartum hemorrhage
- Placenta accreta, increta and percreta

- Malpresentations
- Cesarean section
- Postpartum hemorrhage
- Disseminated intravascular coagulopathy
- Massive transfusion
- Infective hepatitis due to transfusion of infected blood.
- Maternal death.

Symptoms

Asymptomatic patients may have incidental diagnosis of placenta previa during routine ultrasound examination.[6] In the symptomatic patient, characteristically painless per vaginal bleeding occurs; however, 34 percent of placenta previa patients do not bleed. Hemorrhage may occur without warning and there may be no exacerbating cause, for example coitus, exercise. Painless "warning" small hemorrhages may precede a major episode of bleeding. Once labor ensues and with the onset of contractions and cervical dilatation severe hemorrhage will occur. The lower segment where the placenta previa lies does not contract and retract well like the upper segment, hence bleeding might be torrential in the third stage of labor post-cesarean section. This is especially so if placenta accreta, increta or percreta is present and attempts at piecemeal removal of the placenta has occurred in these circumstances. Patients with risk factors like previous placenta previa or previous cesarean section need special evaluation even if asymptomatic.

Signs

A high unengaged presenting part, anterior displacement of presenting part or difficulty in palpating presenting part, an abnormal lie, painless per vaginal bleeding or unstable lie should make one suspect the presence of placenta previa.

Investigations

Basic investigations include hemoglobin estimation and rhesus status. If the cervix had not been examined in early pregnancy a speculum examination (once the patient is stable) will help to rule out a cervical lesion; a Pap smear can also be done if there is no bleeding and there is no recent record of a smear. Patients with rare blood groups and uncommon antibodies for example anti-Lewis and anti-S need the hematologist's attention. Patients with religious affiliations (Jehovah's witness) need special counseling as they decline blood transfusion.

The availability of ultrasound has changed the way placenta previa is diagnosed. Modalities such as soft tissue placentography, thermography and technetium scanning done in the past have been superceded by ultrasonography. Transabdominal imaging is of value in the presence of a good bladder window. However, it can be limited in the presence of a high maternal BMI (body mass index), a posterior previa, acoustic shadowing from the fetus and confusion with local myometrial thickening. Transvaginal ultrasound (TVS) in the properly selected patient in experienced hands is more accurate especially in posterior previas and in the obese patient. TVS affords better resolution with closer proximity of the probe to the area in question. Antepartum diagnosis of placenta percreta have been reported by TVS Doppler, 3-dimensional ultrasound and Magnetic Resonance Imaging (MRI).[7] This is important for management purposes.

Management

The patient who is stable and has no further loss requires conservative management[8] with adequate blood bank support, hematinic supplementation and close observations (pad chart if there is some bleeding) in a tertiary hospital with good neonatal support. The aim is to prolong pregnancy till as near term as possible; thus reducing the inherent risks of prematurity to improve fetal outcome without compromising maternal outcome. If she remained well a cesarean section would be performed at 38 weeks period of amenorrhea. Regular hemoglobin estimation is important to maintain a hemoglobin preferably above 11 to 12 gm percent. Blood needs to be crossmatched in readiness for any bleeding. No digital vaginal examination is done. A gentle speculum examination will exclude a lesion in the vagina or cervix.

Repeat ultrasound examinations for fetal growth and possible "migration" of the placenta upward is important especially in the minor previas (type one). Intramuscular betamethasone/dexamethasone 12 mg × 2 doses, 12 hours apart is given to the mother to promote fetal lung maturity if the fetus is at risk of preterm delivery. The issue of tocolysis in the mother with preterm contractions with a placenta previa is controversial[9] and is not generally recommended. Maternal vasodilation and tachycardia that ensues with β(Beta)sympathomimetic use can impair maternal cardiovascular response in the face of moderate-severe hemorrhage.

Financial, social and emotional costs of prolonged hospitalization need to be considered in the counseling of such patients. Counseling should entail the risks of blood transfusion, postpartum hemorrhage and life saving hysterectomy.

The role of outpatient care for the asymptomatic patient[10] as well as the symptomatic patient[11] with placenta previa, needs further evaluation and are currently not considered mainstream management options. Patients who decline blood transfusion from the outset need to be managed with extreme care and the anesthetist needs to be forewarned.[12] There have been reports of autologous blood collection after use of recombinant human erythropoietin in such instances.

In the patient with recurrent but non-progressive small hemorrhages remote from term or viability there may be a need for top–up transfusions; fetal monitoring is important as growth restriction and fetal compromise can occur with recurrent but non-progressive hemor-rhages. Titrated Rhogam administration in the non-isoimmunized rhesus negative patient is important where relevant.

In the asymptomatic patient with placenta previa type 1 anterior or posterior, a trial of vaginal delivery can be allowed in a tertiary setting, provided there is no bleeding and if it has been agreed that a cesarean section will be required, if bleeding occurred.

The role of examination in theater (double set-up in readiness for cesarean section) has been reduced due to skilled use of good resolution ultrasound scanners. However, examination in theater has a role in remote hospitals where proper ultrasound facilities are unavailable or are suboptimal.

In the patient with significant bleeding which does not stop with conservative measures, delivery by cesarean section is required even if the fetus is preterm. The bleeding is principally maternal in origin as opposed to bleeding from a vasa previa. Concomitant acquisition of good large bore intravenous access, blood product support (involvement of a haematologist), anesthetic support, pediatric support and Consultant involvement is crucial.[4] Initial resuscitation is important. Fetal monitoring whilst preparing for an emergency cesarean section must not be forgotten. The surgeon must be aware that the lower uterine segment has reduced ability to contract and retract which will stop bleeding from the vascular sinuses compared to the upper segment.

Choice of anesthesia is controversial but in the patient with profuse bleeding general anesthesia is faster, does not cause further significant hypotension (as opposed to spinal anesthesia) and is probably wiser in patients with placenta accreta. In patients with posterior previas the delivery of the fetus is less difficult as compared to anterior previas. If the placenta was situated anteriorly, skill is needed when entering the amniotic cavity; cutting through the placenta should be avoided by gaining access to the upper edge of the placenta and rupturing the membranes above this. After delivery of the fetus, use of uterine massage, syntocinon infusion and ergometrine is important in the control of hemorrhage. PGF2-alpha (carboprost) may be helpful in cases that do not respond to syntocinon or ergometrine. In patients with placenta increta or percreta an extrafascial hysterectomy is required; an alternative is to leave the placenta *in situ*. Expert experienced hands are needed in placenta previa percreta with bladder involvement; it is wise to perform a careful hysterectomy.

Surgical procedures that aim to conserve the uterus include undersewing of the placental bed, bilateral internal iliac artery ligation, uterine packing, hemostatic multiple square suturing and B-Lynch plication (uterine atony). In patients who belong to the faith of Jehovah's witness, autologous blood transfusions may be an acceptable compromise; if not early hysterectomy is required in the face of torrential hemorrhage. Radiologic uterine artery embolization is an alternative in a stable patient. Cesarean hysterectomy is lifesaving in selected cases, but it must be done early before DIVC and/or irreversible shock has set in. Aortic compression can be used to reduce the pulse pressure while waiting for the arrival of further support.

Placenta accreta/increta/percreta

Placenta accreta occurs when there is morbid adherence of the placenta to the myometrium (Figures 22.2A to D). This is due to an underdeveloped or absent decidua basalis which permits villous invasion of the myometrium. Placenta accreta occurs very often in association with an anterior placenta previa in a patient with a previous cesarean section. Placenta accreta may be partial or total. Partial placenta accreta is associated with difficulty in delivery of the placenta and post partum hemorrhage due to retained fragments of the placenta. In total placenta accreta, placental separation does not occur normally and there is no distinct plane of separation. Cesarean hysterectomy is often lifesaving. Clinical outcome is very dependent on the back-up facilities available, surgeon's skill and experience. Conservative management in cases with no bleeding, where the placenta has been left *in situ* together with vigilant use of methotrexate, has been reported. As the depth of encroachment of the placenta deepens a placenta increta occurs. When the placenta reaches the serosa a placenta percreta occurs.

Frederiksen et al[2] reported that 55 women required hysterectomy at the time of delivery in cases of placenta previa on the scar; an incidence of cesarean hysterectomy of 11 percent. Pathologic examination revealed 20 women (37%) with placenta accreta, 7 women (13%) with placenta increta, 7 women (13%) with placenta percreta and 20 women (37%) were found to have no placental or uterine pathology. Histologically confirmed placenta accreta in women with placenta previa occurred in 34 (6.6 %) of 514 women. Antenatal diagnosis of placenta percreta involving the bladder has been reported.

Postnatal Care

Postpartum care must be meticulous and steps should be taken to avoid further postpartum hemorrhage from uterine atony. Correct disseminated intravascular coagulation (DIVC), fluid overload and dilutional

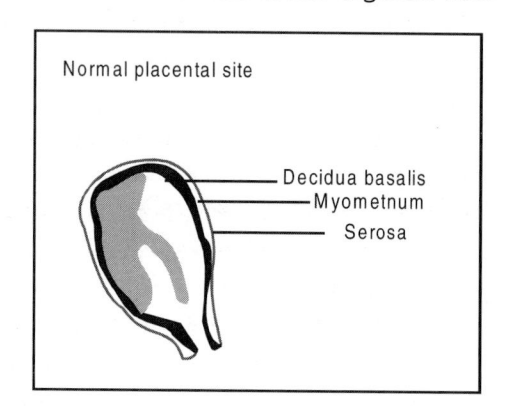

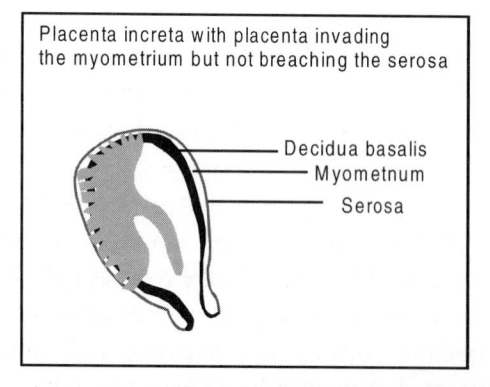

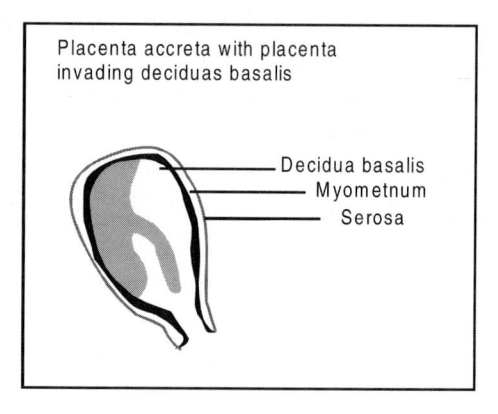

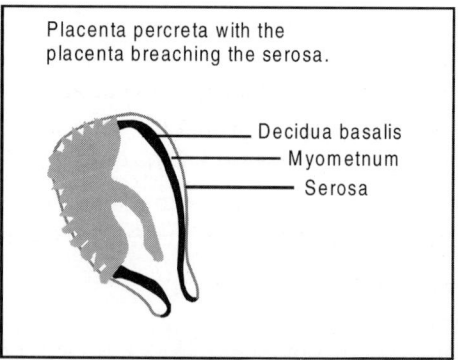

Figures 22.2A to D: Different degrees of adherent placenta

coagulopathy. Observe for renal shutdown, bleeding from the pedicles or vaginal stump in hysterectomised patients. Intra-abdominal drains used must be of adequate size to avoid blockage. Relaparotomies may sometimes be required. Risks of hitherto undetected viral transmissions through blood product usage must be borne in mind. In the hysterectomised patient counseling is important, for example, intact sexual function, but loss of menses and reproductive function.

ABRUPTIO PLACENTA

Definition: Bleeding from the genital tract due to premature separation of the normally sited placenta.[13] The reported incidence is 0.49 to 1.8 percent. Diagnostic precision or rather imprecision will influence reported rates of abruptio placentae. Perinatal mortality is as high as 14.4 to 67.3 percent.[1, 13]

There are two types of abruptio placenta: revealed and concealed. Revealed abruptio placenta occurs when blood tracks down between the membranes and the wall of the uterus; if the blood was to remain within the uterine cavity concealed abruptio placentae would result. The concealed type is more dangerous and is linked to more severe complications. There are four grades of abruptio placenta.[1]

- Grade 0: Asymptomatic. Diagnosed retrospectively when a small retroplacental clot is discovered postpartum
- Grade 1: Vaginal bleeding, uterine tetany and tenderness may be present
- Grade 2: Signs of fetal distress present with or without external per vaginal bleeding
- Grade 3: Persistent abdominal pain, maternal shock and fetal demise present. There is marked uterine tetany with boardlike rigidity. Coagulation defects present in 30 percent. External bleeding may or may not be present.

Risk Factors Associated with Abruptio Placenta

- Direct trauma to the uterus
- Smoking
- Cocaine abuse
- Older women
- Previous abruptio placenta (there is a recurrence risk of 8.3 to 16.7%)
- Hypertension
- Sudden decompression, for example, sudden membrane rupture
- External cephalic version
- Folic acid deficiency (evidence inconclusive)
- Lupus anticoagulant positive.

Symptoms

There is pain, frequent uterine contractions (tetanic more than 5 contractions per 10 minutes) and bleeding per vagina in the revealed type of abruptio placenta. There is usually no period of relaxation in between contractions. There may be difficulty in appreciating fetal movements.

Symptoms of pre-eclampsia may be present. Abruptio placentae is associated with preterm labor, intrauterine growth restriction, congenital malformations, unexpected intrauterine death and a higher perinatal mortality rate. Silent abruption can be diagnosed with a high index of suspicion. Extravasation of blood into the myometrium causes pain.

Signs

Clinical evidence of shock may be present, for example, restlessness, pallor, cold and clammy extremities. Blood pressure may be elevated in the initial stages followed by hypotension. Pallor is present especially in Grades 3 and 4 abruptio placenta associated with maternal tachycardia. The patient would be unduly distressed by pain. In the classical presentation, abdominal examination would reveal *woody hardness,* difficulty in palpating the fetal parts and difficulty in auscultating for the presence of fetal heart. There would be per vaginal bleeding in the revealed variety. Amniotomy would reveal blood stained amniotic fluid.

Often there is associated pregnancy-induced hypertension; thus, in the patient with severe abruption blood pressure may be normal although in the majority it would be low. Overt disseminated intravascular coagulation (DIVC) can be present. In the concealed variety there is no per vaginal bleeding seen. It is not the amount of visible blood loss that is important but the general status of the patient. CTG abnormalities may prompt one to reexamine the patient especially in the patient with minimal signs or symptoms.

The differential diagnosis of abruptio placentae include: other causes of vaginal bleeding (placenta previa, indeterminate antepartum hemorrhage, local causes) and causes of abdominal pain in the second and third trimesters. The latter would include ruptured acute appendicitis, rectus sheath hematoma, red degeneration of uterine fibroid and pyelonephritis among others.

Investigations

Investigations lend support to a diagnosis of abruptio placenta and help assess its severity. A full blood count and DIVC screen is relevant. A urine microscopic examination would reveal no evidence of a urinary tract infection but proteinuria can be present. The hemoglobin level and the platelet count may be low especially if concomitant DIVC has occurred. Ultrasound examination is important to confirm a normally sited placenta. The absence of a retroplacental clot (which appears as a hyperechogenic or iso-echogenic area when compared with the placenta) or a subchorionic hematoma does not rule out an abruptio placenta. Identification of a posterior placenta in the presence of severe backache associated with per vaginal bleeding should make one suspect an abruptio placenta especially in the absence of other indicative signs. The diagnosis of abruptio placente is *clinical*.

Management

The unstable patient with shock and DIVC needs resuscitation to correct the blood loss and the DIVC. Good intravenous access with transfusion of blood product components like fresh frozen plasma and packed red cells are important. Mother's condition should be stabilized. Fetal monitoring is important. If delivery is not imminent and the fetus is alive recourse to delivery by cesarean section is crucial if there are signs of fetal distress. If delivery was imminent especially in a multiparous patient and the CTG trace was reactive, a vaginal delivery can be allowed. Once labor is established it is usually rapid. Amniotomy would release intrauterine pressure and help to avoid extravasation of blood into the myometrium and possible DIVC.

Caution must be excercised when using prostaglandins to induce labor in the presence of a suspected abruptio placentae with a live fetus.

It is controversial as to which came first; preterm labor or abruptio placenta when both are present. The role of tocolysis in these instances and where maturity is not in question is not validated especially in cases with suspected mild abruption. This precept has been challenged.[9] Conservative management, for example waiting, is generally not recommended as even mild abruption is not without risk both for the fetus as well as the mother. Delivery would be wiser. However, a balance must be struck between traditional conservative approach with a resultant low cesarean section rate and a high perinatal mortality versus a more aggressive approach of immediate delivery by cesarean section in all but the mildest cases of abruptio placentae where the fetus was alive.[14] In instances where there is fetal demise, where delivery is not imminent then recourse to an operative delivery may still be required especially if maternal hemodynamic status was compromised.

Cesarean section must be done by an experienced surgeon in the presence of an expert anesthetist with adequate blood bank support. Postpartum hemorrhage due to a poorly contracted uterus must be dealt with accordingly. A Couvelaire uterus (the uterine surface is pale with bluish streaky discoloration due to extravasation of blood) is associated with uterine atony.

Correct management of the third stage of labor is crucial. High dose oxytocic infusion and/or syntometrine usage in the absence of contraindications will help to reduce blood loss.

Examination of the placenta postdelivery would enable quantification of the degree and severity of abruption. A negative rhesus status would require Rhogam to be given in the non-isoimmunized patient in the appropriate amounts based on a Kleihauer test within 72 hours.

Management of more severe complications like severe DIVC and renal shut down would require multidisciplinary management in a high dependency setting. Invasive intravenous central monitoring is controversial in the presence of DIVC. Renal dialysis may be required to overcome temporary renal shut down.

Where *in utero* fetal death has occurred and the patient was in labor, delivery is usually rapid. If labor has not ensued but the patient was stable, onset of labor would usually not be delayed. Adequate bereavement support is important.

Postnatal Care

Hemodynamic stability with normal blood pressure, pulse rate and good urine output are signs of a well resuscitated patient. Recurrence is quoted as 5 to 17 percent after one episode and rises to 25 percent after 2 episodes.[1] Evidence that recurrence can be averted with adequate folic acid intake is not strong. A subsequent pregnancy following one which has had placental abruption is a high risk pregnancy[15] in terms of recurrence, excess risk of preterm birth, small for gestational age (SGA) and pregnancy induced hypertension.[16]

Indeterminate Antepartum Hemorrhage (IAPH)

Indeterminate antepartum hemorrhage (IAPH) is a diagnosis of exclusion after ruling out placenta previa, abruptio placenta, and local genital tract lesions. Its incidence is quoted at 2.23 percent[3] to as high as 5 percent.[17] Recent published studies on this subject are scanty. It is postulated that the origin of the bleeding is due to marginal separation of a normally sited placenta leading to a reduced functional reserve. Morbidity is related to preterm delivery.[3, 18, 19]

The patient classically presents with painless per vaginal bleeding where the placenta is in the upper segment, with no evidence of abruption and there are no local lesions detected. The amount of bleeding is usually not profuse. One needs to perform a clinical assessment to rule out an abruption in the absence of a tense tender irritable uterus with the fetal parts easily palpable and the fetal heart sounds easily heard. A speculum examination needs to be done. An ultrasound examination to assess the site of the placenta and to rule out gross fetal abnormality among others, is important. The absence of retroplacental clots on ultrasound examination does not exclude an abruption.

A full blood count, Group and Screen and a cardiotocographic examination is required. Intravenous access and reassurance is important.

Recurrent episodes of bleeding can occur. Rhogam administration in the appropriate circumstances is important. If the patient remains stable and remote from term conservative management is appropriate.

The controversial issue is: should these patients be allowed past their due dates?[19] Current evidence[3] does not support *routine induction* of labor beyond EDD + 0 days in the absence of other obstetric indications. No doubt close maternal and fetal surveillance is needed. Prognosis is generally good for fetus and mother. In a recently published study[3] there was a reported higher incidence of preterm deliveries and congenital fetal abnormalities without any difference in the incidence of growth restricted fetuses. The perinatal mortality rate was higher in the study group although it did not reach statistical significance. There were significantly more labor inductions in the IAPH group.

Uterine Rupture

Rupture of uterus can occur spontaneously. It can occur in the scarred or unscarred uterus. It can occur antenatally or intrapartum. The fetus usually dies if extruded into the peritoneal cavity. If maternal hypovolemia is significant fetal oxygenation is compromised. Patients with a scarred uterus from previous cesarean section, previous classical cesarean section, previous hysterotomy, previous myomectomy and previous metroplasty are at risk of uterine rupture. Patients with maneuvers done, for example, difficult forceps, version or extraction done are also at risk. There are other causes of uterine rupture: neglected obstructed labor, gunshot wounds, seat belt injuries and inappropriate use of oxytocin or prostaglandins. Prior stabilization of the mother's condition is important. Definitive surgical procedure depends on findings at laparotomy and the need to preserve fertility. If conservative surgery and repair is not possible then a hysterectomy is required.

Vasa Previa

Umbilical vessels course through the membranes in advance of the fetal presenting part characteristically extending across the cervical os; this can occur in patients with a velamentous insertion of the umbilical cord or those with a succenturiate lobe of the placenta. These vessels can tear spontaneously, at spontaneous rupture of membranes or at artificial rupture of membranes. Antenatal diagnosis requires a high index of suspicion. Significant vaginal bleeding, fetal distress, fetal tachycardia with or without sinusoidal fetal heart rate tracings on CTG or variable decelerations on CTG coinciding with membrane rupture must alert one to the presence of a vasa previa.

Fetal exsanguination occurs in the absence of immediate recognition and abdominal delivery. Routine vaginal examination may reveal a pulsatile area in the membranes. It is important to rule out the possibility of vasa previa before an amniotomy. Bleeding is fetal in origin from a disrupted placental circulation. Fetal mortality can approach 50 percent. Apt's test is of help to differentiate the source of bleeding. Prenatal diagnosis is possible by grey scale ultrasound and Doppler examination.[20] In patients diagnosed early, delivery is by cesarean section. In the postdelivery examination of the placenta there is an increased association with velamentous insertion of the cord, bi-lobed placentae, succenturiate lobes and marginal cord insertion.

Apt's Test[1]

Fetal hemoglobin is alkaline stable, whereas adult hemoglobin is not. The Apt test is designed to differentiate fetal from maternal blood that is passed per vagina.
1. A sample of blood is collected per vagina (X). Two ten cc. test tubes with 5 cc. of water each (X and C) is prepared. 2 drops of adult blood (adult volunteer or maternal) is added to one (C), while in the other sufficient X amount of blood is added to match the depth of color as in the control (C).
2. Add 1 cc. of 1 percent sodium hydroxide to each X and C.
3. *Positive for fetal hemoglobin:* X remains pink for longer (fetal hemoglobin is more resistant to alkali denaturation). C tube becomes pink to yellow brown in 2 minutes (as adult hemoglobin is denatured).

Circumvallate Placenta

Patients with circumvallate placenta can present with antepartum hemorrhage. It is associated with prematurity; increased perinatal morbidity and an increased rate of fetal malformations. Bleeding is usually bright red, moderate and is nearly always painless. If remote from term management is expectant. An ultrasound examination is needed to rule out placenta previa. Antenatal ultrasound diagnosis of a circumvallate placenta has been reported[21] but it has been found to be inaccurate.[22] If the patient is in labor and bleeding is persistent or heavy, examination under anesthesia with a view to cesarean section must be arranged. In the absence of other obstetric indications, induction of labor at term is required. Definitive diagnosis is made by examination of the placenta post delivery.

SUMMARY

Antepartum hemorrhage is a very important condition because it entails high maternal and fetal morbidity and mortality. Initial resuscitation of the mother is important. Correct diagnosis will ensure appropriate management. The involvement of a multidisciplinary team in a tertiary hospital that includes a senior consultant obstetrician, a trained anesthetist, a neonatologist and a hematologist is important.

REFERENCES

1. Konje JC, Walley RJ: Bleeding in late pregnancy. In James DK, Steer PJ, Weiner CP, Gonik B (Eds): *High Risk Pregnancy: Management Options.* WB Saunders Co., Fifth printing, Chapter 9, 119-36, 1996.
2. Frederiksen MC, Glassenberg R, Stika CS: Placenta previa: A 22-year analysis. *American Journal of Obstetrics and Gynecology* **180**: 1432–37, 1999.
3. Chan CCW, To WWK: Antepartum Hemorrhage of unknown origin–what is its clinical significance? *Acta Obstetrica Gynecologica Scandinavia* **78**: 186–90, 1999.
4. Report on Confidential Enquiries into Maternal Deaths in the United Kingdom 1991–1993, Department of Health, Welsh Office, Scottish Office Department of Health, Department of Health and Social Services, Northern Ireland, Crown Copyright, Chapter 3, 32-47, 1996.
5. Zhang J and Savitz D: Maternal age and placenta previa: A population based, case control study. *American Journal of Obstetrics and Gynecology* **168**: 641-45, 1993.
6. Hill DJ and Beischer NA: Placenta previa without antepartum hemorrhage. *Australian New Zealand Journal of Obstetrics and Gynecology* **20**: 21–23, 1980.

7. Megier P, Harmas A, Mesnard L, Esperandieu OL, Desroches A: Antenatal diagnosis of placenta percreta using gray scale ultrasonography, color and pulsed Doppler imaging. *Ultrasound Obstetrics and Gynecology* **15**: 268, 2000.
8. Macafee CHG, Millar WG, Harley G: Maternal and fetal mortality in placenta previa. *Journal of Obstetrics and Gynecology British Commonwealth* **69**: 203–12, 1962.
9. Towers CV, Pircon RA, Heppard M: Is tocolysis safe in the management of third trimester bleeding? *American Journal of Obstetrics and Gynecology* **180**: 1572–78, 1999.
10. Rosen DMB, Peek MJ: Do women with placenta previa without antepartum hemorrhage require hospitalization? *Australian New Zealand Journal of Obstetrics and Gynecology* **34**: 130–34, 1994.
11. Cotton DB, Read JA, Paul RH, Quilligan EJ: The conservative aggressive management of placenta previa. *American Journal of Obstetrics and Gynecology* **137**: 687–95, 1980.
12. DeCastro RM: Bloodless surgery: Establishment of a program for the special medical needs of the Jehovah's Witness community–The gynecologic surgery experience at a community hospital. *American Journal of Obstetrics and Gynecology* **180**: 1491-98, 1999.
13. Hibbard BM and Jeffcoate TNA: Abruptio placentae. *American Journal of Obstetrics and Gynecology* **27**: 155–67, 1966.
14. Hurd WW, Miodovnik M, Hertzberg V, Lavin JP: Selective management of abruptio placentae: A prospective study. *Obstetrics and Gynecology* **61**: 467-73, 1983.
15. Rasmussen S, Irgens LM, Dalaker K: Outcome of pregnancies subsequent to placental abruption: a risk assessment. *Acta Obstetrica Gynecologica Scandinavia* **79**: 496–501, 2000.
16. Rasmussen S, Irgens LM, Dalaker K: A history of placental dysfunction and risk of placental abruption. *Pediatrics Perinatal Epideomology* **13**: 9-27, 1999.
17. Chamberlain G, Philipp E, Howlett B, Masters K: Hemorrhage in pregnancy. In: British Births, 1970: a survey under the joint auspices of the National Birthday Trust Fund and the Royal College of Obstetricians and Gynecologists. Volume 2 Obstetric Care. London: Heinemann Medical: 54-79, 1978.
18. Ajayi RA, Soothill PW, Campbell S, Nicolaides KH: Antenatal testing to predict outcome in pregnancies with unexplained antepartum hemorrhage. *British Journal of Obstetrics and Gynecology* **99**: 122–25, 1992.
19. Willocks J: Antepartum hemorrhage of uncertain origin. *The Journal of Obstetrics and Gynecology of the British Commonwealth* **78**: 987–91, 1971.
20. Lee W, Lee VL. Kirk JS, Sloan CT, Smith RS, Comstock CH: Vasa previa: Prenatal diagnosis, Natural Evolution and Clinical Outcome. *American Journal of Obstetrics and Gynecology* **95**: 572–76, 2000.
21. McCarthy J, Thurmond AS, Jones MK, Sistrom C, Scanlan RM, Jacobson SL, Lowensohn R: Circumvallate placenta: Sonographic diagnosis. *J Ultrasound Med* **14**:21-6, 1995.
22. Harns RD, Wells WA, Black WC, Chertoff ID, Poplack SP, Sargent SK, Crow HC: Accuracy of prenatal sonography for detecting circumvallate placenta. *Am J Roentgenol* **168**: 1603-08, 1997.

23. Hypertensive Disorders in Pregnancy

Alokendu Chatterjee
Gita Basu (Banerjee)

PART Two — Feto-maternal Medicine

INTRODUCTION

Hypertensive disorders in pregnancy (HDP) is regarded as one of the most serious medical disorders during pregnancy. It may complicate 5 to 15 percent of all pregnancies, and is responsible for about 15 to 20 percent of maternal mortality in both industrialised and developing countries. There is generalised vasospasm leading to systemic disorders involving all the vital organs of the body. Hence, any vital organ failure can lead to critical illness causing increased mortality. Unfortunately, it cannot be predicted early enough in general pregnant population, except with those with genuine risk factors. Only method to check this menace, is quality antenatal care, judicious use of antihypertensive drugs and early delivery before crisis deepens.

Severity of hypertensive diseases in pregnancy is controllable with proper management in most of the cases and mortality is surely avoidable.

DEFINITION

- *Hypertension*: It is defined as raised blood pressure recorded at least on two occasions at six hours apart, it may be either,
- Diastolic blood pressure greater than 90 mmHg or
- Systolic blood pressure greater than 140 mmHg

During pregnancy blood pressure should be measured in a sitting position (ambulatory patient) or semirecumbent position, 45° head up (hospitalized patient), the right arm should be used consistently and the arm should be in a horizontal position at the level of heart.

In the non-pregnant patient, the fifth Korotkoff sound corresponds to the intra-arterial measurement. Evidences show that Korotkoff sound phase V is closer to true intra-arterial pressure and it is rarely very low or zero as was previously claimed. Phase IV is more difficult to detect and has limited reproducibility.[1] So phase V is used in pregnant patients also.

- *Proteinuria:* Significant proteinuria is defined as 300 mg/ 24-hour in urine sample.

CLASSIFICATION OF HYPERTENSIVE DISORDER COMPLICATING PREGNANCY

Widely known classification of ACOG is as follows:[2]

A. *Pregnancy-induced hypertension (PIH):* Hypertension that develops as a consequence of pregnancy and regresses postpartum. A normotensive woman develops hypertension during pregnancy, which normalizes after delivery.
   Types:
   1. Hypertension without proteinuria—gestational hypertension.
   2. Pre-eclampsia—hypertension with proteinuria.
   3. Eclampsia—pre-eclampsia along with convulsion.
B. *Coincidental hypertension:* Chronic underlying hypertension that antecedes pregnancy or persists postpartum.
C. *Pregnancy aggravated hypertension:* Where underlying hypertension gets worsened by pregnancy.
   1. Superimposed pre-eclampsia
   2. Superimposed eclampsia.

This classification has been recently modified.[3] HDP now is classified as:
- Chronic hypertension
- Pre-eclampsia/eclampsia
- Pre-eclampsia/eclampsia superimposed on chronic hypertension
- Gestational hypertension

CLARIFICATIONS

1. *Normal blood pressure:* Blood pressure normally falls in pregnancy with no change in systolic but diastolic blood pressure is lowered by 10 mmHg with the lowest recording at 14 to 20 week's gestation, before rising toward prepregnancy values by term. The mid trimester fall of blood pressure is due to significant decreases in vascular tone following the cardiovascular alterations, leading to peripheral vasodilatation.
2. *Gestational hypertension:* An exaggerated blood pressure detected first time after mid-pregnancy without proteinuria.
   This non-specific diagnosis covers:
   a. Women who will eventually develop pre-eclampsia, but before they manifest proteinuria.
   b. Women who do not have pre-eclampsia syndrome. The final diagnosis is made at postpartum period. If the blood pressure returns to normal by 12 weeks postpartum it is known as *Transient hypertension.* If raised blood pressure persists even after 12 weeks it is known as *Chronic hypertension.*

   The term gestational hypertension is used only during pregnancy until a more specific diagnosis can be assigned postpartum.
3. *Pre-eclampsia*–A diastolic blood pressure exceeding 90 mmHg on at least two occasions in the second half of pregnancy, where the blood pressure was previously normal, accompanied by significant proteinuria, (>300 mg/24 hr). Traditionally the presence of peripheral edema has been included in the definition, but this is a common finding in normal pregnancy and its absence does not preclude the diagnosis.
4. *Eclampsia:* The occurrence of tonic-clonic convulsions not caused by coincidental neurological disorders in a patient with pre-eclampsia.
5. *Chronic hypertension:* Hypertension which is apparent prior to or in the first half of pregnancy or persisting more than six weeks after pregnancy.

   The definition of superimposed pre-eclampsia in the presence of chronic hypertension can be difficult to make, but is usually associated with a worsening of the hypertension and the development or worsening of proteinuria.
6. *Transient hypertension:* Hypertension that develops after the midtrimester of pregnancy and is characterized by mild elevation of blood pressure that do not compromise the pregnancy. This form of hypertension regresses after delivery but may return in subsequent gestations.

Predisposing factors for the development of pre-eclampsia includes (Table 23.1):
- Conditions where the placenta is enlarged (multiple gestation, diabetes, hydrops)
- Pre-existing vascular disease (such as in diabetes or autoimmune—vasculitis)
- Sickle cell disease.

Table 23.1: High-risk subject

Epidemiology	Abnormal Pregnancy	Medical Disorders
• Nulliparity • Teenage • Elderly • Family history • Past history • Racial • New paternity • Obesity	• Multiple Pregnancy • Hydatidiform mole • Hydrops • Chromosomal anomalies trisomy 13, triploidy	• Essential HT • Renal diseases • Diabetes • Connective tissue disorders • Insulin resistance • Thrombophilia

PRE-ECLAMPSIA

Etiology

Pre-eclampsia is often referred to as the disease of theories with many mechanisms proposed to account for the clinical picture. Current theories of the etiology of PIH center round three mechanisms:

Immunological Mechanism

Immunological mechanism is known that from early pregnancy trophoblastic cells escape into the maternal circulation; this may occur to a great extent in hypertensive pregnancy. Thus an excessive amount of antigens might be released into the maternal circulation and result in the formation of antigen-antibody complexes which are deposited in specific sites like renal glomeruli and placenta. This deposition might be responsible for the development of the hypertension process.

Inadequate trophoblastic invasion: Trophoblast invades the spiral arterioles in the first-half of pregnancy converting them into low-resistance conduits for excess maternal blood flowing into the placenta, leading to adequate exchanges of oxygen and nutrients. If this invasion is inadequate or incomplete, the spiral arterioles have a higher resistance which results in less blood flow, and pregnancy-induced hypertension may be an attempt to compensate for this. Although exact trigger factor(s) are not yet known but a suggestion has been made to understand this theory.

Pathophysiology

Primary cause unknown (? Genetic/? Immunological)
Initial phase: vascular pathology

Failure of second wave trophoblast invasion
↓
↓ Blood flow in spiral art.
↓
↓ Placental blood flow.
↓
Placental bed ischemia
↓
Stimulation of macrophage systems
↓
Liberation of TNFα (Trigger)
↓
Endothelial damage / dysfunction

Liberation of TNF (Tumor necrosis factor) may be the "Trigger" factor, which is released from stimulation of macrophage system due to ischemia.

Altered Vascular Reactivity

In severe PIH there seems to be a reduced concentration of prostacycline (PGI_2) and its metabolites in maternal blood and also in uterine and umbilical vessels. So there is less opposition to the vasoconstrictor action of angiotensin II and the prostanoid thromboxane (TXA_2); placental blood flow is thus reduced.

In normal pregnancy, $PGI_2 > TXA_2$ = vasodilatation
In PIH, $PGI_2 < TXA_2$ = Vasospasm

Coagulation Disturbance

Coagulation disturbance has been postulated that the placenta may release thromboplastin which causes disseminated intravascular coagulation, and that the fibrin deposition in the kidney and placenta results in the development of hypertension and placental insufficiency.

Pathophysiology

There is now ample evidence that the clinical picture of pre-eclampsia is due to an activation or dysfunction of vascular endothelial cells and co-existent platelet activation.

A reduction in the systhesis of vasodilatory nitric oxide (NO) and prostacyclin (PGI_2) and an increased production of endothelin by the vascular endothelium in pre-eclampsia could account not only for the characteristic vasospasm but also for the activation of circulating platelets (NO and PGI$_2$ stabilise these cells).

Vasospasm and endothelial cell dysfunction with subsequent platelet activation and microaggregate formation account for many of the pathological features of pre-eclampsia.

Effects on vital organs
1. *Cerebral lesion*: Vasospasm and cerebral edema have both been implicated in the cerebral manifestations of pre-eclampsia and its progression to eclampsia. There are small hemorrhages scattered throughout its substance. Massive hemorrhage in the brain may cause death.
2. *Eye*: Retinal hemorrhage, exudates and papilledema are characteristic of hypertensive encephalopathy and are rare in pre-eclampsia. Angiospasm seems to be the most common finding.
3. *Kidney*: Characteristic lesion is glomeruloendotheliosis, it consists of endothelial and mesangial cell swelling, basement membrane inclusions but little disruption of renal epithelial podocytes.
4. *Liver*: Subendothelial fibrin deposition is associated with elevated liver enzymes. This can be associated with hemolysis and a low platelet count due to platelet consumption (and subsequent wide-spread activations of the coagulation systems). The presence of these findings is called the HELLP syndrome. The epigastric pain and liver tenderness probably arise from distension of the capsule.
5. *Heart*: Arrhythmia, failure, and pulmonary edema.
6. *Lungs*: Adult respiratory distress syndrome (ARDS), bronchopneumonia, airway obstruction.

Systemic Changes Associated with Pre-eclampsia

1. *Cardiovascular*: Generalized vasospasm. In early phase, cardiac output is high with low peripheral resistance, but as the disease progresses this changes to low cardiac output with high peripheral resistance. There is reduced central venous pressure and pulmonary wedge pressure.
2. *Hematological*
   - Platelet activation and consumptive coagulopathy,
   - Decreased plasma volume, increased blood viscosity
3. *Renal*
   - Proteinuria
   - Decreased glomerular filtration rate, decreased urate excretion.
4. *Hepatic*: Periportal necrosis, Subcapsular hematoma.
5. *Central nervous system*: Cerebral edema, increased intracranial tension, cerebral hemorrhage, hyperemia.

Diagnosis of Pre-eclampsia

1. *Symptoms*—may be asymptomatic, there may be headache, visual disturbances, epigastric pain and progressive edema.
2. *Signs*: Elevated blood pressure, rapid weight gain, non-dependent edema, brisk deep tendon reflexes, and ankle clonus.
3. *Investigations*: (These are repeated at intervals)
   - Urine analysis–24 hour urine collection for total protein and creatinine clearance, quantitative analysis is preferred
   - Full blood count (Platelets and hematocrit)
   - Blood chemistry (renal function, total protein)
   - Plasma urate concentration
   - Liver function tests
   - Coagulation profile
   - Ultrasound—fetal maturity, amniotic fluid volume, Doppler velocimetry, placental maturity
   - NST, biophysical profile
   - Ophthalmologic examination.

Severity of PIH

a. *Mild*: PIH is considered mild if BP < 160-110 mmHg and there is no significant proteinuria.
b. *Severe*: PIH is considered severe when, any one or more of the following are present; even if the DBP is not upto 110 mmHg but if she has any one of the following, she should be treated as a case of severe PIH.
   1. Systolic blood pressure more than 160 mmHg or diastolic blood pressure more than 110 mmHg on at least 2 occasions 6 hours apart.
   2. Proteinuria more than or equal to 5 g in 24 hours.

3. Oliguria less than or equal to 400 ml in 24 hours.
4. Cerebral or visual disturbances.
5. Epigastric pain.
6. Pulmonary edema or cyanosis.
7. Impaired liver function.
8. Thrombocytopenia.
9. IUGR/oligohydramnios

Prediction for PIH

Several tests are proposed, but it is blamed to cause unnecessary alarm in pregnant women when prevention of pre-eclampsia has not yet been proven. Some of the predictive parameters of PIH are:

a. MAP-2: Mean arterial pressure in the 2nd trimester >/= 90 mmHg.
b. Gant's roll over test: In which the patient is first made to lie in the left lateral position and the BP is determined at 5 minutes intervals until stable. Patient is next turned to supine positions and the BP is measured again. If rise of diastolic BP is 20 mmHg or more, test is considered positive.
c. Angiotensin Infusion test: It is more invasive. Women destined to develop PIH lose their refractoriness to an infusion of angiotensin between 28 and 32 weeks of pregnancy. If pressor response occurs with more than 8 ng/kg/min of infused angiotensin, 90 percent of women remain normotensive, as against those who exhibit a pressor response with less than 8 ng/kg/min, of them 90 percent were seen to develop the disease.
d. Uterine artery Doppler waveform study: This test is quick and immediate to detect high resistance vessels or a waveform with a notch that implies inadequate or incomplete trophoblast invasion of the spiral arteries. If performed before 24 weeks, false positive rates will be higher.

Review of world literature of about 100 clinical, biophysical and biochemical tests for predicting PIH, failed to be sufficiently reliable for regular screening. There is no one test which is truly predictive.[4]

Management

1. *Preventive* (Table 23.2): The most widely used preventive therapy is low dose aspirin (60-80 mg daily), which is supposed to inhibit the enzyme cyclo-oxygenase in the platelets and prevents release of thrombaxane A_2. It should begin by 20 weeks of gestation.

Table 23.2: Preventive therapy of PIH

- Preventive
  - Aspirin
  - Fish oil: extensively assessed in last 10-15 years.
  - Calcium
  - Magnesium
  - Dipyridamole
  - Antihypertensive drugs
- Newer development
  - Vitamin C and E (major antioxidants)
  - Nitric oxide donors.

The prevailing opinion is that all women should not be treated, but selective treatment for certain high-risk groups is acceptable. Most clinical trials have resulted in no maternal risks and appears safe for the fetus. In their study, the CLASP(Collaborative Low-dose Aspirin Study in Pregnancy) group concluded that low dose aspirin reduced the incidence of pre-eclampsia by about 12 percent, but no effect in IUGR, still births and neonatal deaths.[5]

2. *Curative:* The ultimate treatment of pre-eclampsia is delivery of the fetus and placenta. The urgency of delivery depends on maternal and fetal conditions.

Treatment of Mild PIH

The urgency for delivery is low. After admission, with no proteinuria, who are not at term, with the facility of follow-up, can be allowed to go home and asked to attend antenatal clinic at least once a week. Role of feto-maternal assessment through Day Care Units is also found to be effective.

What is a Day Care Unit?

It is a comprehensive antenatal care system with standardized protocols of high-risk hypertensive obstetric patients. It is a flexible system with decision making power.[6] The patients who are thought to be at increased risk, along with those who are discovered to have mild to moderate hypertension during pregnancy are all suitable for referral to Day Care Assessment.

Monitoring protocol at Day Care Unit:
- BP 5 times in 3 hours
- Abdominal palpation.
- Uric acid, urea, Hb percent and platelets
- Urine for protein
- CTG
- USG: fetal weight, AFI, Biophysical profile, color Doppler of umbilical artery.

Indication for hospitalization from Day Care Unit
- DBP persistently $\geq$ 100 mmHg
- Uric acid $\geq$ 450 mmol/L
- Platelets < 100 × 109/L
- Proteinuria $\geq$ ++ or $\geq$ 0.3 g/24 hour
- Non-reactive CTG
- IUGR/oligohydramnios.

Other measures
1. *Rest in bed:* Preferably in left lateral position. Despite the lack of data to support its efficacy, bed rest continues to be recommended by many workers.
2. *Diet:* There is perhaps no role for restriction of salt in diet. There is no gain by prescribing low sodium diet. It may, in fact, be hazardous in this group of patients who already have inappropriate intravascular volume contraction.
3. *Sedatives:* It is better avoided. Although they have been used routinely by some, apart from reducing physical activity it is not of much help.
4. *Diuretics:* Contraindicated. A rise in blood urea, uric acid and neonatal thrombocytopenia can be produced by use of thiazide diuretics. There is evidence of decrease in placental function with the use of diuretics.
5. *Antihypertensives:* Its effectiveness in mild PIH is controversial, but we found it useful. In a multicentric trial antiserotonin, calcium channel blocker Nimodipine has been tried, 30 mg four times a day. It showed 73 percent success rate with the patient remaining normotensive throughout rest of pregnancy, labor and puerperium without any perinatal mortality.[7] Atenolol,[8] labetalol,[9] clonidine plus hydrallazine[10] have also been used in such cases, with variable success.

The progress of proteinuric PIH is unpredictable and most obstetricians would admit the patient for closer monitoring of both mother and the baby. But in the absence of proteinuria mild to moderate disease can be managed at home, if there is access to adequate maternal and fetal monitoring.

Maternal monitoring
Blood pressure to be recorded at least twice daily, urinary albumin daily, weekly body weight, weekly biochemical tests of blood. Patients are seen daily and asked for worsening of symptoms.

Fetal monitoring
Daily fetal movement count (DFMC) is noted. NST is performed weekly. Ultrasonography is done 3 weekly to assess fetal growth and amniotic fluid. Patients with controlled mild PIH may be allowed to await spontaneous labor at term, but they are not allowed to go beyond term.

Role of induction of labor
Induction of labor is planned around 40 weeks. If cervix is ripe (Bishop's score >6) low amniotomy followed by oxytocin infusion is used for induction. PGE_2 gel (vaginal or intracervical) or pessary can be used for ripening unfavorable cervix. If induction fails cesarean section is done.

Indications for early delivery
i. Worsening of hypertension, proteinuria and /or signs of vital organ involvement, inspite of rational management.
ii. Gross IUGR or fetal distress.

Intrapartum monitoring
Maternal conditions like blood pressure, pulse rate and urine output are monitored closely. Fetal conditions are better monitored by continuous electronic method otherwise by intermittent auscultation, preferably by 1:1 ratio.

Prophylactic methylergometrine is relatively contraindicated as it may cause a dangerous rise in the BP, 5 unit of oxytocin IV should be used instead.

Treatment of Severe PIH

In severe PIH, there is usually progressive deterioration of the maternal and fetal conditions. If left undelivered, complications like placental abruption, thrombocytopenia, HELLP (Hemolysis, elevated liver enzymes, low platelets) syndrome, eclampsia, acute renal failure, DIC can occur with associated increased perinatal and maternal mortality and morbidity.

The only solution for this condition is delivery. These cases cannot be managed at home and patients should be admitted to hospital having neonatal intensive care facility.

Conservative treatment is started with the aim of buying some time to attain fetal maturity.

Antenatal management of severe PIH/ PE: Admission to a tertiary hospital with rest and appropriate materno-fetal surveillance.

Antihypertensive drugs (Table 23.2): Primary role of antihypertensive drug is prevention of maternal cerebral complications. Target BP should be DBP below 105 mmHg.

Alpha methyldopa (0.5-2 g/day) Nifedipine (10-120 mg/day) and labetalol (30-180 mg/day) are the commonly used antihypertensives. Doses and frequency of antihypertensive drugs will vary.

Prophylactic Magnesium Sulphate (Table 23.4): Parenteral $MgSO_4$ is given with the idea to prevent convulsion in cases of severe PIH. This is especially helpful when steroids are given antenatally for fetal lung maturity. In the UK $MgSO_4$ is used for prophylaxis after the MAGPIE randomized placebo controlled trial. This confirms the earlier study that compared $MgSO_4$ to phenytoin in over 2000 pre-eclamptic women and showed $MgSO_4$ to be superior.[11] The following is the preferred method:

Pritchard Regime:[12] 20 ml of 20 percent $MgSO_4$ (equivalent to 4g) given over 10 minutes. Maintenance therapy consists of 10 ml of 50 percent of $MgSO_4$ (equivalent to 5g) IM in alternate buttocks every 4

Table 23.3: Commonly used antihypertensives

Names	Mode of action	Doses	Common side effects	Remarks
• Alpha methyl dopa	Centrally acting Alpha 2 inhibitor	0.5-2 g/day in 4 divided doses	Hemolytic anemia, sedation, headache, orthostatic hypotension, depression, false+ve Coombs' test	First line of therapy in most cases for long-term treatment.
• Nifedipine	Ca-channel blocker • Increases cardiac output. • Lowers peripheral resistance	10-180 mg in 3 divided doses, orally. In acute condition 10 mg stat, repeat every 30 minute.	Palpitation, flushing, Ankle edema, Hypotension, headache flushing, drowsiness, nausea	Contraindicated in: • Lt.vent.hypertrophy • Gastroesophageal reflux
• Hydralazine	Acts by causing Peripheral vaso-dilatation increases CO and renal blood flow	100 mg/day orally in 4 divided doses. In acute condition IV 5-20 mg, 5 mg boluses, repeat every 20-30 minutes.	Flushing, tachycardia, headache	FHR monitoring to be done during IV therapy
• Labetalol	Combined alpha and beta-blockers.	100 mg orally thrice daily max 2400 mg/24 hr. In acute condition IV 20 mg/hr. Initial bolus 20-50 mg over/minute repeated every 10-15 minutes.	Acute onset of tremulousness or shakiness, postural hypotension.	Advantages: • Reversal of thrombo-cytopenia • Fetal lung maturity increases

hours. Therapeutic blood level of magnesium is 4-6 mg/percent. Before administering next dose following parameters should be checked:
- A urine output of at least 100 ml in the last 4 hours.
- Knee jerk persists.
- Respiration not depressed and is over 16/min.

If any of the above is abnormal, next dose is delayed till normal status is attained. Calcium gluconate IV 1 g (10 ml of 10% solution over 10 mins slowly) and oxygen are given to combat toxicity.

MgSO$_4$ is discontinued 24 to 48 hours afterwards.

Table 23.4: Monitoring during MgSO$_4$ therapy

- *Stop magnesium sulfate if:*
  - Respiratory rate < 16/min
  - Urine output < 25 ml/h
  - Knee jerks are sluggish /absent
- *If magnesium toxicity is suspected*
  - Suggested by the absence of reflexes
  - 1 g IV of calcium gluconate is given

Daily observations of maternal and fetal wellbeing is done; investigations are repeated at intervals. If gestation is less than 26 weeks, maternal counseling is done regarding termination of pregnancy if PIH is uncontrolled.

The conservative line of therapy is continued until there is threat to maternal health or fetal distress or fetal maturity ≥ 34 weeks.

When to Deliver (Table 23.5)

- **Group I** (24-26 wk): If usual management fails to control severity of disease, pregnancy has to be terminated after proper counseling.
- **Group II** (26 to 34 wk): Management depends upon their clinical response during the observation period. Antihypertensives are started; steroids are administered for enhancement of fetal lung maturity. Pregnancy is terminated anytime if monitoring parameters are unfavorable despite treatment.
- **Group III** (> 34 wk): After 34 weeks, if there is worsening of biophysical or biochemical parameters, pregnancy is terminated. Some prefer termination of pregnancy after stabilization of BP at 32 wk.[13] Needless to say that, perinatal mortality will be high, specially if neonatal ICU is not available.

Table 23.5: Management of severe pre-eclampsia

- Group I. (24-26 weeks): if usual management fails
  ↓
  Pregnancy terminated after proper counseling
- Group II (26–34 weeks): conservative management; Antenatal steroids
  ↓
  Pregnancy terminated if monitoring parameters: Unfavorable
- Group III (>34 weeks): worsening of biophysical or biochemical parameters,
  Stabilization of BP
  ↓
  Immediate delivery

How to Deliver

- Induce labor if not contraindicated. Labor can be induced by PGE$_2$ gel or vaginal tablets and ARM and oxytocin if cervix is favorable.
- Cesarean section is indicated when emergency delivery is needed and in cases where induction fails. Epidural anesthesia is encouraged where there is no abnormality in clotting tests (Table 23.6).

Table 23.6: Indication for CS in severe PIH

Elective:
- Associated obstetric indications (CPD, elderly primi, diabetes, etc)
- Worsening maternal condition
- Fetal monitoring not possible
- Vaginal delivery not possible in predetermined time

Emergency:
- Fetal distress
- Failure to progress
- Rapidly worsening maternal condition
- Hepatic capsular distention.

Intrapartum Management

Medical Management

Principles:
- Prophylactic magnesium sulphate—selection of cases is important
- Control of BP (Both SBP and DBP).
- Avoid diuretics.
- Blood must be kept ready.

Methods
- MgSO$_4$ can be given parenterally as prophylaxis to prevent convulsion as per Pritchard's regime

- *Antihypertensives:* When diastolic blood pressure rises above 110 mmHg, higher doses of antihypertensives are used.
  - Hydralazine 5 mg iv bolus is given with additional 5 mg increments a time upto 20 mg.
  - Nifedipine (5 mg) is given sublingually, Nifedipine starts working within 10 minutes. It can be repeated to control DBP and SBP.
  - Labetalol iv drip can also be used when available.
  - Sudden drop of BP should be avoided while using antihypertensives along with $MgSO_4$.
- *Diuretics* should be avoided, unless there is pulmonary edema.
- *Blood* is best kept grouped and cross-matched as these patients are worse affected by PPH due to shrunken intravascular compartment.

Obstetric Management

Principles:
- Induce labor if not contraindicated, by PGE_2 (Gel or pessaries)
- Augment labor as and when necessary by amniotomy and oxytocin
- Fetal monitoring
- Avoid prolonged labor

Fetal monitoring is ideally done by electronic method. Alternatively, intermittent auscultation is done every 15 minutes during 1st stage and after each contraction in 2nd stage.

Progress of labor is documented in partogram. The patient is monitored in the labor ward. $MgSO_4$, if started, is continued for a period of 24 hours after delivery. Emergency cesarean section is performed if induction of labor remains unsuccessful or for any other obstetric indications. Deterioration of maternal condition demands immediate delivery.

Third stage: Prophylactic ergometrine is withheld. Oxytocin and $PGF_{2\alpha}$ can be used in stead.

Immediate postnatal fluid therapy: This should be as per the fluid therapy following delivery in eclamptic women (Table 23.7).

Table 23.7: Maternal sequelae of severe hypertension in pregnancy

- Cerebrovascular accident
- Occipital lobe blindness
- Abruptio placentae
- Convulsions
- Pulmonary edema
- Aspiration syndrome
- Hemolysis, elevated liver enzymes and low platelets (HELLP)
- Hemorrhage from gut, liver, retina
- Renal failure
- Deep venous thrombosis.

Caution: Majority of maternal mortality following PE/eclampsia syndrome occurs *after delivery.*

ECLAMPSIA

Eclampsia may be antepartum, intrapartum, postpartum or rarely intercurrent, when the patient seems to recover after her convulsion and pregnancy continues.

The typical eclamptic seizure is described in 4 phases:
- Phase 1: Initial or prodromal phase. There may be an aura, followed by convulsive movements that begin around the mouth.
- Phase 2: Tonic phase. The entire body becomes rigid, the face becomes contorted and suffused. The arms are flexed and fists clenched. Respiration ceases. This phase lasts for 15 to 20 seconds.
- Phase 3: Clonic phase. Jerky movements starting from the facial muscles, which then involve the entire body. There is frothing of sputum at the mouth. It stays for about 1 minute.
- Phase 4: Recovery. The convulsive movement subsides slowly, respiration resumes and the patients passes into a coma of variable duration.

Principles of Treatment

General Measures

The patient should receive individualized nursing care in an isolated room with adequate monitoring facility. Patient is kept in a railed cot. Two large bore IV lines are established. Usually Ringer's lactate is the ideal fluid. Emergency investigations like full blood count, platelets, liver and renal function tests, arterial blood gas, serum electrolytes, coagulation profile are asked for. One of the effects of pulmonary edema following eclampsia is poor oxygen saturation, so one of the best methods of monitoring fluid status is continuous measurement of oxygen saturation with a pulse oxymeter.[14] Blood must be cross-matched and kept ready. Patient is nursed in left lateral position and oropharyngeal suction is done as necessary. Bladder is catheterized with continuous drainage to facilitate measurement of urine output. It is essential to maintain a strict intake-output chart.

1. *Anticonvulsants:* Magnesium sulfate remains the anticonvulsant of choice in any type of set-up. Magnesium causes relaxation of smooth muscle by competing with calcium for entry into cells at the time of cellular depolarization. It is speculated to work as an anticonvulsant by causing CNS depression and suppressing neuronal activity. Either of the following regimes can be started:
    i. Pritchard regime—mentioned in the antenatal management of severe PIH (Figure 23.1).

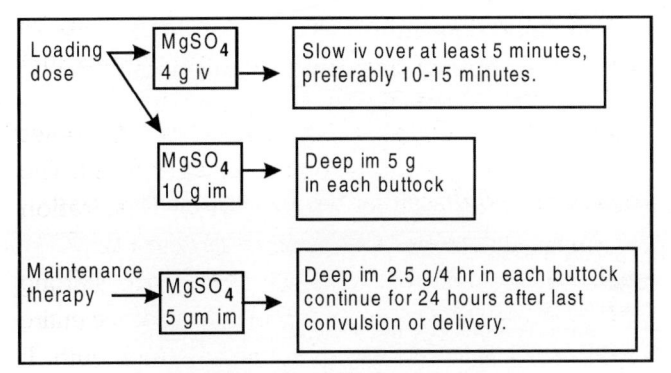

```
Loading dose → MgSO₄ 4 g iv → Slow iv over at least 5 minutes, preferably 10-15 minutes.
           → MgSO₄ 10 g im → Deep im 5 g in each buttock
Maintenance therapy → MgSO₄ 5 gm im → Deep im 2.5 g/4 hr in each buttock continue for 24 hours after last convulsion or delivery.
```

Figure 23.1: Modified Pritchard regime

ii. Zuspan regime[15]—a loading dose of 4 g is to be followed by an infusion of 1gm/hr for 24 hr (Figure 23.2).

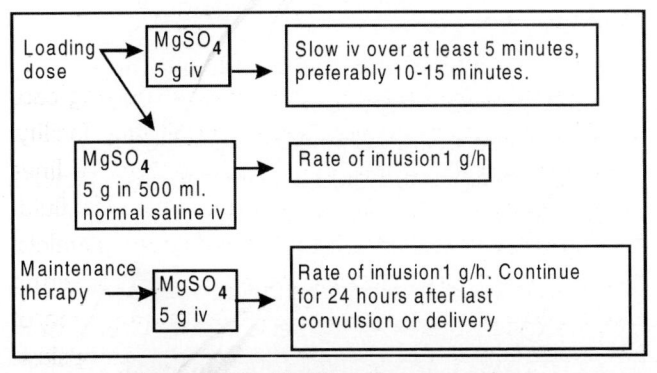

```
Loading dose → MgSO₄ 5 g iv → Slow iv over at least 5 minutes, preferably 10-15 minutes.
           → MgSO₄ 5 g in 500 ml. normal saline iv → Rate of infusion 1 g/h
Maintenance therapy → MgSO₄ 5 g iv → Rate of infusion 1 g/h. Continue for 24 hours after last convulsion or delivery
```

Figure 23.2: Modified Zuspan regime

If convulsion recurs (in both regimes) a further 2 to 4 gm is given IV over 5 min.

Other alternative anticonvulsants which are in use, where $MgSO_4$ is not available are as follows:
- *Diazepam therapy:* It is given as described by Lean and co-workers. A loading dose of 10 mg iv over 2 min, repeated if convulsions recurred, is to be followed by an intravenous infusion of 40 mg in 500 ml normal saline for 24 hr. The rate of infusion is titrated against the level of consciousness. Patients should be drowsy but arousable.
- *Phenytoin therapy:* Phenytoin is only recommended for prevention of convulsions, so diazepam 10 mg is to be given as required for immediate control of seizures.

Magnesium sulphate is the drug of choice for routine anticonvulsant management of women with eclampsia, rather than diazepam or phenytoin. Other anticonvulsants should be used only within the context of randomised trials; and until better evidence is available, magnesium sulphate should be the standard against which these are measured.[16]

2. *Antihypertensives:* These are used for acute control of blood pressure. Hydralazine and nifedipine are used as described earlier. But one should be aware that $MgSO_4$ itself has got variable hypotensive effect.
3. *Antibiotics:* Usually a broad spectrum parenteral antibiotic is prescribed to prevent systemic infection.

Obstetric Management

Cesarean section in eclampsia: It is done for the following conditions:
   i. Fits are not controlled even after 6-8 hours of $MgSO_4$ therapy.
   ii. BP is too high (>180/120 mmHg) and is not responding to maximum doses of Nifedipine or any other suitable antihypertensive. The BP should be controlled and stabilized at least for a short period prior to cesarean section.
   iii. Vaginal delivery is not possible in predetermined time. The shorter the convulsion delivery interval, the better the prognosis for the mother.

iv. Hepatic capsular distention.
v. Any other obstetric indication for elective CS.

Expedite delivery: In rest of the cases, once the condition of the patient is stable and fits are controlled induction of labor is done, preferably by amniotomy followed by oxytocin infusion. If there is failure of induction or delay in progress of labor within 6 to 12 hours of admission cesarean section is done.

Postpartum fluid management: It is very important to prevent circulatory overload. Colloids and Ringer's lactate are preferred fluids in this period. Volume of fluid to be infused is the sum of hourly need of 50 ml + previous hour's output. Volume expansion is done by crystalloids, for example Ringer's lactate, dextrose is avoided. Colloids are infused if there is oliguria or sudden fall of BP.

Blood transfusion is given to treat PPH or to combat hypotension. If patient is in positive balance of over 2 lit., 40 mg frusemide followed by 20G of mannitol given. Oliguria, if any, is mostly corrected (in one-third of cases) on its own. In rest of the cases detailed stepwise investigations for acute renal failure is carried out and treated conservatively awaiting spontaneous resolution. Hemodialysis is indicated for few selected cases.

$MgSO_4$ is continued for 24 hours after delivery or after the last convulsion in case of postpartum eclampsia.

Treatment of Complications

Eclamptic women are prone to develop complications like pulmonary edema, thromboembolism, DIC or hepatic failure and they require intensive supportive treatment.

Once the patient is recovered, psychological support is very important for the patient and her partner to overcome the stress of childbirth.

Mortality: Maternal mortality following eclampsia is mainly due to delayed management. Mortality is found in about 4.7-13.5 percent of cases of eclampsia in developing countries.[17]

Chance of recurrence: Overall 25-30 percent of women with PIH in first pregnancy will have recurrent hypertension in the subsequent pregnancy. If she had PE, her risk of recurrent PE is about 7-10 percent. This risk is increased in women with early onset of the disease, eclampsia or HELLP syndrome. So, measurement of late postnatal BP is essential for determining the future risks. If the BP returns to normal she can use oral contraceptive pills, but her BP should be checked whilst she is on it.

CHRONIC HYPERTENSION IN PREGNANCY

Causes of Chronic Hypertension (Table 23.8)

1. Essential hypertension (in 90% of cases)
2. Renal diseases: Glomerulonephritis, polycystic disease, diabetic nephropathy, renal artery stenosis.
3. Collagen vascular diseases: Systemic lupus erythematosus, sclerodema
4. Coarctation of aorta
5. Pheochromocytoma.

If the blood pressure is elevated for the first time in pregnancy, appropriate investigations should be performed to exclude renal, cardiac and auto-immune disease.

Table 23.8: Risk factor for developing superimposed PE

- Renal disease
- Maternal age > 40 years.
- Diabetes.
- Connective tissue disorder, e.g. SLE
- Coarctation of aorta.
- Blood pressure > 160 mmHg in early pregnancy.

There is increased incidence of abruptio placentae, congestive heart failure, malignant hypertension, cerebrovascular accident, and renal damage.

Management

1. *Preconceptional evaluation*: Ideally the women having chronic hypertension should be evaluated prior to conception. Change of antihypertensives like ACE-inhibitors and diuretics are necessary. Advice should be given regarding diet, lifestyle, smoking habits, etc.
2. *Investigations*: Investigations should aim at detecting treatable causes of hypertension. Creatinine, electrolytes, urates, liver function tests, 24-hour

urinary creatinine clearance, renal scan, autoantibody screen, complement studies are recommended. ECG and echocardiography are recommended in any case of pre-existing hypertension.

The fetus must be evaluated regularly with ultrasound for growth, non-stress test, kick charts and clinical growth parameters.

Antihypertensive Drugs

Low risk group (BP >140/90 to 170/109 mmHg): If antihypertensives have not been stopped prior to conception, review is done after 12 weeks, when BP may fall within normotensive range due to physiological drop at mid trimester. Patients are seen regularly to monitor BP, renal function, urate levels, evidence of IUGR and pre-eclampsia. Antihypertensives like alpha-methyldopa or nifedipine are started when necessary. Patients with chronic hypertensions are followed to term and uncomplicated cases are expected to have normal vaginal delivery in the absence of any obstetric contraindication. If pre-eclampsia is superimposed, management will be the same as in a patient of pre-eclampsia.

High-risk group (BP>170/109 mmHg): Counseling of the patient is very important about continuing the pregnancy, because there is a very high rate of maternal and fetal morbidity. These patients are often hospitalized early for extensive maternal and fetal surveillance and meticulous control of BP. The management protocol is in the same line as severe PE.

Postnatal Counseling

Counseling of the patient and her husband is important for future planning of family size. These patients are advised not to have many pregnancies as it may affect the chronic disease process adversely.

CONCLUSION

Etiology of PIH is yet ill understood but pathophysiology is almost known to us. The basic management of hypertensive disease in pregnancy is comprehensive antenatal care. In many parts of the world, the women present herself at the hospital with headache, increasing edema or convulsion.

Monitoring of the mother and fetus is very important to assess the severity of the disease. Delivery is the only ultimate cure of the condition. As timing of delivery affects the outcome for both mother and baby, continuation of pregnancy, with suitable antihypertensive drugs, is of paramount importance. The developing countries lack the facility of any concept of Regional Hypertension Centers—hence the majority of cases of Hypertensive disorders in pregnancy, are better delivered at a tertiary level hospital and all cases, irrespective of their severity, must be under care of a senior specialist obstetrician. In those patients with severe PE/eclampsia or who are critically ill demanding intensive care; once stabilization of BP and/or convulsions is achieved, a decision of when and how to deliver is taken. Continued vigilance is required for 24 to 48 hours after delivery. Severity of HDP can be controlled in most cases and mortality from this condition is surely avoidable.

REFERENCES

1. Walker SP, Higgins JR, Brennecke SP: The diastolic debat: is it time to discard Korotkoff phase IV in favor of phase V for blood pressure measurement in pregnancy? *Med J Aust* **169:** 203-05, 1998.
2. Hughes EC (Ed): *Obstetric-Gynecology Terminology,* Philadelphia: FA Davis, 422-23, 1972.
3. Report of national high blood pressure education programme working group on high blood pressure in pregnancy. *Am J O and G* **183:** S1-S22, 2000.
4. Dekker G, Sibai B: Primary, secondary and tertiary prevention of pre-eclampsia. *Lancet* **357:** 209-15, 2001.
5. CLASP (Collaborative low dose aspirin study in pregnancy collaborative Group) A randomized trial of low dose aspirin for the prevention and treatment of pre-eclampsia among 9364 pregnant women. *Lancet* **343:**619, 1994.
6. Walker JJ: The case for early recognition and intervention in preg-induced hypertension. In eds. F Sharp, EM Symonds (Eds): *Hypertension in Pregnancy,* Proceedings of the Sixteenth study group of the Royal College of Obstetricians and Gynecologists. Perinatology Press, NYP 289-99, 1987.
7. Chatterjee A, Mukherjee J, Mitra S, Saha S: Clinical Trial with Nimodipine in the Management of PIH. *J Obstet Gynecol India* **49:** 48-50, 1999.
8. Rubin PC, Clark DM, Sumner DJ et al: Placebo controlled trial of atenolol in treatment of pregnancy-associated hypertension. *Lancet* **i:**431-34, 1983.

9. Pickles CJ, Symonds EM and Broughton Pipkin F: The fetal outcome in a randomized double blind controlled trial of labetalol versus placebo in pregnancy induced hypertension. *Br J Obst Gyne* **96:** 38-43, 1989.
10. Phippard AF, Fischer WE, Horvath JS *et al:* Early Blood Pressure control improve pregnancy outcome in primi gravid women with mild hypertension. *Med J Aust* **154:** 378-82, 1991.
11. Lucas NJ, Leveno KJ, Cunningham FG: *N Engl J Med* **333:** 201, 1995.
12. Pritchard JA, Cunningham FG, Pritchard SA: The Parkland Memorial Hospital protocol for treatment of eclampsia: evaluation of 245 cases. *Am J Obstet Gynecol* **148:**951-63, 1984.
13. Paruk F, Moodley J: Treatment of severe pre-eclampsia eclampsia syndrome. In Studd J (Ed): *Progress in Obstet Gyne*, Churchill Livingstone, **14:** 102-19, 2000.
14. Walker JJ: Care of the patient with severe pregnancy induced hypertension. *Eur J Obstet Gynecol Reprod Biol* **65:** 127-35, 1996.
15. Zuspan FP: Problems encountered in the treatment of pregnancy induced hypertension. A point of view. *Am J Obstet Gynecol* **131:** 591-97, 1978.
16. Duley L; Which anticonvulsant for women with eclampsia? Evidence from the Collaborative Eclampsia Trial. *The Lancet* **345:** 1455-63, 1995.
17. Affandi B: Eclampsia. In S Ratnamm, B Rao, Arulkumaran (Eds): *Obstetrics and Gynecology for Postgraduates*, vol. 2, Orient Longman 73, 1994.

24.

Sambit Mukhopadhyay
Sabaratnam Arulkumaran

Gynecological Disorders in Pregnancy

PART TWO — Feto-maternal Medicine

DISORDERS OF THE GENITAL TRACT

Disorders of the genital tract can complicate pregnancy. Some of the common disorders are discussed here.

Retroversion of Gravid Uterus

Retroversion of uterus is not abnormal. Nearly 25 percent of women will have retroverted uterus on bimanual examination. Pregnancy in a retroverted uterus is often uneventful. In majority of cases the uterus rises outside the pelvis by 12 weeks and becomes an abdomino pelvic organ. In minority of cases the uterus remains in the pelvis and as it grows it comes to fill the pelvic cavity completely. The cervix is then directed upward and upward. The uterus then gets incarcerated. The urethra gets elongated and the bladder base is distorted. This results in urinary retention.

Acute retention is painful. If neglected and not properly treated by catheterization overflow incontinence can occur.

Diagnosis

The patient usually presents with difficulty in micturition or with acute retention. This usually occurs between 12th to 16th weeks of pregnancy. On abdominal examination the distended bladder will be palpable and as much as 1–2 liters of urine may be drained by catheterization. Often it may be mistaken for a pregnant uterus.

On vaginal examination the posterior vaginal wall is found to be pushed by smooth elastic swelling which occupies the hollow of the sacrum. The cervix is found to be high up behind the symphysis pubis directed forward and upward. This position of the cervix is very characteristic as it confirms that the swelling in the pelvis is the uterus. Occasionally fibroid in the uterus may give rise to similar symptoms and clinical findings. A pelvic ultrasound scan will help to distinguish between the two conditions.

Treatment

When urinary retention occurs due to retroverted uterus a Foley's catheter is passed immediately and the bladder is drained continuously. As the bladder is emptied the uterus nearly rises above the pelvic brim. When the uterus is palpable abdominally it means the normal bladder anatomy is restored and women will be able to pass urine spontaneously.

Rarely some manipulation of the uterus will be required under anesthesia to correct incarceration.

Prolapse of the Pregnant Uterus

Pregnancy in a completely prolapsed uterus is very rare. The incidence ranges from 1 in 10, 000 to 1 in 15, 000 pregnancies. It can happen in a partially prolapsed uterus. As the uterus grows in size it becomes too large to sink through the pelvic brim, the cervix is gradually drawn up and no longer descends. Minor degree of prolapse requires support by ring pessary until the uterus has grown well up into the abdomen.

Occasionally cervix may be protruding outside the introitus. The cervix can then become thick and edematous and may fail to dilate during labor. If it is detected in the antenatal period, the woman should be kept in bed for some days and the cervix kept inside the vagina to allow the edema to subside.

Women can become pregnant after operation for prolapse. Most gynecologists would recommend elective cesarean section for delivery. However, pregnancy itself is a risk factor for damage to the pelvic floor and recurrence of prolapse.

Successful continence surgery for urinary incontinence in the past is an absolute indication for elective cesarean section.

Uterine Fibroids

Most pregnancies associated with fibroids progress uneventfully. The incidence of clinically detectable fibroid in pregnancy is 1 in 1000. It is somewhat higher in Negroid population.

Effects of Pregnancy on Fibroids

The following changes can occur during pregnancy

Increase in size

The fibroid becomes larger due to hypertrophy of the muscle fibers. There is increased vascularity and edema making it softer.

Red degeneration of fibroid

Red degeneration is typically associated with pregnancy. It is caused by obstruction of the venous flow as the fibroid enlarges during pregnancy. The cut surface shows a reddish purple color. Symptom of red degeneration includes acute pain at the site of the fibroid in the pregnant uterus. It can be associated with mild fever and sometimes vomiting. Differential diagnosis includes acute appendicitis, concealed abruption, and torsion of an ovarian cyst or pedunculated fibroid. Treatment of red degeneration of fibroid is always conservative with analgesia and rest.

Effects of Fibroids on Pregnancy

Miscarriage

Most pregnancies associated with fibroids proceed uneventfully. However, there is an increased risk of miscarriage and preterm labor. Therefore pregnancies accompanied by fibroids should be treated as high risk.

Labor

Fibroids commonly occur in the body of the uterus. Therefore, it is drawn out of the pelvis once the uterus grows in pregnancy. Therefore, they do not obstruct labor generally. Cervical fibroids may prevent the head engaging and cause malpresentation and obstructed labor.

In the presence of a submucosal fibroid the myometrium may not contract efficiently in the third stage and postpartum hemorrhage may occur. Often a submucous fibroid can get infected and separation of infected tumor can cause late postpartum hemorrhage.

Treatment

Most women with fibroids pass through the pregnancy without any difficulty. As mentioned earlier treatment of red degeneration of fibroid is conservative. Symptoms may be quite severe to require hospital admission for analgesia and rest. Myomectomy is unnecessary and dangerous. Apart from causing miscarriage it can cause severe hemorrhage.

Torsion of a pedunculated fibroid can cause severe abdominal pain and vomiting and calls for an urgent laparotomy and removal. This is the only situation when removal of a fibroid from a pregnant uterus is ever justified. There are two rare conditions, which can cause diagnostic confusion. They are torsion of the pregnant uterus itself and intraperitoneal hemorrhage from ruptured vein on the surface of the fibroid.

As mentioned earlier pregnancy with fibroid should be regarded as high risk and therefore all pregnant women with fibroid should be delivered at the hospital. The great majority will achieve a vaginal delivery even when the fibroid seems to lie below the fetal head before the onset of labor. Only in few cases obstruction may happen and this will be detected by the inability of the presenting part to engage and descent through the pelvis. Cesarean section is indicated. No attempt should be made to perform myomectomy at the time of cesarean section as it carries serious risk of hemorrhage. Fibroids decrease in size after delivery. A review should be done at 3 to 4 months after delivery and definitive treatment if any should then be planned.

Ovarian Cysts

Any type of ovarian cysts can occur during pregnancy but simple cysts and dermoid cysts are common. Ovarian cysts during pregnancy are usually benign but around 10 percent of cysts below 30 years are malignant and this proportion actually rises with age. It is detected incidentally at the antenatal clinic or during routine ultrasound scan.

Torsion is more likely to occur during early second trimester or puerperium when there is relatively more space in the abdomimal cavity.

Pregnancy is usually undisturbed by the ovarian cyst unless torsion or other complications supervene. Labor is unaffected unless the cyst is deeply impacted in the pelvis thereby causing obstruction.

Treatment

An ovarian cyst may undergo torsion or rupture during the pregnancy and can cause acute abdominal symptoms. When the patient presents with acute symptoms laparotomy should be undertaken regardless of the duration of the pregnancy. If the ultrasound features suggest complex mass with high suspicion of malignancy laparotomy should be undertaken as soon as possible. If an asymptomatic cyst is discovered it is prudent to wait until after 14 weeks gestation before removing it. This avoids the risk of removing a corpus luteal cyst upon which the pregnancy might still be dependant at an earlier stage. Often it is possible to keep a close eye by serial ultrasound examination during the pregnancy and plan surgery at 6 to 8 weeks after delivery.

Carcinoma of Cervix

Invasive carcinoma of cervix is rare during pregnancy. Cervical intraepithelial neoplasia (CIN) is more common as it affects the younger age group. Screening for cervical cancer with cervical smear from the age of 20 to 60 is routine in many western countries. Therefore, it is not unusual to encounter pregnant patients with abnormal smear of varying degree of severity. Colposcopy is indicated if severe degree of abnormality (CIN3) is detected but treatment is usually carried out 6 to 8 weeks after the delivery. Colposcopic biopsies may be indicated to rule out possibility of invasive cancer. It has to be borne in mind that cervical biopsies during pregnancy can cause heavy bleeding, infection and can precipitate miscarriage. Less severe abnormalities, i.e CIN2 and CIN1 require follow up at 6 to 8 weeks of delivery with repeat smear or colposcopy.

Invasive carcinoma of cervix during pregnancy is rare. The disease progression is same as in non-pregnant women. It presents with vaginal bleeding or purulent discharge from a friable or ulcerated lesion from the cervix. Biopsy is indicated when there is high clinical suspicion.

Treatment depends on the stage of the pregnancy. At an early gestation therapeutic termination of pregnancy should be carried out and cervical cancer should be treated with either surgery or radiotherapy according to the stage of the disease. In later pregnancy cesarean section (classical) should be performed and may be combined with Wertheim's hysterectomy.

Prematurity of the fetus often becomes a major issue when the diagnosis is made at midpregnancy. In such circumstances a delay of few weeks may be acceptable for allowing the fetus to grow and gain lung maturity with a hope of survival but this should be done in close consultation with the patient and her partner and possibly with the multidisciplinary cancer team.

BIBLIOGRAPHY

1. Chamberlain G: Abnormal Pregnancy. In: Chamberlain G (Ed): *Obstetrics by Ten Teachers*. Arnold, London, 1999.
2. Soutter WP: Benign Tumours of the ovary In: Shaw R, Soutter P, Stanton S (Eds), *Gynecology*, Churchill Livingstone, 1992.

25. Multiple Pregnancy and Polyhydramnios

Suchitra N Pandit
Sanjay B Rao

INTRODUCTION

The problems of multiple pregnancy and polyhydramnios pose a unique challenge in the practice of obstetrics. This chapter describes the incidence, etiopathology and the clinical diagnosis of each of the two conditions. The practical problems encountered in the management strategies have also been outlined. The successful outcome of these high-risk pregnancies requires that the clinician coordinate with an experienced group including anesthetists and neonatologists. Despite difficulties, with modern treatment modalities the maternal and perinatal outcomes are good, in most cases.

DEFINITION

When more than one fetus simultaneously develops in the uterus, it is called multiple pregnancy. The simultaneous development of two fetuses—termed twins is the most common. More rarely, the development of three fetuses—triplets, four fetuses-quadruplets, five fetuses—quintuplets or six fetuses—sixtuplets, may occur.

INCIDENCE

Hellins law propounds the following rates of multiple pregnancy:
- Twins   1:80
- Triplets $1:80^2$
- Quadruplets $1:80^3$
- Qunituplets $1:80^4$

The study of twins is a part of the new branch of science named **gemellology**.

The frequency of twinning is highest among the Black race and consistently lower among the Orientals. The incidence of twin gestation increases with maternal age upto 35 to 39 years, and parity. The chances of twin gestation doubles if conception occurs within 1 month after discontinuation of a long-term use of oral contraceptives. Another important factor increasing the incidence of multiple gestation is the use of ovulation induction in infertile couples. The incidence of multifetal pregnancies after induction of ovulation is between 6.8

and 17 percent. Following the use of gonadotropins, the risk of multifetal gestation varies between 18 and 53 percent.[1]

Genesis of Twins

1. *Monozygotic twins*—They originate by fertilization of a single ovum by a single sperm.

   In uniovular (identical or monozygotic) the twinning may occur at different periods after fertilization. This markedly influences the process of implantation and the formation of the fetal membranes.

   Most commonly the stage at which the separation occurs, is after the formation of the inner cell mass (between the 4th to 8th day). Two embryos develop and are enclosed by a single chorion. There is a single placenta and two separate amniotic sacs, resulting in diamniotic monochorionic twins.
   Rarely, the following possibilities occur:
   - *Diamniotic-dichorionic*: The division takes place within 72 hours after fertilization and the resulting embryos will have two separate placenta.
   - *Monoamniotic–monochorionic*: The division occurs after the 8th day of fertilization, when the amniotic cavity has already formed; embroys will share one placenta and one amniotic sac.
   - *Conjoined twins*: Very rarely, the division occurs after the development of embryonic disc resulting in conjoined twins.

2. *Dizygotic twins*: Binovular or dizygotic twins, result from fertilization of two ova which have most probably ruptured from two distinct graafian follicles, usually of the same or one from each ovary, by two sperms. Here, the babies bear only fraternal resemblance to each other and are also called fraternal twins.[2]

   In rare cases, dizygotic twins result from matings with two different fathers within the same menstrual cycle (superfecundation). The fertilization and implantation of ova from different menstrual cycles (superfetation) does not occur in humans.
   - Weinberg's rule states that the number of dizygous twins in any population is twice the number of twins of different sex, the remainder are monozygous.

The most frequently used method to determine the zygosity of twins is the examination of the placenta at birth. However, variations exist in monozygotic placentation. Microscopic examination of a piece of the septum dividing the two fetal cavities is therefore most important. In diamniotic-dichorionic placentae there is chorionic tissue present between the two amnions. In monochorionic-diamniotic placentae, the septum consists of two amnions layers without interposing chorions (Tabe 25.1).

Table 25.1: Differentiating features of monozygotic and dizygotic twins

Different features	Monozygotic	Dizygotic
• Ovum	• Single	• Two
• Sperm	• Single	• Two
• Sex	• Same	• Opposite or same
• Similarity	• Identical	• Fraternal resemblance (similarity between two-brothers or sisters)
• Placenta	• Single(43%) or double	• Double, sometimes fused at margin
• Communicating vessel	• Present	• Absent
• Intervening membrane	• Absent in monochorionic and monoamniotic twin	• Present
• Thickness of intervening membrane	• <2 mm(82-89%)	• >2 mm (95%)
• Twin pig sign	• Absent (44%)	• Present (97.3%)
• Genetic feature	• Same	• Different

The finding of a monochorionic placenta is unequivocal proof of monozygosity.

However, it may be difficult in some cases to decide whether a single placenta is monochorionic-diamniotic or whether it is a fused dichorionic-diamniotic placenta, which variety may be found in both dizygotic and monozygotic twins. Other methods which have been used to determining twin zygosity include study of blood groups, genetic fingerprinting using DNA probes or differences in restriction fragment length polymorphism present in highly polymorphic areas of the genome.[3]

Diagnosis

On history taking, the use of ovulation inducing agents for the treatment of infertility should be recorded. A family history of twins especially the maternal side may also be present.

The symptoms experienced in the first trimester include excess nausea and vomiting. In the later trimester cardiorespiratory discomfort could manifest as breathlessness or palpitations. There is a tendency for swelling of the lower limbs and varicosities. An undue enlargement of the abdomen and excessive fetal movements may be perceived.

On abdominal examination the uterus may appear barrel-shaped; the height is more than the period of amenorrhea. The abdominal girth usually exceeds 100 cm which is more that the average value at term. Multiple fetal parts are palpated. A finding of two fetal heads or three fetal poles confirms the clinical diagnosis. On auscultation, two distinct fetal heart sounds should be located at separate spots with a silent area in between by two observers, and the difference in heart rates is at least 10 beats per minute. Polyhydramnios may occasionally complicate the twin pregnancy. Per vaginal examination may detect premature opening of the internal os. It helps to confirm the presenting part of the fetus.

A straight X-ray of the abdomen only helps to confirm the diagnosis by demonstrating two fetal heads and two fetal spines. It may occasionally identify conjoined twins. Ultrasonography is vital in the confirmation of twins, for the diagnosis of chorionicity and accurate measurement of gestational age. It also helps to diagnose intrauterine growth restriction, discordant twins, twin to twin transfusion syndrome, and intrauterine fetal death (Table 25.2).

Table 25.2: Diagnosis of multiple pregnancy

- **History**: Family history, h/o taking ovulation inducing drugs.
- **Symptoms**: Excessive nausea/vomiting, leg swelling, varicose veins and hemorrhoids get worse; cardio-respiratory embarrassment from undue enlargement of abdomen.
- **Signs**:
  - Anemia, edema, raised BP, abnormal weight gain
  - Height of fundus and girth of abdomen—more than the corresponding period of gestation,
  - Two or more fetal heads
  - Three or more fetal poles
  - Two distinct FHS heard by two observers with at least a difference of 10 beats per minute.
- **Investigations**: USG or X-ray is confirmatory.

Maternal Complications

Maternal morbidity is increased from 3 to 7 times in multiple pregnancy. Anemia is more common in twin pregnancy because of increased iron and folate requirements by the two fetuses. Deficiency of vitamin B_{12} and folic acid causes megaloblastic anemia or dimorphic anemia. There is a 25 percent risk of development of pre-eclampsia as compared to a normal pregnancy.

Polyhydramnios is more common in uniovular twins and usually involves the second sac. Increased renal perfusion and a corresponding increase in urinary output may be coexistent with hypervolemia in the larger twin. Due to a larger placental size, the incidence of placenta previa is more. Multiple risk factors also predispose to antepartum hemorrhage-these include pre-eclampsia, polyhydramnios, megaloblastic anemia and sudden decompression of the uterus following the delivery of the first twin.[4]

There is a high incidence of fetal malpresentation at the time of delivery in twin gestation. The frequency of different fetal presentations reported are as follows:[5]
- Vertex-vertex   : 39.6 percent
- Vertex-breech   : 27.7 percent
- Vertex-transverse : 7.5 percent
- Breech-vertex   : 9 percent
- Breech-breech   : 6.7 percent
- Breech-transverse : 2.6 percent
- Other combinations : 6.9 percent

Malpresentations are more common in the second baby. During labor, early rupture of membranes and cord prolapse are likely to occur due to a higher prevalence of malpresentations. There is increased risk of incordinate uterine activity and a higher risk of operative interference. Due to excessive stretching of the myometrium, postpartum hemorrhage is more common and aggressive use of oxytocics is required to reduce third stage blood loss (Table 25.3).

Fetal Complications (Table 25.4)

1. *Preterm labor* is the single largest factor associated with fetal and neonatal mortality and morbidity in twin gestation. An overdistended uterus,

Table 25.3: Maternal risks in multiple pregnancy

- Miscarriage
- Increased symptoms of early pregnancy
- Increased minor ailments of pregnancy
- Anemia
- Hypertension
- Hydramnios
- APH
  - Placenta previa
  - Accidental hemorrhage.
- Pre-term labor
- Ineffective labor.
- Increased risk of operative delivery
- PPH
- Postnatal problems

Table 25.4: Fetal risks in multiple pregnancy

- Single fetal death
- Pre-term labor and delivery
- IUGR
- Stillbirth
- Congenital abnormality
- Conjoined twin
- Monoamniotic twin
- Twin-twin transfusion syndrome
- Twin reversed arterial perfusion
- Stuck twin
- Asphyxia
- Neonatal death
- Operative vaginal delivery (espcially 2nd baby)
- Twin entrapement.

polyhydramnios and intrauterine infections are the leading causes of preterm labor. Premature opening of the os and exposure of the fetal membranes to the bacterial flora of the vagina lead to amnionitis and in severe cases premature rupture of the membranes.[6]

2. *Discordant growth causes* a difference in the weight of the twins, with a discrepancy of 20 percent or more. It affects 15-29 percent of twin pregnancies.[7] An unequal placental mass and genetic syndromes are the causes of discordancy. In most patients, discordant growth is noticed after 24 weeks. A 5 percent difference in head circumference, a difference of 20 mm in abdominal circumference or a difference of 15 to 25 percent in estimated fetal weight on ultrasonography are the criteria used to diagnose discordant twin growth.

3. *Twin to twin transfusion syndrome* affects 5 to 17 percent of monochorionic twin pregnancies. The problem occurs due to an abnormal artery-to-vein vascular anastomosis. The diagnosis is confirmed when the differences in hematocrit and birth weight is greater than 20 percent. The "stuck twin" is the sonographic appearance of an extreme form of twin-to-twin transfusion syndrome. The donor twin is markedly smaller in size and surrounded by scanty amniotic fluid. It appears stuck against the uterine wall. In contrast, the recipient twin is large and has a polyhydramniotic sac.

The overall mortality is approximately 60 to 70 percent. The recipient twin develops cardiomegaly and congestive cardiac failure and may even die in the uterus. The donor twin has retarded somatic growth, oligohydramnios and a high output cardiac failure. The perinatal mortality improves with serial amniocentesis in the larger twin. Some investigators have occluded the vascular anastomosis between the twins using Nd-YAG laser coagulation through the fetoscope.[8] Since preterm delivery is necessary in a large majority of patients with twin-to-twin transfusion, corticosteroids should be used to accelerate fetal lung maturity at the earliest. The incidence of cerebral palsy and neurologic abnormalities is high in pregnancies affected by twin-to-twin transfusion.

4. *Monoamniotic twin pregnancies* are rare, occurring once in every 12, 500 births. The main factors associated with perinatal mortality are umbilical cord entanglement, congenital abnormalities, preterm delivery and twin to twin transfusion.

Sonographic diagnosis is based in the absence of a dividing amniotic membrane and twins of the same sex with the presence of a single placenta. Color Doppler examination is valuable in detecting umbilical cord entanglement. Presence of variable decelerations is also suggestive of cord entanglement. The optimal route of delivery is by cesarean section, to avoid umbilical cord problems.

5. *Single fetal demise* occurs in monochorionic twin pregnancies. A fetal demise before 14 weeks does not increase the risk on the survivor twin. However, after 14 weeks there is a risk of neurologic damage of the survivor, resulting from transfer of thromboplastin from the dead twin producing

thrombotic arterial occlusions.[9] As a result, occlusions of the anterior and middle cerebral arteries cause multicystic encephalomalacia. The mother is at a risk of developing consumptive coagulopathy usually after a period of 3 weeks. With careful monitoring of the patient, it may be better to deliver the patient after 30 weeks to minimize the complications of preterm delivery.

6. *Congenital anomalies* occur more frequently in twins of the same sex and in monochorionic twins. Neural tube defects and congenital heart diseases occur more frequently in twins.

   Conjoined twins affect 1 in every 200 monozygotic twins. Conjoined twins are mono-ovular and have the same sex and karyotype. The different types of conjoined twins are:
   i. Thoracopagus: fusion at the chest (40%)
   ii. Omphalophagus (Xiphopagus): fusion at the anterior abdominal wall (33%)
   iii. Pyophagus: fusion at the buttocks (18%)
   iv. Ischiopagus: fusion at the ischium (6%)
   v. Craniopagus: fusion of heads (2%)

   The outcome of conjoined twins is poor and is dependant largely on the feasibility of surgical separation.[10]

7. *A cardiac twinning* is a unique anomaly where one twin has no cardiac structures. Circulation for both babies is maintained by the other twin's heart. Eventually the normal twin succumbs to high output cardiac failure. The management is difficult. Research is under progress for selective removal of the acardiac twin or insertion of a thrombogenic coil in the umbilical artery of the acardiac twin.[11]

8. *Umbilical cord problems* are more frequent in twin pregnancies—these include single umbilical artery and velamentous insertion of the cord. Cord entanglements, cord prolapse and torsion due to focal absence of Wharton's jelly are more common in monoamniotic twins.

Antenatal Management

Antenatal care in multiple pregnancy should be directed towards prevention of preterm delivery, evaluation of fetal growth and deciding the optimum mode of delivery.

Dietary advice should be toward adequate caloric intake to meet the increased demands. Supplementary iron (upto 60-80 mg per day), vitamins, calcium and folic acid should be initiated. Elective hospitalization provides physical rest, improves uteroplacental circulation and may have a quiescent effect on myometrial contractility. Reduced pressure on the cervix is useful to prevent preterm labor. However, randomized trials have shown no benefit. Until definitive research conclusions are available, prophylactic tocolytic drugs should be used selectively in those patients with increased uterine activity. Antenatal visits should be every 2 weeks or more frequent if necessary to detect anemia or PE at the earliest. Any infection of the urinary tract, cervix and vagina in patients with twins must be treated aggressively. Close antepartum fetal surveillance is needed to monitor fetal growth. Corticosteroids should be administered when there is a strong possibility of preterm labor.

Management during Labor

Patients with twin pregnancy should be preferably confined in tertiary health care centers with anesthesia services and intensive neonatal care unit.

During labor precautions to be taken include:
1. The patient should be kept nil by mouth to avoid anesthesia complications in the event of operative interference.
2. Adequate caloric supplementation with intravenous fluids.
3. Blood should be cross-matched and preserved ready.
4. Continuous intrapartum fetal monitoring is preferable to detect any signs of fetal distress.
5. Pain relief if required can be done by epidural anesthesia.
6. Two neonatologists should be present preferably at the time of delivery.

Delivery of the First Twin

The delivery of the first baby is conducted as in normal labor. A liberal episiotomy should be made under local perineal infiltration. An outlet forceps if needed should be done preferably under pudendal block. Intravenous ergometrine should be withheld with delivery of the anterior shoulder of the first baby. The cord should be clamped at two places and cut in between and at least 8 to 10 cm of length should be left for administration of drugs or transfusion if required. The baby is handed over to the neonatologist and labeled as the first twin (Figure 25.1).

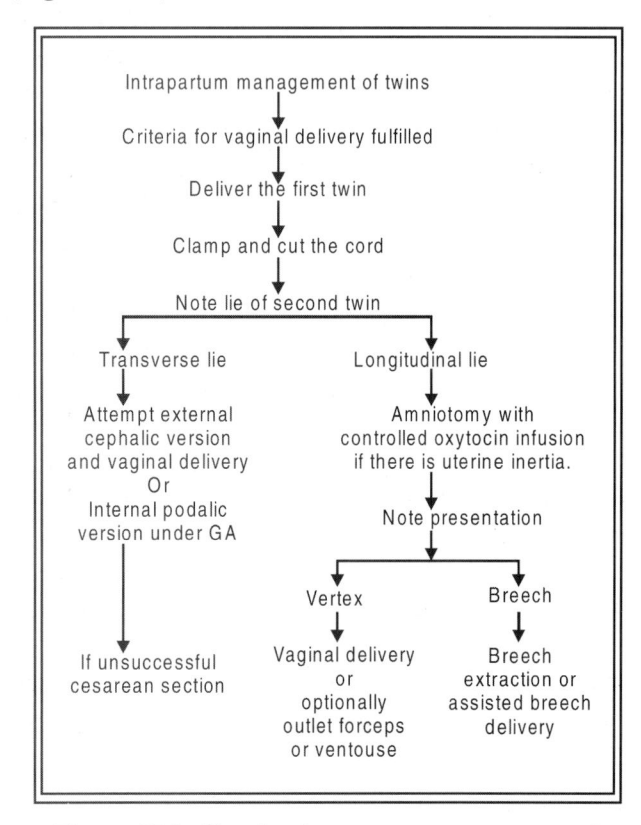

Figure 25.1: Showing intrapartum management of twins during labor

Delivery of the Second Twin

Following the birth of the first baby, the lie, presentation and fetal heart sounds of the second baby should be ascertained. A vaginal examination should be done to confirm abdominal examination findings and to exclude cord presentation or prolapse. The status of the membranes is also noted.

When the lie is longitudinal, a low rupture of membranes is done when the presenting part is fixed to the brim of the pelvis. If there is uterine inertia, a controlled intravenous oxytocin infusion can be used to augment labor. In 80 percent of cases, the second twin is born within 30 minutes of the first. As long as the fetal heart rate remains normal, there is no reason to expedite delivery. If vaginal bleeding occurs suggesting abruptio placentae or there are late decelerations indicating fetal distress, delivery should be immediate by forceps or cesarean section or breech extraction. When the lie is transverse, it should be corrected by external version into a longitudinal lie preferably cephalic; if it fails, to a podalic presentation. If all attempts for external version fails, an internal podalic version may be done under general anesthesia, followed by breech extraction. *An internal version done for the transverse lie of the second twins is the only accepted indication for internal version in modern obstetric practice, to be done only by an expert.*

Management of the Third Stage of Labor

The risk of postpartum hemorrhage can be minimized by administration of 0.25 mg ergometrine or 0.2 mg methyl ergometrine (methergin) intravenously with the delivery of the anterior shoulder of the second baby. The placenta is delivered by controlled cord traction.

The uterus should be massaged continuously and intravenous oxytocin infusion drip should be administered simultaneously. The use of 15-methyl prostaglandin F_2 alpha is largely preferred immediately after delivery of the placenta. A blood loss of more than average should be observed carefully and if it is of concern should be replaced by blood transfusion.

Cesarean Section Delivery (Tables 25.5 and 25.6)

When the first baby is in transverse lie, cesarean section is the only option. If the presentation is breech, most obstetricians favor cesarean delivery. Other associated

Table 25.5: Indication of elective cesarean section

- 1st baby in noncephalic, specially shoulder presentation
- Conjoined twin
- Congenital abnormality precluding safe vaginal delivery
- IUGR in dichorionic twin
- Chronic twin-twin transfusion syndrome in monochorionic twin
- Monoamniotic twin
- Placenta previa
- Contracted pelvis
- Previous cesarean section.
- Severe pre-eclampsia

Table 25.6: Indication of emergency CS

- Fetal distress
- Cord prolapse in 1st baby
- Non-progress of labor
- Collision of both twins.
- 2nd twin transverse, version failed after delivery of 1st twin

indications for a cesarean delivery are contracted pelvis, placenta previa, severe pregnancy-induced hypertension or cord prolapse of the first baby.

Epidural anesthesia administered by an experienced anesthetist is preferable. It allows delivery of the babies without hypoxia or depression which could be caused by transplacental passage of general anesthetic agents. Maternal hemodynamic parameters should be closely monitored.

A monoamniotic placentation requires cesarean delivery due to a high fetal mortality due to cord prolapse or entanglement.

Locking of Twins

Locking of twins is a rare situation in which one baby impedes the descent and delivery of the other. It is more common in primigravidae and in smaller babies.[12]

The four varieties of locking are as follows:
1. *Collision*: The contact of any fetal parts of one twin with those of its cotwin, preventing the engagement of either.
2. *Impaction*: The indentation of any fetal parts of one twin onto the surface of its cotwin, permitting partial engagement of both simultaneously.
3. *Compaction*: The simultaneous full engagement of the leading fetal poles of both twins filling the pelvis. This prevents further descent or disengagement of either twin.
4. *Interlocking*: The intimate adhesion of the inferior surface of a twin's chin with that of its cotwin above or below the pelvic inlet. True locking occurs only in the second stage of labor and treatment must be instituted before there are irreversible complications. If there is collision of twins or suspicion of interlocking, a cesarean section should be performed.

When there is collision, impaction or compaction, strong traction and fundal pressure must be avoided. An attempt is made under anesthesia, to push the second twin out of the pelvis before traction is applied to the first twin and the baby is delivered. If this method fails, cesarean section is performed. When there is a chin-to-chin interlocking, an attempt is made to unlock the chins so that the second twin can be pushed away, allowing the first to be born.[12]

If the first baby is dead, decapitation of the first baby, pushing up the decapitated head followed by delivery of the second baby is done. Thereafter the decapitated head is delivered. If it is associated with infection, a cesarean section is avoided because of the risk of spreading sepsis from the vulva and vagina into the peritoneal cavity. In situations with no infection and less experience with such procedures, a cesarean section may be safer for the mother.

Management of High-order Multiple Pregnancies

Cesarean section is more common with triplets and quadruplets, mainly because of difficulties in ensuring adequate monitoring in labor. The fetal mortality and morbidity is closely related to the fetal weight, birth order and fetal position.

In the recent years, selective reduction of high order multifetal pregnancies has developed as an alternative. Between 9 and 12 weeks under ultrasound guidance, the chosen fetuses receive intracardiac injecton of potassium chloride. However, there is a 30 percent likelihood of losing one of the fetuses.[13]

Conclusion

The incidences of multiple pregnancies are on the increase mainly due to assisted reproductive technology. Both antenatal and intranatal management of any multiple pregnancy requires expertise. As such it is essential for these patients to be looked after either at a tertiary hospital or at a district hospital with senior obstetrician and neonatologist in attendance. Preterm labor and IUGR are both common sequelae in multiple pregnancies. To reduce perinatal mortality and morbidity—a good Neonatal Unit is essential.

POLYHYDRAMNIOS

Definition

Polyhydramnios is a pathological condition characterized by an excessive accumulation of amniotic fluid, usually more than 2000 ml. On the basis of an ultrasound examination, an amniotic fluid pocket measuring 8 cm or more in vertical diameter is suggestive of polyhydramnios.[14] An amniotic fluid index greater than 25 cm is also an ultrasonographic finding in polyhydramnios.[15]

Incidence

Polyhydramnios affects approximately 0.4 to 1.5 percent of all pregnancies.[16] The dynamics of amniotic fluid production and turnover are complex, requiring a delicate balance between maternal and fetal factors. The alteration of any factor that regulates the feto-maternal equilibrium *in utero* may abnormally increase the fluid volume, causing polyhydramnios. The factors involved in this regulation are fetal swallowing, micturition, respiratory movements and uteroplacental blood flow. The composition of amniotic fluid in polyhydramnios is usually not different from that in a normal case.

Acute versus Chronic Polyhydramnios

The differentiation between acute versus chronic polyhydramnios depends on the week of onset, rate of uterine growth and period of delivery.

Traditionally, acute polyhydramnios occurs usually before 24 weeks of gestation. It accounts for less than 2 percent of cases and is characterized by a rapid accumulation of amniotic fluid over a short time.[17] Maternal symptoms like pain, dyspnea, edema of the abdomen and lower extremities, nausea and vomitting are profound. In majority of cases preterm labor occurs before 28 weeks of gestation and the fetal prognosis is guarded.

Chronic polyhydramnios is more common and accounts for 98 percent of the cases. It manifests insidiously in the third trimester with gradual accumulation of amniotic fluid. Maternal symptoms develop over a longer period and become distressing. The neonatal prognosis is dependent on the underlying cause.

Etiopathology of Polyhydramnios

The conditions associated with polyhydramnios include maternal (15%), fetal (18%) or placental (<1%) causes. *In the vast majority of the cases (65%) the etiology is idiopathic.*

Maternal Factors

Polyhydramnios occurs in 1.5 to 66 percent of all diabetic pregnancies.[15] Fetal hyperglycemia can cause polyuria and increased osmolarity of the amniotic fluid. Though Rh isoimmunization could lead to excessive production and accumulation of the amniotic fluid, the use of prophylactic anti-D immunoglobin has reduced the incidence of severe hydrops associated with polyhydramnios.

Placental Factors

Placental Chorioangiomas and the circumvallate placenta could cause polyhydramnios.

Fetal Factors

Polyhydramnios can occur in 25 percent of the cases of the monozygotic twin in a twin-to-twin transfusion syndrome in the recipient.

Fetal anomalies account for 12.7 percent of the cases of polyhydramnios.[15] Abnormalities of the central nervous system include anencephaly, encephalocele, spina bifida and microcephaly. Polyhydramnios occurs in 35 percent of the cases of anencephaly. It may occur due to absent fetal swallowing reflex or as a transudate from the exposed meninges into the amniotic cavity. Another theory in the etiology states that excessive urination due to absence of antidiuretic hormone causes polyhydramnios.

Gastrointestinal fetal anomalies producing polyhydramnios include esophageal atresia, diaphragmatic hernia, and omphalocele and midgut volvulus. Ureteropelvic renal obstruction could lead to polyhydramnios. Skeletal malformations, congenital cystic lung malformations and congenital heart diseases can also account for polyhydramnios. Down syndrome, severe chromosomal abnormalities, intra-uterine infections and hematological disorders like alpha thalassemia are other etiological factors.

Diagnosis

Clinical Features

The patient presents with an undue enlargement of the abdomen with difficulty in ambulation. Breathlessness, fatigue and palpitations can occur. Due to rampant accumulation of fluid there may be edema and varicosities of the lower limbs. Per abdominal examination reveals a disproportionately enlarged uterus. The abdominal skin appears tense, glistening and stretched. The flanks are full and fluid thrill would be evident. It may be difficult to palpate fetal parts, ascertain the presentation or auscultate the fetal heart sounds. Per vaginally, the cervix could be prematurely open with a bulging bag of membranes through the internal os.

Investigations

A baseline hematological profile should include complete blood count, blood group and Rh type. Liver and renal function tests should be done if necessary. It is vital to detect abnormal blood sugars and if required a glucose tolerance test should be done. Glycosuria can be detected by urine examination.

Though an X-ray of the abdomen may detect the fetal shadow, it may appear hazy. A level II ultrasound should be performed on every patient with polyhydramnios to detect congenital and placental abnormalities. In individualized cases, the fetal karyotype must be obtained using amniocentesis, cordocentesis or placental biopsy. The amniotic fluid index (AFI) is the clinical standard in the sonographic evaluation of polyhydramnios. The AFI is calculated by adding the vertical cord-free amniotic fluid pocket depths in each of the four quadrants of the uterus.[18]

Complications

There is an increased risk of fetal and maternal morbidity and mortality associated with polyhydramnios. The increased amniotic fluid volume and overstretched myometrium increase the risk of complication.

Antepartum maternal problems include the risk of developing pregnancy-induced hypertension, preterm labor and prelabor rupture of membranes. There may be marked cardiorespiratory embarrassment.

The para-amnio hippuric acid dye dilution technique provides an accurate measurement but is an invasive technique and thus limited for research studies.[19] Intrapartum complications include placental abruption, cord presentation and cord prolapse. There is an increased risk of operative interference. There is also a higher risk of postpartum hemorrhage due to uterine over distension and the possibility of amniotic fluid embolism through the paracervical veins. During puerperium there is more risk of subinvolution and sepsis could occur due to operative interference.

The fetal outcome is often guarded. The risk of preterm delivery is higher and fetal distress occurs more often due to cord prolapse or abruptio placentae. The major causes of mortality are congenital abnormalities incompatible with life.

Management

For every case of polyhydramnios, a diagnostic work-up is crucial to identify the etiological factor. Hospitalization is often necessary to relieve maternal distress. After exclusion of major congenital fetal anomalies, conservative management is the initial approach. The patient should have frequent periods of modified bed rest with bathroom privileges. A high protein, salt restricted diet should be initiated. In cases of severe edema, diuretics may be considered but they are generally contraindicated because they deplete the vascular volume of the maternal and fetal circulation. Associated conditions like pre-eclampsia and diabetes should be promptly treated.

When no fetal abnormality is detected and expectant management fails to relieve discomfort a slow decompression therapeutic amniocentesis is indicated. The bladder is evacuated before the procedure. Using ultrasonographic guidance the placenta is localized. With adequate aseptic precautions local anesthesia is infiltrated along the proposed point of introduction of the needle. A fine bore needle used for amniocentesis is then introduced into the amniotic sac and the outflow of liquor is controlled by the regulator of an infusion set. Usually about 400 to 500 ml of liquor is aspirated per hour. Following amniocentesis, preterm labor can ensue in 50 percent cases.

An alternative medical treatment is the use of prostaglandin synthetase inhibitors. *Indomethacin* has been proven effective in reducing the quantity of amniotic fluid.[20] It probably acts by reducing the fluid reabsorption via the lungs. The dose recommended is 2.2 mg/kg/day orally every 6 hours. It should be stopped at 32 weeks to avoid premature closure of ductus arteriosus and serious neonatal hemodynamic complications. It also has other complications detrimental to the fetus and hence not recommended.

Polyhydramnios with Fetal Congenital Anomaly

Tense polyhydramnios associated with a congenitally malformed fetus could be first relieved by a slow decompression amniocentesis followed by induction of labor with cervical ripening and use of oxytocics. Care should be taken to avoid abruptio placentae. The use of Drew-Smythe catheter for high rupture of membranes has declined in the practice of modern obstetrics.

Intrapartum Management

During labor, there is a risk of uterine inertia. The obstetrician should be vigilant to detect cord prolapse and malpresentations. The third stage of labor should be monitored carefully to prevent atonic postpartum hemorrhage, which could result due to uterine over distention. To prevent blood loss, intravenous ergometrine 0.25 mg, methergin 0.2 mg or 15 methyl-PGF$_2$ alpha 250 μgm intramuscularly should be given with the delivery of the anterior shoulder.

The neonatologist should evaluate the newborn to exclude congenital anomalies, especially, esophageal atresia by the passage of a soft rubber catheter into the stomach.

REFERENCES

1. Schenker JG, Yarkonis S, Granat M: Multiple pregnancies following induction of ovulation. *Fertility and Sterility* **35**:105-23, 1981.
2. Allen MS, Turner UG: Twin birth, identical or fraternal twins? *Obstetrics and Gynecology* **37**: 358, 1971.
3. Kovacs B, Shahbahrami B, Platt LD et al: Molecular genetic prenatal determination of twin zygosity. *Obstetrics Gynecology* **72**:954-56, 1988.
4. Kovacs B, Kirschbaum TH, Paul RH: Twin gestations. Antenatal care and complications. *Obstetric and Gynecology* **74**: 313-17, 1989.
5. Farooqui MO, Grossman JH, Shannon RA: A review of twin pregnancy and perinatal mortality. *Obstetrics and Gynecology Survey* **28**:144, 1973.
6. Naye RL, Tapari N, Judge D et al: Twins: Causes of perinatal death in 12 United States cities and one African city. *American Journal of Obstetrics and Gynecology* **131**:267-72, 1978.
7. Erkkola K, Ala Mellos, Piroinen O, et al: Growth discordancy in twin pregnancies. A risk factor not detected by measurements of biparietal diameter. *Obstetrics Gynecology* **66**: 203-06, 1985.
8. De Lia JE, Cruickshank DP, Keye WR: Fetoscopic Neodymium-YAG laser occlusion of placental vessels in severe twin-twin transfusion syndrome. *Obstetrics Gynecology* **75**:1046-53, 1990.
9. Enbom JA: Twin pregnancy with intrauterine death of one twin. *American Journal of Obstetrics and Gynaecology* **152**: 424-29, 1985.
10. Kling S, Johnston RJ, Michalyschyn B et al: Successful separation of xiphopagus-conjoined twins. *Journal of Pediatric Surgery* **10**: 267-71, 1975.
11. Porreo RP, Barton SM, Haverkamp AD: Occlusion of umbilical artery in acardiac, acephalic twins. *Lancet* **337**: 326-27, 1991.
12. Nissen ED: Collision, impaction, compaction and interlocking. *Obstetrics and Gynecology* **11**: 514, 1958.
13. Berkowitz RL, Lynch L, Chitkara V et al: Selective reduction of multifetal pregnancies in the first trimester. *New England Journal of Medicine* **318**:1043-47, 1988.
14. Chamberlain, PF, Manning FA, Morrison L, et al: Ultrasound evaluation of amniotic fluid volume–II. Relationship of increased amniotic fluid volume to perinatal outcome. *American Journal of Obstetrics and Gynecology* **150**: 250, 1984.
15. Carlson D, Platt L, Medearic A et al: Quantifiable polyhydramnios: Diagnosis and management. *Obstetrics and Gynecology* **75**: 989, 1990.
16. Queenan J, Gadow E: Polyhydramnios; Chronic versus acute. *American Journal of Obstetrics and Gynecology* **108**: 349, 1970.
17. Queenan JT: Recurrent acute polyhydramnios. *American Journal of Obstetrics and Gynecology* **106**: 625, 1970.
18. Phelan JP, Aha ML, Smith CR et al: Amniotic fluid measurements during pregnancy. *Journal of Reproduction Medicine* **32**: 601, 1987.
19. Charles D, Jacoby H: Preliminary data on the use of Sodium aminohippurate to determine amniotic fluid volumes. *American Journal of Obstetrics and Gynecology* **95**: 266, 1966.
20. Cabrol D, Handesman R, Muller J, et al: Treatment of polyhydramnios with prostaglandin synthetase inhibitor (indomethacin). *American Journal of Obstetrics and Gynecology* **157**: 422-26, 1987.

26.
Preterm Labor and Prelabor Rupture of Membranes

Tan Peng Chiong

PART TWO — Feto-maternal Medicine

INTRODUCTION

In the developed world, preterm birth is the biggest contributor to neonatal mortality and a leading cause of pediatric morbidity. Preterm birth is often preceded by spontaneous preterm labor or preterm prelabor rupture of membranes.

Effective methods of preventing spontaneous preterm labor or preterm prelabor rupture of membranes remain elusive. There is no current effective method of stopping established preterm labor. The primary aim in the current management of preterm labor is of optimizing the condition of the fetus and provision of neonatal facilities.

Preterm labor and delivery may have physical advantages for the mother.

The decision whether to treat preterm labor requires careful balancing of the possible benefit to the fetus of prolonging pregnancy against the possible harmful effect to the mother of any treatment.

PRETERM LABOR

Definition of Preterm Labor

Preterm labor is defined as labor occurring with a potentially viable fetus to 36 weeks 6 days gestation. For statistical purposes some authorities use 20 weeks gestation or 400 gram birth weight as the lower limit of viability. WHO has recommended 22 weeks and 500 gm as the lower limit of viability.

Labor is defined as the birth process where painful uterine contractions cause cervical effacement and dilatation, descent of the presenting part into the birth canal and the eventual delivery of the fetus.

Labor is established when regular painful uterine contractions result in an effaced cervix of at least 3 cm dilatation.

Other Definitions

1. A *stillbirth* is defined as a potentially viable fetus that showed no sign of life at birth.
2. *Perinatal mortality rate* is defined as the total of stillbirths + deaths within the first week of life per thousand total births (i.e. live births + stillbirths).

3. *Neonatal mortality rate* is defined as deaths within the first 4 weeks of life per thousand live births.
4. *Infant mortality rate* is defined as deaths within the first year of life per thousand live births.

Incidence of Preterm Birth

Preterm births account for 5-10 percent[1-3] of all births and the majority is preceded by spontaneous preterm labor. Preterm labor and delivery rates vary considerably between different areas due to different population risk factors.

Table 26.1 shows the weekly delivery rate of singleton livebirth from 24 weeks gestation in the state of Virginia, USA in 1991-1993.[3] In this population, the preterm singleton livebirth rate is just over 7 percent. Preterm birth before 32 weeks comprises <2 percent of births but it accounts for 74 percent of perinatal mortality.[1]

Table 26.1: Weekly delivery rate

Gestation (weeks)	No. livebirths	% livebirths	Cumulative % livebirths
24	194	0.07	
25	228	0.08	0.15
26	294	0.11	0.26
27	303	0.11	0.37
28	369	0.13	0.5
29	378	0.14	0.64
30	479	0.17	0.81
31	589	0.21	1.02
32	962	0.35	1.37
33	1225	0.44	1.81
34	2205	0.8	2.61
35	3771	1.36	3.97
36	8487	3.06	7.03
37	16737	6.04	13.07
38	37162	13.4	26.47
39	58556	21.11	47.58
40	104725	37.76	85.34
41	32116	11.58	96.92
42	8545	3.08	100

• Data derived from a paper by JW Seeds and T Peng[3] describing a complete birth cohort of 277325 live births in Virginia, USA between 1991-93.

Etiology of Preterm Labor

The exact cause of preterm labor remains elusive and is likely to be multifactorial.

Table 26.2 enlists the risk factors for preterm labor and birth.

Table 26.2: Risk factors for preterm labor and birth

- Socioeconomic factors
  - Lower socioeconomic class
  - Young maternal age (less than 16 years)
  - Unmarried or unsupported
  - Underweight (body mass index less than 19)
  - Smoking
- Preterm premature rupture of membranes
- Multiple pregnancy
- Previous preterm delivery
- Intrauterine death
- Short cervix
- Positive fetal fibronectin
- Genital tract infection or colonization with
  - *Chlamydia trachomatis*
  - *Neisseria gonorrhoeae*
  - Bacterial vaginosis
  - *Trichomonas vaginalis*
  - Group B *Streptococcus*
  - *Gardnerella vaginalis*
- Asymptomatic bacteriuria
- Systemic febrile infections
- Cervical incompetence
- Polyhydramnios
- Fetal abnormalities
- Uterine abnormalities
- Iatrogenic (medical indications for preterm delivery)
  - Preeclampsia
  - Intrauterine growth retardation, fetal distress
  - Symptomatic placenta praevia
  - Abruptio placentae
  - Chorioamnionitis
  - Severe maternal disease e.g. cardiac, renal, malignancies

Maternal Consequences of Preterm Labor and Birth

Preterm labor and delivery probably constitute no increased physical danger to the mother. Delivery of the smaller, preterm baby is less likely to cause pelvic floor damage or to result in obstructed labor. It saves the mother the discomfort of advanced pregnancy. A shortened pregnancy may arguably reduce the risk of major complications like preeclampsia and venous thromboembolism.

Physical harm to the mother can arise due to interventions such as medical treatment of preterm labor and from the increased risk of cesarean section.

However, maternal psychological stress often arises due to worries about the ill preterm infant. Mothers are also concerned about financial, personal and family consequences in the care of a possibly disabled child afterward.

The preterm newborn often needs to be separated from their mothers due to requirement for medical care.

Fetal Consequences

At gestation of ≤32 weeks, 36.7 percent of fetuses that are alive at the beginning of labor died either during labor or shortly after birth before they could be admitted to a neonatal unit.[4] Preterm birth has severe fetal consequences.

Neonatal Consequences

Preterm delivery is associated with a whole range of major adverse consequences for the infant.

Table 26.3 shows the risks associated with preterm delivery.

Table 26.3: Major risks of preterm birth

- Death
- Disability and handicap
- Respiratory distress syndrome
- Intraventricular hemorrhage
- Infection
- Necrotizing enterocolitis
- Hypothermia
- Hypoglycemia
- Jaundice
- Feeding difficulties
- Retinopathy of prematurity
- Bronchopulmonary dysplasia

Survival and Mortality

The survival rate of very preterm infants has improved dramatically. At 27 weeks in 1966-69 neonatal survival was just above 20 percent but by 1991-94, this increased to almost 80 percent.[5]

The sophistication and availability of neonatal intensive care is the major factor in ensuring survival in early preterm births. It is essential when counseling parents to use data that is current and locally applicable.

Table 26.4 shows the correlation between survival and gestation for preterm infants delivered at ≤32 weeks gestation in Trent region of the United Kingdom between 1994 and 1997.[4]

Survival increases sharply as gestation approaches 32 weeks. The biggest leap in survival occurs between 24 to 28 weeks with predicted survival increasing from about 20 percent to approaching 90 percent.

Table 26.4: Survival and gestation for preterm infants*

Gestation (weeks)	European infants (95% confidence interval)	Asian infants (95% confidence interval)
22	2 (1-4)	3 (1-6)
23	6 (4-10)	8 (4-15)
24	16 (12-20)	20 (13-30)
25	33 (29-37)	40 (28-52)
26	54 (50-58)	61 (49-72)
27	72 (68-76)	78 (68-85)
28	84 (81-87)	88 (81-93)
29	91 (89-93)	93 (89-96)
30	95 (93-96)	96 (93-98)
31	97 (95-98)	98 (95-99)
32	98 (96-99)	98 (97-100)

Median Predicted Survival (%) (of fetuses alive at the start of labor and survived to be discharged from the neonatal unit)

Data derived from Draper ES et al[4] of a study involving 3760 infants born at 22-32 weeks gestation.

At more than 32 weeks gestation with modern neonatal care, death from complications attributable to prematurity is not a significant contributor to the perinatal mortality rate. Indeed, at ≥29 weeks, stillbirths consistently outnumber neonatal deaths.[3]

Table 26.5 shows predicted survival for selected gestations and the influence of birth weight on survival.[4]

Survival of the preterm infant is also related to birth weight. The influence of gestation on survival is more profound than birth weight at gestations ≤32 weeks. Growth retarded fetuses ≤15 centile birth weight consistently do less well.[3] Very large for dates fetuses also have increased mortality. This is probably due to underlying pathology influencing birthweight.

Table 26.5: Median predicted survival of infants admitted to the neonatal unit (Asian infants)

Birth weights (grams)	Predicted Percentage survival (95% confidence interval) 24 weeks	26 weeks	28 weeks	30 weeks
250-499	16 (12-21)	32 (26-39)	46 (35-56)	*
500-749	25 (21-31)	50 (4-55)	69 (64-74)	77 (69-84)
750-999	32 (26-38)	63 (58-67)	82 (79-85)	90 (87-93)
1000-1249	34 (27-43)	69 (63-74)	88 (86-91)	95 (94-97)
1250-1499	*	69 (61-77)	91 (88-93)	97 (96-98)
1500-1749	*	*	91 (86-94)	98 (96-99)
1750-1999	*	*	*	98 (96-99)
2000-2249	*	*	*	97 (94-99)
2250-2499	*	*	*	95 (92-99)

Data derived from Draper ES *et al*[4] of a study involving 3760 infants born at 22-32 weeks gestation

Female sex, multiple gestation, Asian or African-American origin, pre-eclampsia and antenatal corticosteroids are positively correlated with survival in preterm births.

Pediatric Morbidity

Over a recent period 1983-1994, survival at extreme prematurity (i.e. 22-27 weeks) continues to improve but the disability rate amongst survivors was unchanged.[5] Overall, 25 percent of survivors had severe disability. In 10 percent of survivors the disability is so severe that a life of total dependency is anticipated. In this study, there is also no reduction in the proportion of disabled survivors as gestation increases to 27 weeks.[5] This implies that as the number of survivors increases with better care, the number of survivors with major disability do not correspondingly decrease.

At very preterm gestations, it is vital to involve parents in decision-making regarding labor management and resuscitation of the newborn. The ethics of resuscitation are particularly difficult. Ultimately, care must be individualized.

Assessment of Gestational Age

Accurate pregnancy dating is crucial in the management of preterm labor. Menstrual dates can be unreliable. In a large study of preterm survival, 36 percent of gestation ages were corrected after a dating scan at <20 weeks gestation.[4]

In ideal circumstances, a dating scan should be performed in all pregnancies. The ideal dating scan is at 8 to 11 weeks, using fetal crown-rump length measurement. Ultrasound assessment at ≤20 weeks is accurate for dating.

Symptoms and Signs of Preterm Labor

Symptoms

Preterm labor in its early stages is difficult to diagnose. Placebo control arms in trials of tocolytic drugs typically has over 60 percent of recruits not delivering within 48 hours[2] implying that in almost 2 out of 3 cases, the diagnosis of preterm labor was wrong.

Table 26.6 lists the symptoms of preterm labor.

Table 26.6: Symptoms of preterm labor

- Uterine activity, e.g. contractions or frequent tightening
- Passage of a show
- Lower abdominal pain or cramping
- Sensation of vagina pressure
- Increased vaginal discharge
- Vaginal bleeding

False labor is a diagnosis that can only be made in retrospect.

Signs of Preterm Labor

Table 26.7 lists the signs of preterm labor.

Table 26.7: Signs of preterm labor

- Cervical effacement
- Cervical dilatation
- Rupture of membranes
- Engagement of the presenting part
- Show (maybe bloodstained)
- Bulging membranes
- Palpable uterine activity

Established labor is usually unmistakable. Rarely, even in supposedly established labor, contractions may spontaneously stop or be inhibited by tocolytics for prolonged periods.

Physical Examination and Investigations in Preterm Labor

A thorough assessment of the patient is required as the risk factors and causes of preterm labor are so varied. If a specific reason is highly suspected to be the cause of preterm labor, e.g. malaria, assessment must be targeted accordingly.

Table 26.8 enlists the routine physical assessments in cases of suspected preterm labor.

Table 26.8: Routine physical examination in preterm labor

- Routine pulse, temperature, blood pressure measurement and dipstick urinalysis
- Abdominal examination
- Vaginal speculum assessment to assess cervix, membranes status, for swabs taking
- Digital assessment of the cervix maybe useful but is not always necessary
- Assess uterine activity and fetal viability—a cardiotocograph (CTG) is ideal for this purpose

Table 26.9 lists the investigations usually undertaken in preterm labor.

Table 26.9: Routine investigations for preterm labor

- Urine for microscopy and culture
- Swabs
  - High vaginal for gram staining and culture
  - Endocervical for *Neisseria gonorrhoeae* culture
  - Endocervical for *Chlamydia*
  (If genital infection is suspected, urethral and anorectal swabs are indicated)
- CTG
- Ultrasound fetal assessment (dating, fetal anomalies, presentation, liquor assessment, estimating fetal weight)—clinical assessment of presentation is often inaccurate at early gestations

Recent postulated investigations
- Swab from cervico-vaginal area for fetal fibronectin
- Transvaginal ultrasound assessment for cervical length and funneling at internal os

Fetal Fibronectin

Fetal fibronectin is an extracellular matrix glycoprotein produced by fetal membranes and decidua. Its likely function is maintaining adhesion between the decidua and the chorion. Disruption of the choriodecidual interface causes the release of fetal fibronectin, which can be detected in cervico-vaginal secretions. Fetal fibronectin in high concentrations (≥50 ng/ml) in cervico-vaginal secretions is associated with preterm delivery.

In a meta-analysis, a positive fetal fibronectin test amongst symptomatic women predicts preterm delivery within the next 7 days with a sensitivity of 89 percent (95% confidence interval 80-97%) and a specificity of 86 percent (95% confidence interval 81-91%).[6]

For delivery within 7 days in symptomatic women, the positive predictive value ranged from 6-40 percent and the negative predictive value ranged from 98-100 percent.[7] As the negative predictive value is close to 100 percent, a negative test is interpreted by some as a reassuring sign.

Fetal fibronectin is not a diagnostic test for preterm labor. It is a useful clinical aid, reducing unnecessary treatment without adversely affecting outcome.[7] Established labor, recent sexual intercourse, antepartum hemorrhage and rupture of membranes make the test less reliable.

Transvaginal Ultrasound Cervical Assessment

Transvaginal ultrasound is the best modality to assess cervical length and detect dilatation at the internal os. There is an inverse relationship between cervical length and risk of preterm delivery.

Optimal cutoff values for using cervical length as a marker for preterm delivery in symptomatic women ranged from 18 to 30 mm; at these cutoff values, sensitivity is from 68 to 100 percent and specificity is from 44 to 79 percent[8] for preterm deliveries. Using dilatation or funneling at the internal os as a marker for preterm delivery, the sensitivity is 70 to 100 percent and specificity is 54 to 75 percent.[8]

The clinical utility of transvaginal ultrasound is probably inferior to that of fetal fibronectin amongst symptomatic women for predicting delivery within 7 days.

Sequential or combined transvaginal ultrasound and fetal fibronectin has been proposed with slight improvement in utility.

Management of Preterm Labor

Neonatal Facilities and in utero Transfer

Liaison with the neonatologists is important for the timely mobilization of resources. They also provide an invaluable input in counseling couples and in managing expectations.

If local facilities are inadequate to treat the preterm infant, an *in utero* transfer is preferred to *ex-utero* transfer as the uterus is the best transport incubator. *Ex-utero* transfers may be unavoidable if delivery is imminent or if the woman is too ill to transfer.

It is helpful for couples to visit the neonatal unit pre-delivery. Although the unit is often an intimidating environment, the couple will not get a shock later on when they see their child in that environment.

Corticosteroids for Fetal Benefits

Corticosteroids administered antenatally to mothers are of proven efficacy in reducing neonatal mortality, respiratory distress syndrome and cerebral intraventricular hemorrhages by between 40 to 60 percent.[2,9,10]

The positive effect of antenatal corticosteroids is apparent soon after administration, maximal 24 to 48 hours later and lasts for up to 1 week.[2]

Corticosteroids should be administered to women at imminent risk of preterm delivery. Delivery should not be delayed just for corticosteroid effect if the clinical condition of the mother or fetus warrants immediate delivery.

The RCOG (UK) guideline[10] suggests corticosteroids for preterm births from 24 to 36 weeks. There is general consensus on administering antenatal corticosteroids between 24 to 34 weeks gestation.

At extreme prematurity of 22 to 23 weeks gestation, given that 20 percent of infants at 23 weeks gestation admitted to a neonatal unit now survive,[4] it is logical to expect some fetuses to benefit from antenatal corticosteroids but benefit is unproven.

At more than 34 weeks, almost all infants survive. It is estimated that 94 women had to be treated for one fetus to benefit.[10] Benefit is therefore marginal.

In ideal circumstances, delivery should occur 24 to 48 hours following the administration of corticosteroids. In spontaneous preterm labor, this delay is often not achievable without tocolysis.

Table 26.10 lists the recommended corticosteroids regimes.[9,10]

Table 26.10: Regimes for administration of maternal corticosteroids in pregnancies at risk of preterm birth within the next 7 days

1. Betamethasone – 2 doses of 12 mg intramuscularly 24 hours apart
2. Dexamethasone – 4 doses of 6 mg intramuscularly 12 hours apart

The above regimes are of proven efficacy in trials.
1. Dexamethasone – 2 doses of 12 mg intramuscularly 12 hours apart is a regime commonly used though whether it is as effective is unknown.

No adverse maternal or fetal effects have been noted with regard to a single course of corticosteroids.[9]

Repeat courses of corticosteroids

i. Corticosteroids are sometimes administered on a weekly basis in cases where there is ongoing high risk of preterm delivery, e.g. in expectantly managed pre-eclampsia.
ii. Recent evidence suggests that multiple courses may have adverse effects, e.g. maternal sepsis, neonatal sepsis and death, reduced birth weight and reduced fetal head circumference.
iii. However, multiple courses of corticosteroids are also shown to reduce respiratory distress syndrome and neonatal patent ductus arteriosus.[20]
iv. On balance, whilst awaiting the result of clinical trials, routine weekly courses should be avoided.

A repeat course of "rescue" corticosteroids maybe reasonable in certain circumstances e.g. where a first course was given say at 24 weeks and later at 27-32 weeks, preterm delivery again appeared imminent.

Contraindications to corticosteroids: Corticosteroids are contraindicated in chorioamnionitis, maternal tuberculosis and porphyria.[10]

Maternal diabetes: In diabetes mellitus, the benefit of antenatal corticosteroids is uncertain. The hyperglycemic effect of corticosteroids may retard lung maturation, neutralizing its beneficial effect. Tocolysis with sympathomimetic agents will also exacerbate hyperglycemia.

Multiple pregnancies: There is no direct evidence that corticosteroids are beneficial in preterm multiple pregnancies due to the small number recruited in trials. There is no plausible biological reason why it should not be effective.

Other pregnancy complications: Corticosteroids are beneficial in preterm prelabor rupture of membranes, pre-eclampsia, antepartum hemorrhage and intrauterine growth restriction where iatrogenic preterm delivery is anticipated.

Tocolysis: Tocolytics are available to inhibit uterine activity but none are effective at stopping established labor. In early preterm labor, tocolysis can delay delivery for up to 48 hours.[11]

Meta-analysis of trials of tocolysis against placebo has shown no significant positive effect on neonatal mortality or serious neonatal morbidity.[2,11] Tocolysis have not been shown to reduce preterm birth.

Indications for tocolysis: There are 2 main indications for tocolysis in preterm labor:
- To delay delivery by 24 to 48 hours for corticosteroids to take effect
- To delay delivery for safer *in utero* transfer

Tocolysis maybe used between 20 to 35 weeks gestation including cases of membrane rupture.[11]

Preterm labor itself (if not for giving steroids) is not an indication for tocolysis with current evidence.

Contraindications to tocolysis
- Fetal maturity
- Any indication for expedited delivery, e.g. fetal compromise
- Imminent delivery
- Maternal disease, e.g. cardiac

Antepartum hemorrhage is a relative contraindication to tocolysis.

Tocolysis appears to be safe in symptomatic placenta previa[12,13] and results in pregnancy prolongation and increased birth weight.[12] In non-previa bleeding (i.e. potential abruptio), tocolysis also appears to be safe.[13] However, it has to be used with caution, as it may disturb the hemodynamic response of the mother should there be severe bleeding.

If uterine contraction starts in cases of minor antepartum hemorrhage which are otherwise suitable for expectant management, tocolysis maybe used to delay delivery for corticosteroids to take effect or for *in utero* transfer.

Tocolytic drugs
The following classes of drugs are in current usage for tocolysis:
- Beta sympathomimetic agents, e.g. ritodrine
- Calcium channel blockers, e.g. nifedipine
- Cyclo-oxygenase inhibitors, e.g. indomethacin
- Oxytocin receptor blockers, e.g. atosiban
- Nitric oxide donors, e.g. glyceryl trinitrate
- Magnesium sulfate

Beta-sympathomimetic drugs: The most common tocolytic in current usage are betamimetics.[14,15] Ritodrine has the largest published database.[11]

Betamimetics have severe side effects including hypotension, myocardial ischemia, cardiac failure and pulmonary edema. These unwanted effects are exacerbated by concurrent corticosteroids administration. Maternal fatalities though rare have been regularly reported.

Intravenous betamimetics should only be used with the women under close supervision. Infusion volume should be minimised.[11]

A dilution and infusion regime for ritodrine suggested by the RCOG (UK) is shown on Table 26.11.[11]

Table 26.11: Preparations for ritodrine infusion in preterm labor

Syringe pump Add 3x5ml ampoules (150 mg) ritodrine to 35 ml of dextrose		Controlled infusion device Add 3x5ml ampoules (150 mg) ritodrine to 500 ml of 5% dextrose	
Doses	Rates	Doses	Rates
50 microgram/min	1 ml/hr	50 microgram/min	10 ml/hr
100 microgram/min	2 ml/hr	100 microgram/min	20 ml/hr
150 microgram/min	3 ml/hr	150 microgram/min	30 ml/hr
200 microgram/min	4 ml/hr	200 microgram/min	40 ml/hr
250 microgram/min	5 ml/hr	250 microgram/min	50 ml/hr
300 microgram/min	6 ml/hr	300 microgram/min	60 ml/hr
350 microgram/min	7 ml/hr	350 microgram/min	70 ml/hr

Derived from RCOG clinical guideline Beta-agonists for the care of women in preterm labor[11]

Infusion should start at the lowest dose and increased at 15-minute intervals until contractions are inhibited or the maximum dose of 350 microgram per minute is reached. An alternative regime using an initial starting dose of 200 microgram/min as a loading dose has been found to require less dose adjustments without increasing maternal side effects.[11]

Monitoring during tocolysis: Table 26.12 illustrates a monitoring regime recommended for women on betamimetic tocolysis by the RCOG (UK).[11]

Table 26.12: Risk factors for PPROM

- Socioeconomic factors
  - Lower socioeconomic class
- Previous PPROM
- Short cervix
- Presence of fetal fibronectin
- Multiple pregnancy
- Intrauterine death
- Genital tract infection or colonisation with
  - *Chlamydia trachomatis*
  - *Neisseria gonorrhoea*
  - Bacterial vaginosis
  - *Trichomonas vaginalis*
  - Group B *Streptococcus*
  - *Gardnerella vaginalis*
- Cervical incompetence
- Polyhydramnios
- Fetal abnormalities
- Iatrogenic
  Invasive procedures e.g. amniocentesis, fetal blood sampling

Fetal wellbeing must also be regularly determined. A CTG is useful for monitoring both the fetus and uterine activity.

When to stop tocolysis: Table 26.13 is a list of indications for stopping tocolysis. Intravenous tocolysis can be stopped abruptly if uterine quiescence has been demonstrated for several hours.

Nifedipine: A meta-analysis comparing nifedipine to ritodrine has shown nifedipine to be more effective in delaying delivery and reducing perinatal morbidity, with fewer maternal side effects.[16] Nifedipine can be given orally with an initial dose of 20 mg to be repeated 6 to 8 hourly as required to suppress contractions.

Other tocolytic agents
Atosiban, an antioxytocic, appears to be a promising agent. With its targeted effect, maternal and fetal systemic effects should be minimal. However, preterm labor is not solely oxytocin mediated.

Indomethacin has profound effects on fetal circulation. It is also used in the treatment of polyhydramnios and neonatal closure of patent ductus arteriosus. Concerns about the fetal effects of indomethacin have limited its use despite its tolerability.

Glyceryl trinitrate is also not widely used due to limited data though the principle of using nitric oxide donors in effecting myometrial relaxation has solid scientific credential.

Magnesium sulfate infusion for tocolysis is mainly used in North America. There are doubts about its effectiveness as a tocolytic. There is also recent concern about its safety in neonates.

Maintenance tocolysis: Maintenance tocolysis following primary inhibition of contractions is not of any demonstrable benefit according to a recent meta-analysis.[17]

Prophylactic antibiotics: Prophylactic antibiotics have no role to play in preterm labor with intact membranes. In the ORACLE II[15] trial involving 6241 symptomatic women, neither prophylactic co-amoxiclav alone, erythromycin alone nor combination co-amoxiclav and erythromycin was shown to be of any benefit in reducing neonatal mortality or serious neonatal morbidity.

Group B Streptococcus: Benzylpenicillin or ampicillin should be given in established preterm labor as prophylaxis against early onset neonatal sepsis due to Group B *Streptococcus* in those with a known carrier

Table 26.13: Routine physical examination in PPROM

- Routine pulse, temperature, blood pressure measurement and dipstick urinalysis.
- Palpation for fetal size, presentation, liquor volume, uterine tenderness, multiple gestation
- Vaginal speculum assessment to
  - Confirm pooling of amniotic fluid in the upper vagina
  - Demonstrate gushing of amniotic fluid from the cervical os
  - Allow swab taking
  - Exclude cord prolapse
  - Collect amniotic fluid for further studies
- Digital assessment of the vagina and cervix is to be avoided
- Assess uterine activity and fetal viability—a CTG is ideal for this purpose but palpation and auscultation will suffice.

status. In cases of penicillin allergy, clindamycin can be substituted. Ideally, it should be administered at least 4 hours prior to delivery.

Rescue Cervical Cerclage

In cases where uterine contractions have ceased, at gestations ≤28 weeks, there is a limited role for a cervical cerclage to support a dilated cervix. Cerclage is more for those with 'silent' dilatation of the cervix without uterine contractions.

However, cerclage often fails as labor usually restarts even with tocolysis.

Mode of Delivery in Preterm Labor

Cephalic presentation: With cephalic presentation, vaginal delivery is anticipated. Cesarean section should only be performed for specific indications.

Breech presentation: The randomised term breech trial involving 2083 women has reported that planned cesarean section is better than planned vaginal delivery for neonatal outcome with no increase in serious maternal complications.[18] It is debatable whether this finding is applicable to preterm gestations.

At gestations where survival is expected e.g. ≥ 26 weeks), many obstetricians favor cesarean section despite the lack of convincing evidence of benefit.

Cesarean section at ≤ 28 weeks gestation is technically more challenging with consequent higher maternal complications. As the lower uterine segment is frequently poorly formed, a vertical uterine incision maybe needed. Classical sections are associated with an increased risk of scar rupture in subsequent pregnancies.

The decision on whether to perform cesarean section in preterm breech labor must be individualized and requires consultation with the woman.

Abnormal lie: With transverse or oblique lie at ≥26 weeks, cesarean section is indicated.

At below 26 weeks, as extreme prematurity is the overwhelming determinant of survival, it may be reasonable to allow vaginal delivery in an initially abnormal lie. The lie usually corrects as labor progresses. Even if abnormal lie persisted, obstructed labor is not anticipated, as the fetus is so small. In developed countries, because of better survival statistics as a result of better care, a cesarean section is preferred. However, the decision must be individualized.

Algorithm for the Management of Preterm Labor (Figure 26.1)

Prevention of preterm labor

Screening for infection: In high-risk cases, there is evidence that screening for and treating bacterial vaginosis and trichomoniasis in the second trimester reduces the risk of preterm delivery. Screening of the general pregnant population does not appear to prevent preterm delivery.

Bacteriuria should also be screened for and treated if identified.

Chlamydia or *Gonorrhoea* if identified during screening should be treated and contact tracing of sexual partners should occur.

Social intervention: Interventions tailored to support individuals with social risk factors for preterm labor have not been found to be effective in reducing preterm birth.[1]

Transvaginal cervical assessment: Transvaginal ultrasound of the cervix in the second trimester can identify women at high risk for preterm birth. However, prophylactic cervical cerclage is of uncertain efficacy in preventing preterm delivery in this situation.

Cervicovaginal fetal fibronectin: In the second trimester, the presence of high concentrations of fetal fibronectin in asymptomatic women is associated with preterm delivery. As no effective treatment is currently available, identifying such women is of limited clinical use and may increase maternal anxiety.

PRETERM PRELABOR RUPTURE OF MEMBRANES

Definition

Preterm prelabor rupture of membranes (PPROM) is defined as spontaneous membrane rupture occurring before 37 weeks gestation (preterm) in the absence of uterine contractions (prelabor).

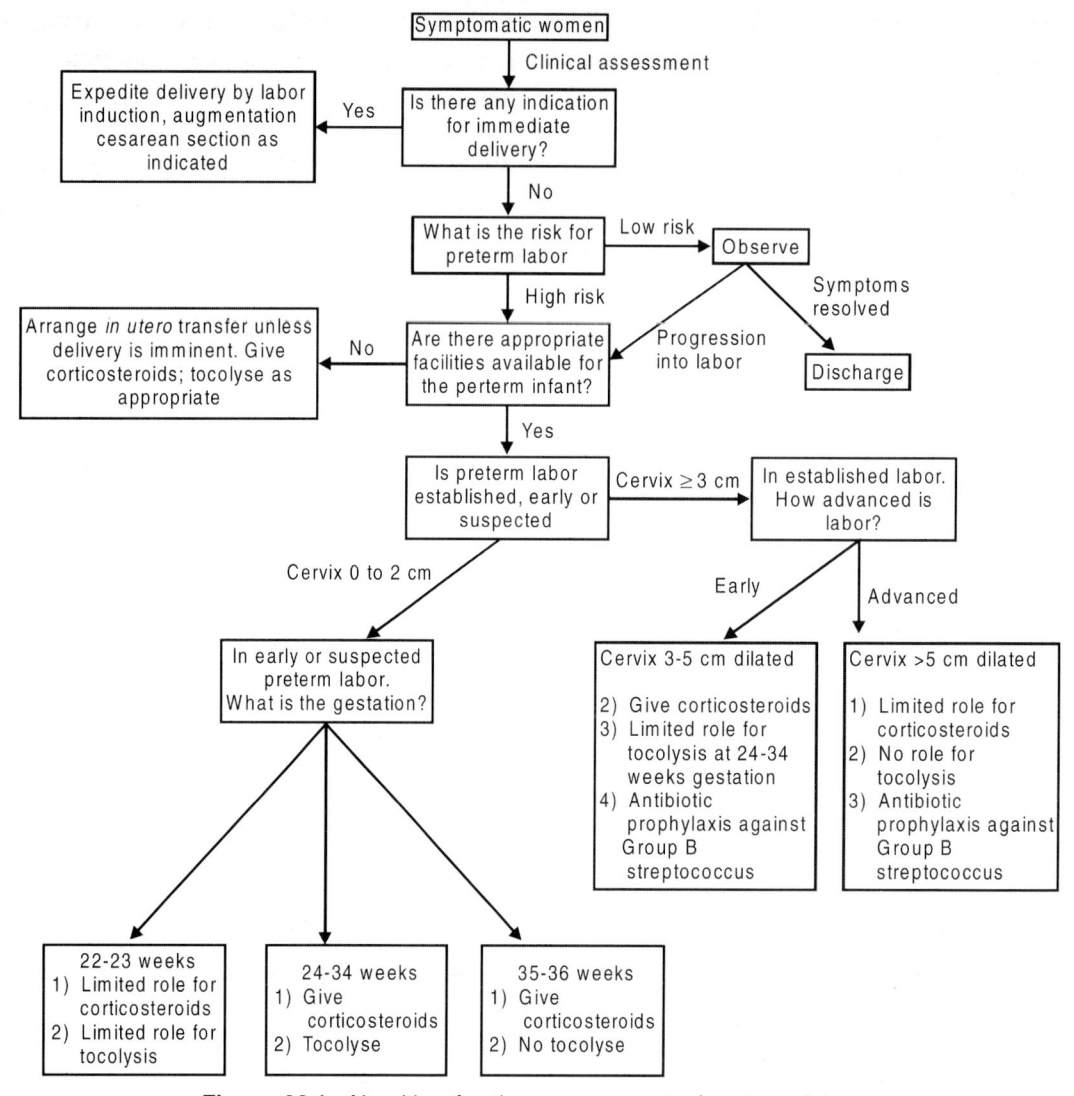

Figure 26.1: Algorithm for the management of preterm labor

PPROM is preterm prelabor rupture of membranes and has replaced the term preterm premature rupture of membranes.

Incidence

PPROM occurs in about 3 percent of pregnancies. PPROM rates vary considerably between different areas due to different population risk factors. PPROM precedes about 30-40 percent of spontaneous preterm labor.[14] 30-40 percent of PPROM will deliver within 48 hours and 56-63 percent within 7 days.[14]

In comparison, prelabor rupture of membranes (PROM) occurs in 10 percent of term pregnancies and 86 percent of such cases labor within 24 hours.

Etiology

The etiology of PPROM is multifactorial but infection plays a significant role. Risk factors for PPROM are very similar to those of preterm labor.

Table 26.12 lists the risk factors for PPROM.

Consequences

The consequences of PPROM include
- Preterm labor and birth
- Chorioamnionitis
- Pulmonary hypoplasia due to severe oligohydramnios
- Skeletal and joint deformities due to compression

- Fetal infection
- Maternal infection

Pulmonary Hypoplasia

Pulmonary hypoplasia is usually due to severe oligohydramnios. Pulmonary hypoplasia is common if PPROM results in severe oligohydramnios ≤ 22 weeks gestation and is rare if PPROM occurs >26 weeks.

Presentation of PPROM

Symptoms

The classic symptom of PPROM is leakage of fluid from the vagina. This fluid is usually colorless. At later gestations, it may contain vernix. Amniotic fluid leakage maybe exacerbated by erect posture and straining of abdominal muscles. Amniotic fluid loss is persistent as amniotic fluid is periodically replenished by fetal urination.

Uterine contractions commonly follow PPROM.

Maternal urinary incontinence is common. Incontinent pregnant women often mistakenly present with complaint of vaginal fluid loss.

Vaginal discharge can also be mistaken for amniotic fluid.

Signs of PPROM

PPROM is diagnosed when vaginal leak of amniotic fluid is demonstrated.

Physical Examination and Investigations

A thorough assessment of the patient is required as the risk factors and causes of PPROM are varied.

Table 26.13 lists the examination expected in the assessment of suspected PPROM.

Amniotic fluid is alkaline. Vaginal secretions and urine are usually acidic. Nitrazine stick and pH paper tests make use of these observations to discriminate between amniotic fluid and vaginal secretions. These tests are prone to give false-positive results especially if blood or infection is present and should not solely be relied upon to diagnose PPROM.

The best physical evidence for PPROM is clear fluid trickling through the cervix and pooling in the upper vagina. A moist upper vagina with a positive nitrazine or pH test is best classified as suspicious. Subsequent leakage resulting in wet sanitary towels confirms PPROM. If no further leakage is demonstrated and amniotic fluid volume is normal on ultrasound assessment, it is unlikely that PPROM has occurred. Diagnosis delayed for upto 24 hours engenders no significant risk, as the management of PPROM is generally expectant in the absence of other complications.

It is difficult to definitively refute a diagnosis of PPROM once it has been made. The diagnosis of PPROM has profound consequences on management for the remainder of pregnancy. Women with PPROM are usually managed as an inpatient. It is therefore important that a false positive diagnosis is avoided.

Table 26.14 lists appropriate investigations in PPROM.

Table 26.14: Investigations for PPROM

- Urine for microscopy and culture
- Swabs
  - High vaginal for Gram staining and culture
  - Endocervical for *Neisseria gonorrhoeae*
  - Endocervical for *Chlamydia*
  (If genital infection is suspected, urethral and anorectal swabs are indicated)
- Ultrasound examination for fetal assessment and amniotic fluid measurement
- Collected vaginal fluid for
  - Microbiological culture
  - Demonstrate ferning to confirm amniotic fluid
  - Fetal lung maturity studies, e.g. lecithin/sphingomyelin ratio

Other tests
- Amniocentesis to provide uncontaminated amniotic fluid for:
  - Microbiological culture (this is the best indicator of chorioamnionitis)
  - Fetal lung maturity studies, e.g. lecithin/sphingomyelin ratio

Amniotic fluid tests to determine fetal lung maturity are not widely available.

Management of PPROM

If the history is highly suggestive but clinical findings are not diagnostic; it is reasonable to admit the woman for a period of observation. If PPROM is confirmed, inpatient management is usual initially.

Expectant Management

Uncomplicated PPROM is usually managed expectantly at gestations <34 weeks.[19]

The main risk of expectant management is of ascending infection causing chorioamnionitis and fetal infection. In the presence of proven infection, urgent delivery is indicated as antibiotic treatment is usually ineffective whilst the pregnancy is ongoing.

Table 26.15 lists the routine monitoring in expectantly managed PPROM.

Table 26.15: Routine monitoring in expectant management of PPROM

Maternal markers of infection
- Temperature measurements 4 times a day
- Maternal pulse 4 times a day
- 3 x weekly white cell count
- 3 x weekly C reactive protein (CRP)
- Daily note of vaginal loss (for detection of purulent discharge)

Fetal wellbeing
- 2-3 weekly growth scan
- Up to weekly amniotic fluid assessment depending gestation
- Fetal biophysical profile (including CTG) is of limited value in detecting fetal infection

Delivery is indicated when any of the following circumstances arises:
- Chorioamnionitis
- Onset of spontaneous labor
- Fetal compromise
- Fetal maturity is achieved
- Maternal disease that may be affected by consequences of PPROM.

There is evidence that with good neonatal care facilities, for PPROM ≥34 weeks, a policy of expediting delivery results in less neonatal infection, maternal infection and in a shorter hospital stay without adversely affecting other neonatal or maternal outcome.[19]

Antenatal Corticosteroids

In uncomplicated PPROM, antenatal corticosteroids should be administered.[9,10]

Prophylactic Antibiotics

The ORACLE I trial[14] which involves 4809 women suggests that prophylactic oral erythromycin 250 mg four times a day should be administered for 10 days or until delivery (whichever is sooner) to singleton pregnancies with PPROM.

This regime reduces adverse composite primary outcome (comprising of combined complications of neonatal mortality, abnormal cerebral ultrasonography and chronic lung disease). Erythromycin when compared to placebo significantly reduces adverse composite primary outcome from 14.4 to 11.2 percent. However, a statistically significant result was only obtained on a secondary analysis, which excludes multiple pregnancies. There were also reductions in the use of surfactant and in blood culture proven sepsis.

Antibiotic choice is extremely important as co-amoxiclav did not improve the composite primary outcome and is in fact associated with increased risk of necrotising enterocolitis.[14]

Compared to antenatal corticosteroids, benefits from prophylactic antibiotics in PPROM are less pronounced.

Tocolysis

PPROM is not a contraindication to tocolysis.[11] Tocolysis should be used for the same limited indications as in preterm labor with intact membranes.

Amniotic Fluid Infusion

Amnio-infusion may be useful in some cases of very early onset PPROM.

If PPROM occurs at <24 weeks gestation and resulted in severe oligohydramnios, infusion of normal saline into the amniotic cavity has been shown to reduce pulmonary hypoplasia. This happens only in the cases where amnio-infusion resulted in a measurable and sustained increase in amniotic fluid volume.

Induction of Labor

If vaginal delivery is to be expedited in PPROM, labor may be induced with either vaginal prostaglandins (e.g. dinoprostone) or oxytocin infusion. In uncomplicated PPROM, where the cervix is unfavorable, dinoprostone is on balance the drug of choice; oxytocin infusion can be used if there is no response after 1-2 doses of dinoprostone.

Mode of Delivery

With cephalic presentation, vaginal delivery is anticipated. In breech presentation or abnormal lie, the same controversies apply as in preterm labor with intact membranes.

With PPROM, cord prolapse is relatively common as the incidence of non-cephalic presentation is high. At ≥26 weeks, the response is the same as cord prolapse at term, i.e. stabilize the situation and expedite delivery (usually by cesarean section). At <26 weeks, as intact survival is low and cesarean section carries higher maternal complication rates, an expectant approach maybe appropriate following consultation with the couple.

The number of vaginal examinations should be kept to the minimum during labor to reduce infective morbidity.

Group B Streptococcus

With PPROM, the risk of neonatal Group B streptococcal sepsis is increased—both preterm delivery and PPROM are independent risk factors for Group B streptococcal sepsis.

Prophylatic benzylpenicillin or ampicillin is indicated at first presentation and again intrapartum.

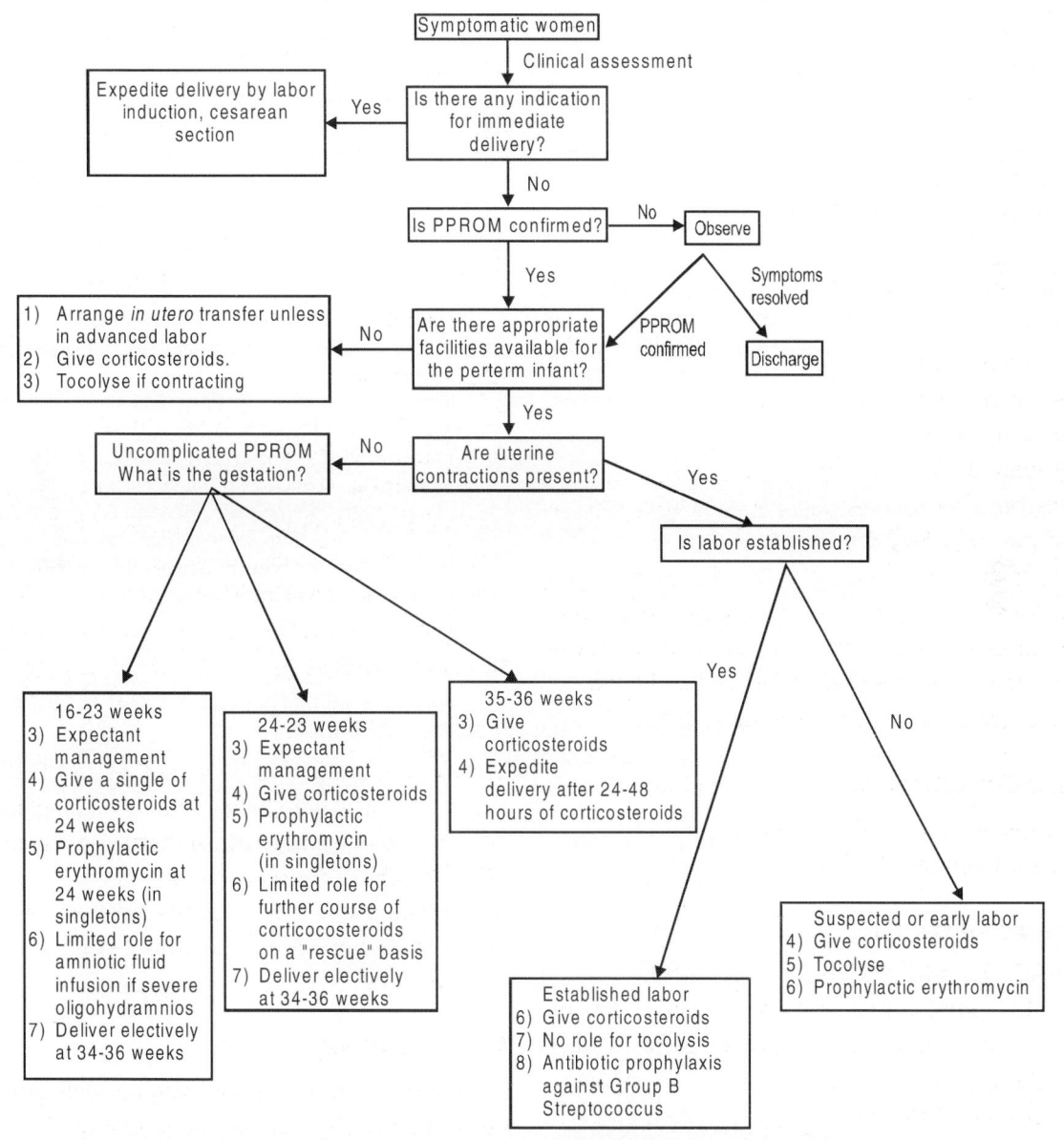

Figure 26.2: Algorithm for the management of preterm premature rupture of membranes

PPROM with in situ Cervical Suture

In this scenario, suture removal can be delayed till uterine contractions are experienced or at least until antenatal corticosteroids have taken effect if there is no other indication for immediate delivery.

Algorithm for PPROM (Figure 26.2)

Prevention of PPROM: PPROM shares similar etiology to preterm labor. Preventative strategies are similar. They are aimed at treating genital infections and reinforcing the cervix with cerclage. The impact of these strategies in preventing PPROM is disappointingly limited.

REFERENCES

1. Keirse MJNC: New perspectives for the effective treatment of preterm labor. *American Journal of Obstetrics and Gynecology* **173**: 618-28, 1995.
2. Steer P, Flint C: ABC of labor care. *British Medical Journal* **318**:1059-62, 1999.
3. Seeds JW, Peng T: Impaired growth and risk of fetal deaths: Is the tenth percentile the appropriate standard? *American Journal of Obstetrics and Gynecology* **178**: 658-69, 1998.
4. Draper ES, Manktelow B, Field DJ, James D: Prediction of survival for preterm births by weight and gestational age: retrospective population based study. *British Medical Journal* **319**:1093-97, 1999.
5. Tin W, Wariyar U, Hey E: Changing prognosis for babies of less than 28 weeks gestation in the north of England between 1983 and 1994. *British Medical Journal* **314**: 107, 1997.
6. Leitich H, Egarter C, Kaider A, Hohlagschwandter M, Berghammer P, Husslein P: Cervicovaginal fetal fibronectin as a marker for preterm delivery: A meta-analysis. *American Journal of Obstetrics and Gynecology* **180**:1169-76, 1999.
7. Lopez RL, Francis JA, Garite TJ, Dubyak JM: Fetal fibronectin as a predictor of preterm birth in actual clinical practice. *American Journal of Obstetrics and Gynecology* **182**:1103-06, 2000.
8. Leitich H, Brunbauer M, Kaider A, Egarter C, Husslein P: Cervical length and dilatation of the internal os detected by vaginal ultrasonography as markers for preterm delivery: a systematic review. *American Journal of Obstetrics and Gynecology* **181**:1465-72, 1999.
9. Crowley P: Prophylactic corticosteroids for preterm birth. *Cochrane Database of Systematic Reviews* **(2)**: CD000065, 2000.
10. Antenatal corticosteroids to prevent respiratory distress syndrome. Royal College of Obstetricians and Gynecologists (UK). *Clinical Guidelines Review* Dec. 2002.
11. Beta-agonists for the care of women in preterm labor. Royal College of Obstetricians and Gynecologists (UK). *Clinical Guidelines Review* Feb 2000.
12. Besinger RE, Moniak CW, Paskiewicz LS, Fisher SG, Tomich PG: The effect of tocolytic use in the management of symptomatic placenta previa. *American Journal of Obstetrics and Gynecology* **172**:1770-78, 1995.
13. Towers CV, Pircon RA, Heppard M: Is tocolysis safe in the management of third-trimester bleeding? *American Journal of Obstetrics and Gynecology* **180**:1572-78, 1999.
14. Kenyon SL, Taylor, DJ, Tarnow-Mordi W: Broad-spectrum antibiotics for preterm, prelabor rupture of membranes: The Oracle I randomised trial. *Lancet* **357**:979-88, 2001.
15. Kenyon SL, Taylor, DJ, Tarnow-Mordi W: Broad-spectrum antibiotics for spontaneous preterm labor: The Oracle II randomised trial. *Lancet* **57**:989-94, 2001.
16. Oei SG, Mol BWJ, de Kleine MJK, Brolman HAM: Nifedipine versus ritodrine for suppression of preterm labor; a meta-analysis. *Acta Obstet Gynecol Scand* **78**:783-88, 1999.
17. Sanchez-Ramos L, Kaunitz AM, Gaudier FL, Delke I: Efficacy of maintenance therapy after acute tocolysis: A meta-analysis. *American Journal of Obstetrics and Gynecology* **181**:484-90, 1999.
18. Hannah ME, Hannah WJ, Hewson SA, Hodnett ED, Saigal S, Willan AR: Planned cesarean section versus planned vaginal birth for breech presentation at term: randomised multicenter trial. *Lancet* **356**: 1375-83, 2000.
19. Naef RW, Allbert JR, Ross EL, Weber BM, Martin RW, Morrison JC: Prelabor rupture of membranes at 34 to 37 weeks: Aggressive versus conservative management. *American Journal of Obstetrics and Gynecology* **178**:126-30, 1998.
20. Abbasi S, Hirsch D, Davis J, Tolosa J, Stouffer N, Debbs R, Gerdes JS: Effect of single versus multiple antenatal corticosteroids on maternal and neonatal outcome. *American Journal of Obstetrics and Gynecology* **182**:1243-49, 2000.

27.
Intrauterine Growth Restriction

Muralidhar V Pai

INTRODUCTION

It was not till recently that we recognized fetal intrauterine growth restriction (IUGR) was a human phenomenon. In 1961, Warkany[1] and co-workers reported normal values for infant weights, lengths and head circumferences and defined fetal growth restriction.

The minimum fetal age beyond which survival is anticipated is not very clear as yet. But Piper et al,[2] reported that growth restricted preterm infants have increased rates of perinatal morbidity and mortality than appropriately grown preterm infants. This makes it essential that every effort be made to detect and treat IUGR.

DEFINITION

Retardation implies abnormal mental function hence the author prefers to use the term 'restriction'. Intrauterine Growth Restriction (IUGR) is the term applied to an infant whose growth velocity as a fetus was less than expected.

Definitions have been based upon birth weights below 10th percentile (Battaglia and Lubchenco[3]) or 5th percentile (Seeds[4]) for their gestational weight. Usher and McLean[5] proposed that fetal growth standards should be based upon mean values with normal limits defined by ± 2 standard deviations. This definition would limit IUGR to 3 percent of births but from a clinical standpoint, this appears to be most meaningful, because most poor outcomes are in those infants with birth weights below the 3rd percentile (Manning[6]). Moreover not all infants with birth weights less than 10th percentile are growth restricted, 25 to 60 percent of infants conventionally diagnosed to be small for gestation were in fact appropriately grown.[8]

In all of the above definitions fetuses are compared to their peer and that may not be the most appropriate way to assess a given fetus's growth velocity because not all cases of IUGR are small for dates (SFD). For instance, if the baby was "programmed" to be 4.5 kg at delivery (according to its initial growth velocity) and was only 3.7 kg it would be not be SFD compared to its peer but would be growth restricted and could be expected to have all the problems associated with IUGR. Hence, it appears appropriate to have "Programmed Weight Chart" for each fetus based on its initial growth velocity to assess its growth.

INCIDENCE

Incidence ranges from 3-7 percent of all deliveries and 12-47 percent of twins.

TYPES OF IUGR

Traditionally two types of IUGR have been described symmetrical and asymmetrical. But in reality there seems to be abnormalities ranging between these two phenotypes. A combined type of intrauterine growth restriction has also been identified by Alkalay,[9] where there may be some skeletal shortening and an associated reduction in the soft tissue mass.

Symmetrically Small Infants

These babies are perfect miniatures, in that they are correctly proportional but are small. In most cases they represent the lower end of the normal range, i.e. they are genetically determined to be small and are not, therefore, abnormal. However, some will be small because of chromosomal, infective or environmental factors that exert an influence early in pregnancy.

Asymmetrically Small Babies

These infants are long and thin at birth. They have a head size that is appropriate for gestational age but have wasted bodies. They look as though they have been starved. This is true because in most cases their size is the result of "uteroplacental insufficiency".

ETIOLOGY

Fetal growth is not thought to be linear but occurs in a stepwise progression, with the fetus undergoing periods of accelerated growth interspersed with periods of slower growth. Normal fetal growth patterns undergo three major stages. Alkalay[9] has described these as:
- Stage 1: From 4 to 20 weeks gestation is characterized by cell hyperplasia and rapid mitosis
- Stage 2: From 20 to 28 weeks gestation is characterized by cell hyperplasia and hypertrophy with declining mitosis and an increase in cell size
- Stage 3: From 28 to 40 weeks gestation is characterized by rapid increase in cell size and accumulation of fat, muscle and connective tissue.

Any growth inhibition during stage 1 will produce a fetus with fewer cells but normal cell sizes, thus presenting as symmetrical IUGR. Intrinsic factors like chromosomal anomalies and gene defects seem to cause this type (Table 27.1).

Table 27.1: Causes of symmetrical IUGR

- Genetic including constitutional, chromosomal and single gene defects
- Inborn errors of metabolism
- Congenital anomalies
- Intrauterine infections
- Substance abuse
- Cigarette smoking
- Therapeutic irradiation (accidental exposure)

Growth inhibition during stages 2 and 3 will cause a decrease in cell size and a reduction in fetal weight. There is less effect on the total number of cells and fetal head circumference and length are maintained. This presents as asymmetrical IUGR (Table 27.2) or combined type of (Table 27.3) IUGR. Uteroplacental insufficiency seems to be the major cause of asym-

Table 27.2: Causes of asymmetrical IUGR

- Chronic hypertension
- Pre-eclampsia
- Chronic renal disease
- Cyanotic heart disease
- Anemia
- Hemoglobinopathies
- Vasculopathies
- Extensive placental infarctions
- Chronic partial separation
- Placenta previa
- Abruptio placenta
- Velamentous insertion of the umbilical cord
- Circumvallate placenta
- Multiple gestations
- Altitude
- Substance abuse
- Cigarette smoking

Table 27.3: Causes of combined type of IUGR

- Substance abuse
- Cigarette smoking
- Abruptio placenta
- Infarct
- Velamentous insertion of umbilical cord
- Circumvallate placenta
- Multiple gestations

metrically small infants, which in turn is due to maternal causes like malnutrition, multiple gestation, anemia, pre-eclampsia, high altitude, smoking, vascular disease and primary placental causes like extensive placental infarctions, chronic partial separation, placenta previa.

PATHOGENESIS

A healthy placenta is the single most important factor in producing a healthy baby. The placenta, which is in fact part of the fetus, is critical for all aspects of pregnancy from implantation to delivery. The primary function of the placenta is the effective transmission of nutrient substances to the fetus. Fetal growth may be affected by changes in the maternoplacentofetal transport of nutrients, energy producing substrates and oxygen. The functional anatomy of the maternal-fetal circulation is characterized by profound hemodynamic changes in the uterine and fetal circulations in early pregnancy. The cytotrophoblast cells migrate through the decidua and into the myometrium. The media layer of the spiral artery is then invaded resulting in the destruction of the medial elastic, muscular and neural tissue and the incorporation of trophoblast cells in the vessel wall. These intravascular changes create a low resistance arteriolar vascular system, which allow a dramatic increase in blood supply to the developing fetus. There seems to be absence of invasion of media of spiral arteries in placenta of growth-restricted fetuses.

A recent study by Krebs *et al*,[10] suggested that in growth-restricted fetuses, the placenta exhibited 'reduced cytotrophoblastic proliferation, increased syncytial nuclei and poor placental blood vessel development with straight unbranched capillaries and serious impairment of placental angiogenesis'.

In the early stages of hypoxia, the fetus uses adaptive techniques such as growth reduction, decreased fetal movement and vascular redistribution to reduce its oxygen requirements, in an attempt to prevent hypoxic injury. Hypoxia is an extremely important cause of cell injury and death, with ischemic and free radical cellular damage being the most common causes. There is emerging evidence that the role of oxygen free radicals in the mechanism of fetal brain injury due to sustained hypoxia or asphyxia is significant.

A decrease in fetal activity and decrease in fetal movements that is also seen with fetuses suffering from intrauterine growth restriction is thought to be a compensatory mechanism to hypoxia.

Fetuses suffering IUGR are thought to stimulate erythropoiesis, resulting in an increase in concentration of fetal hematocrit.

As the hypoxia continues the fetus may demonstrate reduced cerebral oxidative metabolism to reduce its oxidative needs. As the fetus becomes increasingly hypoxemic, there may be a decrease in flow to other organs and a corresponding increase in fetal blood flow to the brain, heart and adrenals. This is commonly known as the *brain sparing effect*.

COMPLICATIONS

When the placenta begins to fail, its ability to supply nourishment declines before its ability to supply oxygen. Detecting failure of growth is, therefore, an early warning that the oxygen supplies to the fetus will decline in the near future.

All fetuses build up reserves of energy so that they can withstand labor. These reserves are stored as a complex sugar (glycogen) in the fetal liver. During uterine contractions the oxygen and glucose supply to the fetus is effectively shut off and the fetus survives these times by using its liver glycogen to supply energy. The fetus decreases its general need for oxygen such that its brain can use most of the available oxygen. If the fetus has no glycogen stores then the brain becomes starved of "energy" and "brain damage" in the form of cerebral palsy or major handicap will occur even without major deprivation of oxygen. If the reduction in oxygen to the brain increases, the fetus will die.

Fetuses that have little or no glycogen stores are those that are preterm and asymmetrically small. In the case of preterm infants, labor occurs before the fetus has been able to complete its stores of glycogen. In asymmetrical small infants the fetus has used its stores of glycogen to allow its brain to continue to grow. Table 27.4 lists the potential problems of symmetrical and asymmetrical small infants.

There is increased risk for perinatal asphyxia, meconium aspiration, electrolyte imbalance from

Table 27.4: Problems associated with symmetrical and asymmetrical IUGR

Problems associated with symmetrical IURG
- Chromosomal anomaly
- Intrauterine viral infection
- Reduced intellect and learning difficult
- Short stature
- Increased incidence of death in the first year

Problems associated with asymmetrical IUGR
- Stillbirth
- Antenatal and/or perinatal asphyxia, leading to cerebral palsy
- Hypoglycemia
- Hypocalcemia
- Polycythemia
- Necrotizing enterocolitis
- Neonatal pulmonary hemorrhage
- Preterm delivery

metabolic acidosis and polycythemia. Fetuses who suffer from IUGR are known to have more adverse perinatal outcomes than fetuses of normal growth. There is 6 to 8 folds increase in intrapartum and neonatal deaths. Delays in neonatal growth, behavioral and cognitive development have also been identified.

SCREENING AND IDENTIFICATION OF IUGR

Unfortunately there are no available data on which to base decisions concerning the number of examinations needed and the menstrual ages at which such examinations should be made. However, since IUGR has been detected as early as 17 weeks, an initial examination in the second trimester would seem appropriate. For high risk (Table 27.5) patients, a reasonable procedure would be to date the pregnancy at 10 to 12 weeks, then evaluate growth at 3-week internals between 28 weeks and delivery. If abnor-

Table 27.5: Women at particularly high risk for IUGR

- Maternal weight less than 10th percentile for height (or under 40 kg as rough guide)
- Previous infants with IUGR
- Maternal vascular diseases
  - Essential hypertension
  - Pre-eclampsia
  - Diabetes mellitus
  - Collagen disorder
- Maternal cardiac disease
- Heavy smokers
- Alcoholics and drug addicts
- Women with sickle cell disease
- Women with recurrent APH
- Women with a raised MSAFP but a structurally normal fetus

malities are seen, the interval between examinations should be shortened but due to measurement errors and growth rates, intervals of less than 2 weeks are not likely to give reliable data.

It is clear from the studies of newborn infants that IUGR can manifest as a decrease in weight, length, head, chest, abdominal circumference, subcutaneous tissue and muscle mass, singly or in various combinations. For this reason, evaluation of a growth profile would be required if IUGR in all its form was to be detected.

The assessment of fetal growth requires an accurate knowledge of the menstrual age of the fetus. Before the introduction of obstetric ultrasound, the determination of the menstrual age of the fetus was established by the patient's medical history, hopefully confirmed by the fundal height assessment during pregnancy, and reviewed in the postnatal period by a physical examination of the neonate. These parameters are variably inaccurate.

The assessment of ultrasound estimated fetal weight is most useful when applied to growth charts that reflect 'normal' fetal growth. It is advisable that each center has its own growth charts that are based on their patient population. Figures 27.1 to 27.6 demonstrate the charts used at Katurba Medical College Hospital, Manipal. Serial fetal growth assessments are used to evaluate the rate of fetal growth and to assess the degree of any growth restriction.

Fetal morphometric ratios like HC/AC and AC/FL allow the assessment of body proportionality, which may be abnormal in some growth, restricted fetuses. HC/AC ratio has been shown to be useful in differentiating "symmetric" and "asymmetric" IUGR.

Unfortunately these methods are unable to account for the constitutionally small but otherwise healthy fetus.

One method currently under investigation is the use of "ideal fetal weight" predictions. Rossavik[11] pioneered the technique in 1986 and uses individual growth curves for a particular fetus, based a mathematical model of biological growth. Ott et al,[12] used Rossavik's technique to assess for fetal growth restriction and found that fetuses with growth restriction were 51 percent lighter than their predicted ideal weight.

Intrauterine Growth Restriction

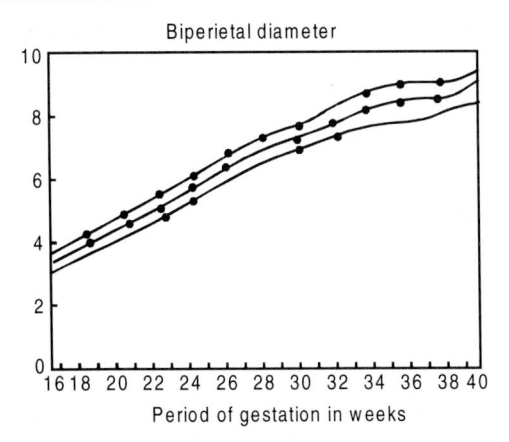

Figure 27.1: Normogram for biparietal diameter

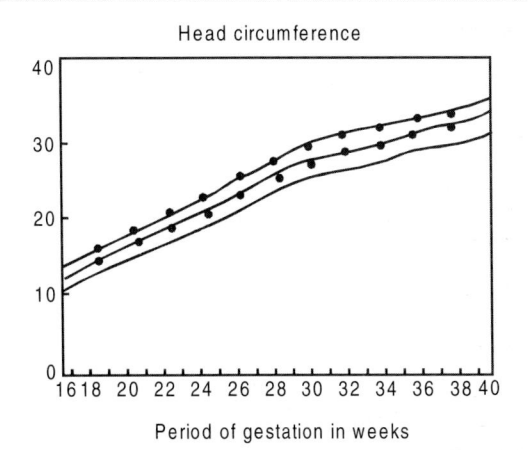

Figure 27.2: Normogram for head circumference

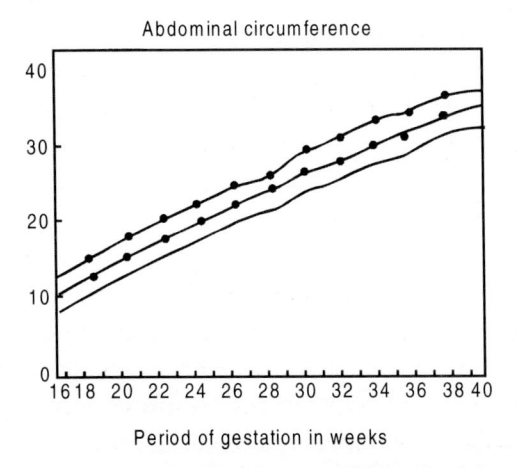

Figure 27.3: Normogram for abdominal circumference

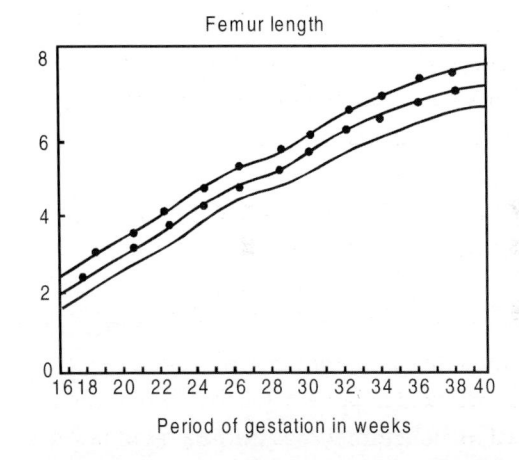

Figure 27.4: Normogram for femur length

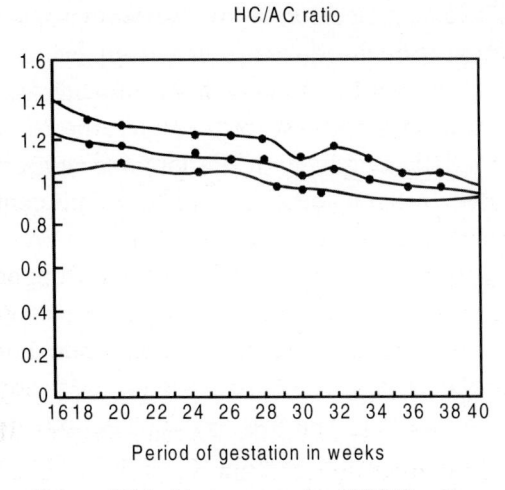

Figure 27.5: Normogram for HC/AC ratio

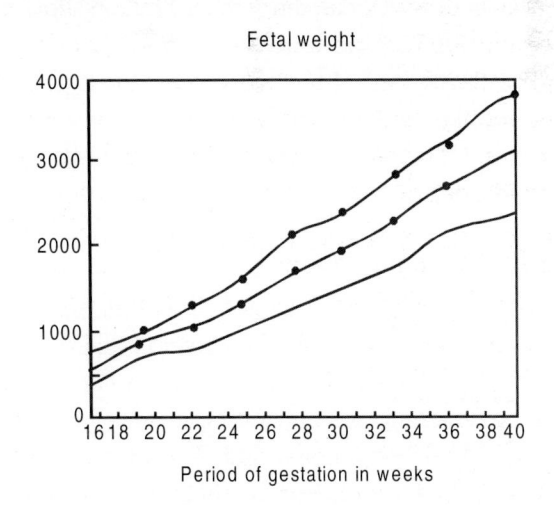

Figure 27.6: Normogram for estimated fetal weight

Other studies to assess for fetal growth restriction have used the assessment of subcutaneous adipose tissue and other soft tissues like cheek to cheek diameters, thickness of the calf, thigh or abdominal wall, and estimations of liver size, volume and weight. There appears to be some clinical utility in these parameters. However, further research in this area is needed to determine their usefulness.

The introduction of realtime ultrasound allowed the accurate monitoring of not only biometric data but also fetal biophysical activities. Introduction of Doppler allowed assessment of blood flow in the umbilical artery followed by various vessels in the fetus.

Fleischer et al[13] found that the umbilical artery systolic/diastolic ratios were significantly higher for babies below the twenty-fifth percentile, than for larger babies. Gramellini et al,[14] 1992, have reported the use of the cerebral-umbilical Doppler ratio as having a high sensitivity and specificity for fetal flow redistribution in the presence of intrauterine growth restriction.

A prospective study on placental laterality done at Kasturba Medical College Hospital Manipal[15] showed that the finding of unilateral placenta by real time ultrasonography may herald the development of PIH and IUGR hence may be used as predictive screening test. Another prospective study[16] on uterine artery resistance conducted at the same institution showed that pregnancies with abnormal outcome, pre-eclampsia and/or IUGR, are characterized by: (a) low diastolic flow, (b) high resistance index which persists throughout the pregnancy, (c) presence of diastolic notch in the uterine artery.

Newer Screening Tools

Tongsong T et al[17] have suggested that the sonographic fetal Transverse Cerebellar Diameter (TCD)/AC ratio as a gestational age-independent method can be helpful in antenatal diagnosis of IUGR, especially in pregnancy with uncertain gestational age. The best cut-off value of the TCD/AC ratio for predicting IUGR was 15.4 percent, Sattar N et al[18] have proposed, that low LDL-cholesterol in the third trimester may be of use in identifying mothers with, or at risk of, a pregnancy complicated by IUGR. Rondó et al[19] found that higher maternal levels of ferritin (>50 micrograms/L) were more common in IUGR than in AGA mothers ($P < 0.001$).

Anticardiolipin antibodies (ACA) could be one of the causes of IUGR. According to Wang Z et al[20] determination of serum ACA would offer a new clue to diagnosis and treatment of IUGR.

MANAGEMENT

The role of antenatal testing has been traditionally considered to aid the obstetrician in managing the pregnancy to enable an optimal outcome, if possible, for both mother and baby.

As there is no specific treatment to improve the placental function, the following have been tried with variable success alone or in combination; bed rest in left lateral position, early antiplatelet therapy with low-dose aspirin, correction of malnutrition and balanced diet.

Lampariello et al,[21] have found positive results with use of L-arginine. This amino acid improves GH-RH secretion, with consequent increase of plasma GH influencing somatic growth. L-arginine is the obligatory precursor for nitric oxide (NO) enzymatic synthesis. NO helps the relaxation of smooth muscle and, consequently improves placental blood circulation. The need for treatment of specific obstetric complication cannot be over emphasized.

The crucial decision in the management of IUGR is the timing of the delivery. When an IUGR fetus is diagnosed prior to 34 weeks, if the amniotic fluid index and fetal wellbeing tests are normal, one can wait to achieve fetal lung maturity. Prompt delivery is likely to afford the best outcome for the fetus that is considered growth restricted at or near term. In the presence of severe oligohydramnios and abnormal Doppler parameters, delivery may be contemplated earlier than term. The baby might do well outside than inside the uterus. Cesarean section may be considered for severe IUGR with or with out abnormal cardiotocography and fetal distress. If cardiotocography is normal, labor may be induced with low rupture of membranes followed by oxytocin.

Throughout the labor, whether spontaneous or induced, fetuses should be closely monitored for evidence of fetal distress. It can be anticipated that the infant may need expert neonatal assistance after birth.

Intrauterine Origins of Adult Disease

Barker's Hypothesis[22]

Based on data available from British cohort studies, *in utero* malnutrition could also result in an increased risk of cardiovascular, endocrine and metabolic diseases in adulthood. Underweight infants at 1 year of age had 3 times the risk of premature death (in their fifties and early sixties) from coronary artery disease compared with infants of normal weight.

Fetal Growth Restriction in Subsequent Pregnancies

The risk of recurrent fetal growth restriction is increased in pregnant women who have previously had this complication.[23] This is particularly true in women with a history of fetal growth restriction and a continuing medical complication.[24]

REFERENCES

1. Warkany JB, Monroe Sutherland BSS: Intrauterine Growth Retardation. *Am J Dis Child* **102**:24, 961.
2. Piper JM, Xenakis EMJ, Mcfarland M, Elliot BD, Berkens MD, Langer O: Do growth retarded prmature infants have different rates of perinatal morbidity and mortality than appropriate-grown preterm infants? *Obstet Gynecol* **87**: 169, 1996.
3. Battaglia FC, Lubchenco LO: A practical classification of newborn infants by weight and gestational age. *J Pediatr* **71**:159, 1967.
4. Seeds JW: Impaired fetal growth: Definition and clinical diagnosis. *Obstet Gynecol* **64**:303, 1984.
5. Usher R, McLean: Intrauterine growth of live Caucasian infants at sea level: standards obtained from measurements in 7 dimensions of infants born between 25 and 44 weeks gestation. *J Pediatr* **74**:901, 1969.
6. Manning FA: Intrauterine growth retardation. In *Fetal Medicine. Principles and Practice.* Norwalk, CT, Appleton and Lange, 317, 1995.
7. Manning FA, Hohler C: Intrauterine growth retardation: diagnosis, prognostication and management based on ultrasound methods. In Fleisher AC, Romero R, Manning FA, Jeanty P, James AE (Eds): *The Principles and Practices of Ultrasonography in Obstetrics and Gynecology,* 4th ed. Norwalk, CT, Appleton and Lange, 331, 1991.
8. Gardosi J, Chang A, Kalyan B, Sahota D, Symonds EM: Customized antenatal growth charts. *Lancet* **339**:283,1992.
9. Alkalay AL, Graham JM Jr, Pomerance JJ: Evaluation of neonates born with intrauterine growth retardation: review and practice guidelines. *J Perinatol* **18(2)**:142-51 (Review), 1998.
10. Krebs C, Macara LM, Leisure R, Bowman AW, Greer IA, Kingdom JC: Intrauterine growth restriction with absent end-diastolic flow velocity in the umbilical artery is associated with maldevelopment of the placental terminal villous tree. *Am J Obstet Gynecol* **175(6)**:1534-42, 1996.
11. Rossavik IK, Torjusen GO, Deter RL, Reiter AA: Efficacy of mathematical methods for ultrasound examinations in diabetic pregnancies. *Am J Obstet Gynecol* **155(3)**:638-44, 1986.
12. Ott WJ: The diagnosis of altered fetal growth.*Obstet Gynecol Clin North Am* **15(2)**:237-63 (Review), 1988.
13. Fleisher A, Guidetti D, Stuhlmuller P: Umbilical artery velocity waveforms in the intrauterine growth retarded fetus. *Clin Obstet Gynecol* **32(4)**:660-08 (Review), 1989.
14. Gramellini D, Folli MC, Raboni S, vadora E, Merialdi A: Cerebral-umbilical Doppler ratio as a predictor of adverse perinatal outcome. *Obstet Gynecol* **79(3)**:416-20, 1992.
15. Muralidhar V Pai, Rebecca Lama: Placental location and pre-eclampsia–what is the connection? *Obs and Gyne Today* **6(4)**:2001.
16. Muralidhar V Pai and Jyoti Sachdev: Improved prediction of PIH and IUGR by 2 stage screening of uterine artery Doppler velocimetry. *Indian Journal of Ultrasound,* June-July, 2001.
17. Tongsong T, Wanapirak C, Thongpadungroj T: Sonographic diagnosis of intrauterine growth restriction (IUGR) by fetal transverse cerebellar diameter (TCD)/abdominal circumference (AC) ratio. *Int J Gynecol Obstet* **66**:1 1-15, 1999.
18. Sattar N, Greer IA, Galloway PJ, Packard CJ, Shepherd J, Kelly T, Mathers A: Lipid and lipoprotein concentrations in pregnancies complicated by intrauterine growth restriction. *J Clin Endocrinol Metab* **84(1)**:128-30, 1999.
19. Rondo PH, Tomkins AM: Maternal iron status and intrauterine growth retardation. *Trans R Soc Trop Med Hyg* **93(4)**:423-26, 1999.
20. Wang Z, Fan Y, Wu G: Relation between fetal intrauterine growth retardation and anticardiolipin antibodies. *Chung Hua Fu Chan Ko Tsa Chih* **32(10)**:623-25, 1997.
21. Lampariello C, De Blasio A, Merenda A, Graziano E, Michalopoulou A, Bruno P: Use of arginine in intrauterine growth retardation (IUGR). Authors' experience. *Minerva Ginecol* **49(12)**: 577-81, 1997.
22. Barker DJ: The long-term outcome of retarded fetal growth. *Schweiz Med Wochenschr* **6; 129(5)**:189-96 (Review), 1999.
23. Bakketeig LS, Bjerkedal T, Hoffman HJ: Small for gestational age births in successive pregnancy outcomes: results from a longitudinal study of births in Norway. *Early Hum Dev* **14**:187, 1986.
24. Patterson RM, Gibbs CE, Wood RC: Birth weight percentile and perinatal outcome: Recurrence of intrauterine growth retardation. *Obstet Gynecol* **68**:464, 1986.

28. Prolonged Pregnancy

Matthews Mathai
B Subhasri

INTRODUCTION

This chapter deals with the common problem of prolonged pregnancy and will familiarize the readers with the definition and epidemiology of prolonged pregnancy. The risks associated with this condition and the controversies in the management of prolonged pregnancy are also discussed.

Prolonged pregnancy is a common clinical problem today. It is associated with significant increase in perinatal morbidity and mortality and is therefore a common indication for induction of labor.

DEFINITION

Several terms are used, often interchangeably, to describe prolonged pregnancy. Post-dates, post-term and post-maturity are some commonly used terms. None of these terms however is clearly defined and a better option is "prolonged pregnancy". The World Health Organization and the International Federation of Gynecology and Obstetrics (FIGO) define prolonged pregnancy as a pregnancy that has completed 42 weeks or 294 days, as calculated from the first day of the last menstrual period. However, the American College of Obstetrics and Gynecology defines prolonged pregnancy as a pregnancy which has gone two weeks beyond the expected date of delivery.

The term "post-mature" should be restricted to the description of a neonate who has clinical features of pathologically prolonged pregnancy. These features include wrinkled, peeling skin, little lanugo hair, overgrown nails, well developed palmar and plantar creases, decreased subcutaneous fat and an alert wizened old man appearance.

INCIDENCE

The reported incidence varies greatly but is generally reported to be between 4 and 14 percent with an average of 10 percent. Several factors influence the incidence of prolonged pregnancy. Reliability of menstrual data is crucial. Where menstrual data are not reliable, the incidence of prolonged pregnancy and interventions for this condition are likely to be high. The routine use of ultrasound for confirmation of dates in early pregnancy reduces the number of inductions for suspected prolonged pregnancy.

The definition of prolonged pregnancy used may vary and therefore the incidence of this condition. There are variations in duration of pregnancy among various ethnic groups.

For example, in a cohort of Indian women whose dates had been confirmed by ultrasound scans in early pregnancy, the median gestation at delivery was the 39th week. In contrast the median gestation at delivery reported from Britain is the 41st week.[1] It is possible therefore that most babies in India are born before the 42nd week resulting in a lower incidence of prolonged pregnancy as defined earlier.

Lastly, management policies and practices vary. For example, a policy of routine induction of labor beyond a specific length of gestation, say 41 weeks, will necessarily result in reduction in the incidence of prolonged pregnancy. It is unlikely therefore that the true incidence of prolonged pregnancy will be known.

PROBLEMS ASSOCIATED WITH PROLONGED PREGNANCY

Prolonged pregnancy is reportedly associated with increased risks for both the baby and the mother. The risk of occurrence of stillbirth increases with gestational age when this risk is expressed as the number of stillbirths per 1000 fetuses undelivered at the beginning of each week of gestation. For example, data from Vellore in 1993 showed that the risks of stillbirth per 1000 fetuses undelivered at 37 weeks, 39 weeks and 41 weeks were 1.35, 2.1 and 5.6 respectively (unpublished data).

Placental function may fail in prolonged pregnancy. Failing placental perfusion may result in reduced renal perfusion and oligohydramnios. Reduced amniotic fluid volume and the resultant cord compression are associated with fetal heart rate decelerations. Late and prolonged decelerations and fetal death may also occur in some of these cases.

Meconium passage occurs in late pregnancy and is considered to reflect increasing fetal maturity. The occurrence of meconium stained liquor at amniotomy as a proportion of 1000 undelivered fetuses in Vellore increased from 19 at the beginning of 37 weeks to 88.9 at the beginning of 41 weeks (unpublished data). Furthermore in prolonged pregnancy, meconium passed remains largely undiluted because of the reduction in amniotic fluid volume. The risk of meconium aspiration is increased under these circumstances.

On the other hand, the fetus can continue to grow *in utero* even after 40 weeks. This may result in fetal macrosomia. Macrosomia is associated with increased risk of birth trauma. After exclusion of congenital malformations, the reported increases in perinatal mortality and morbidity in prolonged pregnancy are due largely to asphyxia and less often to birth trauma.

Prolonged pregnancy causes increased anxiety to the mother and her family. However, most problems for the mother because of prolonged pregnancy are related to therapeutic interventions. Induction of labor is commonly practised as an option in the management of prolonged pregnancy. Failed induction may occur in some of these cases. Cesarean delivery may also be required for fetal distress in labor. The occurrence of cesarean delivery for fetal distress for every 1000 undelivered fetuses in Vellore rose from 8.3 at the beginning of 37 weeks to 34.5 at the beginning of 41 weeks (unpublished data). Operative delivery and anesthesia increase the risk to the mother. Delivery of a macrosomic baby can also result in increased maternal trauma.

PREDICTORS OF PROLONGED PREGNANCY

Several factors determine the length of gestation. However, none of these has been conclusively proven to cause prolonged pregnancy. A woman who has had a prior pregnancy that was prolonged is likely to have another prolonged pregnancy. If the woman's mother had a prolonged pregnancy, she may have a slightly higher risk than the general population. Increasing maternal age and parity may be associated with prolonged pregnancy. Among fetal factors, anomalies like anencephaly especially in the absence of polyhydramnios, and adrenal hypoplasia result in prolonged pregnancies.

PRINCIPLES OF MANAGEMENT

Confirmation of Length of Pregnancy

Confirmation of the length of gestation as early as possible in pregnancy should be part of routine antenatal care. Determination of uterine size by clinical examination is more reliable in early pregnancy than in late pregnancy. Ultrasound confirmation of dates can be done when the menstrual history is unreliable. Routine ultrasound in early pregnancy reduces the number of inductions for prolonged pregnancy (Odds ratio 0.68; 95 % CI 0.57-0.82).[2] However, ultrasound in late pregnancy cannot be used reliably for confirming dates.

To Deliver or not to Deliver

Given the presumed increase in perinatal morbidity and mortality associated with prolonged pregnancies on the one hand and the presumed increase in maternal morbidity related to interventions for prolonged pregnancy on the other, there are two options in the management of this condition: induction of labor at a specified period of gestation or expectant management with close monitoring of fetal wellbeing.

Under the first option, labor is induced usually at or beyond 41 weeks of gestation. Pre-induction ripening of the cervix with prostaglandins will increase the number of successful inductions. However, failed induction may still occur. Cesarean deliveries for failed induction (and for any other indication) increase risk to the mother.

In the second option, fetal wellbeing is closely monitored. Methods of monitoring used include fetal movement counts, (non-stress) cardiotocography, assessment of biophysical profile and Doppler flow velocimetry of fetal vessels. Cardiotocography and liquor volume estimation are perhaps the most commonly used methods for fetal assessment in prolonged pregnancy. Most tests for fetal wellbeing have high negative predictive values, i.e. when the test result indicates that the fetus is well, the chance that it is indeed well is high. On the other hand, the positive predictive values for most tests of fetal wellbeing are low. Thus, if a test result indicates that the fetus is not well, the chances that it is indeed sick are not high. Interventions for fetal ill health are more likely in these situations. However, there are reports of fetal demise in prolonged pregnancy occurring within a short while of a "normal" test suggesting that one cannot entirely rely on these tests for successful outcomes.

Several studies have compared labor induction with expectant management using antepartum fetal testing in the management of prolonged pregnancy. The Canadian multicenter trial[3] randomized 3407 women with uncomplicated pregnancies at 41 weeks or more to either labor induction or expectant management with antepartum fetal testing. Tests included fetal movement counts, and thrice weekly non-stress tests and assessments of amniotic fluid volume. Women in the latter arm were delivered if the test results showed evidence of fetal compromise.

Among the 1701 women in the induction group, 360 (21.2%) underwent cesarean section compared to 418 (24.5%) of the 1706 women in the expectant management group. This statistically significant difference in cesarean section rate resulted from a significantly lower rate of cesarean section performed because of fetal distress in the induction group (5.7%) compared to the expectant management group (8.3%). There were two stillbirths in the expectant management group and none in the induction group. There was no difference in the neonatal morbidity between the two groups.

The National Institute of Child Health and Human Development Network of Maternal-Fetal Medicine Units embarked on a multicenter study[4] to compare induction of labor versus expectant management in prolonged pregnancy. The target number of subjects for the study was estimated to be 2800. However at the end of 18 months, only 440 women had been recruited and the trial was stopped. Analyses of data from these women showed that the adverse perinatal outcomes in both the groups were comparable. The researchers concluded from these data that either management scheme is acceptable.

When the overall perinatal mortality rates are low, a trial to detect differences in mortality would require very large numbers of subjects. This is not feasible. However results of several small to medium sized trials can be pooled together and a meta-analysis performed. Results of meta-analysis of data suggest that induction of labor at 41 weeks when compared to expectant management of prolonged pregnancy is associated with lower risk of perinatal mortality (Odds ratio 0.2, 95% CI 0.06-0.70).[2]

Thus a policy of induction of labor at 41 weeks and beyond is associated with lower cesarean section rate and lower perinatal mortality. When the costs of tests of fetal wellbeing are also included, induction of labor becomes a more cost-effective option in the management of prolonged pregnancy.

Preparing the Cervix for Induction

Successful induction of labor depends on parity and the pre-induction cervical score. The risk of failed induction for a nullipara with a cervical score of less than 3 is almost 50 percent. Ripening the cervix before induction of labor can significantly reduce this risk.

Prostaglandins have been used successfully in softening the unripe cervix and making easy induction possible. Commercially available preparations of prostaglandins for induction of labor are sensitive to tropical climate and expensive. Misoprostol, a prostaglandin E_1 analogue has been used successfully in many trials for induction of labor. This preparation is stable in tropical climate and is less expensive. However, the optimum dose of this drug and the frequency and route of administration are still under study. Until reports on the safety of this drug are available from larger studies, it should be used only in the context of well designed clinical trials.

The Foley's catheter inserted through the cervix and placed in the extra-amniotic space has also been used successfully for ripening the cervix. This may be considered in situations where prostaglandins are not available for cervical ripening.

Stripping/Sweeping the Membranes

Another non-pharmacological method that has been used to reduce the rate of prolonged pregnancy is stripping/sweeping of membranes at term. A meta-analysis of trials on the efficacy of this intervention found that stripping/sweeping of membranes as a general policy at term reduced the duration of pregnancy.[5] The frequency of pregnancy continuing beyond 41 weeks was reduced by more than half. After stripping/sweeping of the membranes, there was a reduction by 17 percent in the use of more formal methods for labor induction.

There was no difference in the mode of delivery or in the risk of infection. Discomfort during vaginal examination and other adverse effects (bleeding, irregular contractions) were more frequently reported by women allocated to stripping.

Monitoring in Labor

The fetus is at high risk during labor when pregnancy is prolonged. This is because of the associated oligohydramnios and meconium stained amniotic fluid. Any woman with prolonged pregnancy who comes in labor should be considered for continuous electronic fetal monitoring if this facility is available.

Amnioinfusion with normal saline should be considered if there is meconium stained liquor in early labor and fetal heart rate patterns do not warrant immediate delivery. Monitor progress in labor using the partograph. Fetal macrosomia may be associated with poor progress in labor and shoulder dystocia. The baby may be asphyxiated, may suffer from birth trauma or other neonatal problems. Arrange for appropriate care of the baby in the immediate newborn period.

OUR PRACTICE

During the first visit to the antenatal clinic, we attempt to confirm gestational age. Where the gestational age is unsure, an ultrasound scan is done to estimate gestation. Women often ask when they should expect to have the baby. Most babies are not born on the estimated date of confinement. The only assurance we give is that if all is well, the woman will not remain undelivered beyond a week after the estimated date of confinement.

If there is no other fetal or maternal problem, we carry out stripping/sweeping of the membranes in the 40th week. An appointment is then made for the woman to get admitted for induction toward the end of the 41st week of pregnancy if she is still undelivered.

We do a pre-induction assessment of the fetus by non-stress cardiotocography. If the non-stress test is reactive, a pelvic examination is carried out to assess the cervix. If the cervix is less than 2 cm long and less than 2 cm dilated, we use prostaglandin E_2 gel to ripen the cervix. Twelve hours later, amniotomy is done and is followed by oxytocin infusion.

The progress of labor is monitored closely using a partograph. We use continuous electronic fetal monitoring if fetal heart rate abnormalities are noted on intermittent auscultation and when liquor is meconium stained. In the absence of fetal heart rate abnormalities that warrant immediate delivery, we use amnioinfusion whenever there is meconium stained liquor. We also carry out oropharyngeal suction as soon as the head is born. Failed induction and perinatal deaths in prolonged pregnancy are now rare events.

PRACTICE POINTS

Prolonged pregnancy is associated with an increase in the incidence of perinatal morbidity and mortality.

While managing this condition, aim to prevent perinatal morbidity and mortality by either elective induction of labor or expectant management with close monitoring of fetal wellbeing. Elective induction of labor at 41 weeks is associated with a better maternal and fetal outcome and is cost effective.

Cervical ripening agents reduce the risks of failed induction.

Stripping/sweeping of the membranes at term reduces the incidence of prolonged pregnancy.

Labor in a woman with prolonged pregnancy needs close monitoring of the fetal condition. Amnioinfusion should be administered in the presence of meconium in the amniotic fluid, if urgent delivery is not warranted.

REFERENCES

1. Mathai M, Thomas S, Peedicayil A, Regi A, Jasper P, Joseph R: Growth pattern of the Indian fetus. *Int J Gynecol Obstet* **48:** 21-24, 1995.
2. Crowley P: Interventions for preventing or improving the outcome of delivering at or beyond term. (Cochrane review) In: The Cochrane Library, Issue 2. Oxford: Update Software, 2000.
3. Hannah ME, Hannah WJ, Hellmann J, Hewson S, Milner R, Willan A: Induction of labor as compared with serial antenatal monitoring in post-term pregnancy. A randomized control trial. *N Engl J Med* **326:** 1587-92, 1992.
4. The National Institute of Child Health and Human Development Network of Maternal-fetal Medicine Units. A clinical trial of induction of labor versus expectant management in postterm pregnancy. *Am J Obstet Gynecol* **17:** 716-23, 1994.
5. Boulvain M, Irion O: Stripping/sweeping the membranes for inducing labor or preventing post-term pregnancy (Cochrane review). In: The Cochrane Library, Issue 2. Oxford: Update Software, 2000.

29. Thalassemia and Rhesus Isoimmunization

Jamiyah Hassan
Sofiah Sulaiman

INTRODUCTION

Hemoglobinopathy is one of the most common causes of anemia in certain parts of the world like Mediterranean countries, Middle East, Africa and southern Asia. In countries where there is a high rate of immigrants like the United Kingdom this is a common health problem. In some of these countries pre-marital screening has been incorporated into the medical services in order to reduce the medical cost of managing such problems.

The thalassemia syndromes are the most common group of hemoglobinopathies. These genetic disorders are inherited defects of hemoglobin as a result of globin synthesis. The presentation can be varied and even undetected in mild forms and will be unmasked during pregnancy. They usually present with various degrees of anemia.

The syndromes are divided into two main groups, the alpha and the beta thalassemias depending on whether the alpha or beta chain synthesis of adult hemoglobin is depressed, viz.:
  i. Alpha thalassemia where one to four of the alpha genes are deleted.
  ii. Beta thalassemia where one to two of the beta genes are deleted.

NORMAL HEMOGLOBIN

It is important to understand the normal structure of hemoglobin (Figure 29.1) so that one is able to identify the problems that can occur in a pregnancy where the couple is affected by this genetic disorder. The normal hemoglobin has four globin chains each of which is associated with a heme complex. Each globin chain is controlled by a separate gene. In humans there are three normal hemoglobins, namely HbA, HbA_2 and HbF and each of these consists of two pairs of globin chains. There are four globin chains; alpha (α), beta (β), gamma (γ) and delta (δ). HbA constitutes 95 percent of the total adult circulating hemoglobin and it contains a pair each of α and β chains. α chain is common to all three hemoglobins and it is controlled by four genes with two genes inherited from each parent. Whereas the beta chain is controlled by two genes and one gene is inherited from each parent.

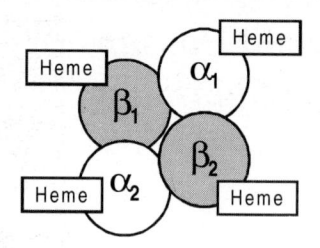

Figure 29.1: Normal hemoglobin

ALPHA THALASSEMIA

The alpha genes play a very important role in the genetic make-up of the normal circulating adult hemoglobin. In the normal individuals they have four functional alpha genes. Therefore, the absence of either one or all of the alpha genes will result in varying degrees of anemia. In alpha thalassemia trait there will be either three normal alpha genes (a$^+$) or two normal alpha genes (a°). In this group of individuals they are usually asymptomatic or may present with mild anemia. HbH disease or an intermediate form of alpha thalassemia has only one normal alpha gene. These individuals usually present with moderate anemia and may require blood transfusions. Alpha thalassemia major has no functional alpha genes and this will result in no alpha chain synthesis. Therefore, the fetal hemoglobin (HbF $\alpha_2\delta_2$) will form together with tetramers of γ chains which are known as hemoglobin Barts (γ_4) (Figure 29.2). This condition will lead to severe anemia. This condition is incompatible with life and the pregnancy usually ends prematurely in a hydrops.

Investigations

Full blood count is usually carried out in suspected cases. In alpha thalassemia there is no abnormal hemoglobin being made. The common findings include smaller red cells (low MCV) and a reduced individual cell content of hemoglobin (low MCH). They usually have a normal mean cell hemoglobin cell concentration (normal MCHC) unlike iron deficiency anemia. Confirmatory diagnosis can be made by globin chain synthesis studies or DNA analysis of nucleated cells in the case of gene deletion.

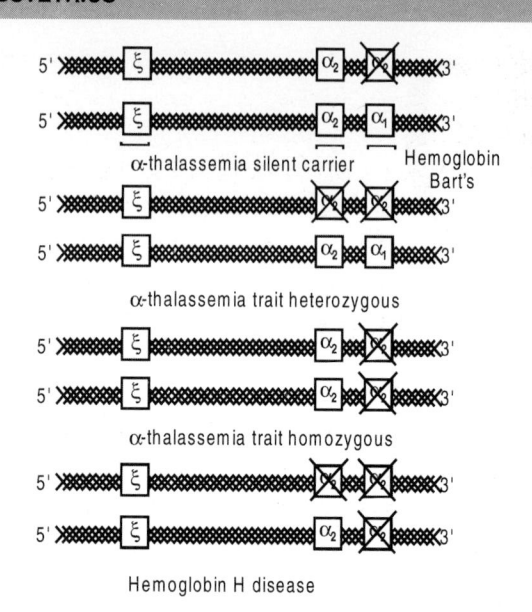

Figure 29.2: Different forms of alpha-thalassemia

Management

The demands of pregnancy can lead to anemia and in women with alpha thalassemia trait, oral iron and folate supplements can be given throughout the antenatal period. However, parenteral iron is contraindicated. In HbH disease or thalassemia intermedia they usually will present with moderate anemia. Their iron contents are usually normal but iron supplements can be given if the serum iron is low. They will however need oral folate supplements throughout pregnancy. Blood transfusion is indicated if the hemoglobin level is inadequate.

In alpha thalassemia the status of the partner should be identified prenatally because of the possibility of carrying a fetus with hemoglobin Barts (γ_4). These pregnancies will result in a hydropic fetus and can be associated with severe pre-eclampsia in the mother. In these cases, termination of pregnancy should be offered.

BETA THALASSEMIA

Beta thalassemia can be divided into beta thalassemia trait or major (homozygous). In beta thalassemia trait the individuals are usually asymptomatic. They commonly present later than two years of age with mild clinical picture of anemia. The hemoglobin value may be between 7 to 10 gram percent.

Homozygous thalassemia or thalassemia major is when the individual inherited a defective beta globin gene from each parent. This condition is usually fatal within a few years of life without regular transfusions. They require hypertransfusion regime (i.e. maintaining the hemoglobin level at 12 g%) to treat the anemia which is caused by enhanced red blood cell destruction. Hypertransfusion regime has been shown to reduce the anemia's morbidity and add up to a marked improvement in the quality of life. These repeated transfusions may cause iron overload resulting in hepatic, endocrine and cardiac dysfunction. Sometimes survival is possible without regular transfusion but this usually results in severe bone deformities due to massive expansion of marrow tissue. Pregnancy is very rare in women with beta thalassemia major but is more likely in those with less iron overload.

Management

In beta thalassemia trait the women may develop anemia during the antenatal period. As in alpha thalassemia, the indices in full blood count reveal low MCV and MCH with a normal MCHC. The diagnosis can be confirmed by finding a raised concentration of HbA_2 ($\alpha_2\beta_2$) and HbF ($\alpha_2\delta_2$) as there are excess alpha chains combined with either delta or gamma chains. They will require the usual oral iron and folate supplements in the antenatal period. Oral iron for a limited period will not result in significant iron loading, even in the presence of replete iron stores but parenteral iron should never be given. Transfusion is indicated to achieve adequate hemoglobin in preparation for delivery at term.

Pregnancy is a rare occurrence in women with beta thalassemia major. However, with the advances in medical technology this may not be a rarity in the future. In this group of women extrafolate supplements should be given daily but iron in any form is contraindicated. Anemia should be treated with transfusion during the antenatal period. Complete iron overload depletion may be achieved with phlebotomies or 6 to 12 monthly treatment with desferrioxamine.

The only radical cure for thalassemia is to correct the genetic defect by bone marrow transplantation.

Prenatal Diagnosis

When both parents are affected, they should be counseled and offered prenatal diagnosis. The options available include chorionic villous or fetal blood sampling and amniocentesis. At the moment the screening procedures for carrier status are often not carried out on the couple until women are pregnant. This means that early prenatal diagnosis by DNA analysis of a chorion biopsy is not possible in most cases.

Chorionic Villous Sampling

This is the method of choice for fetal diagnosis of hemoglobinopathies. The fetal loss rate is less than 2 percent which compares favorably with other methods used in prenatal diagnosis. However, limb reductions associated with this technique continue to give some cause of concern. This had been described in association with chorionic villous sampling done in a pregnancy of less than 10 weeks gestation and hence such a procedure should be advised after that gestation. It is thought to have a vascular etiology related to either decreased fetal perfusion or thrombosis of the sampling site.

Fetal Blood Sampling

The fetal blood would be obtained from the fetal umbilical cord by an ultrasound guided needle which is introduced through the maternal abdominal wall. This technique which is also called cordocentesis or percutaneous umbilical blood sampling usually targets the umbilical vein at the insertion of the cord into the placenta. Other sites which can be used include the intra-abdominal umbilical vein, free loop of cord and the fetal heart. Fetal blood sampling carries a risk of fetal loss of 1 to 3 percent. Nowadays, with better equipment and expertise, it has now largely been superseded by other methods which can be done at earlier gestational age with a lower risk of fetal loss.

Amniotic Fluid Fibroblast

Amniocentesis is safer than fetal blood sampling and possibly safer than chorionic villous sampling. The usage of this technique is made possible by the possibility of amplification of DNA using the Polymerase Chain Reaction (PCR) techniques. The PCR technique allows rapid results without the need of lengthy culturing procedures. However, the PCR technique is not widely available and it is also expensive.

RHESUS ISOIMMUNIZATION

Rhesus factor is a protein on the surface of red blood cells and 15 percent of women in South East Asia are rhesus negative. Rhesus negative mothers who have become sensitized to the D antigen with a rhesus positive fetus develop anti-D antibodies. This can cross the placenta and attack the blood of rhesus positive fetuses in subsequent pregnancies. This will lead to destruction and removal of rhesus positive fetal red blood cells in maternal and fetal circulations. This condition is usually referred to as rhesus isoimmunization; this remains a relatively less common cause of perinatal mortality and morbidity and the general outlook of a rhesus isoimmunized pregnancy is quite optimistic today as newer approaches to diagnosis and treatment have evolved.

The sensitization may occur by blood transfusion, abortion, fetal rhesus positive cells crossing the placenta during invasive procedures, for example amniocentesis, antepartum hemorrhage, external cephalic version or even delivery.

The most common rhesus antigen is D; others such as antigen C, E, c and e, can also produce similar disease. For the child of rhesus negative mother to be rhesus positive, its father must be rhesus positive. If the father is homozygous (DD) all of his children will be rhesus positive. If he is heterozygous rhesus positive (Dd) there is a 50 percent chance of the child becoming rhesus positive.

Pathophysiology

Classically rhesus disease occurs because maternal anti-D antibodies cross the placenta and hemolyse rhesus positive fetal red blood cells. The antibodies are IgG in configuration and are capable of crossing the placental barrier. The fetus is rarely affected before 16 weeks gestation as the antibodies do not cross the placenta until then.

Antibodies will attach to the surface of the fetal red cells and the affected red cells are cleared by reticuloendothelial system. These will lead to fetal anemia and increased erythroblasts in circulation, fetal hepatosplenomegaly and increased bilirubin in amniotic fluid. The fetus may have cardiomegaly with high output cardiac failure leading to fetal edema, ascites and hydrothorax (fetal hydrops).

Management

All pregnant women who are rhesus negative should have serum antibody screen at booking and if they are negative, this should be repeated at 32 and 37 weeks gestation. If the antibodies are positive, then the husband's genotype should be checked if it is not known. Maternal serum antibodies dilution titers or antibodies concentrations should be done every 2 weeks. It is generally accepted that antibodies titer at or below 1:16 are unlikely to produce serious fetal disease.

Amniocentesis should be performed at 10 weeks before the previously affected fetus (death, hydrops, transfusion) and repeated every 4 weeks then on.

Fetal Evaluation

The use of amniotic fluid bilirubin concentration to evaluate rhesus disease was described in early 1960's. Bilirubin is quantified by spectroscopic analysis at a wave length of 450 nm and the optical density difference OD (optical density) plotted on the Liley's chart (Figure 29.3). Treatment is indicated when the bilirubin level crosses the action line. The form of the treatment will depend on the maturity of the pregnancy.

Fetal ultrasound examination allows the detection of early ascites and the biophysical profile may be used to monitor fetal wellbeing. Doppler wave form analysis of blood velocity in fetal vessels is used in centers to suspect fetal anemia.

Fetal Management

The decision to treat the fetus may be based on ultrasound evidence of ascites, a rising amniotic fluid

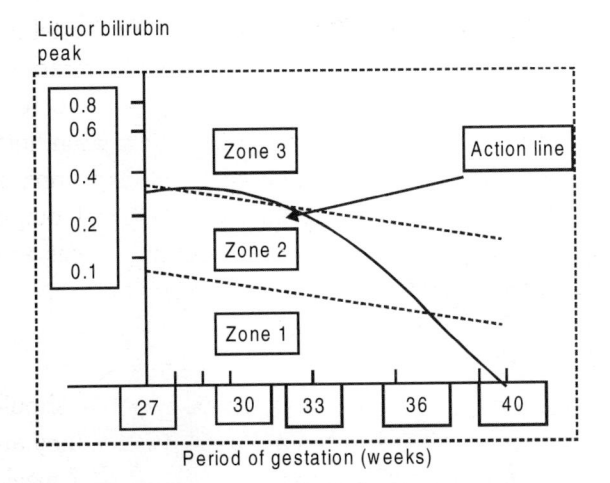

Figure 29.3: Whitfield modification of Liley's prediction graph

bilirubin content or hematological evidence of fetal anemia.

Intrauterine fetal transfusion is the most successful fetal therapy to treat anemia. The fetus would be transfused every 2 weeks as there is an approximate drop of about 1 to 2 percent per day of the hematocrit. The transfusions are continued until 34 to 36 weeks gestation when delivery of the fetus is then considered. Intrauterine intravascular transfusion is usually carried out through either the free loop of umbilical cord or the intra-abdominal portion of the umbilical vein. Intrauterine intraperitoneal fetal blood transfusions were earlier used but rarely successful when the fetus has had hydrops as the lymphatics through which blood is absorbed and transported are water logged.

Plasma exchange of mothers for antibodies removal for the treatment of anti-D isoimmunization has been reported to have good effects, but this is temporary. It is employed as an alternative when the sensitization occurs very early in pregnancy and when the problem of expertise hampers safe intrauterine intravascular transfusions.

Prevention of Rhesus Disease

All eligible rhesus negative mothers should receive anti-D immunoglobulins within 72 hours of delivery, abortion or invasive intrauterine procedures. The amount of anti-D immunoglobulin actually required is proportional to the size of fetomaternal bleed.

For events occurring before 20 weeks gestation it has been traditional to give 250 IU (50 μg) of anti-D immunoglobulin. Later in pregnancy and after delivery the usual dosage is 500 IU (100 μg). This should be increased if a Kleihauer test on the mother's blood shows more than 1 fetal cell per 500 adult red cells (equivalent to 4-5 ml of packed fetal red cells). An additional 150 IU of anti-D immunoglobulin is given for each ml of the transplacental bleed that exceeds 4 mls of packed fetal red cells.

It is now recommended that women who are not sensitized should be offered anti-D immunoglobulins antenatally at 28 and 32 weeks gestation. Rhesus negative mothers whose babies are rhesus positive or whose blood group is unknown should also be given anti-D immunoglobulins.

BIBLIOGRAPHY

1. Burton BK, Schulz CJ, Burd LI: Limb anomalies associated with chorionic villous sampling. *Obstet Gynecol* **79**:726-30, 1992.
2. Crowther CA: Anti-D administration in pregnancy for preventing Rhesus alloimmunisation. The Cochrane Library. Oxford: Update software, 1999.
3. De Sanctis V, Urso Lm: Multicenter study on prevalence of endocrine complications in thalassemia major. *Clin Endocrinol* **2**:5814, 1995.
4. De Sanctis V, Wonke B. Growth in Thalassemia. *Farmaci* (supplement): 145, 1994.
5. Ghidini A, Sepulveda W, Lockwood CJ, Romero R: Complications of fetal blood sampling. *Am J Obstet Gynecol* **168**:1339-44, 1993.
6. Lee D: Recommendations for the use of anti-D immunoglobulin for Rh prophylaxis. *Transfuse Med* **9**: 93-99, 1999.
7. Letsky E: Blood Volume, Haematinics, Anemia. In De Swiet M (ed): *Medical Disorders in Obstetric Practice*, 3rd. edn. Blackwell Science, London, 1995.
8. Old JM, Fitches A *et al*: First trimester fetal diagnosis for hemoglobinopathies. Report on 200 cases. *Lancet* **ii**: 763-67, 1986.
9. Rebulla P, Modell B: Management of beta Thalassemia major. *Cur Pediatr* **4**:3842, 1994.
10. Robson SC, Lee D, Urbaniak S: Anti-D immunoglobulin in Rh D prophylaxis: Revised guidelines for use in the United Kingdom. (Commentary) *Br J Obstet Gynecol* **105**: 129-34,1998.

30. Medical Disorders in Pregnancy (Cardiac, Respiratory and Endocrine Disorders)

Hira Lal Konar

PART TWO — Feto-maternal Medicine

INTRODUCTION

Medical disorders complicating pregnancies are not uncommon. Cardiac, respiratory and endocrine disorders can alter the course of a pregnancy. Similarly, they have significant impact both in terms of maternal and perinatal outcome. Individual medical disorder can affect the specific organ function primarily. Physiological alterations induced by pregnancy often make the diagnosis difficult. For example, it is essential to differentiate cardiovascular symptoms of a normal pregnant woman from those that indicate a cardiac disease in a pregnancy. Dyspnea of normal pregnancy due to hormonal changes (raised serum progesterone, must be differentiated from airway obstructive disease (asthma).

Multidisciplinary involvement and management in a referral center are often required to improve the outcome. Such a medical disorder may pre-exist or may develop during pregnancy for the first time. However, early detection of the abnormality is a key to the management.

CARDIAC DISEASES IN PREGNANCY

There is significant alterations of the hemodynamic system during normal pregnancy. This is in terms of blood volume, pulse rate and cardiac output. Cardiac load increases during pregnancy. Women with cardiac disease may not be able to withstand such physiological changes during pregnancy.[1] So it is essential that while managing heart disease in pregnancy obstetrician, cardiologists and the anesthesists should identify the high risk factors, anticipate the complications and manage the problems faced during pregnancy, labor and puerperium.

Incidence

The overall incidence of heart disease in pregnancy is less than 1 percent amongst the hospital deliveries. In the developing countries, Rheumatic cardiac lesion is common as opposed to congenital one as seen the developed world. Fortunately with improved health care there is a gradual decline in the incidence of rheumatic heart disease in the developing world.

Risk of Cardiac Disease in Pregnancy (Table 30.1)

1. *Maternal*: Maternal mortality is a major risk. In rheumatic heart disease the risk is low compared to other congenital heart disease like Eisenmenger syndrome.
2. *Fetal*: There is increased risk of preterm delivery and intrauterine growth restriction. Perinatal mortality is high. Congenital heart disease run a high risk (two folds) of recurrence of heart disease in the fetus.

Table 30.1: Cardiac disease and pregnancy

Effect of heart disease on pregnancy
- Preterm delivery
- IUGR
- Increased perinatal morbidity and mortality

Effect of pregnancy on heart disease
- Increased chances of cardiac failure.

New York Heart Association Functional Classification System[4]

- Class I: Patients have no limitations of physical activity
- Class II: Slight limitation of physical activity. Patients are comfortable as at rest but ordinary physical activity causes discomfort
- Class III: Marked limitation of physical activity. Less than ordinary activity causes discomfort to the patient
- Class IV: Patients are unable to carry out any physical activity without discomfort.

Clinical Features

A patient with cardiac disease presents with the features of hyperdynamic circulation. The neck veins are engorged and often pulsatile. The pulse may be irregular due to atrial or ventricular ectopic beats. Apex beat may be shifted outward due to the enlarged heart. Chest pain may be associated in a patient with ischemic heart disease or with severe mitral stenosis. One should be careful to detect the signs of heart failure when auscultation is done. The systolic murmur over the second intercostal space is a well known innocent murmur during pregnancy.

Investigations include chest X-ray, ECG, and echocardiography. Chest X-ray should be performed with adequate shielding of the uterus. Echocardiography is very helpful and it is a non-invasive method. It can be repeatedly used when indicated with minimal risk to the mother and fetus.

Rheumatic Heart Disease

It is the common type of cardiac lesion observed in developing countries. Pregnancy has no permanent deleterious effect on rheumatic diseases. Prognosis is good when compared to a cyanotic group of congenital cardiac disease.

Congenital Heart Disease (CHD)

Currently increasing number of women with CHD are seen during pregnancy. Majority of the women with acyanotic group of heart diseases tolerate pregnancy well. CHD when associated with pulmonary hypertension (primary or secondary) is associated with high maternal death. Commonly seen congenital heart diseases are atrial septal defects (ASD), patent ductus arteriosus (PDA), ventricular septal defects and coarctation of aorta. Eisenmenger's syndrome and Fallot's tetralogy in pregnancy are rarely encountered.[5]

Other Cardiac Diseases

Myocardial infarction, pericardial disease and cardiomyopathy are the others. These complications are rarely encountered in pregnancy.[6]

Management

All patients with heart disease in pregnancy should be managed jointly by the obstetrician and the cardiologist. Medical management is optimized following assessment of the functional class of the heart disease (NYHA classification).[4]

Antenatal Management

Routine antenatal visits to obstetricians and cardiologists are a must where all vital signs are evaluated. The patient is routinely examined for signs and symptoms of cardiac failure. Fetal wellbeing is assessed as a routine. The patient is warned against any infection of the respiratory tract or any dental infection. Anemia if present should be promptly corrected. Presence of breathlessness or any arrhythmia should be throughly investigated (Table 30.2).

Table 30.2: Antenatal management

- Prevent anemia, infection and cardiac failure
- Fetal monitoring
- Early detection and management of cardiac failure.

Termination of Pregnancy

It is not generally advised. Pregnancy may be terminated in conditions like inoperable cyanotic heart disease, primary pulmonary hypertension or with Eisenmenger's syndrome. It is preferably done before 8 weeks.[5]

1. *Cardiac surgery* is not contraindicated in pregnancy but generally it is delayed until the postpartum period.
2. *Antenatal admission in hospital* is helpful but not all patients with heart disease need to be admitted antenatally. Patients with high risk factors (infection, anemia or arrhythmias) should be admitted early. Best management can be offered at a tertiary center with facility of ICU jointly by the obstetricians and cardiologists.

Management of Labor

Generally the patients with heart disease deliver vaginally following spontaneous onset of labor. Induction of labor is less frequently indicated. Surgical induction by artificial rupture of membranes is better avoided to minimize the risks of infection. Patient should be covered with antibiotics during the course of labor.

Ampicillin plus Gentamicin are the antimicrobial chemotherapy recommended against bacterial endocarditis.[7] Parenteral fluid infusions are strictly monitored to avoid any overload. Labor pain is adequately controlled preferably with epidural analgesia, with measures to avoid hypotension.[8] Duration of second stage of labor is cut short with the use of prophylactic outlet forces or ventouse. Ergometrine should not be routinely given in the third stage of labor. In case of excessive bleeding-prostaglandin may be tried. During labor, patient should have electrocardiographic monitoring when indicated (Table 30.3).

Table 30.3: Intrapartum care

- Close supervision
- Antibiotic coverage
- Control labor pain
- Cut short second stage
- Avoid ergometrine in third stage.

Management of Cardiac Failure

It is an emergency situation which should be managed immediately. Sudden cardiac failure, in an otherwise asymptomatic woman, may occur shortly after the delivery, due to an increased intravascular blood volume diverted from uterine and pelvic vessels.

The principle of management of CCF are the same as in a patient without pregnancy. Oxygen is administered with the patient in a propped up position. Intravenous morphine, aminophylline and frusemide are administered to reduce pulmonary edema. Digoxin is started to improve myocardial efficiency if she was not digitalized before.

RESPIRATORY DISEASES IN PREGNANCY

Physiological changes in the respiratory system during pregnancy results in increase in ventilation and oxygen consumption. There is reduction in residual lung volume. A healthy woman can tolerate such changes in pregnancy, whereas a woman with some respiratory disease in pregnancy must be seen by the obstetrician in collaboration with a physician with particular interest in pregnancy (Table 30.4).

Table 30.4: Respiratory diseases and pregnancy

1. *Effect of pregnancy on respiratory disease*
   Deteriorate   (30%)
   Improved   (20%)
   Unchanged   (50%)
2. *Effect of respiratory disease on pregnancy*
   - Preterm delivery
   - Hypertension
   - IUGR

Asthma in Pregnancy

Asthma is due to airway obstruction causing shortness of breath, cough, wheeze and chest tightness. It is a chronic inflammatory condition whose cause is ill understood. Immunological, infection and emotional factors are common. Overall incidence in pregnancy is 1-2 percent.

Risks of Bronchial Asthma in Pregnancy

Preterm delivery and maternal hypertension are the known risks.[10]

The risk of the child developing asthma in latter life is high when compared to the child of an unaffected couple.

Management of Bronchial Asthma in Pregnancy

The most widely used drug for prophylaxis is inhalation of disodium cromoglycate, which is safe in pregnancy.[11] The long-acting beta agonist, salbutamol, is commonly used for an attack (rescue therapy) of asthma. It can be given by inhalation (preferred) or orally and by nebulizer for a severe attack.

Betamethasone by inhalation can also be used in cases not responding to beta agonist alone.

Theophylline (aminophylline) is given intravenously in severe asthma. Prednisone 25 mg/day may have to be given in cases with severe asthma. Prednisone is not contraindicated in pregnancy and is not teratogenic.[12]

Epidural anesthesia is preferred to general anesthesia to avoid the risk of atelectasis and infection.

Breastfeeding is not contraindicated in a patient with bronchial asthma while on medication.[13]

Acute Bronchitis in Pregnancy

It is an acute inflammatory condition of the tracheobronchial tree sparing the alveoli. The causative agent may be bacterial, viral or chemical (pollutants). Clinically it is manifested as cough, expectoration and fever. In a mild case supportive care is sufficient. In a worse situation antibiotic therapy is started. Amoxycillin and/or erythromycin can be prescribed for 5 to 7 days without any risk to the fetus.

Chronic Bronchitis and Bronchiectasis in Pregnancy

It is relative uncommon in pregnancy. In the presence of bronchiectasis, the patient's condition deteriorates during pregnancy. Chest infection and airway obstruction is managed in consultation with a physician. Physiotherapy and postural drainage are maintained. Fetal growth restriction has been observed. Pulmonary hypertension and hypoxemia are the two predictors of success for pregnancy outcome.

Pulmonary Koch's Infection

Pulmonary Koch's infection during pregnancy is observed in less than 1 percent. Before the use of antituberculous drugs, the outcome of pregnancy complicated by tuberculosis was poor.

Diagnosis

Depending on the severity of the disease the patient may present with the following symptoms like cough with a without expectoration, hemoptysis, fever, weight loss or chest pain. The diagnosis is based on the chest X-ray and Mantoux test. The Mantoux test becomes positive 4-12 weeks after the initial infection.

Management

The drugs that are extensively studied and found safe in pregnancy are isonizd, rifampicin and ethambutol. Ethambutol has replaced para-amino salicylic acid (PAS). Pyrazinamid can also be used. Treatment should be continued for a period of six to nine months as in the non-pregnant patients.[14] Transplacental risk of infection to fetus is very rare. Detection of congenital lesion is difficult. In congenital tuberculosis lesion must be detected in the liver. When the mother suffers from open infection, the infant should be isolated. Treatment to an infected infant is similar to that in adults.

Breastfeeding

There is no contraindication to breastfeeding. Antitunberculous drugs are secreted in the breast milk, but the concentrations of the drugs are too low to cause any toxicity in the infant.

THYROID DISORDERS IN PREGNANCY

Thyroid disorders are not uncommon in the women of reproductive age. Physiological changes in pregnancy may mimic thyroid dysfunction. An obstetrician, in collaboration with a physician, should see a patient with laboratory tests for complete evaluation of thyroid function.[15]

Hyperthyroidism

Over all incidence of hyperthyroidism is about one per thousand pregnancies. Autoimmune disorder (Graves' disease) is the most common.[16]

Risks of Hyperthyroidism in Pregnancy

Maternal: Cardiac failure is life-threatening. This is due to the effects of T4 on the myocardial muscles. Pre-existing anemia, infection or cardiac disorder may aggravate the complication.[17]

Fetal: Increased incidence of preterm deliveries, low birth weight babies and stillbirths are observed.[18] Perinatal mortality is increased.

Thyroid Nodule during Pregnancy

Isolated thyroid nodule during pregnancy raise the suspicion of malignancy. Goiters during pregnancy are generally diffuse in character. Ultrasonography can be useful to evaluate a thyroid nodule. Fine needle aspiration biopsy can be safely performed in pregnancy when necessity arises.[19]

Diagnosis of hyperthyroidism must be confirmed by measuring free T4 and T3 levels. Radioactive iodine uptake tests are avoided during pregnancy.

Management

Medical therapy is commonly used for control of hyperthyroidism. Propylthiouracil (PTU) or carbimazole can be used with good result. The commonly accepted dose of propylthiouracil is 300 to 450 mg/day and that of Carbimazole is 30 to 45 mg/day. Depending on the response dose may have to be reduced gradually. Beta blockers may be used for relief of toxic symptoms.

Thyroidectomy is rarely indicated during pregnancy. Malignancy must be excluded by ultrasonography or fine needle aspiration before surgery.

Hypothyroidism

Hypothyroidism may be due to hypothalamopituitary dysfunction. More commonly it is due to autoimmune disorders or due to surgical ablation.

Risks of Hypothyroidism in Pregnancy

Women with hypothyroidism commonly suffer from infertility. If they become pregnant, the fetal effects are increased, e.g. miscarriage, stillbirth and congenital anomalies.[20]

Diagnosis: Clinical diagnosis is made by presence of fatigue, dry skin, coarse hair, constipation and weight gain. It must be confirmed by laboratory tests by measuring the values of free thyroid index and free T4 (Table 30.5).

Table 30.5: Endocrine disorders and pregnancy

1. *Effect of hyperthyroidism on pregnancy*
   - Maternal weight loss
   - Preterm delivery
   - Small for gestational age (SGA) baby.
   - Increased perinatal morbidity and mortality
2. *Effect of hypothyroidism on pregnancy*
   - Anemia
   - Miscarriage
   - Preterm labor
   - Intrauterine death (IUD)

Management: Patient once diagnosed as hypothyroid, replacement with thyroid hormone is started. Levothyroxin 0.10-0.20 mg/day is continued. Therapy should be monitored with re-evaluation of serum level of T3 and free T4 levels.

CONCLUSION

Cardiac, respiratory or endocrine disorders during pregnancy increase maternal morbidity and the possibilities of maternal mortality. The patients with any of the conditions described above should be managed at a tertiary level hospital jointly by the senior obstetrician and medical specialist. These patients may become critically ill within a short period, hence it is essential to monitor them very closely. Immediate postpartum period seems to be the worst time especially for women with heart diseases, so a very close watch is mandatory in the labor room.

REFERENCES

Cardiac Diseases in Pregnancy

1. Sadmantz A. Kocheril AG, Emaus SP *et al:* Cardiovascular changes in pregnancy evaluated by two-dimensional and doppler echocardiography. *American Journal of the Society of Echocardiography* **5**:253-58, 1992.
2. Rose V, Gold RJM, Lindsay G. Allen MA: Possible increase in the incidence of congenital heart defects among the offspring of affected parents. *Journal of American College of Cardiology* **6**: 376-82, 1985.
3. Chesley LC: Severe rheumatic cardiac disease and pregnancy: the ultimate prognosis. *American Journal of Obstetrics and Gynecology* **136**:552-58, 1980.
4. Criteria Committee of the New York Heart Association Nomenclature and Criteria for Diagnosis of Disease of the Heart and Great Vessels, 6th edn. Boston. MA: Little Brown, 1964.
5. Patton DE, Lee W. Cotton DB et al: Cyanotic maternal heart disease pregnancy. *Obstetrical and Gynecological Survey* **45**:594-600, 1990.
6. Veille JC; Peripartum cardiomyoplathies: a review. *American Journal Obstetrics and Gynecology* **148**: 805-18, 1984.
7. Seaworth BJ, Durach DT; Infective endocarditis in Obstetric and Gynecology practice. *American Journalof Obstetrics and Gynecology* **154**:180-88, 1986.
8. Ostheimer GW, Alper MH: Intrapartum anesthetic management of the pregnant patient with heart disease. *Clinical Obstetrics and Gynecology* **18**:81-97, 1975.

Respiratory Diseases in Pregnancy

9. Fleming DM, Cromble DL: Prevalence of asthma and hi fever in England and Wales. *British Medical Journal* **294**: 279-83, 1987.
10. Doucette JT, Bracken MB: Possible role of asthma in the risk of preterm labor and delivery: *Epidemiology* **2**: 143-50, 1983.
11. Moore-Gillon J: Asthma in Pregnancy: *British Journal of Obstetrics and Gynecology* **101**:658-60, 1994.
12. Dykes MHM: Evaluation of an anti asthamatic agent cromolyn sodium (aarare, Intal). *Journal of the American Medical Association* **277**:1061-62, 1974.
13. Saarimen UM, Kajosaari M: Breast feeding as prophylaxis against stopic disease: prospective follow-up study until 17 years old. *Lancet* **346**: 1065-69, 1995.
14. Snider DE, Layde PM, Johnson NW *et al*: Treatment of tuberculosis during pregnancy: *American Review of Respiratory Disease* **122**:65-68, 1980.

Thyroid Disorders in Pregnancy

15. Beeks GP, Burrow GN: Thyroid disease pregnancy. *Medical Clinics of North America* **75**:121-50, 1991.
16. Clavel S, Madee AM, Bornet H, *et al*: Anti TSH receptor antibodies in pregnant patients with autoimmune thyroid disorder. *Br Jr Obst Gynecol* **97**:1003-08, 1990.
17. Thomas R, Reid RL: Thyroid disease and reproductive dysfunction a review. *Obstetrics and Gynecology* **70**:789-98, 1987.
18. Mestman JH: Thyroid disease in pregnancy. *Clinics in Perinatology* **12**: 651-67, 1985.
19. Hod M, Sharony R, Friedman S *et al*: Pregnancy and thyroid carcinoma a review of incidence, cause and prognosis. *Obstetrics and Gynecological Survey* **44**:744-49, 1989.
20. Lancet editorial, Thyroid dysfunction in utero. *Lancet* **339**: 155, 1992.

31.

Onnig Tamizian
Sabaratnam Arulkumaran

Principles of Drug Use in Pregnancy

EPIDEMIOLOGY

In the UK about 35 percent of pregnant women take medication (excluding vitamins and iron) at least once in pregnancy, although only 6 percent in the first trimester.[1] This does not include drugs used in labor. The proportion of women taking medication in pregnancy has dropped from around 80 percent in the 1960's, along with a significant reduction in the percentage of women taking self administered drugs from 64 percent to around 9 percent over the same period.[1] Similar consistently high levels of drug use are found in North America and Europe.[2] The reduction in drug use in pregnancy is probably driven by the continued attention in the news media to drug-induced fetal abnormality.

At least half the pregnancies in North America are unplanned,[3] and therefore each and every year hundreds of thousands of women expose their fetuses to a range of drugs before they know they are pregnant. Another important feature is that with the increasing age at which women elect to have children, more women are already on long-term medication for chronic conditions at the time they embark on pregnancy. Women suffering of certain medical conditions that were considered in the past to be incompatible with pregnancy (SLE, certain types of heart disease), now have the opportunity of motherhood due to dramatic improvement in pregnancy outcome.[4]

Congenital defects are present in 2 to 3 percent of babies at birth. The majority (2/3rd) of the defects are of unknown etiology, with a quarter having a genetic cause, while 3 to 5 percent may be due to intrauterine infections, and a similar number due to underlying maternal disease such as diabetes. Only a small proportion, around 1 to 2 percent of the total, is thought to be associated with drug treatment.[5]

TIMING OF EXPOSURE AND PREGNANCY OUTCOME

Medication taken in pregnancy can harm the unborn child through teratogenic effects. Teratogenesis is defined as dysgenesis of fetal organs, either in terms of structural integrity or function.[6] Teratogenic effects may take the form of malformations that occur during the period of organogenesis or subsequently by causing alterations in the structure or function of organ systems formed during organogenesis. Other manifestations of teratogens include

Principles of Drug Use in Pregnancy

growth restriction or fetal death and carcinogenesis. In addition, some drugs such as retinoids, which are high-grade teratogens, may exert their effect for upto 2 years after the last dose.[7]

The timing of exposure to a particular drug treatment is a critical factor in assessing the nature and extent of any adverse effects. Three important phases are recognised in human development:[7]

1. *Pre-embryonic phase:* This extends from conception to 17 days post-conception (or 3 days after the first missed period). During this period of implantation and blastocyst formation, any adverse effect is an 'all or non phenomenon' and the result of an insult will either be death and abortion/resorption or intact survival through multiplication of the totipotential cells.
2. *Embryonic phase:* This period extends from post-conception day 18 to day 55 and is the most crucial period of organogenesis. It is the period of greatest theoretical sensitivity and risk of congenital malformation with rapidly differentiating tissues, so that any damage becomes irreparable. The earlier in this period the insult occurs, the more marked is the likely effect. The following lesions have been identified with time of exposure[8] (days post-conception); anencephaly—day 24, limb reduction defects—days 12 to 40, transposition of great vessels—day 34, cleft lip—day 36, ventricular septal defects—day 42, syndactyly—day 42, hypospadias—day 84.
3. *Fetal phase:* This phase runs from post-conceptional age of 8 weeks through to term. The impact of drugs that can cross the placenta affect fetal growth and development rather than causing gross structural malformations.

PRESCRIBING PRINCIPLES

When prescribing in pregnancy it is important to consider the following principles:

a. Drugs should be prescribed only for clear indications and where the benefits (usually for the mother) outweigh the potential risks (usually to the fetus). Question the need for any drug in pregnancy.
b. If possible it is better to try and avoid all drugs (including nonprescription medications) in the first trimester.
c. Medication should be used in the smallest effective dose for the shortest period of time required.
d. It is preferable to prescribe medication that has been widely used in pregnancy and has a good safety track record, rather than newer agents that may have theoretical though as yet unproved advantages.
e. All women of reproductive age are at risk of pregnancy.
f. Most drugs with a molecular weight of less than 1500 are capable of crossing the placenta[9] and therefore of potentially affecting the fetus, but very few drugs have been conclusively shown to be teratogenic.
g. Encourage preconceptual counseling in all patients with chronic medical disorders and in particular those on long-term drug therapy. If this has not been possible, review all drug regimens as early in pregnancy as possible avoiding polypharmacy as far as possible.

PHARMACOKINETICS

Pharmacokinetics refers to the absorption, distribution, metabolism and excretion of a drug; variables that can be influenced by maternal physiological adaptation to pregnancy.

Gastrointestinal transit time is prolonged due to slower emptying of the stomach and reduced gut motility, hence the rationale of parenteral administration of drugs in labor.[9] Molecular distribution of a given drug is affected by its lipid solubility and protein binding. Another physiological adaptation to pregnancy involves increase in the total body water and plasma volume (and hence volume of distribution), along with a fall in plasma proteins such as albumin. Drugs that have low lipid solubility and are predominantly bound to plasma proteins will thus have a greater plasma concentration of the unbound drug, which would be both available for distribution out of the circulation, and for elimination. The total level of a drug such as phenytoin may thus fall but the free drug concentration remains unchanged,[9] and this should be examined if levels are being monitored.

Drugs that are water soluble are generally eliminated unchanged. In pregnancy, renal plasma flow, glomerular filtration rate and creatinine clearance all increase, which in turn leads to more rapid elimination of water soluble drugs, such as Lithium and ampicillin,[10] which are excreted unchanged.

Lipid soluble drugs are further metabolised prior to elimination. The process of drug metabolism may involve the maternal liver, the placenta or the fetal liver and fetal adrenal gland. Although blood flow to the liver is unchanged in pregnancy, certain metabolic pathways are induced such that, where the rate of elimination of a drug such as phenytoin by the liver is dependent on hepatic enzyme activity, there may be significant falls in serum concentration of the drug.[10] On the other hand, where the rate of elimination of the drug is dependent on hepatic blood flow, pregnancy does not affect clearance of the drug.[10]

The placenta is essentially a lipid barrier between the maternal and fetal circulations. Lipid soluble, un-ionized, low molecular drugs will cross the placenta faster than their water soluble and polar counterparts but given time both groups will achieve similar concentrations in the maternal and fetal circulation.[9,10] Exceptions include heparin, insulin and curare.

BREASTFEEDING

The vast majority of drugs cross into breast milk. In general terms the doses of drugs reaching the baby are clinically insignificant when one considers dilution of the drug in the mother and the small volumes of milk the neonate feeds on.

Drugs can be considered in three broad categories with respect to breastfeeding:
a. Drugs that cannot be detected in the baby, examples include the anticoagulant warfarin and the group of antibiotics known as aminoglycosides, which are not absorbed from the gastrointestinal tract of normal infants.
b. Drugs that are detectable in the baby in clinically insignificant amounts, such as nonnarcotic analgesics, nonsteroidal anti-inflammatory drugs, penicillins, cephalosporins, antihypertensive drugs, bronchodilators and most anticonvulsants except barbiturates.
c. Drugs that reach the neonate in sufficient amounts to cause fetal side effects. Examples in this group include benzodiazepines reported to cause lethargy, barbiturates causing drowsiness, amiodarone with a theoretical risk of hypothyroidism, tetracyclines and potential risk of discoloration of teeth, combined OCP and risk of diminishing milk supply and reduction in nitrogen and protein content, ephedrine associated with irritability, cytotoxic drugs and immune suppression/neutropenia, and aspirin with risk of Reye's syndrome.[10]

DRUGS USED IN PREGNANCY

Antibiotics

Pregnant women appear to handle antimicrobial agents differently from non-pregnant patients and serum levels of ampicillin in pregnant women were 50 percent of the values in the same women when not pregnant.[11] Adverse effects have been proven with very few antibiotics and therefore treatment of pregnant women should be with standard adult doses for adequate duration as dictated by the underlying condition.

The fluoroquinolones (ciprofloxacin, ofloxacin, etc) are best avoided, although no human data on teratogenesis is available; there are reports of irreversible arthropathy from animal studies.

Treatment of tuberculosis should be similar to the non-pregnant individual in terms of duration. Ethambutol and isoniazid appear safe.[11] Rifampicin has a two- to three-fold higher congenital abnormality rate than ethambutol and isoniazid, while streptomycin is best avoided in pregnancy as it causes deafness.[11] Treatment is best carried out in conjunction with a respiratory physician specializing in tuberculosis treatment.

In the treatment of chlamydial infections, doxycycline should be replaced with erythromycin 500 mg 6 hourly for 7 days. If erythromycin is not tolerated, alternatives in pregnancy include amoxycillin or clindamycin but these have lower cure rates (98% and 93% respectively). Contact tracing for the past 30 days and appropriate counseling and treatment is essential.

The antiviral agent acyclovir is the drug of choice for treatment of herpes virus infection such as primary genital herpes or varicella. There is no evidence of increase in infant malformations or adverse fetal outcome when used in pregnancy, but its routine use in pregnancy is not recommended for women with genital herpes.[13] There is, however, a role for its use in overwhelming varicella infection. Topical acyclovir results in negligible systemic levels and therefore can be used for genital and orolabial herpes infection. There is no information regarding the use of amantadine in pregnancy, while ribavirin is contraindicated in pregnancy based on animal studies showing teratogenesis.[13]

In terms of breastfeeding, chloroamphenicol is best avoided in breastfeeding due to the risk of grey baby syndrome, while tetracyclines should also be avoided due to the risks of dental discoloration.[11, 12] If isoniazid is used, both mother and baby should be given folic acid supplements,[11] while metronidazole, although safe, does affect the taste of breast milk.[11]

Anticoagulants

Heparins (both unfractionated and low molecular weight) do not cross the placenta, therefore have no teratogenic effects and are generally the anticoagulant of choice in the antenatal period, probably with the exception of patients with mechanical valves.[14] Heparins are, however, associated with reversible loss of bone mineral density on prolonged use and in certain individuals may cause thrombocytopenia. Low molecular weight heparins have the advantage of once daily dosage, more predictable bioavailability and less risk of loss of bone mineral density. An alternative to heparin for thromboprophylaxis in pregnancy in lower risk individuals may be low dose aspirin,[14] but patients with recurrent venous thromboembolism, inherited clotting abnormalities or antiphospholipid syndrome would warrant heparin for thromboprophylaxis.

Oral anticoagulants such as warfarin have been associated with a number of problems when used in pregnancy.[12,14] These include an increased rate of spontaneous miscarriage giving an overall miscarriage rate of around 25 percent. Warfarin is also known to be teratogenic and when used in the first trimester, a syndrome of warfarin embryopathy has been described including shortening and stippling of long bones (chondrodysplasia punctata) and nasal hypoplasia. The incidence quoted in the literature varies between 10 and 25 percent.[12, 14] The third group of abnormalities is associated with use of warfarin in later pregnancy. These are abnormalities of the central nervous system under the collective term dorsal midline dysplasias, which encompass absence of corpus callosum, Dandy-Walker syndrome and encephaloceles. Nevertheless, warfarin has a clear role in the management of cardiac patients in pregnancy, such as those with metalic valve replacements, pulmonary hypertension and atrial fibrillation. The aim would be to maintain the INR not much above three to minimize the teratogenic effects of warfarin without significantly increasing the risk of venous thromboembolism.

Anticonvulsants

Phenytoin, primidone, phenobarbitone, carbamazepine and sodium valproate all cross the placenta and are potentially teratogenic. The risk of malformation increases with the number of anticonvulsant drugs taken simultaneously, therefore the aim should be monotherapy.[15,16] The incidence of congenital malformations in mothers with epilepsy on a single anticonvulsant is around 6 percent compared to the background rate of 2 percent. Well over 90 percent of mothers on anticonvulsants will have a normal pregnancy and deliver a healthy infant.

Several major malformations caused by anticonvulsants have been reported.[13, 15, 16] They are:
1. Neural tube defects: Sodium valproate (1-2%) and carbamazepine (0.5-1%)
2. Orofacial clefts: Phenytoin
3. Congenital heart defects: Phenytoin and valproate

Minor malformations associated with anticonvulsant use in pregnancy known as the 'fetal anticonvulsant syndrome' include dysmorphic features (V-shaped eyebrows, low-set ears, broad nasal bridge and irregular teeth), hypertelorism and hypoplastic nails and distal digits.[15, 16]

It is advisable that patients on anticonvulsants take high dose folic acid (5 mg/day as opposed to 400 mcg) periconceptually and throughout the first trimester of pregnancy, as one mechanism of teratogenesis is thought to be folate deficiency through the interference of anticonvulsants with folate metabolism.[16] Prenatal screening for neural tube defects and congenital malformations with maternal serum alphafetoprotein and detailed ultrasound at 18-20 weeks should be offered, along with a further ultrasound at 22 weeks if cardiac abnormalities are suspected on the earlier scan. Vitamin K, at a dose of 10 mg/day, should be prescribed for all pregnant epileptic women on treatment during the last 4 weeks of pregnancy.[16] This is to reduce the risk of hemorrhagic disease of newborn in the offspring, as hepatic enzyme inducing drugs may result in reduced levels of vitamin K dependant coagulation factors. Breastfeeding whilst on anticonvulsants is safe.

Antihypertensive Drugs

Drug treatment may be required for pre-existing hypertension as well as for treatment of high blood pressure in pregnancy-induced hypertension and pre-eclampsia. Methyldopa, although it crosses the placenta, is considered a safe drug in the treatment of pre-existing and pregnancy-induced hypertension throughout pregnancy.[17] Beta blockers are also considered safe in pregnancy and may be better tolerated than methyldopa. Beta blockers cross the placenta producing a harmless reduction in fetal heart rate, but not the reactivity on CTG monitoring. If treatment is commenced before 28 weeks there is a gestationally adjusted reduction in birthweight but subsequent infant growth is unaffected.[17] In general, if treatment is commenced before 28 weeks, methyldopa may be a better first choice.

Calcium channel blockers effectively control antenatal and postnatal hypertension. Nifedipine is also used to inhibit pre-term labor and delivery. The main maternal side effects are facial flushing, headache and edema. Thiazide diuretics, though safe in terms of adverse effects, their role in pregnancy is limited to treatment of heart failure and not hypertension.

Angiotensin converting enzyme inhibitors often prescribed to the young patient with essential hypertension or diabetics with microalbuminuria (owing to its additional renoprotective effect) are contraindicated in pregnancy.[13, 17] Intrauterine death in animal studies, oligohydramnios, fetal anuria and stillbirth in humans, later in pregnancy, have been reported.

Analgesics and Anti-inflammatory Drugs

Paracetamol is safe in pregnancy and lactation.[13, 18] For headaches (tension headaches, migraine) paracetamol and codeine are the drugs of choice.[18] Aspirin and non-steroidal anti-inflammatory drugs may be used but are best avoided in the third trimester.[19] Non-steroidal anti-inflammatory drugs used in pregnancy and lactation should be those with a short half-life and inactive metabolites such as ibuprofen, to minimize effects on the fetus. Babies born preterm after exposure to indomethacin given to delay preterm delivery, have a higher neonatal morbidity, with necrotising enterocolitis, intracranial hemorrhage and patent ductus arteriosus.[18] Sulphasalazine has been shown to be safe in pregnancy and lactation but folate supplementation is recommended as it impairs folate absorption.[20]

Immunosuppressants and Corticosteroids

Generally used in patients with autoimmune conditions such as rheumatoid arthritis and SLE and following organ transplantation. Increasing number of normal pregnancies have been reported in women taking azathioprine, though some infants have had lymphopenia, growth restriction and an increase in chromosomal breakages.[13, 20] Cyclosporin appears safe in pregnancy but breastfeeding is not recommended.[13,20] Corticosteroids such as prednisolone are safe in pregnancy and lactation, though additional peripartum doses are required to cover delivery.[20]

Psychotropic Drugs

Neuroleptics are unlikely to be prescribed in pregnancy, but women on long-term treatment or prophylaxis for functional psychosis may present with pregnancy. The high lipid solubility of these drugs and their active metabolites, mean that stopping these drugs in someone already pregnant will make little, if any, immediate difference to the environment of the fetus.[21] Prochloperazine, more commonly used as an antiemetic, has been found to be safe in large scale surveillance studies.[13] Chlorpromazine, due to its hypotensive effects, is best avoided immediately before and during delivery.[21] Neuroleptic drugs enter breast milk in clinically insignificant amounts and sedation is the most common effect in the neonate.

Tricyclic antidepressants are structurally very similar to neuroleptics, hence considerable overlap in their pharmacological effects.[21] A withdrawal reaction has been reported in some neonates born to mothers who received tricyclic antidepressants in the last month of pregnancy,[21] including abdominal cramps, restlessness, insomnia and fever. Often dose reduction toward term is aimed for, planning to restart medication immediately postdelivery. In the management of depression, tricyclic antidepressants appear to be the drugs of choice along with fluoxetine as an alternative.[13, 21]

Lithium carbonate is used in the treatment of manic depressive illness, a disorder of young adults which by definition includes women of childbearing age. Lithium is known to be teratogenic in the first months of pregnancy, with a risk of around 7 percent.[13, 21] The cardiovascular system appears to be the main organ system affected. Lithium clearance doubles during pregnancy and dose increase may be required, to maintain serum concentration at therapeutic levels, remembering to dose reduce immediately postdelivery as the abrupt fall in clearance may precipitate toxic levels. Breastfeeding is contraindicated as levels of lithium in breast milk approach adult serum therapeutic levels.[21] Patients using lithium in the second and third trimesters should be routinely assessed by ultrasound for increased amniotic fluid volume.[13] Alternatives to lithium in the treatment of mania or bipolar affective disorder in pregnancy are chlorpromazine and haloperidol.

Monoamine oxidase inhibitors such as tranylcypromine, phenelzine and isocarboxazid are contraindicated in pregnancy due to the potentially fatal interaction between these drugs and those normally used in anesthesia.[9]

In terms of anxiolytics and hypnotics, benzodiazepines are the only agents that should be considered, barbiturates now being obsolete for these purposes. Abrupt withdrawal in pregnancy is not justified, due to the incapacitating nature of withdrawal reaction with distorted sensory perceptions. Withdrawal is likely to be worse if the initial benzodiazepine is shorter acting.[21]

Antiretroviral Agents

The antiretroviral drugs used in the management of HIV infection and AIDS, zidovudine and lamivudine (Nucleoside reverse transcriptase inhibitors) have been assessed and appear to be safe for use in pregnancy.[22] There is at present insufficient evidence to establish a causal relationship between exposure to antiretroviral drugs and a small number of cases (8 cases of children) with mitochondrial dysfunction.[22] Safety of neviparine (a non-nucleoside reverse transcriptase inhibitor) also appears safe[22] but efanvirez is contraindicated in pregnancy.[22]

TREATMENT OF MINOR AILMENTS IN PREGNANCY

The Table 31.1 summarises drugs that are safe for treatment of minor ailments in pregnancy.[9,18,19]

Table 31.1: Minor ailments in pregnancy and their treatment

Complaints	Treatment options
• Acne	• Topical erythromycin, clindamycin or tretinoin
	• Systemic erythromycin
• Pruritus, itching	• Depends on underlying cause.
	• *Topical agents* such as moisturising creams and ointments, zinc oxide cream, aluminium acetate, calamine lotion, glucocorticoid ointments, local anesthetic ointments. Alternatively.
	• *Systemic agents* hydroxyzine, glucocorticoids, diphenhydramine.
• Constipation	• Sodium docusate, lactulose, magnesium hydroxide, glycerine, bisacodyl. High fiber and water intake.
• Nausea, vomiting	• Metoclopramide, cyclizine, chlorpromazine, diphenhydramine
• Heartburn, reflux, dyspepsia	• Antacids, magnesium or aluminium hydroxide, ranitidine
• Hay fever/allergic rhinitis	• *Topical*: Decongestants, glucocorticoids, cromolyn, phenylephrine.
	• *Systemic*: Diphenhydramine, astemizole
• Cough	• Diphenhydramine, codeine

Table 31.2: Common drugs and their teratogenic affects

Categories	Drugs	Teratogenic effects
• Antibiotics	• Aminoglycosides	• Deafness, vestibular damage
	• Tetracycline	• Anomalies of teeth and bone
	• Quinolones	• Animal studies only- irreversible arthropathy
	• Sulphonamides	• Hyperbilirubinemia, kernicterus
• Anticholinergics		• Neonatal meconium ileus
• Anticoagulants	• Warfarin	• Skeletal and CNS defects, Dandy-Walker syndrome
• Anticonvulsants	• Carbamazepine	• Neural tube defects
	• Phenytoin	• Growth retardation, CNS defects
	• Valproic acid	• Neural tube defects
	• Paramethadione, Trimethadione	• CNS and facial abnormalities
• Antidepressants	• Lithium carbonate	• Ebstein's anomaly, hypotonia, reduced suckling, hyporeflexia
• Antihypertensives	• Angiotensin converting enzyme inhibitors	• Prolonged renal failure in neonates, decreased skull ossification, renal tubular dysgenesis.
	• Beta blockers	• Growth restriction, neonatal bradycardia and hypoglycemia
• Antithyroid drugs	• Propylthiouracil,	• Fetal and neonatal goitre and hypothyroidism.
	• Methimazole	• Aplasia cutis. Fetal and neonatal goitre and hypothyroidism
• Cytotoxic drugs	• Aminopterin, methotrexate	• CNS and limb malformations
	• Cyclophosphamide	• CNS malformations, secondary cancer
• Diuretics	• Frusemide	• Decreased uterine blood flow, hyperbilirubinemia
	• Thiazides	• Neonatal thrombocytopenia
• Hypoglycemics		• Neonatal hypoglycemia
• NSAIDs	• Indomethacin	• Premature closure of ductus arteriosus, necrotising enterocolitis, neonatal pulmonary hypertension
	• Salicylates	• Hemorrhage
• Prostaglandin analogues	• Misoprostol	• Moebius sequence
• Recreational drugs CNS	• Ethanol	• Fetal alcohol syndrome (pre- and postnatal growth restriction, anomalies, characteristic facial features.
	• Cocaine	• Growth retardation, placental abruption, uterine rupture
• Systemic Retinoids	• Isotretinoin, etretinate	• CNS, craniofacial, cardiovascular and other defects
• Sex hormones	• Danazol and other androgenic drugs	• Musculinization of female fetuses
	• Diethylstilbestrol	• Vaginal carcinoma, genitourinary defects in male and female offsprings
• Sedatives	• Thalidomide	• Limb shortening and internal organ defects
• Psychoactive drugs	• Barbiturates, opioids, benzodiazepines	• Neonatal withdrawal syndromes when drugs taken in late pregnancy
	• Phenothiazines	• Neonatal effects of impaired thermoregulation, extrapyramidal effects

MANAGEMENT OF PREGNANCY AND POTENTIAL TERATOGENESIS

The risk of teratogenesis is present in two broad groups of patients.[5] In the first group are patients on long-term medication for a chronic condition, who ideally should be counseled prior to pregnancy and made aware of the risks of fetal malformation and how these risks could be reduced. Often however this has not been the case. The second group are those patients taking a single course of treatment unaware of early pregnancy.

The management of exposure to potential teratogens in pregnancy relies on accurate determination of the history of exposure including the gestational age at exposure, as well as, up to date information on the teratogenic potential of the agent in question at the particular gestation of exposure. Accurate dating of pregnancy is essential and this can be performed by a combination of early dating scan, menstrual and conception history. Fetal malformations associated with teratogens affect the CNS, cardiovascular system, arms and legs, orofacial clefting and multisystem defects. The majority of major malformations are detectable on detailed ultrasound scanning at 18 to 20 weeks. Where cardiac abnormality is suspected from an earlier scan a repeat scan around 22 weeks may be helpful. In cases where neural tube defects are one of the manifestations of exposure to a particular teratogen, maternal serum alphafetoprotein estimation may also be of value. Further management will depend on the established risks from exposure to the given teratogen at a particular gestation time along with the wishes of the couple after comprehensive counseling, preferably by experts in the field.

Drugs with Proven Teratogenic and Fetal Effects in Humans

Table 31.2 summarises teratogenic and fetal effects of common medication.[5, 8, 10, 13, 19]

CONCLUSION

Fetal safety is a major concern, so effective drugs that have been in use for long periods are preferable to new alternatives, which, although may be more specific and have fewer adverse effects in adults, their safety in fetuses is less likely to be known. In order to minimize fetal risk, drug doses at the lower end of the therapeutic range should be prescribed in pregnancy, accepting that due to altered pharmacokinetics in pregnancy, higher than normal adult doses may sometimes be required. Counseling is imperative before prescribing and women should be discouraged from taking over the counter medication. Counseling will need to take into consideration many factors, among them the risk versus benefit of using a certain drug and the stage of pregnancy. For teratogenesis to be ascribed to a particular drug, certain patterns of defects should be seen when exposed to at a particular gestation time, the evidence being stronger if the defect caused has a biologically plausible mechanism of teratogenesis and/or proven on animal models. Alongside the risk of teratogenesis, there is however also the risk of misinformation about teratogenesis and the potential for unnecessary terminations or avoidance of much needed therapy. Women and their unborn offspring need to be protected from both these risks. Most drug labels will have the warning 'not to be used in pregnancy unless benefits outweigh risk', putting heavy responsibility on the physician and reluctance by the woman to take the prescribed medication. One should always be prepared to consult colleagues or experts in the field if in doubt.

REFERENCES

1. Rubin PC, Craig GS, Gavin K, Sumner D: Prospective survey of use of therapeutic drugs, alcohol and cigarettes during pregnancy. *BMJ* **292**: 81-3, 1986.
2. Bonati M, Bortolus R, Marchetti F, Romero M, Tognoni G: Drug use in pregnancy: An overview of epidemiological (drug utilisation) studies. *Eur J Clin Pharmacol* **38**: 325-28, 1990.
3. Better news on population. *Lancet* **339**: 1600, 1992.
4. Newton ER (Ed): Medical disorders of pregnancy. *Med Clin North Am* **73**:517-752, 1989.
5. Hanretty K, Whittle M: Identifying abnormalities. In Prescribing in Pregnancy, 2nd edition. Edited by Rubin PC. BMJ Publications, 1995.
6. Moore KL: The developing human: Clinically oriented embryology. 4th edition. Philadelphia: WB Saunders: 131, 1988.
7. Geiger JM, Baudin M, Saurat JH: Teratogenic risk with etretinate and acitretin treatment. *Dermatology* **189**:109-16, 1994.
8. Arulkumaran S: Prescribing for the pregnant patient—Is any drug safe? Update on Obstetrics and Gynecology. Mont Elizabeth Hospital 13th Annual seminar. November, 1999.
9. Ledward RS: Drugs in pregnancy. In J Studd (Ed): *Progress in Obstetrics and Gynecology*, 12th edn. Churchill Livingstone, 1996.
10. Rubin PC: General principles. In Rubin PC (Ed): *Prescribing in Pregnancy*, 2nd edn. BMJ Publications, 1995.
11. Wise R: Antibiotics. In Rubin PC (Ed): *Prescribing in Pregnancy*, 2nd edn. BMJ Publications, 1995.
12. Sampson JE, Gravett MG: Other infectious conditions in pregnancy. In James DK, Steer PJ, Weiner CP, Gonik B (Eds): *High Risk Pregnancy - Management Options*, 2nd edn. W B Saunders, 1999.
13. Gilstrap LC, Little BB; Medication during pregnancy. In James DK, Steer PJ, Weiner CP, Gonik B (Eds): *High risk Pregnancy- Management Options*, 2nd edn. W B Saunders, 1999.
14. De Swiet M: Anticoagulants. In Rubin PC (Ed): *Prescribing in Pregnancy*, 2nd edn. BMJ Publications, 1995.
15. Sawle G: Epilepsy and anticonvulsant drugs. In Rubin PC (Ed): *Prescribing in Pregnancy*, 2nd edn. BMJ Publications, 1995.
16. Nelson-Piercy C: Neurological problems. In *Handbook of Obstetric Medicine*. ISIS Medical Media Ltd. Oxford, 1997.
17. Hopkinson HE: Treatment of cardiovascular diseases. In Rubin PC (Ed): *Prescribing in Pregnancy*, 2nd edn. BMJ Publications, 1995.
18. Howden CW: Treatment of common minor ailments. In Rubin PC (Ed): *Prescribing in Pregnancy*, 2nd edn. BMJ Publications, 1995.
19. Koren G, Pastuszak A, Ito S: Drug therapy. Drugs in pregnancy. *New England Journal of Medicine* **338(16)**: 1128-37, 1998.
20. Byron MA: Treatment of rheumatic diseases. In Rubin PC (Ed): *Prescribing in Pregnancy*, 2nd edn. BMJ Publications, 1995.
21. Loudon JB; Psychotropic drugs. In Rubin PC (Ed): *Prescribing in Pregnancy*, 2nd edn. BMJ Publications, 1995.
22. Drugs and Therapeutics bulletin. **37(9)**: 1999.

32.

Devendra Kanagalingam
Sabaratnam Arulkumaran

Acute Abdomen in Pregnancy

An acute abdomen is defined as any intra-abdominal process characterized by pain, tenderness and muscular rigidity for which emergency surgery must be considered. Although the approach to pregnant women with acute abdomen is very similar to that of non-pregnant individuals, factors are present which make management more challenging. These are as follows:
- Physiological changes in pregnancy may alter the clinical presentation, interpretation of physical signs and investigations in these women
- Intra-abdominal pathology may be unrelated to pregnancy, be associated or predisposed to be pregnancy or be complications of pregnancy
- Management of these conditions may differ in pregnant women and delivery of the fetus may need to be considered.

EFFECT OF PHYSIOLOGICAL CHANGES IN PREGNANCY

The clinician relies on symptoms in arriving at a diagnosis. Nausea, vomiting, constipation, increased frequency of micturition and abdominal discomfort are frequently experienced in normal pregnancies. It is useful to ask the woman who presents with an acute event if there has been a change in these symptoms from what she regards as usual for her pregnancy. The most noticeable physiological change in pregnancy is seen in the uterus which increases from its average non-pregnant weight of 70 to 1110 gm. This almost 20-fold increase in mass causes lifting and stretching of the abdominal wall. The ovaries become abdominal organs and come to lie posterior to the uterus, making the palpation of ovarian masses difficult. Other abdominal organs such as bowel and omentum are displaced superiorly, laterally or posterior to the uterus from their usual position. The underlying inflammatory process has no direct contact with the parietal peritoneum overlying the anterior abdominal wall. This prevents the muscular response in the form of tenderness and muscular rigidity or guarding. These clinical signs, which are regarded as the hallmark of the surgical abdomen, may thus be absent or develop much later in the pregnant woman. This is well illustrated by the presentation of acute appendicitis in pregnancy. In the non-pregnant individual, the base of the appendix is beneath the McBurney's point which is located one-third of the way on an imaginary line drawn between the anterior superior iliac spine and the umbilicus. Tenderness at this point in association with abdominal pain and fever is the classical presentation of acute appendicitis. In late pregnancy, the appendix is displaced upward and laterally to lie in close proximity to the gallbladder. This results in a confusing clinical picture in which pain from an inflamed appendix is felt in the upper abdomen. Tenderness and guarding may not be present leading to a delay in diagnosis and treatment.

Some very commonly used laboratory tests have altered reference ranges in pregnancy. The white blood cell count rises progressively in pregnancy. The upper limit of the accepted range in pregnancy is 16×10^9 but may be as high as 40×10^9 at the onset of labor. The count only returns to normal prepregnancy levels by the sixth postpartum day. Therefore, leukocytosis may not be helpful in detecting the presence of an infective or inflammatory process. Although the number of red blood cells increases in pregnancy, there is a relatively greater increase in plasma volume. This results in a physiological hemodilution in pregnant women. The accepted lower limit of the normal range for hemoglobin concentration in pregnancy is 11 g/dl which should be taken into consideration when evaluating women with suspected intra-abdominal bleeding. In addition, the platelet count may be physiologically low in pregnancy (gestational thrombocytopenia) and alkaline phosphatase levels as measured by liver function tests are often elevated.

DIFFERENTIAL DIAGNOSIS

Conditions Unrelated to Pregnancy

The recognition that the cause of acute abdomen in a pregnant woman overlaps specialities is important. The obstetrician must involve surgeons and physicians when the cause is suspected to be incidental or unrelated to pregnancy. A list of the more commonly seen of these conditions is shown in Table 32.1.

Table 32.1: Acute abdomen from conditions unrelated to pregnancy

- Acute appendicitis
- Acute pancreatitis
- Ovarian cyst accidents
- Peptic ulcer
- Abdominal trauma
- Intraperitoneal hemorrhage

The incidence of acute appendicitis in pregnancy is 1 in 1500 pregnancies which is similar to that found in the non-pregnant population. However, there is an increased morbidity and mortality from acute appendicitis in pregnant women which is largely related to a delay in diagnosis and treatment. The alteration of clinical symptoms and signs in these women is described at the beginning of this chapter. The clinician must, therefore, have a high index of suspicion for this condition when no other cause for the abdominal symptoms can be found. Surgery may have to be undertaken when appendicitis is suspected even when clinical signs are equivocal. The negative laparotomy rates, i.e. cases in which a normal appendix is found, in these women may be as high as 35 percent but this is justified on the basis that delaying treatment in genuine cases would lead to considerable maternal and fetal morbidity and mortality. The altered location of the appendix requires that an appropriate surgical incision be used. The incision commonly used in non-pregnant women is known as a grid-iron muscle splitting incision which is placed at McBurney's point. This is clearly unsuitable in pregnancy and a midline or paramedian incision should be used. As a rule the appendicitis is managed and the pregnancy left undisturbed.

The predominant symptoms and signs of acute pancreatitis are not altered by pregnancy. The most common presentation is of nausea, vomiting and severe non-colicky epigastric pain radiating to the back which is relieved by leaning forward. When acute pancreatitis occurs in the first trimester, the diagnosis may be missed as these symptoms are often attributed to the physiological changes in pregnancy. The principle laboratory test, serum amylase, tends to be low in pregnancy. In view of this, even modestly elevated levels of serum amylase may be significant. Amylase in the serum is rapidly excreted so a urinary diastase estimation must always be ordered concurrently. The disease is generally self-limiting and responds to bed rest, parenteral fluids and pain relief.

Bleeding may sometimes occur spontaneously from a corpus luteum which is physiologically present in the first trimester of pregnancy. Rarely, bleeding may be considerable leading to hypovolemia and shock. In these women, surgical intervention for hemostasis will be necessary. In early pregnancy, this can be achieved by laparoscopy and diathermy of the bleeding vessel. The corpus luteum should not be removed as it is necessary for hormonal support of the pregnancy and a miscarriage may occur if this is done. Neoplastic ovarian cysts may be found in pregnant women, the most common being a benign cystic teratoma or dermoid cyst. These may be identified incidentally during a first trimester ultrasound scan. As the pregnancy progresses and the uterus enlarges, the ovaries lie freely suspended by their ovarian ligaments and are prone to torsion. The incidence of torsion of ovarian cysts in pregnant women may be as high as 22 percent. Early intervention when torsion is suspected is important to enable the ovaries to be conserved. Delay may result in gangrene of the ovary which necessitates removal of the entire affected adnexa.

Peptic ulcer disease (PUD) is infrequent in pregnancy and a remission rate of 90 percent in women with pre-existing PUD has been reported. Nevertheless, the acute complications of PUD in the form of a bleeding or perforated ulcer are important as they carry significant maternal and fetal risk. In perforated ulcers, free gas can often be identified under the diaphragm on an erect chest X-ray. This can be safely performed in pregnancy with an abdominal shield to protect the fetus. Radiation from a single chest X-ray has not been shown to result in harmful fetal effects. Bleeding peptic ulcers must be dealt with aggressively as maternal hypovolemia is dangerous to both mother and fetus.

Abdominal trauma in pregnant women is frequently a result of motor vehicle accidents. Apart from other visceral injuries, there is a risk of placental abruption which must be excluded whenever there is a history of closed abdominal trauma. Pregnant women should always use a seat belt with the straps correctly positioned "above and below the bump and not over it". Spontaneous intraperitoneal hemorrhage is rare but hepatic rupture which may be seen with pre-eclampsia and rupture of a splenic artery aneurysm are seen more frequently in pregnant women than their non-pregnant counterparts.

Conditions Associated with Pregnancy

Table 32.2 enlists causes of acute abdomen to which pregnant women are predisposed to as a result of the anatomical and physiological changes in pregnancy.

Table 32.2: Conditions associated with pregnancy

- Urinary tract infections
- Ureteric stones (Urolithiasis)
- Acute cholecystitis
- Acute fatty liver of pregnancy
- Red degeneration of a fibroid
- Rupture of the rectus abdominis muscle
- Torsion of the pregnant uterus

In pregnancy, there is dilatation of the ureters and pelvicalyceal system resulting in urinary stasis in the form of increased "dead space". This makes the pregnant woman susceptible to urinary tract infections (UTI). Asymptomatic bacteriuria, which is the presence of pathogens in a urine culture specimen in the absence of clinical signs of infection, should always be treated with antibiotics in pregnant women as 30 percent of such cases will progress to clinical UTI. In acute cystitis, the infection is confined to the bladder and is characterized by suprapubic pain, dysuria, frequency, urgency and hematuria. Oral antibiotics in the form of ampicillin or amoxycillin is effective. When the infection involves the upper urinary tract (kidney and ureters), the presentation is of acute pyelonephritis. The classical symptoms are fever, rigors and loin pain and the woman is constitutionally unwell. Acute pyelonephritis may predispose to preterm labor and delivery and must be treated aggressively with intravenous antibiotics. A perinephric abscess is a rare fulminant variety of pyelonephritis for which surgical drainage is sometimes necessary. Physiological dilatation of the urinary tract predisposes to passage of renal calculi down the ureters. This is manifested by ureteric colic which is characterised by severe, colicky "loin to groin" pain. Nausea, vomiting and gross or microscopic hematuria may also be present. Treatment is dependent on the size of the stone although most stones are small and will be passed out spontaneously. Hydration and pain relief should be instituted. Minimally-invasive procedures such as ureteroscopic retrieval of stones can be considered.

Extracorporeal shock-wave lithotripsy (ESWL), the use of sound waves to fragment urinary tract calculi, has not been approved for use in pregnancy.

Acute cholecystitis is more common in pregnant women. The physiologically increased serum cholesterol levels and delayed emptying of the gallbladder are predisposing factors. Pre-existing asymptomatic gallstones are present in 3 percent of pregnant women and is the cause of acute cholecystitis in most cases. The classical signs and symptoms are nausea, vomiting, acute right hypochondrial pain, tenderness and guarding. Murphy's sign, the presence of tenderness on deep inspiration in the right subcostal margin, is less commonly elicited in pregnancy. In addition, the evaluation of tenderness and guarding can be difficult in the third trimester because of the large uterus. Acute cholecystitis is generally managed conservatively by intravenous hydration, nasogastric suction, and appropriate use of analgesia and antibiotics. Complications such as perforation or empyema of the gallbladder (a collection of pus in the gallbladder) must be treated surgically.

Acute fatty liver in pregnancy (AFLP) is peculiar to pregnancy and has an incidence of 1:10000 pregnancies. The pathogenesis is unknown. The condition is heralded by nausea, vomiting, abdominal pain and jaundice without fever. Pregnancy-induced hypertension is commonly present. There is rapid progression to hepatic coma, disseminated intravascular coagulation (DIC) and renal failure. Mortality in AFLP is high, upto 90 percent in untreated cases. Early recognition and delivery is the only treatment and can result in survival rates of more than 70 percent. Survivors often recover with no residual liver damage and recurrence in subsequent pregnancies is rare.

In red degeneration of a uterine fibroid (leiomyoma), acute infarction occurs during pregnancy in a pre-existing fibroid. This results from rapid growth of the fibroid in pregnancy such that there is inadequate blood supply to the core of the fibroid. Pain, tenderness, low grade fever as well as nausea and vomiting may be present. If a fibroid is palpable, tenderness can usually be localized to it. The name "red degeneration" is derived from the typical appearance of the cut section of these fibroids in a pathological specimen. Treatment must be conservative in the form of analgesia as the condition is self-limiting and surgery for uterine fibroids in pregnancy is contraindicated.

Rupture of the rectus abdominis muscle is rare but is associated with pregnancy. The majority of women are multiparas. The typical presentation is of acute abdominal pain precipitated by a forceful cough. A tender, elongated swelling may be palpable on the affected side of the abdomen. The significance of this condition is the difficulty in differentiating it from other causes of acute abdomen. Treatment is usually conservative though a small number of women may need surgery if the hematoma is enlarging or if other causes of a surgical abdomen cannot be excluded. Torsion of the pregnant uterus is similarly rare and is often discovered incidentally at laparotomy for a suspected placental abruption. The cardinal symptom is severe abdominal pain in the presence of fetal malpresentation or obstructed labor. The uterus may need to be incised on the posterior aspect of the lower segment to effect delivery, after which spontaneous rotation of the uterus to its normal position occurs.

Complications of Pregnancy

Table 32.3 enlists the complications of pregnancy which present as an acute abdomen

Table 32.3: Pregnancy associated complications

- Ectopic pregnancy
- Septic miscarriage
- Acute retention of urine from a retroverted gravid uterus
- Placental abruption
- Preterm labor
- Uterine rupture

The triad of lower abdominal pain, vaginal bleeding and a positive pregnancy test are classical of an ectopic pregnancy. Atypical presentations are not uncommon leading to delay in diagnosis and treatment. A high index of suspicion is important as mortality from this condition, though rare, is still present. The presence of abdominal tenderness and shoulder tip pain indicate the presence of free blood in the peritoneal cavity from rupture of the ectopic pregnancy. A pelvic examination is best avoided when ectopic gestations are suspected as they may provoke bleeding or rupture. The advent of transvaginal ultrasound scanning and quantitative serum beta-hCG estimations have revolutionized the treatment of this condition. The basis of clinical diagnosis is the absence of an intrauterine pregnancy on transvaginal ultrasound in the presence of a serum beta-hCG level exceeding 1500 IU/liter. Treatment is usually surgical. An increasing number of ectopic pregnancies are treated by laparoscopy rather than the traditional laparotomy. A linear salpingotomy (incising the fallopian tube to remove the pregnancy) or salpingectomy (removal of the affected tube) can be performed. In a small group of women with unruptured ectopic pregnancies who are clinically stable, medical treatment in the form of intramuscular methotrexate may allow surgery to be avoided and the fallopian tube conserved.

Septic miscarriage is uncommon today as a result of legalized termination of pregnancy and the eradication of criminal abortion. The condition can also arise following an incomplete miscarriage, the dilated cervical os and the presence of retained products of conception allowing ascending infection to occur. These women are often unwell. Fever, abdominal pain and tenderness may be present. A pelvic examination may reveal a dilated cervix with offensive vaginal discharge. Intravenous broad-spectrum antibiotics followed by surgical evacuation of the uterus under anesthesia should be carried out.

After 12 weeks gestation, the uterus begins to rise out of the pelvis to become an abdominal organ. It is at this time that the weight of a retroverted gravid uterus may cause the cervix to be displaced anteriorly and abut against the urethra and bladder neck. This may lead to acute retention of urine for which passage of a urinary catheter may become necessary. Fortunately, the condition is self-limiting as the uterus soon rises into the abdomen and the retroversion is corrected. The pressure on the urethra and bladder neck is relieved allowing normal voiding to occur.

In later pregnancy, placental abruption may occur. Bleeding occurs in the interface between the placenta and the uterus leading to a partial or complete detachment of the placenta. The condition is also known as accidental hemorrhage, emphasizing that it is unpredictable and can occur in any pregnancy. There is an association with pregnancy-induced hypertension. The typical history is of sudden-onset abdominal pain with vaginal bleeding. The pain is described as being constant and board-like rigidity of the abdomen may be present. In 20 percent of cases, the bleeding is completely concealed. A placental abruption is an obstetric emergency as the lives of both mother and fetus are at risk. In severe placental abruption, fetal death is immediate and the mother is at risk of hemorrhage. Hemorrhage occurs both at the time of the abruption as well as subsequently from disseminated intravascular coagulation (DIC) with which it is associated. The diagnosis of placental abruption is made clinically as ultrasound cannot reliably detect it. The definitive treatment is delivery though resuscitation, detection and correction of coagulopathy are important. Vaginal delivery can often be achieved if there is no fetal distress as labor may ensue following an abruption. If vaginal delivery is not imminent or if fetal wellbeing is compromised, delivery by cesarean section is necessary. Supportive treatment in the form of blood products such as fresh frozen plasma and cryoprecipitate may be necessary after delivery if coagulopathy is present.

In preterm labor, painful uterine contractions and cervical dilatation occur prior to 37 weeks gestation. Preterm labor is an important diagnosis to establish as it is a major cause of perinatal mortality and morbidity. The history of painful uterine contractions is not conclusive as 50 percent of women with this symptom will have spurious labor and the contractions will subside. Serial pelvic examinations may be necessary to detect cervical change. There are no effective interventions to prevent preterm labor. Management is therefore, directed at treatment. The mainstay of this is to administer tocolytics (drugs which cause uterine relaxation), administering steroids to promote fetal lung maturation and ensuring that the laboring woman is transferred to a center with adequate facilities to care for premature neonates. It is important to remember that tocolytic drugs have only been shown to delay delivery by an average of 24-48 hours and that serious maternal side effects from these medications are present.

Uterine rupture is a catastrophic event which carries a high fetal and maternal mortality. The condition is predisposed to by multiparity and the presence of previous uterine scars such as a cesarean section. This occurs in 1:200 women with a previous lower segment uterine scar for which labor is undertaken. Induction of labor with prostaglandin pessaries or augmentation of uterine contractions with an oxytocin infusion is an additional risk factor. These interventions should be avoided or used very cautiously in these women. In women with a previous cesarean section, scar tenderness may manifest when uterine rupture is imminent. Most commonly, fetal heart abnormalities on the cardiotocograph (CTG) are the earliest detected signs. Continuous CTG monitoring during labor in these women is essential as it will allow early intervention. When a uterine rupture does occur, primary repair of the site of rupture may be possible although a hysterectomy is sometimes required.

MANAGEMENT OF THE FETUS

The management of the acute abdomen in pregnant women is made more complex by the need to evaluate fetal well-being and to modify management where appropriate due to fetal concerns. This is especially the case after 24 weeks gestation when fetal survival is possible. An assessment of the fetus must be included in the initial evaluation of these women. Evaluation of the fetal heart beat with a hand-held Doppler device or CTG as well as fetal ultrasound examinations are commonly used. Investigations and drugs used in these women may carry fetal risks. In most circumstances, it is necessary to weigh up the potential advantages of these interventions against their fetal risks. A discussion between the clinician and the pregnant woman is essential in arriving at mutually acceptable decisions.

The need to deliver the fetus should be based on obstetric indications. In conditions incidental to pregnancy, it is usually best to deal with the cause of the acute abdomen and leave the pregnancy undisturbed. An exception may be situations in which the mother is seriously ill and the fetus is judged to be at risk from this. Conversely, in conditions which are complications of pregnancy such as a placental abruption, delivery of the fetus is the definitive treatment and continuation of the pregnancy will be detrimental to both mother and fetus.

33. Antenatal Assessment of Fetal Wellbeing

Narendra Malhotra, Jaideep Malhotra, Amita Singh, Vanaj Mathur, Samiksha Gupta

INTRODUCTION

Assessment of fetal wellbeing is important not only for high risk patients but also for other pregnant women who might develop unexpected complications in the course of otherwise normal pregnancies. This chapter is dedicated to analyzing methods for classifying pregnant females into low risk and high risk group and to methods used for the fetal surveillance. Preconception counseling, preimplantation diagnostic methods and role of molecular biology in antenatal fetal monitoring are also discussed.

A wide range of tests of fetal wellbeing have been introduced during the last thirty years. Both biochemical tests (which monitor the endocrine function of the placenta or the fetoplacental unit) and biophysical methods of monitoring (which provide different information about fetal growth and physiological function) have the theoretical ability to detect changes in fetal wellbeing that may occur over hours, days or weeks.

Antenatal monitoring is clinically useful due to two reasons:
- *Firstly:* These methods can detect or predict fetal compromise.
- *Secondly:* With appropriate interpretation and action they can reduce the frequency or severity of adverse perinatal events and needless interventions.

Tests of fetal wellbeing have been used both as screening tests with the purpose of preventing those otherwise unpredictable fetal problems that occur from time to time, and in specific clinical situations with a high estimated fetal risk. However, it should be understood that no known method of assessment can predict sudden events, such as cord prolapse or placental abruption, which may also cause fetal damage or death.

HIGH RISK PATIENT

A careful elaboration of a medical and obstetrical history not only helps the obstetrician to identify the pregnant patient at high risk but also elaborates the need for referral to a maternal fetal medicine specialist.

Following patients should be referred to a specialist:
1. Cases that may require invasive procedures for fetal diagnosis or fetal therapy:
   a. Rh isoimmunization
   b. Nonimmunologic fetal hydrops

c. Fetal urinary tract obstruction
   d. Fetal congenital heart block
   e. Fetal hydrocephaly and fetal anomalies
2. Cases with medical complications:
   a. Brittle diabetes
   b. Cardiac disease grades III and IV
   c. Artificial heart valves
   d. Systemic lupus erythematosus
   e. Sickle cell disease
3. Cases with bad obstetric history:
   a. Habitual abortion
   b. Failed cerclages
   c. Recurrent stillbirths
   d. Recurrent early rupture of membranes
   e. Recurrent pre-term labor
4. Cases with complications requiring specialized care for management:
   a. Severe pre-eclampsia or eclampsia with renal failure, pulmonary edema, hypertension unresponsive to treatment, intracranial bleeding or severe HELLP syndrome.

METHODS OF FETAL SURVEILLANCE

Clinical Methods

1. *Perabdomen examination:* Measurement of fundal height (distance between the upper border of the pubic symphysis and the uterine fundus) and the measurement of abdominal girth at the level of the umbilicus.

   Fundal height measurement may be useful as a screening test for further investigation—as it has good sensitivity and specificity for predicting low birth weight for gestation. Vertical length of gravid uterus is measured from superior border of symphysis pubis to fundus in cm.

   Abdominal girth measurement has not been adequately evaluated. It is estimated that at 30 weeks, abdominal girth with normal fetal growth comes to 30". One inch increase occurs per week till term. This is an imprecise method and depends on the degree of obesity of each woman.

2. *Fetal movement counting:* Reduction and cessation of fetal movements may precede fetal death by a day or more (Movement Alarm sign), recognition of this reduction, followed by appropriate action to confirm fetal jeopardy and expedite delivery could prevent fetal death. The most commonly used method is to ask the mother to record on a chart daily, the time at which she has noticed 10 kicks (Cardiff count of 10 formula).

   The cause of most antepartum late fetal deaths, however, is unknown. These deaths are unpredictable and the extent to which they can be prevented by current forms of antenatal care is, therefore, limited. Screening by fetal movement, because it can be performed each day, has theoretical advantages over other tests of fetal wellbeing, all of which are either difficult or impossible to perform daily for practical reasons.

Fetal Biometry

Fetal biometry is the most important test for following the high-risk patient. All patients classified as high risk should have serial ultrasound examinations every 4 to 6 weeks to follow fetal growth. If necessary, it can be performed every 2 to 3 weekly. Frequency of testing at shorter intervals may not show adequate growth. It helps the obstetrician to determine the gestational age of the fetus and the adequacy of fetal growth. BPD, FL, HC, and AC are measured and compared with the norms, and deviations from normality can be recognized.

1. *Biparietal diameter (BPD):* Serial measurements of BPD help in detecting impaired fetal growth which can show two patterns, viz *slow growth profile*. There is continuous BPD growth during the entire pregnancy but the measurements remain below the 10th percentile for the gestational age at all times.
   Late flattening profile: There is normal BPD growth during the first two trimesters of pregnancy followed by arrest of growth during the last trimester. This group is more likely to develop antepartum and neonatal problems than fetuses with slow growth profile.

   The main disadvantage of using BPD as a biometric profile to detect intrauterine growth restriction is the low sensitivity and specificity. This is because the head is one of the last organs affected by fetal malnutrition.

2. *Abdominal circumference (AC):* A normal AC practically rules out the possibility of a small for date baby—the negative predictive value of a single measurement of AC is over 90 percent.

The AC should be measured at the level of the bifurcation of the hepatic vein in the center of the fetal liver.

The rate of growth of the abdominal circumference is linear from 15 weeks gestation onward. A growth rate less than 1 cm in 2 weeks identifies most IUGR babies, but it is best to plot serial measurements on a chart.

3. *Estimated fetal weight:* Usually obtained by the formula given by Hadlock *et al*. The margin of error is usually within 5 to 10 percent of the true fetal weight. This method is valuable in diagnosis of small fetuses with a sensitivity of 87 percent and a specificity of 87 percent when the estimated fetal weight is below the 10th percentile for the gestational age.

4. *Head to abdomen circumference ratio (H/A Ratio):* This ratio compares the most preserved organ in the malnourished fetus viz the brain, with the most compromised, the liver and is of significant value in identifying asymmetric IUGR babies. When a baby is small and symmetric, the liver will be preserved and the H/A ratio will be normal. The H/A ratio decreases with the gestational age. Fetal malnutrition should be suspected when the H/A ratio is abnormally high. A small fetus with normal H/A ratio may be symmetric IUGR or may be small and healthy.

5. *Femur to abdomen ratio (F/A ratio):* This method compares the femur length (FL), which is minimally affected by fetal growth impairment, with the abdominal circumference (AC), which is the most affected measurement. This ratio remains constant after 20 weeks. Normal value is 22 + 2. When F/A ratio is abnormally high, fetal malnutrition is suspected. When this ratio is normal, the chances of IUGR are unlikely although the baby may be small and healthy.

6. *Fetal ponderal index (PI):* Obtained by dividing the estimated fetal weight by the third power of the femur length. Normal value is 8.325+2.5 (2 SD) remaining constant through out the second part of the pregnancy. A fetal PI of 7.0 or less should be considered abnormal and strongly suggestive of fetal malnutrition.

7. *Newer parameters:* Thigh circumference and liver volume are being studied.

Detection of Congenital Abnormalities in the Fetus

This has been discussed in Chapter 17 on Prenatal Diagnosis.

AMNIOTIC FLUID INDEX

Amniotic fluid reflects the physiology of the fetus and the two important sources of AF are:
- Fetal urine
- Lung
- Fetal oronasal cavities (to some extent).

AF is removed by:
- Fetal swallowing
- Blood perfusing the fetal surface of placenta

The AF serves to protect the fetus during the pregnancy and AFI (amniotic index representing the fluid volume) gradually increases throughout pregnancy from 60 ml in 1st trimester to around 900 ml at term Wallenburg (1977)[1], Seeds (1980).[2]

Various methods are available for measurement of adequacy of amniotic fluid in the third trimester:
- 1 cm Pocket (minimum), Manning and Platt 1979
- 2 cm Pocket (minimum), Chamberlain *et al* 1984
- 3 cm Vertical pocket (atleast one), Crowley, O' Herlihy 1984
- Four Quadrant method, Phelan *et al* 1987

Method of measuring AFI (Amniotic fluid index)
- Patient should be in supine position
- Uterus is divided into four quadrants using the umbilicus and linea nigra as reference points
- Ultrasound transducer is placed on maternal abdomen in each quadrant in long axis
- Largest vertical AF pocket in each quadrant is measured.

The sum of the four measurements is the AFI in cm. The following criteria of Phelan *et al* for AFI are almost universally accepted:

Amniotic Fluid Index (Phelan)

5 cm or less	Oligohydramnios
5-8 cm	Borderline AFI
8-24 cm	Normal AFI
25 cm or more	Polyhydramnios

Oligohydramnios may be due to:
- Fetal renal agenesis or urinary tract obstruction.
- PIH, essential hypertension and IUGR (alone or together). It indicates *decreased renal perfusion and redistribution* of blood to adrenals, heart and brain. As such oligohydramnios is an indicator of chronic placental insufficiency/chronic fetal asphyxia.
- Post-maturity also causes *decreased placental perfusion.*

Oligohydramnios may lead to:
- Thoracic compression (lung, heart changes)
- Cord compression and hypoxia, amniotic bands
- Limb abnormalities
- Preterm deliveries
- Growth restriction (usually oligohydramnios is the consequence)
- Stillbirth

Polyhydramnios is associated with:
- Anencephaly and spina-bifida
- Upper GI obstruction; for example, esophageal and duodenal atresia
- Multiple pregnancies
- Large placenta
- Maternal diabetes
- Rh incompatibility
- Syphilis and other infection

Oligohydramnios is more important because of its association with fetal hypoxia. AFI assessment is useful in antepartum surveillance along with biophysical profile parameters to determine the proper time of intervention resulting in a good perinatal outcome.
- Low AFI 5-8 cm: Closer daily surveillance is indicated
- Less than 5 cm: Consider delivery by induction or elective cesarean section depending on the clinical situation, fetal maturity and results of the other tests of fetal wellbeing.

Studies show that low AFI is associated with (Divon and Mark (1995),[7] Grubb and Paul (1992),[8] Jayanti Karetal (2000):[9]
- Higher incidence of operative deliveries
- Fetal distress
- Low Apgar score
- High perinatal mortality.

Anand Kumar, Biswas *et al* (1993), Bowen, Chatoor and Kulkarni (1995), Jayanti Kar *et al* (2000) have also reported similar PNM.

PATIENTS WITH ABNORMAL FETAL ULTRASOUND FINDING

Since the frequency of chromosomal disorder associated with fetal malformations is high, karyotyping through amniocentesis or umbilical blood sampling may be required in such cases. These procedures are discussed in Chapter 17 on Prenatal Diagnosis.

Biophysical Tests

Biophysical tests have greatly increased the understanding of fetal behavior and development and have almost completely replaced biochemical tests. These tests include:
- Non-stress test (NST)
- Contraction stress test (CST)
- Fetal biophysical profile (BPP)
- Vibroacoustic stimulation test (VAST)
- Modified biophysical profile (MBPP)
- Umbilical and uterine Doppler ultrasound

Non-stress Test

The evaluation of fetal heart rate patterns, without the added stress of induced contractions, has been widely incorporated into antenatal care for both screening and diagnosis. It is an assessment of immediate fetal condition.

The rationale underlying this is that the presence of spontaneous fetal heart rate accelerations associated with fetal movements (fetal reactivity) is an indicator of fetal wellbeing and vice versa.

The variables that must be evaluated in a NST are:

- *Baseline fetal heart rate* (Normal being 110-160 beats/minute): Alterations of baseline frequency are most commonly due to maternal medications and maternal temperature but fetal hypoxia can be the cause.
- *Variability of fetal heart rate:* Variability (the minor fluctuations of the baseline rate assessed over a minute) depends on the interaction of the fetal sympathetic and parasympathetic systems and is influenced by gestational age, maternal medications, fetal congenital anomalies, fetal acidosis and fetal tachycardia. The normal baseline variability is more than 5 beats.
- *Presence or absence of accelerations:* Presence of accelerations in the FHR associated with fetal movements or in response to fetal stimulation is a reliable sign of fetal health. Presence of accelerations is related to gestational age; occurring more frequently as a pregnancy approaches term.
- A *reactive test* is present when two or more FHR accelerations are clearly recorded during a 20-minute period, each acceleration of 15 or more beats per minute and lasting 15 or more seconds, usually occurring simultaneously with episodes of fetal activity.
- *Presence or absence of decelerations:* Absence of decelerations is reassuring. Although NST is noninvasive easily performed and interpreted and readily accepted by patients, it has high frequency of false-positive results (~ 50-80%).[5] False-negative rate is only 3.2 per 1000, so the likelihood of fetal death or serious fetal morbidity following a negative (reactive) test is extremely low. NST is not an ideal test for primary fetal surveillance because of its inability to recognize early stages of fetal distress.

Contraction Stress Test

Since many fetal deaths occur prior to the onset of labor, the stimulation of contractions with oxytocin and observing fetal heart rate under labor like conditions in pregnancies at risk is known as "oxytocin challenge test" or "contraction stress test".

This test is based on experimental evidence showing that the uteroplacental blood flow decreases markedly or ceases during uterine contractions. Therefore, uterine contractions cause a hypoxic stress that a normal, healthy fetus can tolerate without difficulty. In contrast, a fetus with chronic or acute problems will not be able to tolerate such a decrease in oxygen supply and this will result in decelerations following contractions.

The end point of CST is the presence or absence of late deceleration of the fetal heart rate following uterine contractions induced by intravenous oxytocin or by nipple stimulation. CST has a false-negative rate of 0.4/1000, which is significantly better than NST, and a false-positive rate of 50 percent.

Although CST can detect early stages of hypoxia. It has many disadvantages, viz:

1. Time consuming
2. Requires an intravenous infusion
3. Can cause fetal hypoxia
4. Contraindicated in APH, prelabor rupture of membranes in the preterm period, etc.
5. May cause preterm labor if done in the preterm period.

Fetal Biophysical Profile

It combines five biophysical variables considered to be of prognostic significance, viz. fetal movement, tone, reactivity, breathing and amniotic fluid volume into a score and is an excellent test for the evaluation of fetal wellbeing. These variables are dependent on the integrity of the fetal central nervous system and are affected in situations of fetal compromise.

It is a better predictor of low 5-minute Apgar scores than the non-stress test and is both more sensitive and more specific in predicting overall abnormal outcome than the non-stress test. This test has no contraindications, and involves no risk for the mother or the fetus. An additional advantage of the biophysical profile over the non-stress test is that it permits assessment of the possibility of major congenital anomalies. This may be important as detection of a serious anomaly may on occasion help to avoid a cesarean section when the baby is clearly abnormal.

False-negative rate of BPP is 0.7/1000 and false-positive rate is 30 percent—better than that of NST or CST.[7]

Physiology: The BPP variables are dependent on the activity of certain areas of the fetal central nervous system that become functional at different gestational ages.
- *Fetal tone and movement* appear between 7 and 9 weeks and require activity of the brain cortex.
- *Fetal breathing movements* begin at 20 to 21 weeks and depend on centers in the ventral surface of the fourth ventricle.
- *Fetal heart rate reactivity* appears between 28 and 30 weeks and depends on function of the posterior hypothalamus and nucleus in the upper medulla.

The sensitivity of each of these centers to hypoxia is different, and those that become functional earlier in fetal development are more resistant to acute changes in fetal oxygenation. Hence, the interpretation of the biophysical profile results should be made by separate analysis of each of the individual components of the test. Also decreased body movement and tone are found only when the fetal compromise is severe.

Manning score[12,13]—Each variable is allotted a score of either 0 or 2.
- A score of more than 8 is normal
- A score of 6 to 8 is suboptimal
- A score of less than 6 needs intervention

1. *Fetal breathing movement:* 30 seconds of sustained breathing movement during a 30-minute observation period.
2. *Fetal movement:* Three or more gross body movements in a 30-minute observation period.
3. *Fetal tone:* One or more episodes of limb motion from a position of flexion to extension and a rapid return to flexion.
4. *Fetal reactivity:* Two or more FHR accelerations associated with fetal movement of at least 15 bpm and lasting at least 15 seconds in 20 minutes.
5. *Fluid volume:* Presence of a pocket of amniotic fluid that measures at least 1 cm in two perpendicular planes (with no cord in the pocket). The predictive value in terms of perinatal mortality is better if this measurement is more than 2 cm. Many centers adopt 2 cm as the cut off.

A normal BPP corresponds to a score of 8 or greater, but this value must include a normal amniotic fluid volume. The program of BPP is poor if the score for amniotic fluid is 0.

Modified Biophysical Profile

It is one of the best tests available for fetal surveillance. It combines the observation of an index of acute fetal hypoxia, NST with or without VAST, and a second index indicative of chronic fetal problems viz. the amniotic fluid volume.

1. If both tests are normal, weekly fetal surveillance with MBPP is continued.
2. If both tests are abnormal (non-reactive NST, decreased amniotic fluid volume) and pregnancy is more than 36 weeks, patient should be delivered. For less than 36 weeks gestational age, management is individualized depending on the circumstances.
3. If the amniotic fluid volume is decreased but the NST is reactive, a search for chronic fetal conditions, particularly congenital abnormalities is undertaken, and the frequency of MBPP testing is twice weekly.
4. If the amniotic fluid volume is normal and the NST is non-reactive, further testing with contraction stress test or full biophysical profile is indicated.

Vintzelos[14] pioneered the modification of the biophysical profile.

Accoustic Stimulation Test

The NST with the VAST (Vibroaccoustic stimulation test) is substituting the classical NST as the test most commonly used for antepartum fetal surveillance. The use of FAST reduces the number of non-reactive traces by producing accelerations with the stimulus. The use of VAST also reduces the testing time, thereby improving the efficiency of the services.

Methodology

Stimulation with an artificial larynx over the fetal head for 1 to 3 seconds producing a vibratory accoustic stimulus of approximately 80 Hz and 82dB. A healthy fetus will respond with sudden movement (startle response) followed by accelerations of the fetal heart rate.

According to Crade and Lovett,[15] fetuses of less than 24 weeks do not respond to vibroaccoustic stimulation.

Between 24 and 27 weeks of gestation 30 percent of all fetuses will respond between 27 and 30 weeks, 86 percent will respond, and after 31 weeks, 96 percent will respond to artificial larynx.

Accoustic Stimulation Result Criteria

Reactive: If either of following is observed within 15 seconds of stimulation:
1. Two 15 bpm accelerations, each of at least 15 seconds in a 10-minute interval after stimulation.
2. Single prolonged 15 bpm acceleration of greater than 2-minute duration.

Non-reactive:
1. Borderline: 10 to 14 bpm acceleration.
2. Abnormal (poor response): Less than 10 bpm accelerations.
3. Abnormal (non-response): Absence of accelerations.

If VAST is abnormal, it is repeated in 5-minutes—if the response is still poor, a biophysical profile or contraction stress test is performed.

If the fetus does not show movement under ultrasound observation, further evaluation for anomalies, fetal karyotype, TORCH titers and fetal acid-base assessment may be indicated.

VAST is safe, and no evidence of hearing impairment or other abnormality has been reported in neonates exposed to VAST *in utero*.

Several factors may influence the result of VAST viz thickness of the maternal abdominal wall, the amount of amniotic fluid, the pressure exerted by the examiner in holding the artificial larynx against the abdomen and the intensity of the stimulation. Only 2 percent of NSTS are non-reactive following VAST. Of those NSTS that are non-reactive to VAST, 17 percent are followed by positive contraction stress test or by biophysical profiles equal to or less than 4.

Color Doppler

Pulsed Doppler sonography is useful for detection and evaluation of intrauterine growth restriction and other high-risk pregnancy complications. It does correlate well with fetal compromise, often giving earlier warning of fetal distress than other tests.

Normal pregnancy is dependent on the development of an adequate fetal and ultraplacental circulation, which in turn is responsible for maternal fetal transfer of oxygen and nutrients and for the elimination of fetal waste products. Doppler ultrasound is based on 'Doppler effect' described by Christian Johanna Doppler in 1842, which shows the change in observed frequency of sound or light waves when there is relative motion between the source and the observer.

Doppler Spectrum

Single red cells do not produce Doppler echoes on their size is only a fraction of the wavelength of ultrasound. Scattering is more likely to be produced from random changes in the density of red cells in the plasma. Groups of cells close to the vessel wall move slowly whereas cells near the center of the blood vessel have the maximum velocity and produce the largest Doppler shifts.

The width of the Doppler spectrum is dependent upon the flow velocity profile, Plug flow occurs in arteries close to the heart, and as the distance away from the heart increases, flow becomes increasingly parabolic because of slowing produced by the friction of the vessel walls. In the umbilical artery and vein blood flow is probably entirely parabolic.

Doppler Equipment

Doppler signals may be obtained by three types of device:

Continuous wave–Doppler ultrasound equipment: It uses a probe, which emits ultrasound continuously from one crystal, and the back-scattered signals are received by a second crystal. Signals are obtained from all moving structures in the line of the Doppler beam. The main disadvantage is that the vessel being studied cannot be simultaneously visualized.

Pulsed Doppler ultrasound equipment: Here the same transducer is used to transmit and then to listen for returning signals by only allowing the equipment to receive echoes for a short period of time, the depth from which the echoes arise can be precisely determined. The combination of pulsed Doppler and realtime ultrasound is known as a duplex system, and allows simultaneous imaging at low pulse repetition frequency, usually less than 2.5 KHz. The sequence of transmitting and then receiving signals needs to be repeated to build up the Doppler signal. The rate at which pulses of ultrasound are emitted is known as the pulse repetition frequency (PRF). The higher the PRF the more pulses will be available per cycle, thus giving a better quality signal. However, the PRF is limited as there must be sufficient time to collect all echoes from one pulse prior to emitting a further pulse. The minimum PRF allowable must be twice the frequency of the Doppler signal.

Color flow equipment: It is a recent method where conventional realtime images are superimposed with blood flow information, coded in colors, to indicate the direction and velocity of flow.

Color flow mapping displays the direction of blood flow in three different formats; blue, indicating flow away from the transducer; red-orange, indicating flow toward the transducer; and a mosaic pattern of red-orange or blue-green which represents flow in several directions, suggesting turbulence. Vessels in the uteroplacental circulation are more easily visualized the arcuate artery being easily distinguished from the uterine vessels.

Qualitative Flow Analysis

- A/B = A/B ratio
- A-B/A = Resistance index
- A-B/Mean = Pulsatility index

Indications for Umbilical Artery Waveforms

1. Assessment and continued monitoring of the small for gestational age fetus.
2. Assessment of the fetus of a mother with systemic lupus erythematous (SLE) and PET.
3. Assessment of differing sizes or growth patterns in twins.
4. Conjunction with uteroplacental waveforms in the assessment of oligohydramnios.

The role of umbilical artery waveforms is not established in fetuses of insulin dependent diabetics. Fetal death has been reported within 24 hours of obtaining normal umbilical artery waveforms from the fetuses of such women as the cause of demise is likely to be metabolic and can be sudden rather than hypoxia.

Interpretation of the waveforms

1. In the absence of an acute incident such as a placental abruption a small for gestational age fetus with normal umbilical artery waveforms (Figure 33.1, Plate 2) is unlikely to develop loss of end-diastolic frequencies within a 7 day period, so that monitoring may be performed weekly.
2. Only 10 percent of fetuses that are demonstrated to be asymmetrically small for gestational age on real-time ultrasound will demonstrate loss of end-diastolic frequencies at any time during their pregnancy.
3. Loss of end-diastolic frequencies is associated with an 85 percent chance that the fetus will be hypoxic *in utero* and a 50 percent chance that it will also be acidotic.
4. The finding of a symmetrically small fetus with absent end-diastolic frequencies in the umbilical artery but with normal utero placental waveforms suggest the possibility of a primary fetal cause for the growth retardation such a chromosomal abnormality or a TORCH virus infection.
5. Fetuses demonstrating absence of end-diastolic frequencies but which are managed along standard clinical lines have a 40 percent chance of dying and at least a 25 percent morbidity rate from necrotizing enterocolitis, hemorrhage or coagulation failure after birth. The time between loss of end-diastolic frequencies and fetal death appears to differ for each fetus. Following loss of end-diastolic frequencies there are no other reliable changes in the waveform that help in deciding when to deliver the baby.
6. Reversed frequencies in end-diastolic are only observed in a few fetuses prior to death. This finding is a pre-terminal condition; few if any, fetuses will survive without some form of therapeutic intervention.
7. Loss of end-diastolic frequencies precedes changes in the cardiotocograph by some 7-42 days in fetuses that have been shown to be small for gestational age on realtime ultrasound. The occurrence of CTG decelerations not related to

contractions, together with absent end-diastolic frequencies, carries an extremely poor prognosis.
8. In cases of IUGR Wladimiroff and colleagues (1986) described compensatory reduction in vascular resistance in fetal brain during fetal hypoxemia usually called as 'Brain sparing effect' and is the earliest Doppler based marker for IUGR compromised fetus (Figure 33.2, Plate 2).
9. Detection of elevated resistance to flow within fetal descending aorta (Figure 33.3, Plate 2) reflects the increased vascular resistance associated with high-risk pregnancy not only within the placental vascular bed but also within fetal abdominal viscera.
10. Increased resistance in fetal renal arteries with growth restriction has been seen especially with oligohydramnios.
11. Increased resistance in uterine artery as indicated by an elevated index of resistance by persistence of an early diastolic notch often precedes the onset of growth restriction (Figure 33.4, Plate 2).

The future will improve our ability to study both the fetal and the uteroplacental circulation with color flow mapping that allows accurate localization of blood vessels. Knowledge of the balance between the cerebral circulation, aortic blood flow and the renal and mesenteric circulations may allow more precise timing of delivery than the approach of delivery for absence of end-diastolic frequencies.

Biochemical Tests

Biochemical testing in late pregnancy is now only of historical interest. They are not sensitive enough to detect the majority of pregnancies destined to have an adverse outcome. The tests needed the biochemical expertise and the lab, were retrospective and costly. The high false-positive and false-negative rates and the availability of less costly prospective biophysical modes of testing had made biochemical testing redundant.

- *Estriol assays:* The assays were done on blood or on 24 hour urinary collection. The fluctuations from time to time, the wide range and its dependence on urinary output made this test difficult to interpret. There was no evidence to suggest any benefit from estriol assays and hence, it is not used.

- Human placental lactogen: It rises in serum from 0.3 g/ml at 10-14 weeks to 10 g/ml at 36 weeks. It acts like growth hormone. There is little role of human placental lactogen measurements for surveillance of high-risk pregnancy.

CONCLUSION

The fetus growing and developing inside should be considered as a separate individual and not just another maternal organ. Antenatal evaluation of the fetal wellbeing begins right at the time of conception till delivery. A proper clinical antenatal examination will help in recognizing fetus at risk and will help us to use the appropriate tests available to achieve the ultimate goal of a healthy baby.

REFERENCES

1. Hadlock FP, Harrist RB, Sharman RB et al: Estimation of fetal weight with the use of head, body and femur measurements. A prospective study. Am J Obstet Gynecol **151**: 333, 1985.
2. Allen R: The significance of me conium in midtrimester genetic amniocentesis. Am J Obstet Gynecol **152**: 413-17, 1985.
3. Zorn EM, Hanson FW, Greve C, et al: Analysis of the significance of discolored amniotic fluid detected at midtrimester amniocentesis. Am J Obstet Gynecol **154**: 1234-40, 1986.
4. Hanson FW, Hopp RL, Tennant FR et al: Ultrasonography guided early amniocentesis in singleton pregnancies. Am J Obstet Gynecol **162**: 1376-83, 1990.
5. Devoe LD, Castillo RA, Sherline DM: The nonstress test as a diagnostic test: A critical reappraisal. Am J Obstet Gynecol **152**: 1047-53, 1985.
6. Thacker SB, Berkelnan RL: Assessing the diagnostic accuracy and efficacy of selected antepartum fetal surveillance techniques. Obstet Gynecol Surv **41**:121-41, 1986.
7. Vintzileos AM, Campbell WA, Ingardia CJ, et al: The fetal biophysical profile and its predictive value. Obstet Gynecol **62**: 271-78, 1983.
8. Trudinger B, Wiles W, Cook C et al: Fetal umbilical artery flow velocity waveforms and placental resistance: Clinical significance. Am J Obstet Gynecol **92**: 23, 1985.
9. Hardy K, Martin KL, Leese HJ, Winston RmL, Handyside AH: Human preimplantation development *in vitro* is not adversely affected by biopsy at the 8 cell stage. Hum Reprod **5**: 708-14, 1990.
10. Plachot M, Mandel bacem J, Junca AM, Grouchy JD, Sala Baroux J, Colen J: Cytogenetic analysis and developmental capacity of normal and abnormal embryos after IVF. Hum Reprod **4 (Suppl)**: 99-103, 1989.

11. Muggleton-Harris AL, Glazier AN, Pickering JJ: Biopsy of the human blastocyst and polymerase chain reaction (PCR) amplification of the B-globin gene and a dinucleotide repeat motif from 2-6 trophoectoderm cells. *Hum Reprod* **8:** 2197-2205, 1993.
12. Manning FA, Marrison I, Harman CR, *et al:* The abnormal fetal biophysical profile score: V. Predictive accuracy aurding to score composition. *Am J Obstet Gynecol* **162:** 918-24, 1990.
13. Manning FA, Harman CR, Marrison I, *et al:* Fetal assessment based on fetal biophysical profile scoring: IV. An analysis of perinatal scorbidily and mortality. *Am J Obstet Gynecol* **162:** 703-709, 1990.
14. Vintzileos AM, Campbell WA, Nochimson DJ, *et al:* The use and misure of the fetal biophysical profile. *Am J Obstet Gynecol* **156:** 527-33, 1987.
15. Crade M, Lovett S: Fetal response to sound stimulation: Preliminary report exploring use of sound stimulation in routine obstetrical ultrasound examinations. *J Ultrasound Med* **7:** 499-503, 1988.

34. Induction of Labor

Sambit Mukhopadhyay
Sabaratnam Arulkumaran

INTRODUCTION

The mechanism of onset of labor remains one of the most elusive regulatory problems in human reproductive physiology. Recent emphasis has been placed on cervical softening and dilatation. Methods used to induce labor primarily acts by causing cervical softening and dilatation. Failure to induce is not an uncommon problem. This again highlights our ignorance in the understanding of the basic mechanism of onset of labor.

Induction of labor is common in our daily practice. Done for the right reasons and the correct way it confers benefit. Advances in pharmacology and in biophysical methods of monitoring fetuses have made induction of labor a relatively safe procedure. Despite its safety, liberal induction policy due to inappropriate indications carry unnecessary risks of increased maternal morbidity and poor neonatal outcome.

INDUCTION

Induction is the initiation of uterine contractions in a pregnant woman who is not in labor with the intention of achieving vaginal delivery.

Indications for Induction

Induction is indicated when the risk of continuation of pregnancy exceeds the risk associated with induction and delivery. Maternal indications for induction are few as pregnant mother is accessible for examination and investigation. Virtually all cases of induction of labor are for fetal indications. While elective delivery/induction is advantageous to prevent maternal morbidity in severe pre-eclampsia, the advantageous is less clear when it is carried out for 'possible fetal compromise'. Current biophysical tests enable the evaluation of fetal health, but cannot be totally relied upon. The following conditions provide a list of clinical scenario when induction of labor is undertaken after proper evaluation fetal and maternal health. Performance of induction may be prioritized according to the urgency of the clinical situation and availability of resources.

Urgent

- Severe proteinuric hypertension (pre-eclampsia) with escalation of the condition
- Suspected fetal compromise (suspicious CTG, marked oligohydramnios)
- Severe IUGR

- Significant maternal disease not responding to treatment
- Chorioamnionitis
- Significant antepartum hemorrhage.

Semi-urgent

- Prelabor rupture of membranes at term
- IUGR without evidence of fetal compromise
- Poorly controlled diabetes
- Isoimmune disease at or near term.

Elective or Non-urgent

- 'Post-term pregnancy'
- Intrauterine fetal demise
- Logistic problem (location of residence from hospital)
- Gestational diabetes at term
- Suspected fetal macrosomia is a debatable indication for induction of labor. Induction of labor is sometime performed for the convenience of the mother in the absence of any medical reasons or clear health benefit. A request for such social indication under certain circumstances may be acceptable but should be discussed on an individual basis after fully informing the woman and her partner of any potential disadvantages.

Post-term Pregnancy

Post-term pregnancy is defined as a pregnancy continuing for more than 42 weeks or greater than 294 completed days. It occurs in about 6 percent of births. Post-term pregnancy is the most common indication for induction of labor and together with maternal request and social factors it accounts for 70 percent of all inductions. The risk of perinatal morbidity and mortality increases after 42 weeks of pregnancy and there is now good evidence from meta-analysis that induction of labor should be offered routinely to all women whose pregnancies continue beyond 41 weeks of gestation. Induction at 41+ weeks is associated with reduction in cesarean section and instrumental delivery rate, reduced risk of fetal distress, meconium staining, macrosomia and of perinatal mortality (Crowley 1994). If following discussion with the patient induction is not chosen, then fetal surveillance is required.

Contraindications

There are certain contraindications to induction of labor. These include the following:

- Placenta previa or cord presentation
- Abnormal lie (transverse or oblique lie)
- Prior classical or inverted T uterine incision*
- Active genital herpes
- Uterine surgery involving full thickness of the myometrium
- Pelvic structural deformities
- Invasive cervical carcinoma

METHODS OF INDUCTION OF LABOR

A thorough evaluation of mother and fetus is required before labor is induced. Confirmation of the period of gestation is required and ideally this should have been with the use of ultrasound in the first or early second trimester. It is a routine practice in the United Kingdom to offer mid-trimester ultrasound scans between 18 to 20 weeks of pregnancy. Clinical examination should include abdominal examination to confirm lie and presentation and vaginal examination to assess the favorability of the cervix. The cervix should be assessed by means of Bishop score or one of its modifications. The score was subsequently modified by Calder (1979) by substituting the length of the cervix for percentage of effacement. A score of more than 6 is considered favorable and is likely to result in successful labor induction.

Table 34.1: Modified Bishop's score (Calder *et al* 1979)

	Scores			
	0	1	2	3
Cervical dilatation (cm)	0	1-2	3-4	5-6
Cervical length (cm)	>4	3-4	1-2	<1
Cervical consistency	Firm	Medium	Soft	-
Cervical position	posterior	central	anterior	
Station (cm to spines)	−3 above	−2 above	−1 to 0 above	Below spines

If the cervix is unfavorable the need for induction should be reconsidered. Induction with an unfavorable

---

* It is important to review the operative notes of previous cesarean section before deciding the exact mode of delivery in the subsequent pregnancy.

cervix is associated with high rate of induction failure and increased rate of cesarean deliveries (Arulkumaran et al, 1985a). An unfavorable cervix can be made favorable by cervical ripening using either pharmacological or mechanical means.

Cervical Ripening

Important structural and biochemical changes take place in the cervix thereby transforming the cervix from a sphincteric organ acting to preserve and contain the growing fetus to a canal which softens, shortens and dilates to facilitate the passage of the fetus. The methods used for cervical ripening are as follows:

Pharmacological Methods of Cervical Ripening

Prostaglandins

Both PGE2 and PGF2a have been used for this purpose, although PGE2 seems to be more effective than PGF2a. Synthetic prostaglandin analogues have generally been avoided for ripening or induction because of the uncertainties over their effects on fetus and neonate. Prostaglandins may be given via the oral, intravaginal, intracervical or intravenous routes all of which are effective. Intracervical gel and intravaginal preparations have fewer systemic side effects compared with other methods of administration. When compared with placebo or no treatment, the use of prostaglandins for cervical priming does ripen the cervix, reduces the likelihood of not being delivered in 12 to 24 hours, lowers epidural rate and decreases cesarean and operative vaginal delivery rates (Keirse, 1995a). This occurs at the expense of increased gastrointestinal side effects and uterine hypertonus or hyperstimulation in about 7 percent of cases (Keirse 1995b).

1. *Intracervical vs intravaginal prostaglandins:* Recent studies have found that intracervical gel has a higher failure rate than vaginal gel, as well as being more difficult to administer and less efficient at ripening the cervix (Nuntila et al, 1996, Seeras, 1995). Therefore, there are more advantages of using vaginal prostaglandins over intracervical prostaglandins.
2. *Sustained release preparation:* A variety of vehicles have been developed to deliver vaginal prostaglandins. These include lactic acid based pessaries, water-soluble gels and most recently hydrogel polymers. The hydrogel devices allow sustained and controlled release of prostaglandins to the vaginal tissues over the course of several hours. Recent developments allow the hydrogel pessary to be presented in a retrieval system (Propess, Ferring A B, Malmo, Sweden). Therefore, the insert can be removed from the vagina if uterine hypertonus or fetal distress develops. The insert contains 10 mg of PGE2, which is released over 12 hours period. The rate of release of any vaginal prostaglandin preparations may be affected by the pH, moisture, temperature and the presence of infection in the vagina. A high degree of patient acceptability is reported, although the preparation is expensive. Sustained release prostaglandin appears to be an effective cervical ripening agent resulting in change in Bishop score, and increasing rate of vaginal delivery within 12 hours compared to placebo. When compared to Prepidil or intracervical preparation, there is shorter time from induction to delivery with sustained-release form, but higher rate of excessive uterine activity. When compared to misoprostol, sustained-release prostaglandin does not appear to be as effective, as there is a lower rate of delivery in 12 hours and more women requiring oxytocin augmentation (Crane and Bennett, 2000).
3. *Doses of prostaglandin:* Intracervical PGE2gel (Prepidil) 0.5 mg and intravaginal PGE2 gel (Prostin) 1 mg and 2 mg are marketed for cervical ripening. A variety of doses and regimes have been used in different studies. In primigravidae with an unfavorable cervix, an initial dose of 2 mg may be given, followed by further 1mg doses at six hourly intervals to a maximum of 4 mg. In multigravidae or nullipare with a favorable cervix an initial dose of 1mg followed by further 1 mg doses at six hourly intervals to a maximum of 3 mg should be given (Manufacturer's Recommendation).
4. *Monitoring with prostaglandin gel:* At present it is common practice to monitor maternal and fetal wellbeing just prior to and for 30 to 60 minutes following PGE2 gel administration and once the

contraction become established. The pattern of uterine activity after prostin gel suggest that uterine activity usually starts after an hour and can last up to 4 hours. It usually peaks within this first 4 hours. Therefore, an observation ranging from 30 minutes to two hours may be appropriate.

Misoprostol

It is much cheaper and more easily stored than prostaglandins. It is efficacious but questions still remain as to the safest and most effective dose (Wing et al, 1995). Several trials have examined different doses of misoprostol (from 25 to 200 mcg) for induction of labor. Misoprostol appeared to be an effective agent for induction of labor and when compared to placebo. Misoprostol use decreased oxytocin requirements and achieved higher rate of vaginal delivery within 24 hours of induction. It also compares favorably with intra-cervical or intravaginal gel. However, uterine hyperstimulation or tachysystole (defined as 6 or more uterine contractions in 10 minutes in consecutive 10-minute intervals) is more common with misoprostol. There have been reports of uterine rupture following misoprostol use for cervical ripening in patients with previous uterine surgery. Oral misoprostol has also been tried for induction of labor. When compared with vaginal misoprostol there was no significant difference in cesarean section rate, epidural rate or neonatal outcomes. Tachysystole or hyperstimulation was more common in the vaginal misoprostol group (Bennett et al, 1998). Given the current evidence intravaginal misoprostol tablets appear to be effective in inducing labor in pregnant women who have unfavorable cervices; however further prospective studies are required to define optimal doses (ACOG 1999). It is not recommended for patients with prior uterine surgery. Therefore, the use of misoprostol should be confined into clinical trials (RCOG Guidelines 1998).

Other pharmacological agents

Regular uterine contractions achieved with intravenous oxytocin or buccal oxytocin would result in cervical ripening in many cases. Before introduction of prostin this was the usual method in women with poor cervical score. However, it is a laborious process necessitating constant monitoring and may require several 8 to 15 hours sessions spread over number of days.

Estradiol (150-300 mg) in tylose gel has been used extra-amniotically, intracervically or vaginally for effective preinduction cervical ripening (Craft and Yovich 1978, Tromans et al 1981). Mifepristone (Ru-486) at a dose of 200 mg orally for 2 days, 48 hours before formal induction, has been used in France with encouraging results (Frydman et al 1991, Lelaider et al 1994).

Mechanical Methods of Cervical Ripening

Balloon catheters

Foley's catheter is an alternative to prostaglandin cervical ripening. After thorough cleansing of the vagina and cervix, the catheter is inserted into the endocervix and passed above the level of cervical os. The balloon is then inflated with 30 to 50 ml of sterile saline and left in place for 24 hours or until spontaneous expulsion (Barkai et al 1997). The proposed advantages of the Foley's catheter over PGE2 are that it is considerably cheaper and can be deflated and removed immediately should any undesirable side effect occur.

Foley's catheter appears to be significantly more effective than placebo. Some reports suggest that there is no difference in the efficacy between intracervical prostaglandin and intracervical Foley's catheter as measured by changes in Bishop score. Since mechanical agents bring about cervical ripening by local release of prostaglandins there seems little rationale for their use where topical prostaglandin preparations are available.

Hygroscopic Mechanical Dilator

Introduction of hygroscopic tents, such as laminara tents or synthetic hydrophillic polymer rod like Dilapan into the cervical os 12 hours prior to induction of labor has been shown to improve the cervical score. The endocervical methods exert their effect by gradual distention of the cervix and thus hyperstimulation of the uterus is not a concern as with the prostaglandins. Local mechanisms which involve degradation of collagen bundles in the cervical tissue also play a part in softening the cervix. When compared to prostaglandin E2 gel significantly more women in the group who received Dilapan required forewater amniotomy and oxytocin for induction of labor more than 12 hours after priming but there was no difference in other outcome measures like operative delivery for fetal distress or non-progress of labor (Chua et al 1997). Dilapan, mechanical method of cervical ripening is as effective as the more widely accepted method of cervical ripening with prostaglandin gel in achieving vaginal delivery. It does not require a cold chain and is less expensive than prostaglandins. It may therefore be used in places where prostaglandins are not available and in cases where unexpected hyperstimulation of the uterus may cause fetal compromise.

Labor Induction

Sweeping of Membranes

Stripping or sweeping of the membranes were first described in 1810. The technique involves introducing the clinician's finger into the cervical os and mechanically detaching the membranes from the lower uterine segment by circular movement of the examining finger. Sweeping of the membrane probably initiates cascade of events, the exact mechanism of which is not clearly understood. It is believed that local release of prostaglandin may play a significant role. Although there are successful uses of this simple method there are limited reports of its efficacy compared with other methods. Most of the studies included singleton pregnancies and low risk women. Sweeping of the membranes, performed in low risk women at term is associated with a decreased incidence of pregnancy continuing beyond forty-one or forty-two weeks gestation.

Amniotomy

Amniotomy or artifitial rupture of membranes, since its introduction by Thomas Denman more than 200 years ago, has had marked ups and downs in popularity. This is not surprising since the procedure represents one of the most irrevocable interventions in pregnancy and more than any other procedure, calls for a firm commitment to delivery. It is an effective method of labor induction particularly when the cervix is favorable. Special amnihooks are available in the labor ward for fore-water amniotomy. Color and quantity of the amniotic fluid should be recorded and care should be taken whilst rupture of the membranes with high presenting part. Hind water amniotomy with a Drew-Smythe catheter is hardly used in modern obstetrics. In cases with severe polyhydramnios where strong indication for induction exists, hind-water rupture will probably reduce the risk of cord prolapse by controlled release of amniotic fluid. However, the procedure is potentially dangerous and can damage the fetus and placenta.

Amniotomy alone would result in spontaneous labor within 6 to 12 hours in majority of women with favorable cervix. However the main disadvantage is the occasional unpredictable interval between the procedure and onset of regular uterine contractions. Therefore, in current practice amniotomy is usually combined immediately or after a variable interval, with intravenous oxytocin infusion, in order to reduce the induction delivery interval.

Oxytocin

Sensitivity of the uterus to oxytocin increases through out pregnancy but is maximal near term. Concurrent or prior treatment with prostaglandins can enhance or potentiate the action of oxytocin on uterine contractions. Extreme care is needed when oxytocin is prescribed for grandmultiparous woman.

The goal of oxytocin administration is to effect uterine activity that is sufficient to produce cervical change and fetal descent while avoiding uterine hyperstimulation. Many infusion protocols have been proposed to achieve this goal. The amount of oxytocin required to maintain labor is substantially less than that required to initiate it. Most dosage schedule retain the original approach of escalating the dose until effective contractions are established and subsequently maintain the dose until delivery. In the majority desired frequency of uterine contractions can be achieved with doses less than 11mu/min (Steer et al 1985, Arulkumaran et al 1985b). It appears safe to titrate oxytocin starting from 2 to 2.5 mu/min up to 14 to 15 mu/min till a contraction frequency of 4 to 5 in 10 min is reached with each contraction lasting for more than 40 sec. If an adequate response is not observed after reaching

14 to 15 mu/min it is reasonable to increase the oxytocin dose in increments of 4 to 5 mu/min every 30 min (up to maximum of 30 to 40 mu/min) till desired contraction frequency is observed. A longer dosing interval (e.g. 30 min compared to 15 or 20 min) has been shown to be associated with decreased incidence of hyperstimulation (ACOG 1987, Crane and Young 1998).

Various delivery systems have been used for titration of oxytocin during induced or augmented labor. Either gravity fed system with manual compression switch or pumps controlled mechanically or electronically are used. The precision of dose delivery is important as there is substantial risk of hyperstimulation and consequent fetal hypoxia. Electronic pumps are preferred as the gravity fed systems with manual control is less dependable. Automatic infusion pump with feedback from the intrauterine pressure has been used but is not popular because of the cost and due to no distinct advantage over peristaltic infusion pumps.

Apart from the risk of fetal hypoxia secondary to uterine hyperstimulation, oxytocin can cause water retention due to its antidiuretic action. This effect is observed with infusion rates of more than 16 mu/min with a peak effect at 45 mu/min. Mothers with cardiac disease and pregnancy induced hypertension therefore require special consideration. Prolonged infusion can result in maternal and fetal hyponatremia and water intoxication. Maternal complications range from headache, nausea, psychosis and convulsions. Fetal adverse effects include feeding difficulties, apnea, cyanotic spells respiratory distress and convulsions. Neonatal hyperbilirubinemia has also been reported with oxytocin infusion.

Prostaglandins

The successful use of vaginal prostaglandin PGE2 for labor induction in women with favorable cervices has been reported. Women with favorable cervices are more likely to go into labor and deliver following a single dose of prostaglandins. However, in women with good cervical score failed induction is not a problem. For this group of women forewater amniotomy with oxytocin infusion should be the preferred method as it is less expensive and allows better control over uterine contractions than vaginal prostaglandins.

RISKS OF INDUCTION

1. *Failed induction:* Any attempt at initiation of labor is associated with a chance of failure. Failed induction equates to cesarean section. Therefore if indication of labor was unnecessary, the consequence of failed induction would also result in an unnecessary operative delivery. Inadvertent preterm delivery is a risk and therefore estimation of gestational age is a necessary prerequisite.

2. *Uterine hyperstimulation:* Any pharmacological agent used to stimulate the uterus can lead to hyperstimulation. This can give rise to fetal hypoxia, uterine rupture in grandmultipara mothers or scar dehiscence in a uterus with previous cesarean scar. There is no uniform definition of uterine hyperstimulation. Some studies never defined hyperstimulation. Uterine hyperstimulation has been defined as either a series of single contractions lasting 2 minutes or more or a contraction frequency of five or more in 10 minutes. Another definition includes the above definition plus evidence of abnormal FHR pattern on cardiotocography. Fortunately most of the fetuses tolerate hyperstimulation without much adverse effects. Its reversal could be achieved by employing tocolysis with Ritodrine 6 mg iv/10 ml of normal saline or Terbutaline 250 microgram in 5 ml saline intravenously or subcutaneously. Laparotomy is indicated if complications like uterine rupture occurs.

3. *Other risks:* Low amniotomy especially with high presenting part could result in prolapse of the cord. This does not always occur at the time of amniotomy but may become evident when labor starts. Another potential risk of amniotomy is introduction of pathogenic organism and infection. The risk of clinically significant infection is largely dependant on the aseptic procedure practised at the time of amniotomy, cervical infection already present and the interval between amniotomy and delivery. Abruption is a rare but possible complication with amniotomy in cases with polyhydramnios.

INDUCTION OF LABOR IN SPECIAL CIRCUMSTANCES

Previous Cesarean Section

It is important to recognize that pre-existing scar on the uterus represents a potential for trouble. There is very small risk of scar rupture during pregnancy. It is considerably higher during spontaneous labor and is higher still where oxytocic drugs are used. Classical scars, inverted T or unusual scars from difficult operative deliveries carry a higher risk and there is no place for spontaneous labor let alone induction.

In women with one previous section when cervix is favorable, induction of labor with rupture of membranes and oxytocin infusion can be carried out with fair safety. In the presence of poor cervical score PGE2 gel may be used for labor induction. The quoted incidence of scar rupture varies from 0.7 percent to 2.2 percent (MacKenzie 1991). Most of the cases are scar dehiscence when the peritoneum is intact rather than complete scar rupture. The dangers associated with prostaglandin and oxytocin must be borne in mind and used with strict guidelines. Prostaglandin 1mg gel is an appropriate therapy and if no response is obtained in improving Bishop score the use of repeated dose of prostaglandins has to be weighed with caution. Perhaps the same general principle applies to the use of oxytocin to augment slow progress in labor. Constant vigilance should be kept for signs of scar dehiscence; fetal distress, poor progress of labor, vaginal bleeding, tachycardia, hypotension or severe lower abdominal pain or tenderness suggestive of scar rupture. Early resort to cesarean section is advisable when there are signs suspicious of scar rupture.

Prelabor Rupture of Membranes

When the membranes have ruptured spontaneously before the onset of labor there is a risk of cord prolapse, intrauterine infection and increased operative deliveries with induction of labor. A large prospective randomised trial has shown no difference in outcome whether induction was immediate or delayed for 4 days, whether prostaglandins were used or not, regardless of the favorability of the cervix (Hannah et al 1996). Observational studies have suggested that more than 75 percent get established in spontaneous labor within 24 hours and the infective morbidity increases after 48 hours. Based on available information options of immediate induction of labor or delayed induction after 24 hours of membrane rupture should be offered to the women.

Twin Pregnancies

Induction is often necessary in twin pregnancy because of high incidence of maternal and fetal complications. There is very little written in the literature about the use of prostaglandins in twin pregnancy. When cervical score is favorable with the first twin in cephalic presentation, labor can often be induced by forewater amniotomy and oxytocin infusion. A PGE2 gel may be used when the cervix is unripe.

Intrauterine Fetal Death

Intrauterine fetal death (IUFD) at any stage of pregnancy is a tragic event. Special sensitivity is required to conduct the delivery. Induction of labor with a dead fetus is often difficult. It differs from normal term pregnancy in a number of ways. The sensitivity of myometrium to prostaglandin and oxytocin increases with gestational age and therefore it is often difficult to initiate uterine contractions remote from term. Certain methods of induction of labor like amniotomy or intra-amniotic instillation of prostaglandin may be effective but not suitable because of the possible risk of sepsis. Infection, maternal distress and coagulopathy are the three potential problems associated with the retention of a dead fetus. Infection involving the dead fetus particularly by gas gangrene organisms is almost unknown in the western world, but have fatal consequences in the developing world. If membranes are left intact the risk is very low.

The woman's wish should always be taken in account in planning the date and time of induction of labor with intrauterine fetal death.

The risk of coagulopathy with intrauterine death is low. It seems to occur only after the dead fetus is retained *in utero* for more than 4 weeks. In reality this situation is rare as majority of cases would be delivered within 4 weeks of diagnosis of intrauterine death. Expensive coagulation tests like estimation of fibrinogen, fibrinogen degradation products are often not necessary but platelet count should be checked before any intervention is planned.

PGE2 and PGF2a and their analogues have been used via different routes for induction of labor in presence of intrauterine fetal death. *Vaginal* route is the preferred route. Gemeprost 1mg pessaries are widely used for induction of labor with dead fetus. The usual dose is 1mg pessary inserted into the posterior fornix, every 3 hours for maximum 5 doses and the course may be repeated after an interval of 24 hours in cases of failure. Gemeprost need to be stored in the fridge and is expensive (£121.12 for 5 pessaries). Misoprostol has been used for induction of labor with dead fetus. It is cheap (60 tablets =£11.14) and cold chain is not required. PGE2 gel (Prostin gel) may be used in the same way as it is used for induction of labor in the presence of a live fetus.

Other prostaglandin analogue like Sulprostone have been used successfully both intramuscularly and intravenously. Parenteral administration has higher incidence of side effects compared to vaginal administration. The intramuscular preparation has recently been withdrawn from the market because of the reported rare occurrence of anaphylaxis.

Extra-amniotic prostaglandin allows delivery of the drug at the site of response and administration of doses can be effectively controlled. Therefore the side effects are minimised. It is particularly helpful in early gestation when Bishop score is less favorable. A 12 to 14 F Foley's catheter is passed through the cervix and the balloon is inflated with 20-40 mls of saline. An infusion pump is used to administer PGE2. Extra-amniotic solution is available as 10 mg/ml and the infusion is commenced at a rate of 0.5 ml/hr and increased hourly by 0.5 ml increment to a maximum of 3.0 ml/hr. Uterine response is monitored clinically. Oxytocin augmentation is indicated once the catheter is extruded spontaneously via the cervix or the patient remains undelivered for 24 hours. There is significant risk of severe cervical laceration and uterine rupture with simultaneous administration of oxytocin and prostaglandins particularly in advanced gestation and in multiparous patients.

Intra-amniotic prostaglandins is best avoided in the presence of intrauterine death because of the risk of sepsis and erratic absorption of prostaglandin through devitalised fetal membranes. Hypertonic solution in the presence of dead fetus is best avoided.

Oxytocin *per se* may be used near term when cervix is favorable. Controversy exists whether membranes should be left intact. High vaginal swab before induction of labor is a useful step to identify potential pathogens. Artifitial rupture of membranes may be done when the cervix is very favorable and simultaneous oxytocin infusion should be commenced at the same time.

BIBLIOGRAPHY

1. American College of Obstetricians and Gynecologists. Induction and augmentation of labor ACOG technical bulletin 110, 1987.
2. American College of Obstetricians and Gynecologists. Induction of labor. ACOG practice bulletin Washington, DC ACOG, 1999.
3. Arulkumaran S, Gibb DMF, TambyRaja RL, Heng SH, Ratnam SS (a) Failed induction of labor. *Austr NZ J Obstet Gynecol* **25**:190-93, 1985.
4. Arulkumaran S, Gibb DMF, TambyRaja RL, Heng SH, Ratnam SS: (b) Rising cesarean section rates in Singapore. *Sing J Obstet Gynecol* **16**:6-15, 1985.
5. Barkai G, Cohen SB, Kees S *et al:* Induction of labor with use of a Foley catheter and extra-amniotic corticosteroids. [Clinical Trial. Journal Article. Randomized Controlled Trial] American Journal of Obstetrics and Gynecology. **177(5)**:1145-48, Nov, 1997.
6. Benett KA, Butt K, Crane JMG, Hutchens D, Young DC: A masked randomised comparison of oral misoprostol and vaginal administration of misoprostol for labor induction. *Obstet Gynecol* **92**:481-86, 1998
7. Bouvain M, Irion O Stripping sweeping the membranes for inducing labor or preventing post-term pregnancy. (Cochrane Review) In: The Cochrane Library, issue 1, 200 Oxford update software.
8. Chua S, Arulkumaran S, Vanaja K, Ratnam SS: Preinduction cervical ripening: Prostaglandin E2 gel vs hygroscopic mechanical dilator. *J Obstet Gynecol Res* **23(2)**: 171-77, 1997.
9. Craft I, Yovich J: Estradiol and induction of labor. *Lancet* **ii:**208, 1978.

** The simultaneous administration of prostaglandin and oxytocin is associated with iatrogenic damage to the uterus**

10. Crane JMG and Young DC: Meta-analysis of Low-Dose versus High –Dose Oxytocin for Labor Induction. *J Soc Obstet Gynecol Can* **20(13):** 1215-23, 1998.
11. Crane JMG and Bennett KA: A meta-analysis of controlled release of prostaglandin for cervical ripening and labor induction. *J Soc Obstet Gynecol Can* **22(9):** 692-98, 2000.
12. Crowley P: Electve induction of labor at 41 weeks gestation (revised 5th May 1994) In: Enkin MW, Keirse MJNC Renfrew MJ, Neilson JP Crowther C(eds). Pregnancy and Children module In: The Cochrane Database(database on disk and CD ROM) The Cochrane Collaboration; issue 2, Oxford Update software, 1995.
13. Frydman R, Baton C, Leiladier C, Vial M, Bourget P, Fernandez H: Mifepristone for induction of labor. *Lancet* **337:**488-89, 1991.
14. Hannah ME, Ohlsson A, Farine D *et al:* Induction of labor compared with expectant management for prelabor rupture of the membranes at term. TERMPROM Study group. *N Eng J Med* **334:**1005-10, 1996.
15. Keirse MJNC: a) Any prostaglandin/any route for cervical ripening. In the Cochrane Pregnancy and Childbirth Database (1995b, Issue 2), 1995
16. Keirse MJNC 1995. b) Endocervical vs vaginal PGs for cervical ripening /induction. In:The Cochrane Pregnancy and Childbirth Database (1995a, Issue 2).
17. Lelaidier C, Baton C, Benifla JL Fernandez H, Bourget P, Frydman R: Mefipristone for onduction after previous cesarean section, 1994.
18. Mackenzie IZ: Prostaglandin induction and the scarred uterus. Second European Congress on prostaglandins in Reproduction, The Hague 1991, Amsterdam: Excerta Medica 29-39, 1991.
19. Nuutila M, Kajanoja P: Local administration of prostaglandin E2 for cervical ripening and labor induction: the appropriate route and dose. *Acta Obstet Gynecol Scand* **75:**135-38, 1996.
20. Royal College of Obstetricians and Gynecologists: Induction of labor Guideline No 16 July 1998.
21. Society of Obstetricians and Gynecologists of Canada Policy statement on Induction of labor. No. 57 October 1996.
22. Seeras RC: Induction of labor utilising vaginal vs intracervical prostaglandin E2. *Int J Gynecol Obstet* **48:** 163-67, 1995.
23. Steer PJ, Carter MC, Choong K, Hanson M, Gordon AJ, Pradhan P: A multicentric prospective controlled trial of induction of labor with an automated closed loop feedback cotrolled infusion system. *Br J Obstet Gynecol* **92:**1127-33, 1985.
24. Wing DA, Rahall A Jones MM, Goodwin TM, Paul RH: Misoprostol: An effective agent for cervical ripening and labor induction. *Am J Obstet Gynecol* **172:**1811-16, 1995.

35. Mechanism of Labor

Kamala Sikdar
Alokendu Chatterjee

PART TWO: Feto-maternal Medicine

INTRODUCTION

Normal labor is a process by which a mature fetus, presenting by vertex is expelled through the birth passage followed by placenta and membranes at the end of a pregnancy. Traditionally the process of labor is divided into 3 stages. *First stage* extends from the onset of uterine contractions, strong enough to bring about cervical dilatation and effacement, till full dilatation of cervix is achieved. *Second stage* begins with full dilatation of cervix till expulsion of the fetus. *Third stage* is concerned with the separation and expulsion of placenta and the membranes. The total duration of normal labor on an average is about 12 hours in primigravida and that in multigravida is about 6 hours.[1] According to some obstetricians one hour period immediately following 3rd stage of labor may be termed as 4th stage of labor. The mother needs close observation and monitoring of vital signs during this period to avoid some complications of childbirth.

NORMAL LABOR

Components

The components of normal labor include [a] the powers, [b] the passage, [c] the passenger

Powers

The *primary force*—in the first part of labor is derived from the actions of the muscles of the upper uterine segment, which contract, relax as well as retract, i.e. slightly shortened in length compared to pre-contraction state. Uterine contractions probably begin at the cornual regions of the uterus. From there, they spread outward and downward in a circular fashion like a peristaltic wave. They are intermittent in nature followed by a period of relaxation. Gradually their frequency, duration and power increase. During the first stage, contractions are one in every 10 min increasing upto 1 in every 1-3 min or even less during second stage. There is also 1-2 minute's effective relaxation between them. Duration of each contraction ranges from 30 to 90 seconds, averaging about 1 minute. The average intrauterine pressure during labor varies from 20 to 60 mmHg. Retraction facilitates stretching of lower uterine segment, effacement and full dilatation of the cervix and descent of the presenting part to the pelvic floor. It starts near the end of the 1st stage, pronounced in

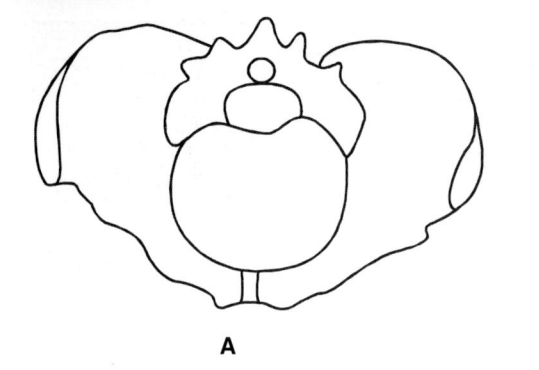

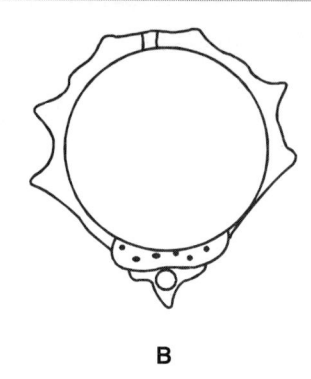

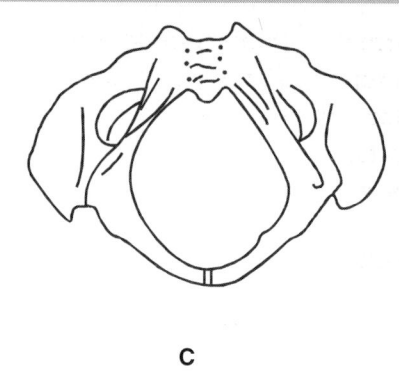

Figures 35.1A to C: Showing (A) pelvic inlet, (B) pelvic cavity, (C) pelvic outlet

second and third stages. It causes permanent shortening of uterine muscles.

The secondary forces—involuntary contraction of the muscles of the diaphragm and anterior abdominal wall also help to expel the fetus. However, mother usually has voluntary bearing down efforts synchronous with the involuntary contractions of these muscles, for more effective outcome.

Passage

The passage through which the baby is expelled during labor include the soft tissues, covering the bony pelvis. But the journey is not always a very easy one. Because, the shape of the pelvic canal is irregular with transversely oval inlet, almost circular cavity and anteroposteriorly oval outlet (Figure 35.1).

The *pelvic inlet* is bounded by anterior margin of the sacral promontory, iliopectineal line of one side, posterior aspect of upper surface of the pubis to opposite side of iliopectineal line.

The diameters of pelvic inlet:
a. *Antero-posterior* or *true conjugate* is the distance between the mid point of sacral promontory and mid point of inner margin of the upper border of symphysis pubis measuring 11.5 cm.[2] But the shortest antero-posterior diameter of obstetrical importance is the *obstetrical conjugate* through which head must pass while descending through pelvic inlet. It is the distance between the mid point of the sacral promontory and prominent bony projection in the midline on the inner surface of the symphysis pubis measuring 10 cm.
b. *Transverse diameter* represents the greatest distance between the linea terminalis on either side measuring 13.6 cm.
c. *Oblique diameter* extends from one of the sacroiliac joint to the iliopectineal eminence on the opposite side of the pelvis and measures 12 cm.

Pelvic cavity, bounded above by inlet and below by plane of least pelvic dimension, is almost round. Anteroposterior diameter measures from the mid point on the posterior surface of the symphysis pubis to the junction of 2nd and 3rd sacral vertebrae. It measures 12 cm. The transverse diameters between the tissues covering the sacrosciatic notches and obturator foramina also measure 12 cm.

Obstetric outlet: It is antero-posteriorly oval space bounded above by the plane of least pelvic dimension and below by the anatomical outlet.
a. Anterior-posterior diameter extends from the inferior border of the symphysis pubis to the tip of the sacrum measuring 12.5 cm.
b. Transverse or bispinous diameter is the distance between two ischial spines measuring 10.5 cm.

Anatomical outlet: It is a linear boundary formed by the lower border of the symphysis pubis, ischiopubic rami, ischial tuberosities, sacrotuberous ligaments and tip of the coccyx.

Posterior sagittal diameter of the outlet extends from the tip of the sacrum to the mid point of the line between two ischial tuberosities. It usually exceeds 7.5 cm.

Normally, there should not be any feto-pelvic disproportion at any level for smooth delivery to take place. At the same time, any tumours of the soft structures of the pelvis or bony anomaly may alter the process of labor.

Passenger

In utero, the fetus usually adopts an *attitude* of flexion, *attitude* of the fetus is the relation of different parts of the fetus to each other. *Lie* of the fetus indicates the relationship of the long axis of the uterus to that of the fetal spine. In longitudinal lie both the axes are either parallel or superimposed. Transverse lie is when fetal spine is transverse to uterine long axis and in oblique lie fetal spine is oblique to that of longitudinal axis of the uterus. *Presentation* is the portion of the fetus which is either in closest proximity to pelvic brim or foremost within the birth canal. It may be either cephalic (cranial end), Podalic (caudal end) and transverse (either shoulder). *Presenting part* indicates the portion of the presentation overlying the internal os or felt through the cervical canal on internal examination. There are 3 types of presenting part in cephalic presentation, e.g. *vertex* (full flexed head), *face* (full extended head) and *brow* (midway between full flexion and full extension of the head). Other presenting parts are *breech* and *shoulder* when buttock and shoulder overlie the internal Os respectively. In normal labor, lie of the fetus is longitudinal and presentation is cephalic. Here the presenting part of the fetus is vertex where the head is in fully flexed attitude, presenting smallest antero-posterior diameter which is ideal for *easy delivery*. *Denominator* is the most identifiable peripheral bony point on the presenting part. In vertex presentation, denominator is the occiput and in face presentation it is the mentum or the chin. *Position* indicates the relationship of denominator to the different quadrants or fixed points of maternal pelvic inlet. When the occiput is directed laterally to the left, it is called left occipitotransverse position (LOT), found in 40% of all labors.[4]

If directed towards right it is called right occipitotransverse position (ROT), found in 20 percent of all labors (Figures 35.2 and 35.3).[3]

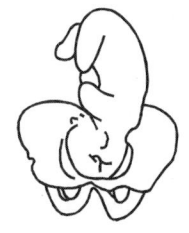

Figure 35.2: Left occipito-transverse position

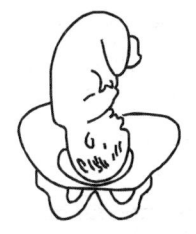

Figure 35.3: Right occipito-transverse position

If occiput lies anteriorly, 450 anterior to the transverse (90°) position against the left iliopectineal eminence, it is called left occipitoanterior (LOA) position or right occipitoanterior (ROA) position when occiput lies against the right iliopectineal eminence (fixed point of the pelvic inlet) (Figures 35.4 and 35.5).

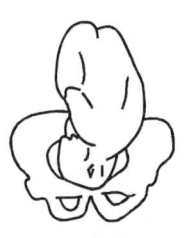

Figure 35.4: Left occipito-anterior position

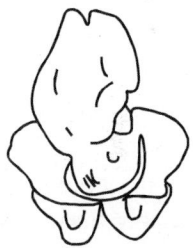

Figure 35.5: Right occipito-anterior position

Less commonly (approximately 20%) the occiput may lie posteriorly against right sacro-iliac joint (right occipitoposterior ROP) position, or left sacroiliac joint (left occipitoposterior, LOP) position (Figures 35.6 and 35.7).

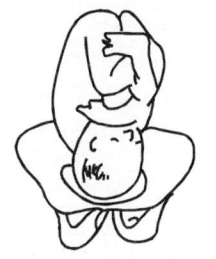

Figure 35.6: Right occipito-posterior position

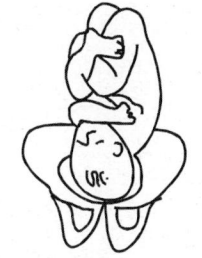

Figure 35.7: Left occipito-posterior position

Posterior positions are associated with a narrow fore pelvis and anterior placentation. Left occipitoanterior and ROP positions are little commoner than ROA and LOP position respectively as the available left oblique diameter of the pelvis is shortened by encroaching rectum.

The shape of the fetal head is more or less oval. The engaging antero-posterior diameter in vertex or occiput presentation is either suboccipitobregmatic (9.5 cm) in fully flexed head or suboccipitofrontal (10 cm) in slightly deflexed head. Further deflexion may present with the occipitofrontal diameter (11.5 cm) commonly seen with OP positions.

It is evident that not all diameters of the presenting part can easily pass through all diameters of the pelvis. So the fetus, during delivery undergoes some passive movements while passing through the birth canal. Although alterations are mostly evident on the presenting part, but the rest of the fetal parts also either participate simultaneously or follow it. The components of these movements are engagement, flexion, descent, internal rotation, extension, restitution, external rotation and lateral flexion. Usually, during first stage of labor engagement, descent and flexion of fetal head occur and movements of internal rotation and subsequent movements occur during the second stage. Main features: (i) descent occurs throughout, (ii) leading part when meets the resistance of pelvic floor flexes and rotates forward until it comes under the symphysis pubis, (iii) Any part emerging from the pelvis will pivot around the pubic bones

Definition in relation to mechanism of labor comprises a series of passive changes in position and attitude adopted by the fetus during expulsion through the birth canal.

In normal labor with vertex presentation, the head usually enters the pelvic brim with sagittal suture in the transverse pelvic diameter. For convenience, the mechanism of normal labor will be described in LOT or LOA position. Although the components of movements of labor will be described separately but in reality the mechanism of labor consists of a combination of movements that occur simultaneously. For instance, the process of engagement includes both flexion and descent of the head. At the same time uterine contractions, after engagement help straightening of the fetus with loss of dorsal convexity and apposition of extremities to the body. Thus, a fetal ovoid is converted into a cylinder with the smallest possible cross-section normally passing through the birth canal.

Mechanism

1. *Engagement* (Figure 35.8)

When the maximum transverse diameter of the presenting part passes through the pelvic inlet it is called engagement. This may occur during the last few weeks of pregnancy, mostly in primigravidae or may not occur until labor commences in multigravidae. During engagement, the sagittal suture in LOT position usually tends to accommodate to the transverse axis of the pelvic inlet, i.e. midway between the symphysis pubis and sacral promontory (Figure 35.9).

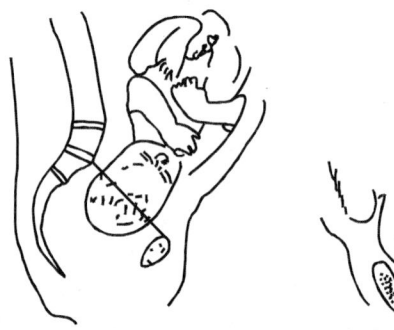

Figure 35.8: Shows engagement

Figure 35.9: Synclitic engagement of the head

In LOA position engagement occurs along the right oblique diameter of the maternal pelvis. Some time sagittal suture may be deflected posteriorly toward the promontory or anteriorily toward the symphysis pubis. Such lateral tilting of the head to a more anterior or more posterior position in the pelvis is called *Asynclitism*. If the sagittal suture lies close to the sacral promontory, more of the anterior parietal bone presents and the condition is called anterior asynclitism or Naegele's obliquity,[4] commonly found in multigravidae (Figure 35.10).

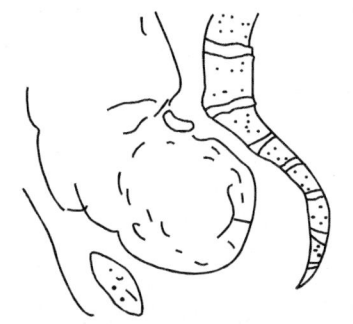

Figure 35.10: Anterior asynclitism (Naegele's obliquity)

If the sagittal suture lies close to the symphysis pubis, more of the posterior parietal bone will present and the condition is called posterior asynclitism, commonly found in primigravidae due to good uterine tone and tight abdominal wall (Figure 35.11). At the extreme of posterior asynclitism posterior ear is in the lower most position and it is called Litzman's obliquity.[5]

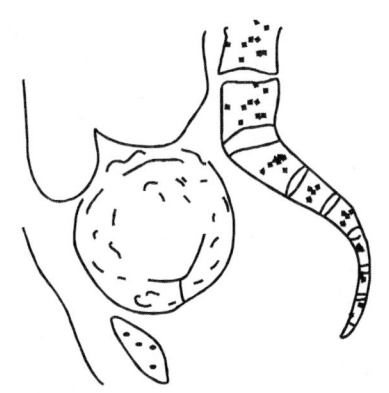

Figure 35.11: Posterior asynclitism

Engagement with asynclitism is called asynclitic engagement. In posterior parietal presentation, posterior lateral flexion of the head occurs during engagement to glide the anterior parietal bone past the symphysis pubis. In anterior parietal presentation, lateral flexion in reverse direction occurs to glide the posterior parietal bone past the secral promontory. Moderate degree of asynclitism is found in normal labor, but if severe, may result in cephalopelvic disproportion.

2. *Descent*
Descent is the first requisite for birth of the fetus. It is a continuous movement provided there is no undue bony or soft tissue obstruction. In primigravida further descent may not follow until the second stage of labor if engagement has occurred before the onset of labor. In multigravida descent follows engagement. Descent is brought about by: (a) uterine contraction and retraction, (b) pressure of the amniotic fluid, (c) contraction of abdominal muscles, (d) straightening of the fetal ovoid.

3. *Flexion*
Some degree of flexion of the head is possible at the beginning of labor but complete flexion is rather common during descent when head meets the resistance of the lower uterine segment, cervix, walls of the pelvis or the pelvic floor. The flexion is explained by head lever action,[6] the fetal head being regarded as a lever. The occipitoatlantoid joint being the fulcrum, short arm extends from the condyles to the occipital protuberance and the long arm extends from the condyles to the root of the nose (Figure 35.12).

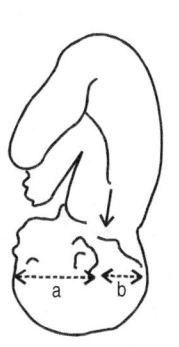

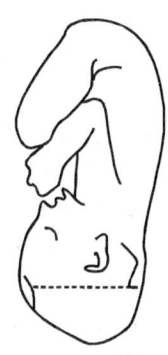

Figure 35.12: Flexion of the head during labor. The arrow indicates the direction of fetal axis pressure

Figure 35.13: The dotted line shows the reduction in diameter after flexion

When resistance is encountered the long anterior arm meets more resistance than the short posterior arm. So the long anterior arm moves upwards and the short posterior arm descends downwards resulting in flexion of the head (Figure 35.13).

Flexion has advantage of bringing the shortest suboccipito-bregmatic diameter (9.5 cm) of the head into engagement and descent. The transverse diameter is the distance between the two parietal eminences which is constant (9.5 cm) with different degrees of flexion if there is no asynclitism.

4. *Internal rotation*
With internal rotation occiput rotates forward from the LOT (90⁰) or LOA (45⁰) position to lie under the subpubic arch (occipitoanterior position 0⁰) when the head meets the resistance of the pelvic floor at the level of ischial spines. The sagittal suture lies in the anteroposterior diameter of the pelvic outlet (Figures 35.14 and 35.15).

Resistance of the pelvic floor is an important factor of internal rotation of the head, which is further facilitated by the gutter shape of the pelvic floor with

Figure 35.14: Beginning of internal rotation in LOT position

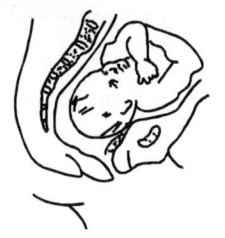

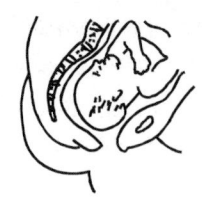

Figure 35.15: End of internal rotation, OA position

its forward and downward slope. According to Hart's rule[1] whichever part of the fetus first meets the lateral half of this slope, will be directed forwards and toward the center. In LOT or LOA position, the occiput during uterine contraction first stretches the left half of the levator ani muscle. As the contraction fades, the pelvic floor rebounds causing the occiput to glide forward. With each uterine contraction and relaxation forward rotation continue till occiput is brought down behind the symphysis pubis. Other factors, which influence the internal rotation, are: (a) forward inclination of the walls of the pelvic cavity, (b) effective uterine contractions.

The internal rotation causes a slight twist in the neck of the fetus as the head is no longer in direct alignment (90°) with the shoulder, which occupies the left oblique diameter of the maternal pelvis (Figure 35.16).

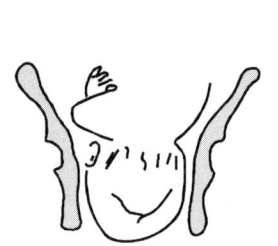

Figure 35.16: Shows shoulders occupying left oblique diameter, occiput in direct anterior position in pelvis

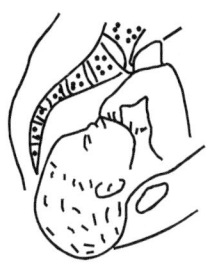

Figure 35.17: Showing crowning

5. Extension

With further descent, the occiput slips beneath the subpubic arch and head extends with the nape of the neck pivoting against the subpubic arch. Extension of the head causes stretching of the anterior part of the perineum gradually, until the moment of crowning (Figure 35.17), when the greatest transverse diameter slips through the introitus but does not recede during uterine relaxation.

At the same time fetal shoulders, now have entered the pelvic cavity with its bisacromial diameter lying along the left oblique diameter of maternal pelvis. The shoulder will undergo similar movements undertaken by the head after its escape from the birth canal.

After crowning further extension allows the forehead, face and chin successively to escape over the perineum (Figures 35.18A and B).

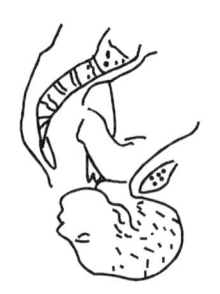

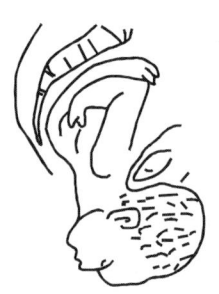

Figures 35.18A and B: Showing extension of head whereby forehead, face, are born successively

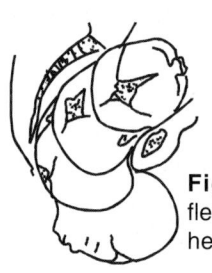

Figure 35.18C: Showing descent, flexion, internal rotation and delivery of head from LOT position

Two forces come into play for extension. The driving force of uterine contraction pushes the head posterior and downward direction. The second force is the resistance of the pelvic floor in the upward and forward direction. The downward and upward forces neutralise. The remaining forward force helps extension of the head.

Immediately following the release of the head, it drops downwards whereby chin lies over the maternal anal region.

6. Restitution (Figures 35.19A to D)

The twist in the neck of the fetus, which resulted from internal rotation of the head, is now corrected by visible passive movement of the head due to untwisting of the neck. The occiput moves by 45° toward the side from which it started internal rotation restoring head to its natural right-angled relation to the shoulders.

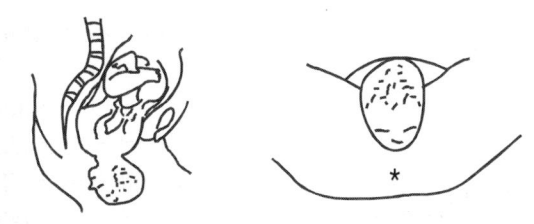

Figures 35.19A and B: Shows lateral and front view of head after birth

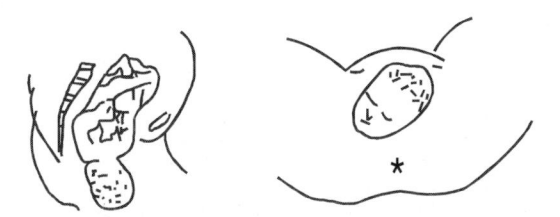

Figures 35.19C and D: Shows restitution lateral and front view

7. *External rotation* (Figure 35.20)

With further descent shoulders advance. The right and anterior shoulder is lower and meets the resistance of the right half of pelvic floor before the left shoulder. The right shoulder rotates towards symphysis pubis, as did the occiput. Along with internal rotation of the anterior shoulder there is external rotation of the head by 45° towards the mother's left thigh in the same direction as restitution. Thereby 90° relationship of head with the shoulder is restored. The shoulders now occupy the antero-posterior diameter of the pelvis.

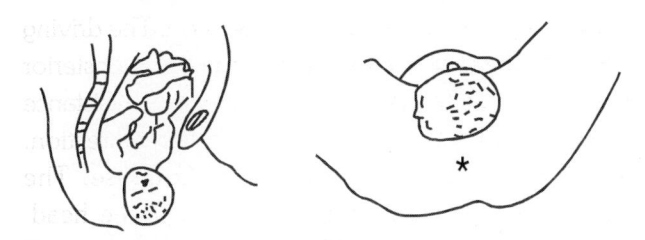

Figures 35.20 and 21: Showing external rotation, lateral and front view

8. *Lateral flexion* (Figure 35.21)

With further descent anterior shoulder escapes underneath the symphysis pubis. Then acute lateral flexion of the body of the baby takes place towards mothers abdomen whereby posterior shoulder slides over the perineum. Rest of the body is born by lateral flexion with arms folded on the chest and hands under the chin.

Mechanism of Normal Labor in Right Occipitotransverse or Right Occipitoanterior Positions

The same description applies for these position but with substitution of right for left and vice versa throughout.

Mechanism of Normal Labor in Occipitoposterior Positions

With an average sized fetus and pelvis, adequate flexion of the head and *effective uterine contractions*, most of the cases of posteriorly positioned occiput undergo identical mechanisms to those of occipitotransverse or anterior varieties except long (135°) internal rotation of occiput compared to 90° and 45° in transverse and anterior position respectively. If rotation is incomplete or if occiput rotates posteriorly in unfavorable circumstances, deep transverse arrest and persistent occipitoposterior position respectively result deviating from normal mechanisms.

Normal Changes in Fetal Head during Labor

During passage along the birth canal an area of edema of few millimeters called the *caput succedaneum* may form in the scalp protruding through the dilating cervix due to its pressure (Figure 35.22).

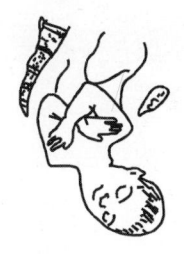

Figure 35.22: Lateral flexion of body

It usually follows rupture of membranes and subsides spontaneously within few days.

Another important change in the fetal skull is called *moulding* due to considerable pressure during passage of head along the birth canal. It is the movement of skull bones near frontanelle and sutures. Usually the edges of the occipital and frontal bones pass under the edges of the parietal bones. The two parietal bones pass one under the other in the region of the sagittal sutures. When the parietal bones meet it is termed moulding +; if one over rides the other but can be reduced to the same level by gentle pressure it is ++; if it cannot be reduced by gentle pressure it is +++. Moulding may cause diminution in biparietal and suboccipito-bregmatic diameter by 0.5 to 1 cm. without causing damage to brain tissue or even more in prolonged labor (Figure 35.23).

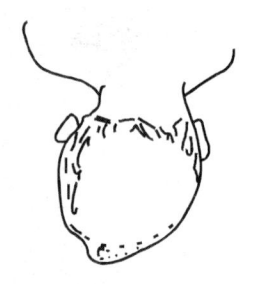

Figure 35.23: Caput succedaneum

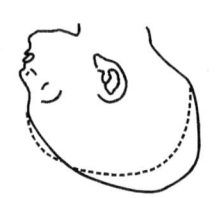

Figure 35.24: Showing moulding. Dotted line

CONCLUSION

Labor is a crucial period at the end of a pregnancy for both mother and the fetus. Journey through the maternal pelvis is the most hazardous of all journeys. Any sort of deviation from the normal process of labor may lead to complications to both of them. So proper understanding of the mechanism of labor helps to guide obstetrician to differentiate normal from abnormal condition during the process of labor so that appropriate intervention may be undertaken, whenever needed, to avoid any complication either to mother and/or fetus.

REFERENCES

1. Dawn CS: *Text Book of Obstetrics and Neonatology*: Edited by C.S. Dawn, Fifteenth edition: Dawn Books; 238-40, 2001.
2. *Dewhurst's Text Book of Obstetrics and Gynaecology for Post Graduates*. Edited by C.R. Whitfield, 5th edn, Blackwell Science. 298, 1995.
3. Caldwell WE, Moloy HC, D'Esopo DA: A roentgenologic study of the mechanism of engagement of the fetal head. *Am J Obstet Gynecol* **28:** 824, 1934.
4. Gardberg M, Tuppurainen M: Anterior placental location predisposes for occiput posterior presentation near term. *Acta Obstet Gynecol Scand* **73:** 151, 1994.
5. Cunningham FG, Mac Donald PC, Grant NF, Leveno KJ *et al*: *Williams Obstetrics,* 20th edn, Prentice-Hall-International, INC; **263:**321, 1997.
6. Obstetrics by Ten Teachers: Edited by GVP Chamberlain, 16th edn. ELBS with Edward Arnold, 175, 1995.

36. Normal Labor

K Sujata

PART Two — Feto-maternal Medicine

INTRODUCTION

During the first 36 to 38 weeks of pregnancy uterus is in a state of contractile unresponsiveness. The final stage of pregnancy is characterized by painful uterine contractions, which force the fetus through birth canal.

1. *Labor*: Events that take place in the uterus and birth canal to expel the viable fetus through the vagina.
2. *Delivery*: Expulsion or extraction of a viable fetus out of the uterus (womb). Normal labor should lead to spontaneous vaginal delivery, but at times delivery may be surgical via an abdominal or vaginal route.
3. *Normal labor (eutocia)*: Labor is considered normal when mature fetus presenting by the vertex delivers by natural efforts, unaided without undue prolongation of labor or complications to mother or baby.
4. *Dystocia*: A difficult labor, which refers to a labor not progressing satisfactorily with possible undue consequences to the mother and fetus.

ONSET OF LABOR

Exact cause of onset of spontaneous labor is still not clear. In humans however it appears that the fetus, placenta and fetal membranes play the major role in initiation and continuation of labor.

Endocrinology of Onset of Labor

Fetoplacental Contribution

Due to unknown factors fetal pituitary is stimulated prior to onset of labor → Stimulates fetal adrenals → cortisol secretion → inhibits progesterone synthesis. Alteration of estrogen and progesterone ratio leads to prostaglandin synthesis (Estrogen promotes synthesis of oxytocin receptors in the myometrium and deciduas and causes lysosomal disintegration resulting in increased prostaglandin synthesis).

Oxytocin

No conclusive proof of increased level prior to labor. However, there is an increase in oxytocin receptors at term, which in turn stimulate prostaglandin synthesis. Oxytocin is important in final stages of labor.

Prostaglandins (PGs)

Prostaglandins play an important role in initiation of parturition. Primary effect of PGs at term is by increase in synthesis and myometrial sensitivity through formation of gap junctions. Gap junctions are cell-to-cell contacts at plasma membranes of adjacent cells, which help in ionic and metabolic coupling between cells. PGs act by inhibiting calcium binding thereby increase in free calcium, which in turn stimulates uterine contraction. Both oxytocin and PGs act synergistically inhibiting calcium binding and stimulate uterine contraction.

PG synthesis reaches its peak in third stage, which help in placental expulsion and control of postpartum hemorrhage. Placenta, fetal membranes, decidua and myometrium are major sites of PG synthesis.

Synthesis is triggered by:
- Rise in estrogen level.
- Altered estrogen and progesterone balance.
- Mechanical stretching
- Stripping of membranes.

Evidence to support prostaglandin's role in parturition:
- Increased production at term.
- Suppression of premature myometrial contraction by PG synthesis inhibitors
- Exogenous PG's stimulate uterus to contract.

Nervous Factor

Labor may also be initiated through nerve pathways. Both α and β adrenergic receptors are present in myometrium. The contractile response is initiated through α receptors of postganglionic nerve fibers in and around cervix and lower part of uterus. This is based on the observation of onset of labor following stripping or low rupture of membranes.

Date of Onset of Labor

Calculation of expected date of delivery, based on Naegeles formula, can only give a rough guide. Based on the formula labor starts on expected date in 4 percent, one week either side in 50 percent, two weeks earlier and one week later in 80 percent.

Stages of Labor

Labor is a continuum, but three stages are generally described, which helps in management. Besides the classic three stages, a period of prelabor and fourth stage are also described

Prelabor Period (Premonitory Stage)

The changes preliminary to onset of labor begin 2 to 3 weeks before the true onset of labor in primigravid and few days before in multigravid. The changes are:
1. Lightening—2 to 3 weeks before term as the baby settles into lower uterine segment, specially in primigravida. It is due to the formation of the lower segment of uterus that allows the presenting part to descend, which results in lowering of the fundal height; a sense of relief for the mother. There may be frequency of micturition and constipation due to pressure by engaged presenting part on the bladder and rectum. Engagement is a welcome sign as it rules out cephalopelvic disproportion
2. Increased vaginal secretions.
3. Cervix becomes soft and effaced.
4. False labor pains occur with variable frequency.

Signs of true labor
- Pain felt in front of lower abdomen
- Painful uterine contractions which increase in frequency and duration, associated with hardening of uterus.
- Blood stained mucus discharge—show
- Progressive effacement and dilatation of cervix.
- Formation of bag of membranes.
- Descent of head.

False labor pains have the harmful effect of tiring the patient so that when true labor begins she is in poor mental and physical state. They may be associated with a loaded rectum or temporary indigestion and appropriate treatment should be provided (Table 36.1).

First Stage (Cervical Stage of Labor)

First stage starts from the onset of true labor pains to full cervical dilatation. Average duration of fisrt stage of labour is 12 hours in primigravida and 6 hours in multigravida.

Table 36.1: Differentiating features of true and false labor pains

True labor pains	False labor pains
• Marks the onset of labor • Are associated with efficient uterine contractions	• Appears days before term • Inefficient contractions of uterus/painful spasm of uterus, bladder and abdominal wall muscles
• Occur at regular intervals	• Irregular intervals
• Increase in frequency and duration	• No change
• Starts in the back and move to the front of abdomen	• Mainly in the front
• Hardening of uterus	• No hardening of uterus
• Bloody show	• No show
• Progressive effacement and dilatation and formation of bag of membranes	• No change in cervix
• Descent of presenting part	• Inefficient to push the presenting part
• Sedation/Enema does not interfere with true labor	• Relieves the pains

Second Stage

Second stage starts from full cervical dilatation to delivery of the baby. Average duration 2 hours in primigravida and 30 minutes in multigravida.

Third Stage

Third stages starts from delivery of the baby to expulsion of placenta and membranes. Its duration is usually 15 minutes in primi or multigravida with active management of the third stage of labor.

Fourth Stage

It is stage of observation after third stage for one hour to detect any postdelivery problems, which are more likely within a short duration after delivery (for example, primary PPH, uterine inversion, vulval hematoma).

PHYSIOLOGY OF NORMAL LABOR

Primary Forces

Primary forces are uterine contractions in labor. Uterus has no pacemaker that is demonstrable anatomically, physiologically or pharmacologically. Contractions start near one cornual region and the wave of contraction spread downward. Cause of pain is due to stretching or ischemia. Pain of uterine contraction is distributed along the cutaneous nerve distribution of T10-L1. Pain of cervical dilatation is referred to the back through sacral plexus. The character of uterine contractions changes with the onset and progress of labor.

1. There is good *synchronization of contractile* waves between upper and lower segment.
2. *Fundal dominance* is shown by strong contractions at the fundus that gradually diminishes as it proceeds down to lower uterine segment.
3. *Contractions* follow a regular pattern. Intrauterine pressure rises beyond 20 mmHg with onset of true labor pains during contraction (palpable uterine contraction and pain).
4. The *baseline pressure* (tonus) during first stage is 8 to 10 mmHg (i.e. intrauterine pressure between contraction).
5. *Intrauterine pressure* rises to 40 to 50 mmHg during first stage and 100 to 120 mmHg in second stage during contraction.
6. *Duration*: In early first stage it would be less than 20 seconds with gradual increase with progress of labor. Conventionally contraction durations are marked as less than 20 seconds, 20 to 40 seconds and greater than 40 seconds. It can be 60 seconds in late first stage of labor to 60 to 90 seconds in second stage.
7. *Interval*: In the first stage, it starts as 1 to 2 contraction/10 minutes and increases to 4 to 5/10 minutes in the late first and second stage of labor.
8. During contraction uterus is pushed forward to make the *longitudinal axis* of uterus in line with that of pelvic axis.
9. In labor uterine muscle exhibits the properties of *contraction/relaxation/retraction*.

10. *Retraction*: It is a special property of upper segment. There is progressive shortening of muscle fibers following contraction. It starts toward end of first stage and continues through to second and third stage of labor. Net effects are changes in the uterus and cervix to effect a normal delivery.
11. *Net effect of retraction*: Formation of lower uterine segment and cervical changes are due to retraction. It helps to maintain the advancement of presenting part. In the third stage decreased surface area of uterus favors separation of placenta followed by effective hemostasis after separation of placenta.

Secondary Forces

Contraction of voluntary muscles of abdominal wall reinforcing uterine contractions to expel the fetus during second stage. This is called Bearing down effort (Figure 36.1). Intra-abdominal pressure is raised thereby augmenting intrauterine pressure. Uterine contraction force on fetus is 1kg/sq cm in first stage and it doubles in second stage of labor.

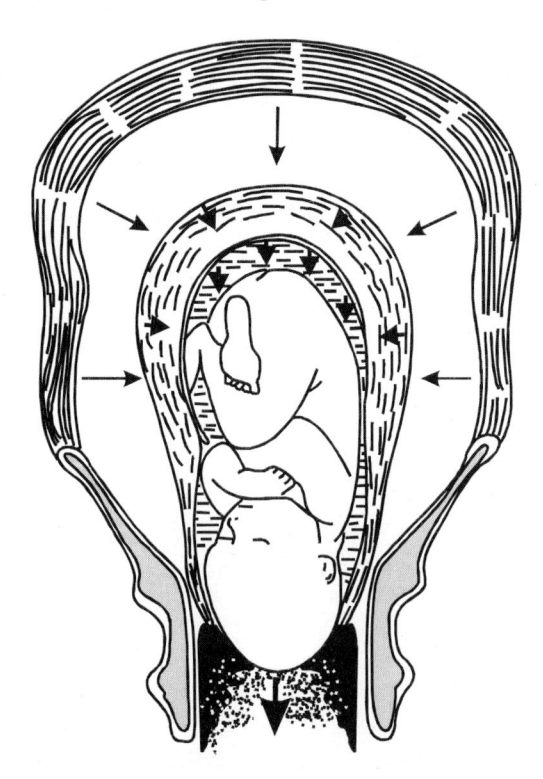

Figure 36.1: Second stage expulsive forces

Metabolic Changes

Considerable loss of energy occurs in second stage of labor due to uterine contraction and bearing down efforts. The resulting metabolic acidosis is well compensated. Normal fetus has got enough reserve to withstand the physiological hypoxic state induced during uterine contractions of labor. Transient fetal acidosis may appear simultaneously with maternal acidosis specially in late second stage.

Events in First Stage of Labor

Main events that occur in the first stage are uterine contractions of true labor pains, dilatation, effacement of cervix, descent of fetus, formation of lower uterine segment, formation of bag of waters and finally rupture of membranes at the end of first stage.

1. *Uterine contractions*: Increase in intensity and duration of 4-5 contractions in ten minutes lasting for 40 to 45 seconds in late first stage. Pain is felt shortly after the contraction and passes off before complete relaxation of uterus.
2. *Bloody show*: This is a plug of cervical mucus mixed with blood discharged as an evidence of start of effacement and dilatation.
3. *Effacement of cervix*: It is the process of thinning out of cervix with gradual shortening of cervix. It is caused by incorporation of cervix with lower uterine segment due to pull of active upper segment. Cervix, which is 2.5 cm in length, will become papery thin when it is 100 percent effaced. Effacement is measured as percent of shortness of cervical canal. In primi effacement precedes dilatation, multi both occur simultaneously (Figure 36.2).
4. *Dilatation of cervix*: Prior to onset of labor there may be certain amount of dilatation of cervix specially in multigravida and some primigravida. Dilatation occurs progressively from internal os to cervical canal and lastly external os. The process is rapid in multigravida as dilatation occurs simultaneously. Dilatation is measured in terms of fingerbreadth but recorded in cm. One fingerbreadth is 1.5 cm. Two fingers equal 3 cm dilatation. Where there is a cervical lip, it can be 7 to 9 cm and when cervical lip is not felt, it is full dilatation.

(A) Primigravida (B) Multipara

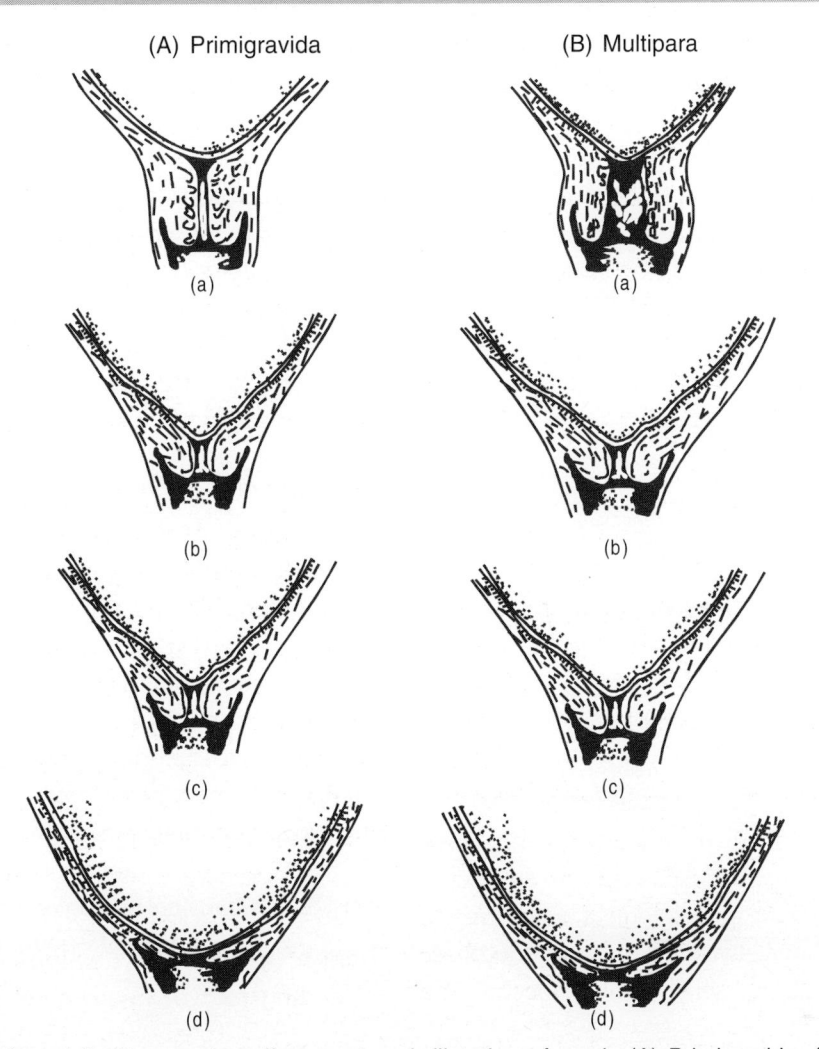

Figures 36.2A and B: Progressive effacement and dilatation of cervix (A) Primigravida; (B) Multipara

Factors responsible for dilatation of cervix are *uterine contraction and retraction*: Longitudinal muscle fibers of upper segment are attached with circular muscle fibers of lower uterine segment and upper part of cervix in a bucket holding fashion. Thus with each contraction cervix is opened and shortened.

5. *Bag of membranes:* Hydrostatic action of bag of forewaters provides ball valve like action with the well flexed head (Figure 36.3)

Fetal Axis Pressure

Straightening of fetal axis allows fundal contraction to traverse through podalic pole via the spinal column to

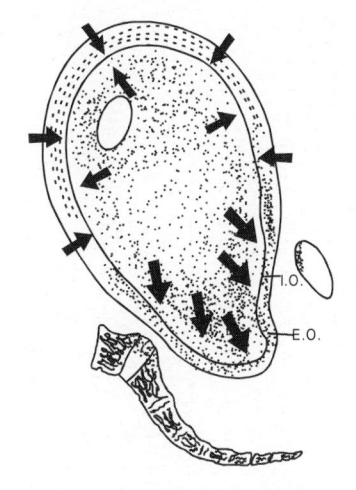

Figure 36.3: Hydrostatic action of membranes in effective cervical effacement and dilatation

the head causing mechanical stretching of lower uterine segment and opening of cervix.

Cervical Dilatation Curve (cervicograph/partograph)

Friedman 1978 described graphical representation of cervical dilatation in cm against duration of labor in hours. It is a sigmoid curve and first stage of labor is divided into the following (Table 36.2):
• Latent phase: upto 3 cm
• Active phase: 3-10 cm

Active phase is further subdivided into:
• Acceleration phase: 3-4 cm
• Phase of maximum slope: 4-9 cm
• Phase of deceleration: 9-10 cm

Table 36.2: Phases of first stage of labor

Phases of first stage	Primi	Multi
Latent phase	6-8 hrs	4-6 hrs
Active phase	4 hrs	2 hrs
Rate of dilatation	1 cm/hr	1.5 cm/hr

Friedman developed the concept of three functional divisions of labor—preparatory, dilatational, and pelvic division—to describe the physiological objectives of each division. Dilatational division corresponds to phase of maximum slope during which dilation occurs at a rapid rate and is not affected by sedation and analgesia unlike in preparatory division or latent phase. Cardinal movements of fetus takes place during pelvic division of labor.

Fetal descent pattern of normal labor show hyperbolic curve where station of head is plotted as a function of duration of labor. Active descent is observed during phase of maximum slope of cervical dilatation.

Cervical dilatation and descent of fetus are best parameters to decide the progress of labor than uterine contractions (Figure 36.4).

Lower Uterine Segment Formation

During labor demarcation of upper segment and relatively passive lower uterine segment is more pronounced. This is pronounced in late first stage especially after rupture of membranes and attains its maximum in second stage. Junction of two segments is marked by raised ridge of rim called *physiological retraction ring*. The ring is prominent in obstructed labor, when it is termed *pathological retraction ring/bandles ring*. Formation is facilitated by contraction and retraction of upper uterine segment and pressure of fetus below causing receptive relaxation.

Station of head: It is palpated by marginal level of leading part of head in relation to ischial spine

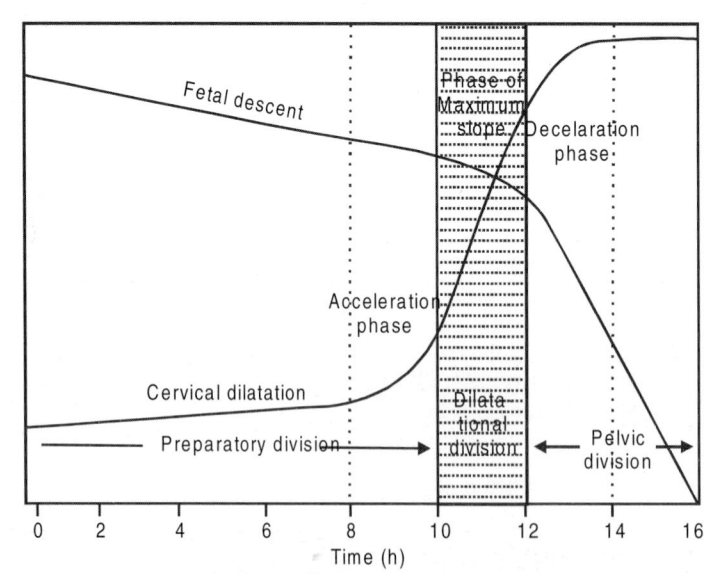

Figure 36.4: Partographic representation of labor showing dilatation of cervix in cm against time and descent of head

enter the intrathecal space. A very small amount of local anesthetic (e.g. 2.5 mg bupivacaine) and narcotic (25 mcg fentanyl) are then injected into the intrathecal space. These drugs introduced into the intrathecal space provide a rapid onset of analgesia for a duration varying from one to three hours. After the introduction of the drugs into the intrathecal space, the spinal needle is removed, a epidural catheter is now introduced through the epidural needle like in the epidural technique and left in place for further administration of low dose local anesthetic and narcotic.

The advantage of this method over the epidural technique is that the onset of analgesia is more rapid and this is particularly useful for parturients presenting in advanced first stage of labor with severe pain.

The combined spinal epidural set is more expensive compared to an epidural set.

3. Spinal analgesia[7]

This method which involves the administration of a small amount of local anesthetic and narcotic into the intrathecal space as a bolus dose is not frequently used for labor analgesia. The local anesthetic provides only 1 to 3 hours of pain relief which may not be adequate to cover the whole duration of labor whilst narcotics alone may not be adequate to cover pain toward the end of the first stage or second stage. It may however, be a very useful option in the absence of other methods of pain relief in a mother in the very advanced first stage of labor and in need of an instrumentation delivery. Administration of drugs into the intrathecal space as part of the CSE is discussed earlier. Another option is to administer either local anesthetics or narcotics or combination of both through a catheter in the intrathecal space throughout labor. However, continuous spinal analgesia through spinal catheters in non-parturients has been associated with cauda equina lesions[8] and hence, is not a popular technique.

Contraindications to Regional Methods

The regional methods are definitely more effective for labor analgesia but they are more invasive as well. Hence, consents must be obtained before they are administered. They are contraindicated in parturients with coagulopathy or are on anticoagulant therapy, hypovolemic parturients, those with infection either around the site of injection or systemic sepsis, those with certain anatomical abnormalities like arteriovenous malformation within the spinal canal and in those parturients who are unwilling to have the method of analgesia or in those units where there is a shortage of skilled anesthetic staff to provide the analgesia.

Complications

Complications can arise from these methods in the form of hypotension, spinal headaches, convulsions, peripheral or central neurological damage.

Hypotension is not uncommon as most of these methods cause some degree of sympathetic blockade. This should be treated with intravenous fluids and putting the parturient in the left lateral tilt position to avoid the supine hypotension syndrome. Compression of the inferior vena cava by the gravid uterus especially in a parturient with sympathetic blockade drastically reduces the volume of blood that can return to the heart from the lower limbs. Oxygen should also be administered via a nasal prong so that oxygenation of the fetus is not compromised during this period of hypotension. Small boluses of intravenous ephedrine 3 to 5 mg may have to be administered to treat the hypotension so as to prevent fetal compromise.

Spinal headaches occur if a large bore needle like an 18 or 16 gauge epidural needle has accidentally penetrated the dura or spinal needles with cutting edges are used. These headaches must be differentiated from other headaches that can occur during the postpartum period especially those associated with meningitis or any space occupying lesion. Spinal headaches can be managed in a variety of ways depending on the severity but the most effective method involves using patient's blood introduced into the epidural space in the technique widely known as "epidural blood patch".

Local anesthetic accidentally introduced into the intravascular space can cause convulsions or even myocardial depression. The emphasis is to ensure that the catheter is in the correct space by using a test dose before the continued administration of drugs for maintenance of analgesia and to fractionate the dose of drugs to avoid an excessive large dose with each administration.

Walking Epidurals[9]

The emphasis on epidurals and CSEs now is to provide just enough to allow the parturients to have analgesia without removing the ability to move the lower limbs and to mobilize. In fact this is the basis of the "walking epidurals" which involve the use of either of these two techniques in such a way that the mother is pain-free but is still able to use her lower limbs to move around for a fair period of time during labor. This ability to walk has to be meticulously checked and she has to be accompanied at all times so that she does not fall whilst given this new found freedom.

Other Regional Methods

1. *Pudendal block*[10]

The pudendal nerve which is derived from the 2nd, 3rd, and 4th sacral nerve is blocked with local anesthetic administered using a special needle via a needle guide. With the parturient in the lithotomy position, the needle can be placed either via the vagina or the perineum with the tip aiming just medial and posterior to the ischial spine. A block needs to be repeated on the opposite site.

A pudendal block is useful for the process of delivery if analgesia is required and if no block has been inserted prior to this for the control of pain. The failure rate however is high, approaching almost 50 percent.

2. *Paracervical block*[10]

The aim in this block is to prevent transmission through the paracervical plexus bilaterally. It involves the placement of a total of 5 to 10 ml of local anesthetic through the lateral vaginal fornix on both sides with the mother in the modified lithotomy position. The block allows the patient to be relieved of pain during the first stage of labor—the relief depends on the success of the block and the duration of action of the local anesthetic.

The drawback is the high incidence of fetal bradycardia that has been reported with several reports of fetal deaths. The block has suffered a decline in use with the more popular use of epidurals and combined spinal epidurals.

Miscellaneous Methods

These are usually described as nonpharmacologic alternatives for obstetric analgesia and include methods like transcutaneous electrical nerve stimulation, hypnosis, natural childbirth and acupuncture. The success rate of these methods varies and hence, they are not very popular.

ANESTHESIA FOR CESAREAN SECTION

Anesthesia for cesarean section can be in the form of a general anesthesia or a regional anesthesia. There is a growing trend[11-13] to use regional anesthesia as maternal mortality audits show that regional anesthesia is safer than general anesthesia. Parturients given general anesthesia has a higher risk of hypoxia and pulmonary aspiration (in the event of a difficult/failed intubation) especially during an emergency cesarean section. Mothers given regional anesthesia are awake and are able to protect their airways at all times. They are also able to participate in the delivery process and this may enhance infant-maternal bonding.

In order to prevent aspiration during anesthesia, most mothers during labor are fasted. There is growing pressure to liberalize oral intake in labor. Due consideration must be given in any feeding policy to make sure mothers at high risk of operative deliveries are fasted and to accommodate the fact that as many as 15 percent of mothers in normal labor may end up with a cesarean section. Chemoprophylaxis must also be undertaken to reduce the acidity and volume of gastric contents. These can be in the form of a H_2 receptor blocker, an antacid, a proton pump inhibitor or metoclopramide or a combination of these.

General Anesthesia

All parturients for cesarean section, more so those who have undergone a period of labor and given narcotic parenterally are considered to have a "full stomach" as they have delays in gastric emptying. These when aspirated whilst they are rendered unconscious during the administration of a general anesthesia can give rise to consequences that can threaten the mother's life. Hence, general anesthesia for cesarean section whether in an elective or emergency situation involves a "crash induction" which is the administration of an induction agent together with a very rapid-acting muscle relaxant whilst cricoid pressure is applied (to prevent aspiration) before the endotracheal tube is inserted and its cuff inflated. Anesthesia is continued with oxygen, nitrous oxide and a low concentration of volatile agent like isoflurane together with a longer acting muscle relaxant. Narcotics are not administered until after the delivery of the baby. Aspiration can occur even after the general anesthesia and it is the onus of the anesthetist to ensure that the parturient is able to protect the airway before she is extubated.

Analgesia for cesarean section after general anesthesia can be in the form of parenteral narcotics administered either by medical staff or by the parturient herself either as bolus doses or continuous infusions. They are usually administered for 1 to 3 days postoperatively.

Regional Anesthesia

Regional anesthesia can either be in the form of a spinal, an epidural or a CSE. The placement of these are no different as for labor analgesia. The concentration of drugs used to provide anesthesia as opposed to analgesia is however, higher. If an epidural or a CSE is already in place for labor analgesia and the parturient needs a cesarean section, a dose of local anesthetic and narcotic of higher concentration is titrated in to provide the necessary level of anesthesia for the operation. In the case of a cesarean section without any of the regional methods in place, the choice between the three methods involves the time taken for performing the anesthetic technique, the rapidity of onset of anesthesia and whether the technique can be used to provide post-operative analgesia. Spinals can be performed in less than 5 to 10 minutes whereas epidurals and CSEs take a slightly longer time. Both spinals and CSEs have a more rapid onset of adequate anesthesia but epidurals take almost 30 minutes. Hence for a parturient with fetal distress, epidurals inserted *de novo* is not an acceptable option. Spinals without the use of catheters cannot be used to provide postoperative analgesia but it is possible for medical staff or the parturient herself to titrate epidurals and CSEs for postoperative analgesia.

REFERENCES

1. Ward MS, Cousins MJ: Pain mechanisms in labor. In Drs David J Birbach, Stephen Gatt and Sanjay Datta (Eds): *Textbook of Obstetric Anesthesia*. Churchill Livingstone, Philadelphia, 3-30, 2000.
2. Chamberlain G, Wraight A, Steer P: Pain and its relief in labor: Report of the 1990 NBT survey. Churchill Livingston, Edinburgh, 1993.
3. Reynolds F: Pain relief in labor. *British Journal of Obstetrics and Gynecology* **100:** 979-83, 1993.
4. Cohen SE: Inhalation analgesaia and anesthesia for vaginal delivery. In Schnider SM, Levinson G (Eds): *Anesthesia for Obstetrics*. 2nd edn. Williams and Wilkins. Baltimore, 142-56, 1987.
5. Paull J: Epidural analgesia for labor. In Drs David J Birbach, Stephen Gatt and Sanjay Datta (Eds): *Textbook of Obstetric Anesthesia*. Churchill Livingstone, Philadelphia, 145-56, 2000.
6. Rawal N, Van Zundert A, Holmstrom B, *et al*: Combined spinal-epidural technique. *Regional Anesthesia* **22:** 406-23, 1997.
7. Gamlins FMC, Lyons G: Spinal analgesia in labor. *International Journal of Obstetric Anesthesia* **6:**161-72, 1997.
8. Rigler ML, Drasner K, Krejcie TC *et al:* Cauda equina syndrome after continuous spinal anesthesia. *Anesthesia and Analgesia* **72:**275-81, 1991.
9. Elton CD, Ali P, Mushambi MC: "Walking extradurals" in labor: A step forward? *British Journal of Anesthesia* **79(5):** 551-54, 1997.
10. Vloka JD, Hadzic A, Drobnik L: Nerve blocks in the pregnant patient. In Drs David J Birbach, Stephen Gatt and Sanjay Datta (Eds) *Textbook of Obstetric Anesthesia*. Churchill Livingstone, Philadelphia, 693-706, 2000.
11. Chan YK, Ng KP: A survey of the current practice of obstetric anesthesia and analgesia in Malaysia. The *Journal of Obstetrics and Gynecology Research* **26(2):** 137-40, 2000.
12. Chan YK, Ng KP: Regional Analgesia in Obstetrics in the Far East. In Felicity Reynolds (Ed): *Regional Analgesia in Obstetrics–a millenium update*. Springer-Verlag. London, 73-78, 2000.
13. Shibli KU, Russell IF: A survey of anesthetic techniques used for cesarean section in the UK in 1997. *International Journal of Obstetric Anesthesia* **9:** 160-67, 2000.
14. Crowhurst JA, Plaat F: Why mothers die—report on confidential enquiries into maternal deaths in the United Kingdom 1994-96. *Anesthesia* **54(3):** 207-09, 1999.

38.
Malposition, Malpresentations and Cord Prolapse

Sudip Chakravarti
Krishnendu Gupta
Sajal Datta

INTRODUCTION

The most common presentation of the fetus in late pregnancy is cephalic presentation. This is not because of the shape of the pelvis or the fetal head, but because of the pyriform-shaped cavity of the uterus (more so in the primigravidae), which allows for more room for lower limb activity in the fundal region. But sometimes, malpositions like occipitoposterior and malpresentations like breech, face, brow and transverse lie occur. In all the malpositions and malpresentations there is a badly fitting presenting part, often associated with poor uterine contractions, early rupture of membranes because of irregular bag of forewaters and risk of cord prolapse. This often causes a significantly higher maternal and fetal risk. These malpositions and malpresentations will be discussed briefly in this chapter.

NORMAL POSITION AND MALPOSITION

Occiput Posterior Position

Nearly 95 percent of fetuses at term present with the vertex (an area subtended by the two parietal eminences and the anterior and posterior fontanelle). With vertex presentation the vast majority progress in labor and have spontaneous vaginal delivery and hence the vertex is called the normal presentation. Any other presentation other than the vertex have difficulties in labor with higher rates of operative deliveries and fetal morbidity and are termed as malpresentations. About 90 percent of the vertex presentation are associated with an occipitoanterior position which usually have a flexed head and pauses little difficulty with labor and hence is called normal position. Anything other than occipitoanterior is termed as malposition, i.e. occipitolateral and posterior.

Definition

In a vertex presentation when the occiput, the denominator, is placed posteriorly in any posterior quadrant of the pelvis or directly on the sacrum then it is called occiput posterior position. These positions are usually associated with a deflexed head and as such present a larger anteroposterior diameter (occipitofrontal—11.5 cm) and this can give rise to dystocia (difficult labor).

Types

The following positions are described:
- ROP or right occiput posterior position, when the occiput is on the right sacroiliac joint
- LOP or left occiput posterior position, when the occiput is on left sacroiliac joint
- DOP or direct occiput posterior position when the occiput is directly on sacrum

Most common position is ROP as dextro-rotation of gravid uterus and presence of the sigmoid colon does not favor LOP position.

Incidence

At the onset of labor the incidence is about 10 percent. It is possibly more in late pregnancy but much less in the 2nd stage of labor as it spontaneously gets corrected to the normal occiput anterior position.

Causes

The shape of the pelvis very often leads to the occiput posterior position. The android type of pelvis favors oblique occiput posterior position, as there is a narrow forepelvis and a roomy hind pelvis, which accommodates the larger occiput. This accounts for almost 50 percent of its incidence. Anthropoid pelvis favors direct occiput posterior position whereas platypelloid pelvis favors transverse position of the occiput. When the placenta is situated anteriorly the back of the head with broader biparietal diameter is pushed to the rear. A relatively large fetus and poor uterine contraction that does not promote proper flexion (deflexion) encourages occiput posterior position. Deflexed head results in failure in rotation and persistence of occipitoposterior position in early labor when normally there should be flexion and descent (Table 38.1).

Table 38.1: Causes of occipitoposterior position

1. Abnormal pelvis
   a. Android
   b. Anthropoid
   c. Platypelloid
2. Anterior insertion of the placenta
3. Large size of the fetus
4. Poor uterine contraction

Diagnosis

1. *During pregnancy:* The following features on abdominal examination indicate the presence of a occiput posterior position (Table 38.2).

   The fetal heart is usually heard muffled in the flanks unless it is direct occipitoposterior position, when the fetal heart is usually heard loud and clear and in the midline near the umbilicus as the fetal chest is directly under the anterior abdominal wall.

Table 38.2: Diagnosis of occipitoposterior position

a. Subumbilical flattening of the abdomen.
b. Difficulty in palpating the fetal back.
c. Easily palpable limbs by the side of the midline.
d. Head appears to be relatively large and high up.
e. Occiput and sinciput appears to be at the same level.
f. Muffled fetal heart sound at the flanks.

2. *During labor:* In early labor the anterior frontanelle is easily felt whereas there is difficulty in feeling the post-frontanelle and it is felt near the sacroiliac joint. The sagittal suture is placed on any one of the oblique plains or anteroposteriorly.
3. *In late labor:* Very often caput formation tends to hide the frontanelles and they are not felt easily. We need to feel the pinna of the ear, which guides us to the position of occiput.

Mechanism of Labor (Figures 38.1A and B)

In Right Occiput Posterior Position

The engaging diameter is occiput frontal (11.5 cm) with the occiput, the denominator, tries to engage along the right oblique diameter of the pelvis and it lies against right sacroiliac joint. The sinciput rests against the left ileopectineal eminence. There is always delay in engagement as the head remains in deflexed attitude. If the uterine contractions are good, the pelvis is adequate and the baby is of reasonable size and the vertex is well flexed, the labor will progress normally in 90 percent cases. In 10 percent cases if the above factors are unfavorable the labor will be arrested in oblique occiput posterior, direct occiput posterior or in the transverse diameter of the pelvis. This is referred to as the deep transverse arrest when it occurs at full dilatation of the cervix.

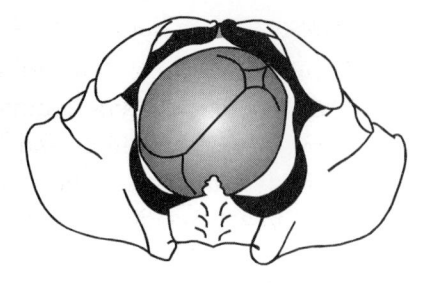

1. Descent and flexion in labor
2. ROP to ROT— Internal rotation
3. ROT to ROA—Internal rotation
4. ROT to ROA—Internal rotation

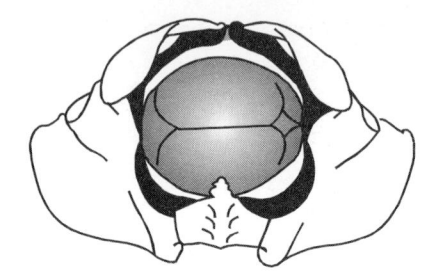

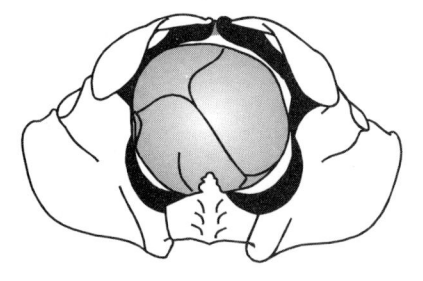

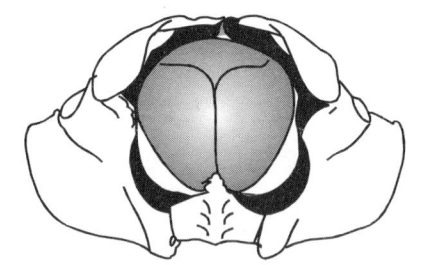

Figure 38.1A: Occipitoposterior position mechanism of labor

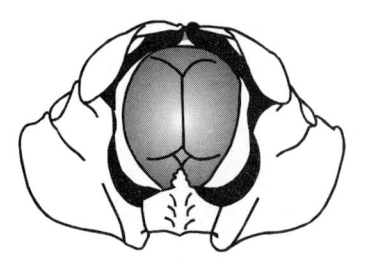

1. Beginning of extension
2. Completed extension
3. OA to ROA—Restitution
4. ROA to ROT—External rotation

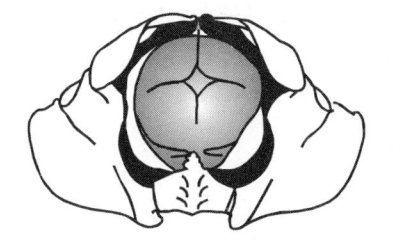

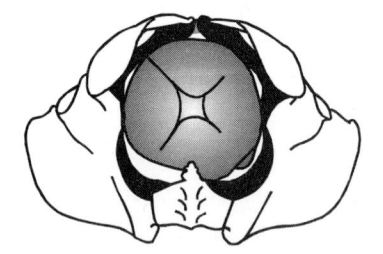

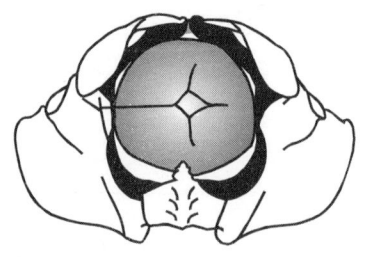

Figure 38.1B: Mechanism of labor in occipitoposterior position
ROP : Long Arc Rotation (contd.) (Favorable outcome)

In favorable situation, further descent and flexion will bring the occiput to touch the right half of pelvic floor first, which will now rotate 3/8th circle anteriorly (long internal rotation of occiput) to come behind symphysis pubis. Before touching pelvic floor shoulder rotates 2/8th of a circle so that neck is twisted by 1/8th rotation. This is not internal rotation of shoulder, as it has not yet touched the pelvic floor. After this rotation shoulder now occupies right oblique diameter of pelvis.

When there is further descent and flexion, the occipital protuberance escapes under the symphysis pubis and crowning starts, i.e. biparietal diameter is at the level of bituberous diameter and the head would not recede in between contraction.

Undoing of flexion attitude of the head will be achieved by extension movement of head so that the head is born. Now there will be restitution, i.e. turning of head to untwist 1/8th of a circle to correct the prior neck rotation. The occiput rotates 1/8th to the right and now there will be internal rotation of shoulder as it touches pelvic floor and 1/8th forward rotation will occur to bring shoulder in antero-posterior diameter of pelvis. External rotation of head is accompanied with internal rotation of the shoulder. The occiput turns further 1/8th of a circle, always in the same direction as restitution, i.e. to mother's right. Trunk and the rest of fetal body will be born by lateral flexion.

Outcome of Labor

1. *Favorable situation*: Flexion of head helps in long rotation and delivery as in case of occiput anterior, but in the 1st stage of labor, if there is descent of the presenting part, without much flexion it creates an unfavorable situation. At times the head can rotate to direct occipitoposterior position and have a face to pubis delivery (Figure 38.2).

1. ROP—Descent and flexion

2. ROP to OP—Internal Rotation

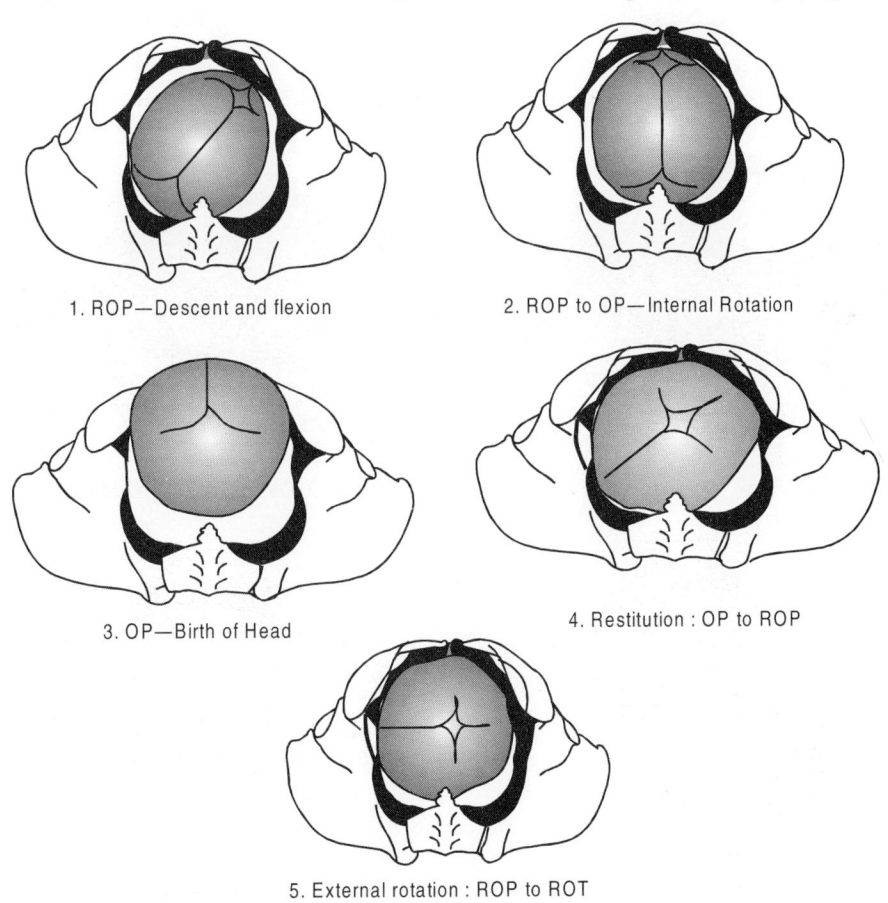

3. OP—Birth of Head

4. Restitution : OP to ROP

5. External rotation : ROP to ROT

Figure 38.2: Mechanism of labor in occipitoposterior position Short Arc Rotation to OP (Favorable outcome)

2. *Unfavorable situation (Figures 38.3A to C):*
   a. *Incomplete rotation:* Occiput rotates only 1/8th of a circle anteriorly at the level of the pelvic floor, instead of 3/8th and there is no further progress of labor. This will lead to occiput posterior arrest in transverse diameter at the level of ischial spines (deep in pelvis) and is called the deep transverse arrest (DTA) (Figure 38.3A).
   b. *Nonrotation:* Both sinciput and occiput touch the pelvic floor at the same time and does not allow further rotation. This lead to oblique occiput posterior arrest (Figure 38.3B).
   c. *Malrotation:* When there is gross deflexion, the occipitofrontal diameter (11.5 cm) presents at the oblique diameter of pelvic brim. Biparietal diameter may get caught at the sacrocotyloid diameter and the descent is retarded. The sinciput becomes the leading part and it touches the pelvic floor first. Then the sinciput rotates 1/8th forward throwing the occiput at the hollow of the sacrum. This is called occiput sacral position. In true sense this is the persistent occiput posterior position (POP). Under favorable circumstances with good roomy pelvis, the labor may progress to a spontaneous delivery (Figure 38.3C), as face to pubis or else there will be occiput sacral arrest (Figure 38.3D).

In Direct Occiput posterior position or Persistent occipitoposterior position (POP)

The engaging diameter occiputofrontal occupies the right oblique diameter of the pelvis. Here sinciput touches the pelvic floor first (instead of occiput) and rotates 1/8th circle anteriorly (internal rotation) and hinges beneath the symphysis.

Now occiput sweeps the perineum and the head is born by flexion instead of extension as face to pubis. Sinciput turns to the left (restitution) and the shoulder enters along the oblique diameter. The anterior shoulder touches pelvic floor first and 1/8 forward rotation takes place. Head rotates another 1/8th circle with sinciput to the left (external rotation of the head).

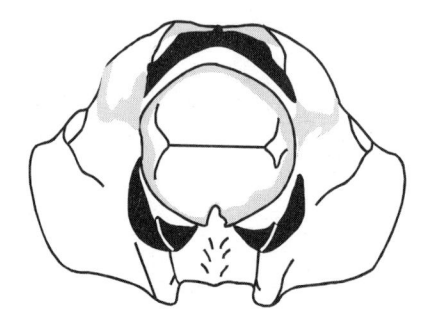

a. Deep transverse arrest

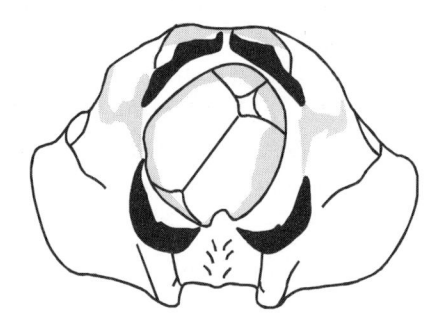

b. ROP to oblique occiput posterior arrest

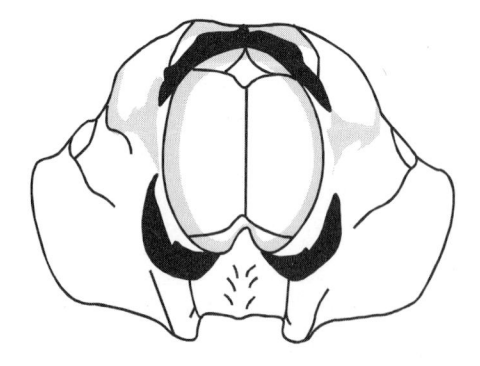

c. Descent in ROP position

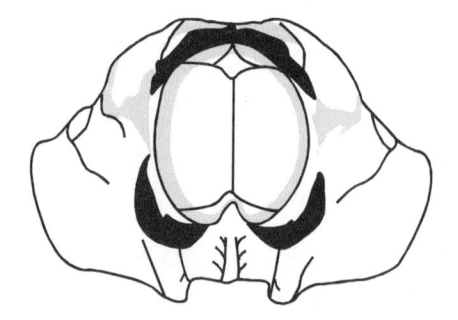

d. Persistent OP arrest of labor

Figures 38.3A to D: Arrested occipitoposterior positions (Unfavorable outcome)

The anterior shoulder escapes under the symphysis pubis and the posterior shoulder sweeps over the perineum and the body is born by lateral flexion (Table 38.3).

Table 38.3: Outcome of labor in occipitoposterior position

Primary occipitoposterior position:
a. Anterior rotation of the occiput → Delivery as that of occiput anterior
b. Incomplete anterior rotation → Arrest of head in transverse diameter → Deep transverse arrest
c. Non-rotation → Arrest of head in oblique occipitoposterior position
d. Malrotation → Sinciput touches the pelvic floor first → Anterior rotation of the sinciput → Occiput at the sacral hollow → Occipito-sacral position
  - Favorable outcome: Spontaneous delivery as face-to-pubis
  - Unfavorable outcome: Occipitosacral arrest.

Management of Labor

When occiput posterior position is detected in early first stage of labor, it is expected to progress normally in 90 percent of cases and to deliver as occiput anterior. This normal progress can only be achieved if uterine contractions are good, the pelvis is spacious, and the fetus is of average size.

Labor may be prolonged and care should be taken to ensure that first stage is not unusually prolonged leading to any maternal and/or fetal morbidity. In presence of high risk and unfavorable factors a decision of early cesarean section is to be taken.

In early 2nd stage of labor an attempt should be made to assess outcome of labor. In persistent occiput sacral position further rotation is unlikely but face to pubis delivery is possible in favorable circumstances. When full dilatation of the cervix is acheived, in presence of good uterine contractions if there is no delivery in the next one hour- arrest of labor is suspected.[1]

Arrest of labor with occiput oblique or transverse position is managed in present day obstetrics by emergency cesarean section or ventouse delivery in favorable circumstances (i.e. station of the presenting part, degree of caput, moulding and size of baby needs to be considered) (Table 38.4).

Alternative methods of delivery sometimes undertaken in current modern practice are:
1. Manual rotation followed by forceps application
2. Forceps (Kielland) rotation and forceps delivery

Table 38.4: Indications for a cesarean section in occipitoposterior position

1. Cesarean section in early labor
   a. Gross CPD
   b. Big baby
   c. Associated maternal complications, e.g. severe PIH, elderly primigravida, post-CS pregnancy, post-dated pregnancy, etc. (relative indications strengthened by poor progress)
2. Cesarean section in late labor
   a. Prolonged labor
   b. Fetal distress
   c. Failed instrumental delivery
   d. Patient not agreeing to difficult vaginal delivery.

Manual rotation and forceps delivery

This method may be useful if the facilities for immediate cesarean section is not available and the obstetrician is well versed in this technique.

1. Procedure may be performed under general anesthesia and patient in lithotomy position.
2. In presence of a large caput, the pinna of the ear is the guiding factor to detect the position of occiput. If it is folded, this guide is not helpful.
3. In ROP or ROT, left hand is introduced and vise versa (whole hand method).
4. Disimpaction (not disengagement), flexion and rotation is tried so that the occiput becomes anterior.
5. Abdominal hand will try to rotate the back simultaneously.
6. When the right hand is used, left blade is applied first.
7. When the left hand is used, the right blade is applied first and then the left blade is applied from underneath the right blade.
8. Direction of the pull is downward first and then forward.

Vacuum Extraction

Vacuum extraction is gaining popularity in our current practice. Most cases of occipitoposterior position requiring instrumental delivery may be managed this way. The principal advantage in this technique is the lower incidence of maternal injury to the perineum and the anal sphincter during the course of operative delivery.

In exceptional circumstances it may be applied through a partially dilated cervix but this is in a multigravid with an occipitoanterior position and no disproportion. It is an ideal choice in non-rotation of the head, typically in transverse and persistent occipito-posterior positions. It requires proper training in technical skills to be always a 'flexing median application', e.g. a posterior cup should be applied for malpositions and the cup application should be on the 'flexion point' which is on the sagittal suture 3 to 4 cm in front of the occiput.

The disadvantages are that the operation takes longer time and has a failure rate closer to 10 percent. When the vacuum cup is applied to the scalp, the delivery has to be completed ideally with bearing down efforts of the mother and pull on the vacuum with three contractions. If not delivered then there should be significant advance and it should be accomplished within 30 minutes. Otherwise there is a chance of necrosis of this scalp tissue. Similarly if the cup slips off (pop off) three times then the situation should be reassessed and if needed the instrument should be abandoned and a CS preferred. Because the instrument is simple and easy to handle and easier to use if one persists it may lead to a cephalhematoma or a serious subgaleal hemorrhage.

Problems with Occiput posterior Position in Labor

1. Prolonged 1st and 2nd stage of labor
2. Increased morbidity due to prolonged labor, i.e.fetal distress, maternal dehydration
3. Increased incidence of operative and instrumental delivery
4. Increased maternal morbidity
5. Increased perinatal morbidity and mortality.

MALPRESENTATIONS

Face Presentation

Definition

Face is an uncommon cephalic presentation where the head is hyperextended, the presenting part being face, and mentum (chin) the denominator. It is the part between the glabella and the chin and the presenting diameter is the submentobregmatic (9.5 cm).

Obstetric boundary of the face

- Above: Supra-orbital ridge
- Below: Chin (mentum)
- Laterally: Malar prominence

Incidence

The commonly reported incidence is 1:500-600 deliveries (0.5-0.6%).

Etiology

Face presentation occurs due to the extreme extension of the head. The common causes are as follows:

1. *Maternal*
   - Multiparity
   - Lateral obliquity of the uterus
   - Contracted pelvis and fetopelvic disproportion
   - Flat pelvis

2. *Fetal*
   - Congenital malformations (15%): Anencephaly; iniencephaly; dolichocephalic head
   - Several coils of umbilical cord around the neck
   - Musculoskeletal abnormalities: Spasm or shortening of the extensor muscles of the neck
   - Tumors around the neck (congenital goiter; Congenital branchocele)

Diagnosis

The diagnosis is rarely made before the onset of labor and it is of little significance if it is made earlier.

Findings on abdominal examination (Figures 38.4 and 38.5)

- Longitudinal lie with the body nearer to mid-axis of the uterus
- Cephalic prominence on the same side as the back on vaginal examination
- Do not expect the face to feel like the newborn baby's face; edema always obscures facial parts
- Supraorbital ridges lead to the bridge of the nose
- Two smaller holes of the nostril where the examining finger cannot be introduced
- Mouth has hard gums and may suck on the examining finger unlike the anus.

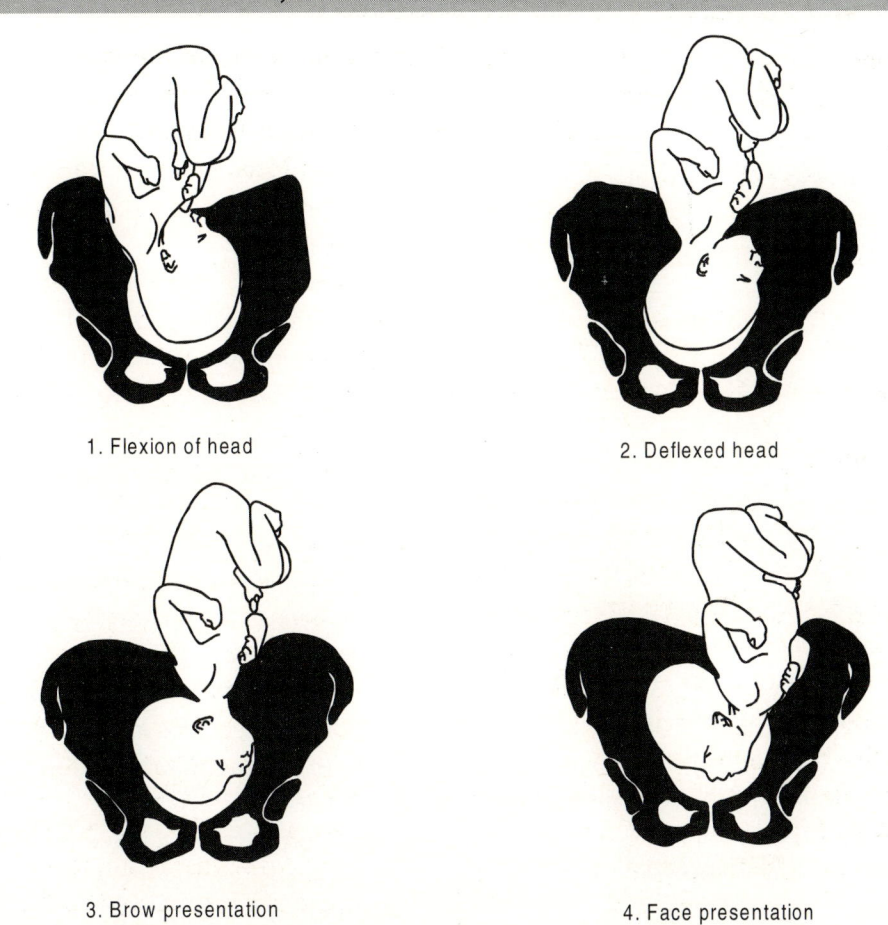

MALPOSITION, MALPRESENTATIONS AND CORD PROLAPSE

1. Flexion of head

2. Deflexed head

3. Brow presentation

4. Face presentation

Figure 38.4: Attitude of the head

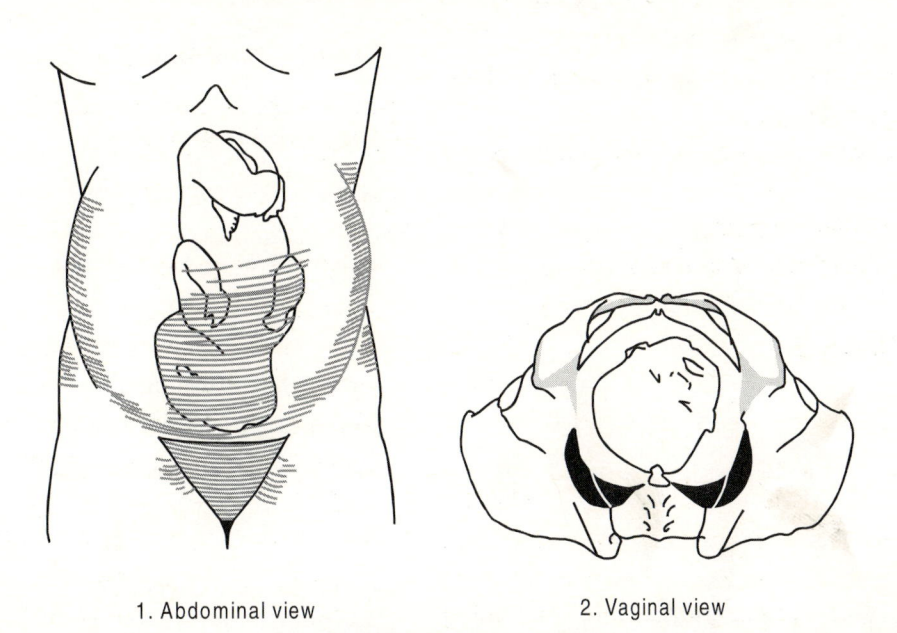

1. Abdominal view

2. Vaginal view

Figure 38.5: Face presentation

Mechanism of Labor

The fetal face may present with the mentum anterior or posterior, in relation to the maternal pelvis. Face presentations are rarely observed above the pelvic inlet. The brow generally presents and it is usually converted into a face presentation after further extension of the head during descent.

Mentum anterior (MA)—left MA or right MA

1. Most common position: Left MA
2. Engaging diameter:
   - Submentobregmatic (9.5 cm) in full extension
   - Submentovertical (11.5 cm) in partial extension

The mechanisms of labor are descent with increasing extension, internal rotation, delivery of the head by flexion, external rotation, restitution and delivery of the trunk by lateral flexion. Face presentation commonly prolongs the second stage of labor due to the poor thrust between the body and the fetal head. It must be remembered that the biparietal diameter (BPD) is usually 7 cm behind the advancing face, so in reality, when the face is distending the vulva (crowning), the BPD has only just engaged. Marked caput and molding is often present.

Mentum posterior (MP)—Right MP or left MP

The mechanisms of labor in MP are like those of occipitoposterior position except that anterior rotation of the mentum occurs in only 45 to 65 percent of cases in the second stage.[2] In cases of persistent MP, the neck is too short to span the 12 cm of the anterior aspect of the sacrum, and the thorax thrusts in to occupy the pelvis with the engaging sternobregamatic diameter of 18 cm. Hence, it is almost impossible for persistent MP to deliver vaginally (unless the fetus is extremely small or one that is macerated).

Risks/Complications

- Perineal tear during delivery of the head.

Management Options

1. Antenatal
   - To rule out congenital abnormalities by ultrasound scan
   - Membranes may rupture early (examine vaginally to exclude prolapsed cord)
   - To check that pelvis is adequate and that the fetus is not 'oversized'. If either feature is present cesarean section (CS) should be considered (Table 38.5).
2. Intrapartum
   - If anterior rotation to MA, a longer labor but spontaneous vaginal delivery will occur in 90 percent of cases. May require forceps to assist last part of second stage
   - If MT, emergency CS is preferred (Table 38.5) and commonly performed, although in the decades bygone manual rotation followed by forceps extraction (Thorn's maneuver), Kielland forceps rotation and extraction have been described with success
   - If MP, it is impossible to deliver vaginally with any normal-sized fetus and hence, CS is always done. It is pertinent to mention here that internal version or conversion to vertex presentation when the head is low are both maneuvers best avoided.
3. Postpartum
   - Prevent postpartum hemorrhage (PPH) with oxytocics.

Table 38.5: Indications of cesarean section in face presentation

---

1. *Early cesarean section in labor*
   a. Mentoposterior position
   b. Associated maternal complications

2. *Late cesarean section*
   a. Persistent mento-transverse position
   b. Prolonged labor
   c. Fetal distress

Brow Presentation (Syn: *Glabella presentation*)

Definition

Brow is the rarest variety of cephalic presentation where the head is partial (halfway) extended; the presenting part being an area between the orbital ridges below, the bregma above and the frontum (forehead) is the denominator. However, the denominator in brow presentation is of little value as there is no mechanism of labor due to the large presenting diameter (mento-vertical—13.5 cm). Many cases of brow become a face or vertex presentation with onset of labor and deliver vaginally. If they persist as a brow presentation a CS should be undertaken for a term live fetus.

Incidence

The reported incidence is 1:1000-3000 deliveries (0.1-0.03%).

Etiology

A brow presentation is commonly unstable and often converts to a face or occiput presentation. The causes of persistent brow presentation are similar to those of face presentation and include anything that interferes with flexion. The common causes and associations are (Fig. 38.6):

1. Maternal
   - Contracted pelvis and fetopelvic disproportion
   - Uterine anomalies (Bicornuate; neoplasm of lower segment)
   - Polyhydramnios
   - Prelabor rupture of membranes (PROM)
2. Fetal
   - Prematurity
   - Congenital malformations
   - Coils of umbilical cord around the neck
3. Placental
   - Placenta previa
4. Iatrogenic
   - External version
5. Idiopathic (30%).

Diagnosis

- Rarely made before labor and of little significance if it is brow presentation in the antenatal period.
- Brow presentation may be detected on a late ultrasound scan when there is a "high head at term".

On abdominal examination

- Head feels big
- Not engaged
- Groove between occiput and back; Head felt on both sides of fetus

On vaginal examination

The forehead presents but the definable features are the supraorbital ridges and base of nose that can be

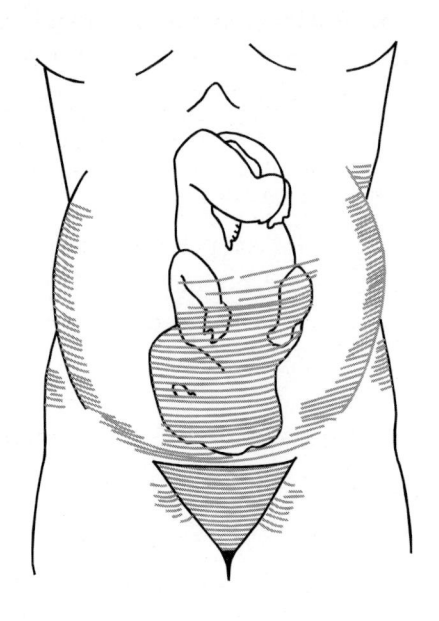

1. Abdominal view

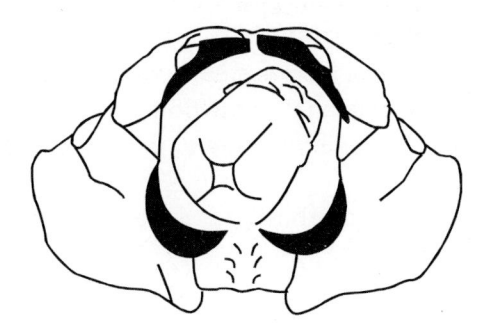

2. Vaginal view

Figure 38.6: Brow presentation

felt at edge of field of examination. Landmarks may be obscured by caput formation in late labor.

Mechanism of Labor

The fetal brow may present as brow anterior or posterior, with the engaging diameter being mentovertical (14 cm). Hence, in a normal-sized fetus and a normal pelvis, there is no mechanism of labor in brow presentation. However, in rare circumstances, with a very small fetus and a large roomy pelvis with good uterine contractions, delivery is possible in anterior brow presentation. There is no mechanism of labor for posterior brow presentation.

Risks/Complications

- Obstructed labor → Rupture uterus (in multiparae).

Management Options

"Any multipara who demonstrates delay in labor with the head above the brim should be suspected of having brow presentation until the contrary is proven".[3]

1. Antenatal
   - Await events; No point in trying to convert to a more favorable presentation
   - Membranes may rupture early (examine vaginally to exclude prolapsed cord)
2. Intrapartum
   - If diagnosed early, one may await events for spontaneous conversion to face (by further extension) or vertex (by flexion)
   - If the brow presentation persists, it will not be possible to deliver, should the fetus be of reasonable size and hence, CS is the preferred and safer treatment
   - If the fetus is dead or there is gross hydrocephaly, craniotomy and vaginal extraction is recommended, after excluding rupture of the uterus
3. Postpartum
   - Higher maternal morbidity associated with operative delivery.

Transverse Lie

Definition

A transverse lie involves the long axis of the fetus lying approximately at right angles (perpendicular) to the long axis of the uterus. Because the shoulder is placed so frequently in the brim of the pelvis, with the head lying in one iliac fossa and the breech in the other, it is often referred to as shoulder presentation, with the back being the denominator. As there is no mechanism of labor with transverse lie–the denominator here is of no consequence.

The long axis of the fetus may lie along the oblique diameter of the uterus. The oblique lie may be only transitory, because either a longitudinal or transverse lie commonly results when labor supervenes. Hence, the presence of an oblique lie after 36 weeks may be an unstable lie if the lie changes from time to time to transverse or longitudinal lie.

Incidence

The incidence is 2 percent in early third trimester but only 0.2 to 0.3 percent (1:200 to 300 deliveries) at term.

Etiology

Anything that prevents engagement of the head or the breech may predispose to transverse lie. The common causes are (Figure 38.7):

1. Maternal
   - Ninety percent of the transverse lie presentations are seen in multiparae because of pendulous abdomen. Grand-multiparae have a ten-fold incidence of transverse lie than nulliparous women
   - Contracted pelvis and fetopelvic disproportion
   - Uterine anomalies (Uterus subseptus; uterus arcuatus; uterus bicornis; neoplasms: fibroids)
   - Polyhydramnios
2. Fetal
   - Prematurity
   - Forty percent of the transverse lie presentations are associated with multiple pregnancy; usually involves the 2nd twin
   - Intrauterine fetal death (IUFD)
   - Congenital malformations
3. Placental
   - Placenta previa
4. Idiopathic (30%)

Malposition, Malpresentations and Cord Prolapse

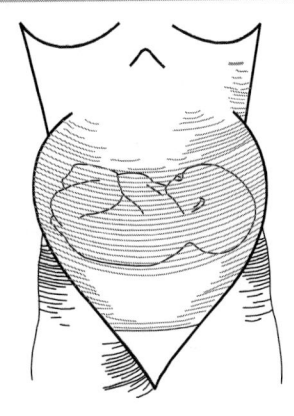

1. Transverse lie : LScP

2. Breech in iliac fossa   3. Head in iliac fossa

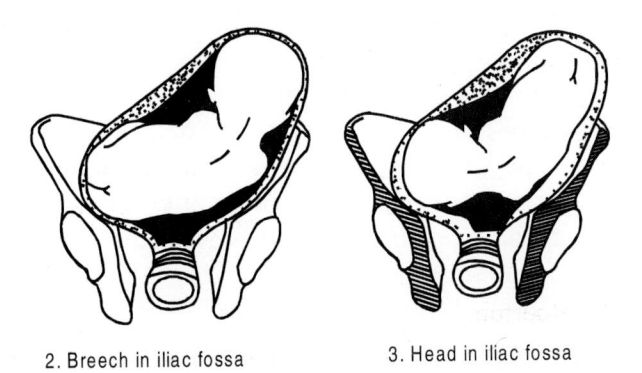

Figure 38.7: Transverse lie

Diagnosis

- Ultrasound scan confirms the diagnosis

On abdominal examination

- Abnormal shape of the uterus (the fundus being lower than expected)
- No fetal pole in the fundus or in the pelvic inlet (Pawlik's grip empty)
- Head is in one flank and the breech in the other. Commonly, the fetus can be rotated to a cephalic presentation quite readily but reverts to the transverse lie
  Fetal heart is usually audible best below the umbilicus but it has no diagnostic significance.

On vaginal examination

- Pelvis is empty with no presenting part (negative finding)
- During labor: Palpation of the side of the thorax, scapula and clavicle; "Grid-iron" feel of the ribs

- If the diagnosis of placenta previa has not been ruled out by prior ultrasound examination, vaginal examination is avoided in transverse lie.
  The presence of placenta previa should be excluded with ultrasound scan of the abdomen.

Mechanism of Labor

Transverse lie may present as dorsoanterior, dorsoposterior, dorsosuperior or dorsoinferior, either left or right in relation to the maternal pelvis.

Most common position: Left dorsoanterior

A persistent transverse lie cannot deliver spontaneously, and if uncorrected impaction takes place. The shoulder is jammed into the pelvis, the head and breech stay above the inlet, the neck becomes stretched, and progress is arrested. Transverse lie must never be left to nature.

The events that usually occur are as follows:

1. *Spontaneous version*: Over 80 percent of all transverse lie in the antenatal period will spontaneously convert (spontaneous correction) to longitudinal by the time the patient presents in labor; This is also called spontaneous version when converted to breech or spontaneous rectification when converted to vertex.
2. *Spontaneous expulsion*: If the fetus is very small (< 800gm) and the pelvis is large, spontaneous expulsion is possible despite persistence of transverse lie by a mechanism known as "birth conduplicato corpore", wherein the fetal head and thorax, and the body of the fetus, which is doubled upon itself, is expelled.
3. *Spontaneous evolution*: Expulsion of the breech and trunk followed by the delivery of the head, in cases with arm prolapse and in the presence of very strong uterine contractions.
4. *Neglected shoulder presentation*: Persistence of transverse lie which when left unattended → Obstructed labor → Rupture uterus (with clinical evidences of dehydration, ketoaciosis, shock, sepsis) → Increased maternal and fetal morbidity and mortality.

Risks/Complications
- PROM → Prolapse of cord/arm
- Neglected shoulder presentation and obstructed labor.

Management Options
Patients with transverse lie should not be allowed to go into labor because of the risks of uterine rupture and cord prolapse.[4]

1. Antenatal
   - Provided the gestational age has been confirmed, a persistent transverse lie should be managed conservatively till 37 weeks
   - External cephalic version (ECV) may be attempted to convert a transverse lie to a longitudinal one (cephalic / breech) and repeated if necessary. If the lie corrects itself or is corrected by ECV and remains longitudinal await spontaneous onset of labor. In early labor the lie should be checked again.
   - Stabilizing induction (explained later).
   - *Elective CS at term (Table 38.6)*
   - **Caution**: Care should be taken while performing elective CS as the lower segment is most often not well formed; Usually the normal transverse incision or a 'J' shaped incision on the lower segment should suffice.
   - Membranes may rupture early (examine vaginally to exclude prolapsed cord/arm) → Perform immediate CS.

Table 38.6: Indications of elective cesarean section in transverse lie

1. Failed external version
2. Associated high-risk factors
3. Compound presentation with transverse lie.

1. Intrapartum
   - *Stabilizing induction* is done by first converting the lie by external cephalic version to a cephalic presentation, and if the fetus stays in the changed position, oxytocin infusion is started with the lie remaining longitudinal. Close observation is maintained and subsequent amniotomy is performed only when the head is fixed in the brim. Labor usually follows in the normal fashion and if there be any problem during labor, immediate CS is performed.
   - Internal podalic version (IPV) has no place in the treatment of transverse lie in labor except for delivery of the second twin in modern obstetric practice.
   - If the fetus is long dead in cases of neglected transverse lie and where avoidance of CS is desirable, due to fulminating peritonitis destructive operations have been recommended. Decapitation with the use of the Blond-Heidler saw (to be used only by skilled obstetricians) or evisceration may be performed, in exceptional cases. It may be still wise to do a CS if no one is experienced in destructive procedures. In such a situation peritoneal toilet and intravenous broad spectrum antibiotics are essential to avoid systemic sepsis.
3. Postpartum
   - Increased maternal morbidity and mortality because of obstructed labor, sepsis and operative interventions.
   - The overall perinatal mortality rate is as high as 25 to 50 percent.

Breech Presentation

Breech presentation is the most common malpresentation encountered in our clinical practice.

Definition
A fetus is said to be in breech presentation when its podalic extremity lies on the pelvic brim and head occupies the fundus of uterus. It is a longitudinal lie with a difference in polarity. The denominator is the sacrum and the fetal pelvis is the leading pole.

Incidence
Incidence of breech presentation at term is around 3 percent whereas at 28 weeks of pregnancy it is as high as 20 to 25 percent and at 34 weeks it is around 5 percent.

Etiology

In the uterine cavity the spacious area is the fundal region. A live mature fetus by natural rule will try to accommodate its widest area, i.e. podalic region into this spacious area and that is why the most common presentation of a fetus is cephalic at or near term. In very preterm pregnancy, the cephalic portion of the fetus is the wider area and this explains the high incidence of breech around 30 to 34 weeks. As the fetus gradually matures, the podalic portion becomes the widest part of the body, so this will tend to position itself, in the fundal region by kicking the wall of the uterine cavity. The head being a heavier pole also promotes gravitation into the lower uterine segment. Once it occupies this space it remains cephalic due to the contour of the lower portion of the uterus. *A fetus with extended legs, i.e. extended knees, cannot kick because flexed knees are pre-conditions for kicking any object. Hence, these fetuses stay as breech presentation.* Any condition that affects this accommodation process (as mentioned above) will lead to a breech presentation and is the cause for the change of polarity (Table 38.7).

Table 38.7: Causes of breech presentation

1. *Maternal*
   a. Multiparity
   b. Polyhydramnios
   c. Oligohydramnios
   d. Uterine anomalies: Bicornuate; septate; subseptate
   e. Contracted pelvis
2. *Placental*
   a. Cornu-fundal implantation
   b. Placenta previa
3. *Fetal*
   a. Prematurity
   b. Multiple pregnancy
   c. Short cord
   d. Fetal anomalies: hydrocephaly; anencephaly
   e. Intrauterine fetal death
4. *Idiopathic* (50%)

Prematurity is said to be the most common cause of breech presentation. At term pregnancy congenital malformation of uterus, e.g. bicornuate or septate uterus, placenta previa, multiple pregnancy, contracted pelvis, cornufundal insertion of placenta are frequently seen as etiological factors. Anencephaly, hydramnios, intrauterine fetal death, short cord can also be etiological factors though in more than 50 percent of cases the etiology remains unknown.

Types of Breech (Figure 38.8)

Recurrent breech: Recurrence of breech presentation in consecutive three or more pregnancies is known as recurrent or habitual breech. Congenital abnormality of uterus is the frequent cause.

Complete or flexed breech: Here both hip and knee remain in a flexed attitude so that the presenting part is external genitalia, buttocks and the feet.

Incomplete breech

This may be of three types:

a. *Frank breech:* Breech with extended legs (80 percent of all breech presentations). Here the legs remain extended from the knee and the thighs remains flexed on the trunk.
b. *Knee presentation.* Thighs are extended and legs are flexed at the knee.
c. *Footling presentation.* Legs and thighs are both extended, so the feet become the presenting part.

In primigravida, frank breech is more common whereas flexed breech is frequently seen in multigravida. Frank breech fits snugly in the lower segment and cervix and hence, it is a better cervical dilator than flexed breech when in labor. Cord prolapse is less frequently seen in frank breech and more frequent in knee and footling presentation. In frank breech the incidence of cord prolapse is almost comparable to cephalic presentation (0.3%). Flexed breech, when in labor has more chances of cord prolapse, PROM, slow dilatation of cervix and prolonged labor.

Clinical Types

Uncomplicated breech: Breech presentation with no maternal or other fetal complications.

Complicated breech: When conditions that can alter prognosis or outcome of pregnancy is found to be associated, i.e. prematurity, placenta previa are associated with breech presentation. Complicated breech delivery and complicated breech presentation are not synonymous.

1. Complete breech

2. Frank breech

3. Fottling breech

3. Kneeling breech

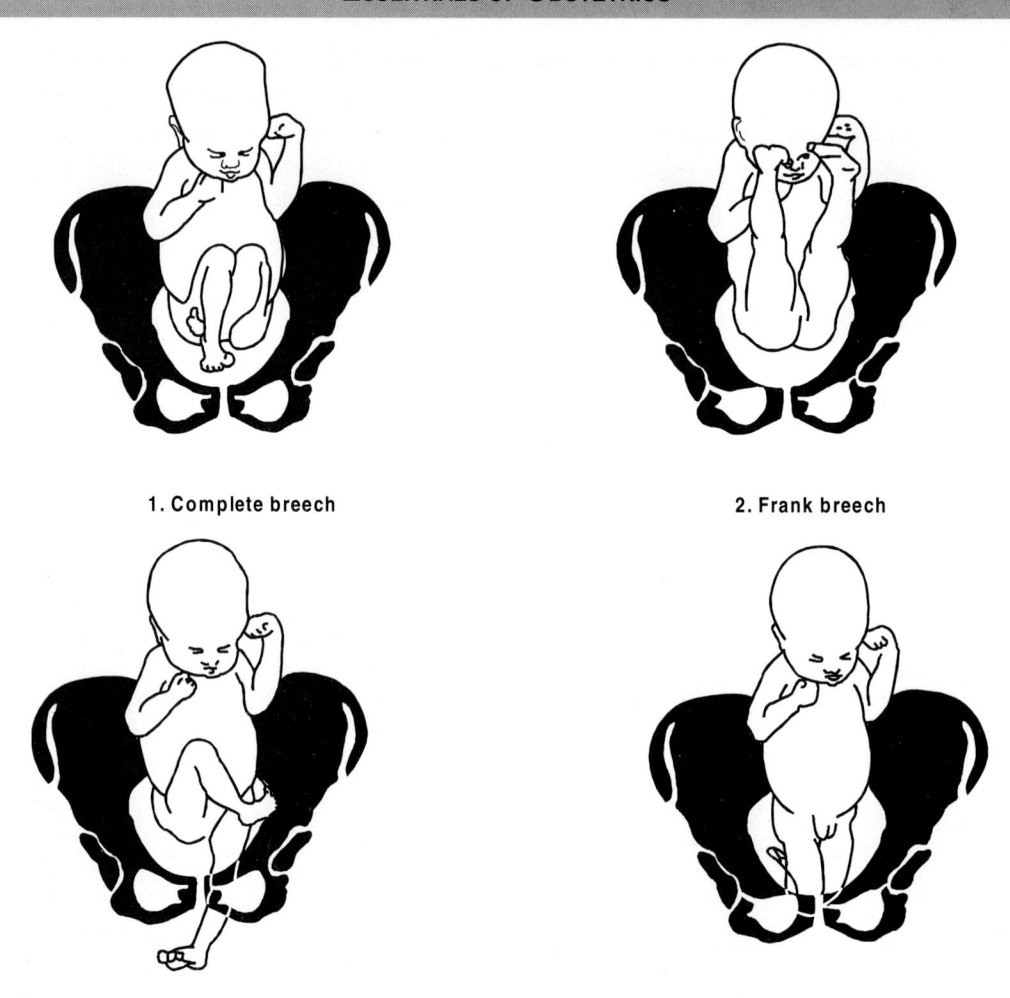

Figure 38.8: Type of breech presentation

Diagnosis

Diagnosis of breech presentation is possible by abdominal and vaginal examination (Table 38.8).

Table 38.8: Diagnosis of breech presentation

1. *Antenatal*
   - Per abdomen
     - Head in the fundus
     - Breech in the lower pole of uterus
     - FHS audible at or above the umbilicus
   - Per vagina: Broad irregular soft mass felt through fornix
   - Confirmation: Ultrasonography
2. *Intranatal*
   - Per abdomen: Same as antenatal examination
   - Per vagina: Presence of anus, sacrum, external genitalia and foot helps to clinch the diagnosis

On abdominal examination

In antenatal period, examination reveals hard, smooth, ballotable head of the fetus occupying fundus of uterus (fundal grip) and soft, broad, irregular non-ballotable mass in the pelvic grip.

FHS is usually heard around or above the umbilicus as the distance of the fetal heart is away from the buttock.

Failure to feel fetal head in pelvic grip would raise the suspicion of breech presentation though on occasions the head may be deeply engaged in the pelvis and is not felt. Non-ballotability of fetal head in breech presentation points toward the possibility of frank breech as the head remains inbetween stretched legs.

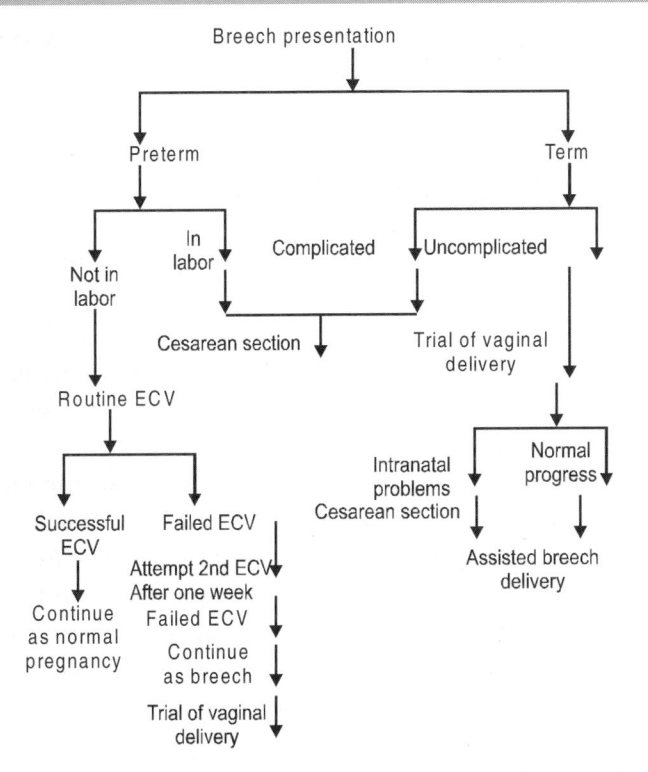

Figure 38.9: Flow chart showing summary of management of breech presentation

2. *Cord presentation:* The cord lies below the level of the presenting part and is felt by the fingers on vaginal examination through the membranes which are intact.
3. *Cord prolapse:* The membranes have ruptured and the cord has prolapsed into the vagina or has emerged out of the vaginal introitus.

Incidence

1:300-400 deliveries (0.3-0.4%).
The incidence varies depending on the presentation:
i. Cephalic: 0.3-0.4%
ii. Breech:
   a. Flexed (Frank): 0.4-0.5 percent (almost that of cephalic)
   b. Complete: 5%
   c. Footling: 15%
iii. Transverse lie: 20%

Etiology

Cord prolapse is associated with anything that prevents the presenting part from fitting closely into the lower uterine segment and thus shutting off the forewaters from the hindwaters.

The *risk factors* associated with cord prolapse are:
1. *Maternal*
   a. Multiparae
   b. Polyhydramnios
   c. Fetopelvic disproportion
   d. Malpresentations (Breech) and abnormal lie–(e.g. Transverse lie)
2. *Placenta and cord abnormalities*
   a. Placenta previa (minor degree)
   b. Battledore placenta
   c. Velamentous insertion of the cord
   d. Unduly long cord
3. *Fetal*
   a. Prematurity
   b. Small baby
   c. Multiple pregnancy
4. *Iatrogenic:* Following amniotomy, version and/or manual rotation of the head

Dangers

The fetus is at immediate risk of hypoxia due to cutting off blood supply:
a. Spasm of umbilical arteries from:
   - Change of temperature (lower temperature outside)
   - Drying (Exposure to outside)
   - Handling
b. Mechanical compression of cord between the presenting part and maternal bony pelvis

Diagnosis

1. *Clinical*
   - *Per abdomen:* Fetal heart may show a sudden alteration in rate or rhythm soon after membrane rupture
   - *Local examination:* Loop of the cord seen at the vulva
   - *Vaginal examination:* Loops of the cord felt in the vagina following rupture of the membranes
2. *Ultrasonography:* Routine scan showing herniation of the membranes with loops of cord below the presenting part (cord presentation) ⟶ sign of

impending cord prolapse on rupture of the membranes.

Management

The essence of good management is anticipation. Prophylactic measures such as the admission of patients to hospital with unstable and transverse lie on completing 37 weeks of gestation, and the avoidance of amniotomy before the fetal pole has become deeply engaged in the pelvis, and the early vaginal examination following spontaneous rupture of the membranes will all go a long way to reduce the mortality and morbidity for the fetus.

Cardinal principle

On diagnosing prolapse of the umbilical cord, do *not* handle the cord too much; Just determine whether the vessels are pulsating or not!! Replace the cord within the vagina to maintain the temperature and moisture content to reduce the chance of cord artery going into spasm.

Fetus is mature and alive

1. Deliver immediately:
   a. If cervix is not fully dilated: Immediate cesarean section (CS)
   b. If cervix is fully dilated with favorable cephalic presentation in a multiparous woman: Vacuum extraction is usually considered; No difficult forceps application is permitted in modern obstetrics; Any associated problems: CS
   c. If cervix is fully dilated with breech presentation in a multiparous woman: Breech extraction can be considered only if vaginal delivery is expected within 10 to 15 minutes; Otherwise, plan for immediate CS

   Note: The fear of performing CS for a dead baby can, should and must be minimized by auscultating the fetal heart immediately before operating.

2. If immediate delivery is impossible (e.g. prolapsed cord occurs outside a properly equipped obstetrical unit):
   a. Send for the obstetric Flying Squad urgently.
   b. Keep cord moist, warm by reducing it into the vagina and do not handle; Do *not* try to put the cord back into the uterus above the presenting part, as each attempt will allow more loops to come down and the additional handling increases spasm.
   c. Prevent compression of cord between the presenting part and bony pelvis:
   - Put the mother in lateral position with pelvis raised on pillows (or exaggerated Sims' position); press up the presenting part with the fingers in the vagina
   - Vago's method: With the patient in a moderate Trendelenburg position, a No. 16 Foley's catheter is inserted into the urinary bladder (balloon inflated with 5 ml of normal saline), following which 500 ml of warm normal saline is rapidly introduced and the catheter clamped thereafter; the distended bladder keeps the presenting part high and relieves pressure on the cord. This allows time for preparation for CS

Fetus is dead

There is no urgency, as there is no immediate increased risk to the mother. Allow events to proceed, as the prolapsed cord will not obstruct labor.

Prognosis

Maternal: Increased morbidity due to risk of operative delivery.

Fetal: Depends where the woman is when the cord prolapse occurs and at what stage of labor:
- If the mother is in hospital and the prolapse occurs in the second stage, the fetal loss is less than 3 percent
- If the mother is at home with a cord prolapse, the fetal loss is as high as 70 percent

REFERENCES

1. Phillips RD, Freeman M: The management of persistent occiputposterior position: A review of 552 consecutive cases. *Obstet Gynecol* **43:**171, 1974.
2. Johanson R: Malposition, malpresentation and cephalopelvic disproportion. In Edmonds DK (Ed): *Dewhurst's Textbook of Obstetrics and Gynecology for Postgraduates,* 6th edn, 277-90, 1999.
3. Malvern J: Abnormal fetal presentations and cephalopelvic disproportion. In Chamberlain G (Ed): *Turnbull's Obstetrics,*

2nd edn, 657-84, 1995.
4. Gemer O, Kopmar A, Sassoon E, Segal S: Neglected transverse lie with uterine rupture. *Arch Gynecol Obstet* **252**:159-60, 1993.
5. Bradley-Watson PJ: The decreasing value of external cephalic version in modern obstetrics practice. *Am J Obstet Gynecol* **123**:237, 1975.
6. Ranney B: The gentle art of external cephalic version. *Am J Obstet Gynecol* **115**:497, 1973.
7. Marcus RG, Crewe-Brown H, Krawitz S, Katz J: Fetomaternal hemorrhage following successful and unsuccessful attempts at external cephalic version. *Br J Obstet Gynecol* **82**:578, 1975.
8. Collea JV, Chein C, Quilligan EJ: The randomised management of term frank breech presentation: A Study of 208 cases. *Am J Obstet Gynecol* **137**:235, 1980.
9. Lyons ER, Papsin FR: Cesarean section in the management of breech presentation. *Am J Obstet Gynecol* **130**:558, 1978.
10. Gimovsky ML, Paul RH: Singleton breech presentation in labor. *Am J Obstet Gynecol* **143**:733, 1982.
11. Rovinksy JJ, Miller JA, Kaplan S: Management of breech presentation at term. *Am J Obstet Gynecol* **15**:497, 1973.

39.
Operative Obstetrics

Silvam Sellappan
V Sivanesaratnam

PART TWO

Feto-maternal Medicine

INTRODUCTION

Operative obstetrics covers a wide range of obstetric procedures from fetomaternal investigations to normal delivery to cesarean hysterectomy. For the purpose of this chapter, discussion will be confined to intrapartum events requiring assistance at vaginal delivery with forceps or vacuum extraction, shoulder dystocia and cesarean section.

Operative obstetrics is a changing art. Many of the earlier concepts and procedures, especially difficult manipulation of vaginal delivery, are currently considered obsolete. Contemporary techniques and strategies are being developed and increasingly accepted. Cost effective practice, patient demands and legal consequences of any serious injury to mother or infant are pertinent in the ideal management plan.

This review of selected obstetric procedures focuses on current trends of operative delivery practice considered safe by the majority of obstetricians.

FORCEPS DELIVERY

Forceps delivery was introduced as an extricating tool to be used in emergency situations to save the life of the mother. The most widely recorded and historically accurate use of forceps for extraction of a living child is credited to the *Chamberlin family* (17th century). After the secret of forceps delivery was released many modifications were made to the original Chamberlin model.

However, use of obstetric forceps has been controversial since their invention. After early use, the use of forceps was almost abandoned by early 19th century. The reasons were that the instrument was used by unskilled practitioners, resulting in injury to the mother and the child, increase in litigation and popularity and over-reliance on cesarean section.

The resurgence in forceps use is attributed to the 'triple obstetric tragedy' (involving Princess Charlotte, her baby and Dr. Richard Craft) in 1818, development of excellent obstetric anesthesia and prophylactic use of forceps. Again with the increasing popularity of cesarean section the more difficult forceps deliveries were abandoned. The apparently favorable results of cesarean section (in term of perinatal morbidity) has led to liberal use of cesarean section in the first stage of labor. This event immensely contributed to a generation of obstetricians who are inexperienced and uncomfortable with the use of forceps.[1]

Adequate knowledge of the instruments, anatomy of the pelvis, physiological changes during labor, an understanding of the mechanics of labor and appropriate selection of cases will ensure minimal morbidity in forceps delivery.

Instrument

Forceps are paired, symmetrical and have matched blades. The left blade is applied to the left side of the maternal pelvis and similarly the right blade to right side. Each blade is divided into 4 parts, i.e.: handle, lock, shank and curved blades. There may be an axis traction bar (Figure 39.1, Plate 3).

1. *Blades* are either open (fenestrated) or solid. Open blades facilitate traction but are prone to injure maternal soft tissue if used for rotation of the fetal head. Solid blades are designed for rotation but there is an increased chance of slippage. After articulation, the forceps present with 2 curves in planes at right angles to each other. First, the cephalic curve is the curve that accommodates to the fetal head; secondly, the pelvic curve that corresponds to curve of pelvis.
2. *Shank* connects the handle and the blades. It may be parallel or may overlap. It is designed to be longer in instruments for midpelvic delivery (e.g. Kiellands forceps)
3. The *locking* mechanism is placed at the shank or where the shank joins the handle. By convention, the lock is built into the left blade. Types of locking mechanism are English type (e.g: Neville-Barnes), sliding lock (Kiellands forceps) and pivot lock (Piper forceps).
4. *Handle* is the distal part of forceps with finger grips and/or lateral flanges.

The forceps can be divided into *classical and specialized types*. The classical forceps (e.g. Neville-Barnes, Figure 39.1, Plate 3) are used more for an outlet or low cavity forceps delivery. These have a pelvic curve directed upward so that when the forceps are applied to the fetal head presenting in an occipito-anterior position, the curve of the instrument approximates the pelvic curve. These forceps are not meant for rotation. The specialized forceps are used for cases of midpelvic arrest or for rotations, e.g. in Kiellands forceps where the pelvic curve is no longer desirable.

Classification of Forceps Delivery

The forceps operation has classically been described according to the station of the fetal bony head in the pelvis. The American College of Obstetricians and Gynecologists classification[2] has clarified a few previous inconsistent definitions. The classification is summarized below:

1. *Outlet forceps:* The scalp is seen at the introitus without separating labia and the fetal head is at the perineum. Fetal skull has reached pelvic floor. The sagittal suture is in antero-posterior diameter. If the head is in ROA or LOA position (the position is less than 45° from anteroposterior axis), rotation must first be performed.
2. *Low forceps:* Leading point of fetal skull is at station > + 2 cm but not on the pelvic floor. Rotation may be less or more than 45°.
3. *Mid forceps:* The head is engaged and is below ischial spines with station less than + 2 cm.
4. *High forceps:* Fetal head is not engaged and is not included in the classification.

Note: The above classification is also applicable for *vacuum delivery*.

Tips for Safe and Successful Forceps Delivery

1. *Correct indications for forceps delivery must be present*
   - Maternal
     - Maternal exhaustion from prolonged labor
     - Maternal disease (e.g. cardiac disease, pregnancy induced hypertension) where use of prophylactic forceps will help to minimize maternal effort.
     - Poor maternal effort
   - Fetal
     - Impending fetal compromise (as evidenced by non-reassuring fetal heart rate patterns)
     - Prolonged second stage of labor (and arrest in progress of labor)
     - 'aftercoming' head of breech delivery
2. *Pre-requisites for safe application of forceps*
   - Cervix must be fully dilated
   - Fetal head must be engaged; ideally it should not be palpable per abdomen

- Head must be in a suitable position for the application of forceps
- Membranes must be ruptured
- Maternal pelvis is adequate for safe vaginal delivery
- Contractions must be present and adequate (4 in 10 min each lasting > 40 secs)
- Empty bladder and rectum
- Appropriate analgesia (pudendal block or epidural)
- Surgical asepsis is observed

3. Prior to forceps delivery *a thorough assessment* of the fetal head must be carried out per abdomen as well as per vagina. The head should preferably be not palpable per abdomen. Vaginal examination will help to determine the exact position and station of the fetal head. *The following points should be noted:*
   - Severe moulding (overlapping of the skull bones) may indicate cephalopelvic disproportion
   - The presence of caput may obscure the fontanelles and sagittal sutures and may make the determination of fetal position difficult ; palpating the fetal ear in this situation is helpful
   - The presence of caput and moulding should also alert the accoucher to the presence of asynclitism or deflexed head

4. A careful reassessment of the pelvic capacity is carried out. *An inadequate pelvis is suspected in the presence of one or more of the following features:*
   - Palpable sacral promontory
   - Prominent ischial spines
   - Narrow greater sciatic notch (suggested by width of sacro-spinous ligament of less than 3 finger breath)
   - Convergent pelvic side walls
   - Narrow sub-pubic arch

5. *Technique of application of forceps*
   - The left blade is held in the left hand and inserted between the left vaginal wall and head by inserting the right hand to guide a sweeping arch-like movement to negotiate the pelvic and cephalic curve. The blade is guided into the correct position with first two fingers of the right hand. As the blade is inserted, the handle is gently and carefully dropped into a horizontal position. The right blade is then held in a similar manner with the right hand and introduced into the right side of the pelvis, with guidance of left hand. Gentle wondering may help to improve the blades position. The blades are then locked
   - Correctly applied blades of forceps will lock easily. If this does not occur it may indicate malposition and possible asynclitism. Remove the blades and reassess the position of the fetal head. The sagittal suture should always be perpendicular to the plane of the shanks. Forcible locking should be avoided as this may invariably result in fetal trauma
   - Apply traction on the forceps only during a uterine contraction to coincide with maternal bearing down efforts; when the contraction has subsided release the lock to avoid prolonged compression on the fetal head.
   - The descent of the fetal head through the pelvis must follow the curve of Carus (pelvic axis). Traction must, therefore, be applied in this direction.
   - Outlet and low forceps deliveries are generally safe. However, mid-forceps deliveries are associated with high morbidity and should be performed by experienced personnel.[3]

Trial of Forceps

Trial usually takes place in the operation theater with the anesthetist being present. Forceps is attempted with the intention of abandoning should there be difficulty. Persistence when delivery is difficult results in increased maternal and fetal morbidity.

VACUUM DELIVERY

The concept of vacuum extraction was first introduced by James Young in 1706.[4] However the practical application of this device became popular only after Malmstrom described his vacuum extractor in mid-twentieth century (Figure 39.2, Plate 3). For the first time a device with a different mechanism of action from forceps was used, i.e. instead of getting hold of the whole head, the vacuum extractor adhered to the scalp through the forces of vacuum and suction.

Steel cup is bell-shaped with a smooth turned in lip and has a diameter of 60 or 50 mm. The dome of the cup is attached to a rubber suction tube through which is passed a traction chain that is anchored in the cup. A traction handle is fixed at the other end of tubing.

Beyond the handle, the tubing is attached to a bottle with vacuum gauge and air pump. By gradual increase in negative pressure, the fetal scalp tissue is sucked into the hollow of the shallow cup to create a caput succedaneum called a 'Chignon' (acts as a traction area for the cup).

Soft Vacuum Extraction Cups (Figures 39.3A and B, Plate 3)

The soft cups made of pliable plastic material were introduced in 1973.[5] Soft cup device resulted in a reawakening of interest in the vacuum extractor. Kobayashi silastic cup with a stainless steel valve on the stem allowed release of a significant amount of the suction force between contractions without loss of cup application to the fetal head. The cup diameter (65 mm) is the largest and it fits over the fetal occiput similar to a skull cap. It offers the advantage of less scalp trauma as it better adapts to the fetal head, required no chignon and has no rigid metal edge.

Overall much less scalp trauma occurred with soft cup than had been cited in several series using the metal cup. Silastic cup extractor effects delivery in a shorter time period but a higher failure rate compared with metal cups has been observed. These cups are most suited for occipitoanterior position. For occipitoposterior and transverse positions, a metal posterior cup or a '"Kiwi" omnicup is needed so as to manipulate the cup to the flexion point, which is on the midline 3 to 4 cm anterior to the posterior fontanelle.

Tips for Safe Vacuum Delivery

- *Indications*
  - The indications are similar to those for forceps.
- *Contraindications*: These include:
  - Cephalopelvic disproportion
  - High station
  - Face presentation
  - Aftercoming head of breech delivery
- The prerequisites (which are similar for forceps) must be fulfilled
- The vacuum system is checked for leaks prior to ventouse application
- A careful vaginal examination is carried out to ensure all the features are appropriate for safe instrumental delivery
- The position and attitude of the head should be carefully ascertained to achieve a flexing median application; this is important as application of the cup without recognizing an abnormal position can lead to a deflexing median or paramedian application and difficult delivery resulting in intracranial injury
- Before application of the cup, identify the sagittal suture, posterior fontanelle and anterior fontanelle When the cup is applied, it should be bisected by the sagittal suture and there should be at least 3 cm between the edge of the cup and the anterior fontanelle (flexing median application)
- Before traction is applied, vaginal examination is carried out to ensure that maternal tissue is not caught within the cup
- Traction is applied only during a uterine contraction together with maternal effort. The direction of traction should be perpendicular to the cup (as far as possible) as oblique traction can result in cup detachment. Placement of the thumb of the non-pulling hand on the dome of the cup and the index finger of the same hand against the fetal skull will help to apply counter-pressure that helps to prevent detachment of the cup. The following points should be taken note of:
  - The birth canal is not a straight line; the axis of the 2 parts (mid-pelvis to pelvic floor and pelvic floor to introitus) are almost $90°$ to each other
  - The soft tissue of the perineum can limit the direction of traction; an episiotomy will allow traction in the right axis
- If the cup is well placed, i.e. flexing median application, traction on the cup will flex the fetal head. By maintaining the traction axis parallel to the axis of the birth canal through which the head is traversing, the head will usually rotate to an occiput anterior position as it encounters the muscular levator ani sling posteriorly

- For metal cup, Bird (1976) modified the instrument by moving the vacuum hose away from the center of the cup to the periphery, but still retaining the traction chain in the center of the cup. This is for easier cup placement when the head is in the occipitoposterior or lateral position. Traction at an acute angle to the plane of the cup is likely to elevate one edge of the cup and for it to 'pop-off'.
- If the properly applied cup slips, it could be due to one of two reasons:
  - Leakage in the system
  - Unrecognized disproportion

Thus, if leakage in the system is excluded, disproportion is likely. Never reapply the cup if the likely reason is disproportion; resort to lower segment cesarean section instead.

Vacuum versus Forceps

Generally vacuum delivery is felt to be simpler and requires less anesthesia. Maternal morbidity and perinatal deaths is lower with vacuum delivery than with forceps. However, there is a higher incidence of non-serious scalp trauma with vacuum-extractor than with forceps.[6]

Although the studies are more favorable for vacuum delivery, reports of fetal complications such as scalp abrasions, caput succedaneum, intracranial bleeding and subaponeurotic or subgaleal hemorrhages suggests that this technique should be practiced with care.

Significant improvement in instrumentation (e.g. posterior cups, soft cups), limiting vacuum extraction to only second stage of labor with full cervical dilatation, proper case selection, limiting duration of procedure to 15 minutes and abandoning the procedure if the cup 'pops-off' (after leakage in the system has been excluded) will make the use of vacuum safe and more attractive than forceps.[7]

CESAREAN SECTION

In the last 2 decades tremendous improvements have been achieved in the technical and safety aspects of cesarean section. A very good outcome is expected from childbirth by the couple. *Therefore, there is no place for vaginal delivery at all cost.* The important factor to consider is minimal birth trauma at either vaginal delivery or cesarean section. About 12 to 25 percent of all deliveries are from cesarean section.[8]

At the end of 19th century cesarean section was one of the most fatal surgical operations due to hemorrhage and infection. Maternal mortality rates decreased steadily with the introduction of blood transfusion, antibiotics and safe anesthesia. Improvement in fetal monitoring with ultrasound, cardiotocograph and fetal blood sampling was a great achievement after 1960. Cesarean section provided the ideal choice of fulfilling both maternal safety (in high risk cases) and reduction in perinatal morbidity and mortality.

1. *Skin incisions* can be either transverse or vertical. Both types have their advantages and disadvantages. Choice of abdominal incision depends on the clinician and clinical situation (Table 39.1).

Table 39.1: Features of transverse and vertical incision

Transverse (Pfannensteil)	Vertical
• More popular due to cosmetic purposes	• Less popular
• Limited exposure	• Rapid entry and good exposure
• Cherny/Maylard modification may be needed, in the presence of previous similar surgery.	• Median/paramedian incision can be made
• Hernia less common (this usually occurs at the angles)	• Post-operative hernia more common (this can occur anywhere along the incision)

2. *Peritoneal* opening usually will be vertical but can be modified to tailor clinical condition.
3. *Uterine incisions*: Three common types:
    i. Lower segment transverse section.
    ii. Lower segment vertical section.
    iii. Classical section.
4. *Lower segment transverse section* is the most widely used incision and ideal for most patients. The incised area is less vascular than other parts, uterine closure is easier and it is easier to advance the bladder peritoneum to cover the incision. The problems are limitation of incisional length by the width of the lower segment and accidental lateral extension may cause bleeding from torn arteries and veins.

Technical Clues

- Peritoneal reflection between bladder and uterus must be identified (uterovesical fold). Uterine dextrorotation must be noted. About 1 cm below uterovesical fold's firm attachment to the uterus, the loose visceral peritoneum is incised laterally toward the round ligament. Blunt (finger) and sharp dissection may be needed.

- Entrance through the entire uterine wall (after initial small transverse incision at midline) can be in 2 ways:
  - Incising with a Mayo scissors
  - Insert 2 fingers and enlarge the incision

  Use of scissors lead to precise termination of lateral margin and gives clean cut edges for closure; but arcuate arteries which run transversely can be cut resulting in bleeding. On the other hand, 'tearing' avoids injury to arcuate arteries but skill and experience is needed to avoid injury to the lateral vessels; the edges of the wound will be ragged.
- Large uterine incision is necessary for an atraumatic delivery. A traumatic delivery through a small incision will increase perinatal morbidity.
- Placing of Green Armitage clamps at incised edges of the lower segment and securing the angles with suture before removal of placenta will reduce blood loss.

  Angle suture placed at uterine muscle must avoid vessel injury.
- Uterine closure: Bladder need to be mobilized sufficiently to avoid suture line. The closure is carried out in two layers; the first layer is a continuous locking suture (excluding the endometrium) and is more hemostatic if each lock is pulled and held tight. A continuous running suture is easily readjustable at the end and more rapid for fast hemostasis. The second layer (continuous running) buries the first layer. The unique features of uterine incision are healing, tissue catabolism and involution; thus, the suture line become loose in a few days. Interrupted sutures may be more useful then continuous sutures, this will, however, take longer to perform.[9]

  Suture type: Heavy suture with large diameter is best (1/0 or 0) because it will not cut through the muscle even though it is tied snugly. The bites should be big enough and carefully pulled straight up. Bleeding along suture line can be controlled with figure-of-eight stitches. One should remember that suturing the uterus is easy but it needs to be done well.
- *Uterine vasculature*—Uterus is supplied by 4 major arteries and 2 ascending vaginal branches of the pudendal arteries. There are numerous anastamoses. Ligation of a specific vessel is impossible and bleeding point is best controlled by placing fairly deep mattress suture around the site of hemorrhage.

Lower Segment Vertical Section

It is useful for the delivery of premature infants and abnormal presentation and in situation where the lower segment is not well-formed and is narrow. Incision can be easily enlarged. However, bladder injury can occur. Upper segment extension may be needed and adhesion along the course of the incision may lead to more difficult repeat cesarean section.[9]

Classical Cesarean Section

The bladder and cervix is not disturbed. It is useful for cases of carcinoma of cervix in pregnancy (prior to performing radical surgery), major placenta previa and transverse lie with back turned downward or after a previous vesico-vaginal fistula repair or extensive bladder adhesion to the uterus.[9] The disadvantages of this operation are more chances of rupture in a subsequent pregnancy, technical difficulty in closing the uterine incision and subsequent adhesion formation. The uterine incision is usually closed with several layers of interrupted sutures.

Cesarean Hysterectomy

Technically difficult operation because of the vascularity and anatomic changes in the pregnant uterus and supporting structures. The most common indication is intractable uterine bleeding that cannot be controlled by other means. The common causes of massive bleeding are atonic uterus, placenta accreta and rupture of uterus. Some useful tips to remember are:

Technical clues

- In non-pregnant women without pelvic relaxation, the broad ligament (fibrous sheet of peritoneum) is taut as it stretches across the pelvis. At postpartum

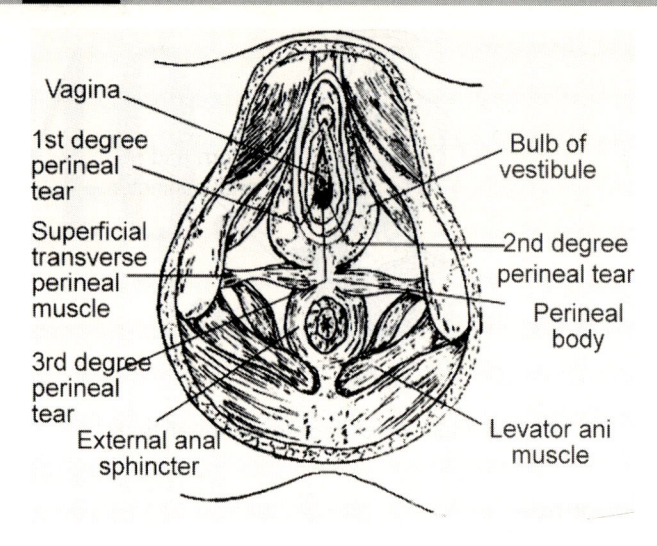

Figure 40.4: Diagrammatic representation of different stages of perineal tear

- The skin may be closed with interrupted transcutaneous sutures or continuous subcuticular suture using an absorbable material (PGA)
- Good hemostasis should be maintained.

Method (Figures 40.4 and 40.5)

1. *First and second degree tear*: The repair is done under local anesthesia with 1 percent lignocaine injected slowly in the surrounding tissues avoiding accidental puncture of veins. First the vaginal mucous membrane is apposed and then the torn perineal muscles, followed by suturing of the perineal skin.
2. *Third degree tear*: This operation is best done with the patient under general or spinal anesthesia. The rectum or anal canal is repaired with 00-chromic catgut or fine PGA suture, knot tied inside the rectum or anal canal. The two ends of the anal sphincter are picked up with tissue forceps and sutured in the middle with two or three, no 1-chromic catgut or PGA suture. The repair is completed as for second degree tear.

Postoperative Care

- The perineal wound is kept cleaned by sterile antiseptic swab after each act of urination and defecation.
- In case of complete tear low residual diet is given for 4 to 5 days and the patient is given a stool softener (Milk of magnesia) from 2nd day on wards.
- Antibiotics and analgesics are added.

If the repair breaks down or if the patient comes after 24 hours of injury, it should be left for 3 months before repair. If pregnancy follows a well healed complete tear, a large episiotomy is needed preferably on the other side during vaginal delivery.

INJURY TO VULVA

Tear of vestibule is common and is the result of over distension during delivery. Tear may be close to the urethral meatus and often associated with brisk hemorrhage, This should be repaired with fine suture material (00-chromic catgut with atraumatic needle) after a catheter is placed inside the bladder to avoid injury of the urethra (Figure 40.6).

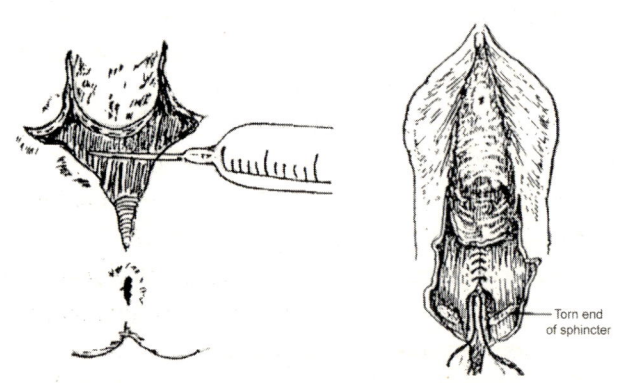

Figure 40.5A: Local infiltration anesthesia

Figure 40.5B: Approximation of mucosa of rectum and anal canal

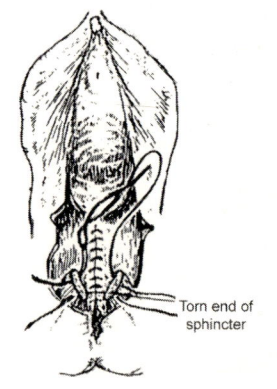

Figure 40.5C: Suturing of anal sphincter

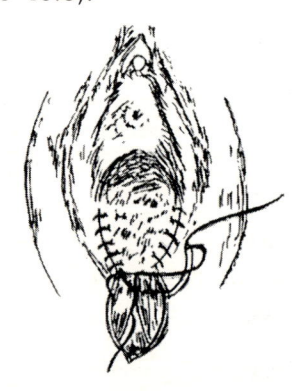

Figure 40.5D: Perineal muscle suture

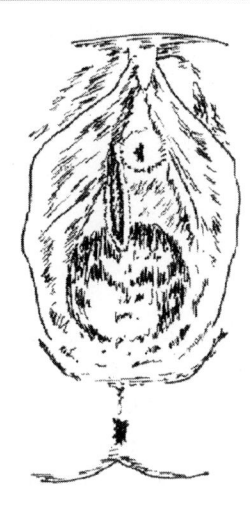

Figure 40.6: injury to vulva (para urethral tear)

VAGINAL INJURY

These are commonly accompanied by perineal tear. The tears often extend upwards for a variable distance in posterolateral sulcus of one or both sides. Injury to upper third of vagina may be an extension from cervical tears and need to be carefully examined. Injury to lateral vaginal wall, at the site of ischial spine may be possible due to faulty application of forceps. Vaginal tears in the upper third are better repaired under general or regional anesthesia with good exposure and assistance by 0-chromic catgut or PGA suture with good hemostasis.

Types

Vesicovaginal fistulae are uncommon injuries nowadays. They may be traumatic or ischemic following prolonged compression of the vaginal wall and bladder between fetal head and the symphysis pubis. This type of injury will be discussed elsewhere.

Colporrhexis (Rupture of Vaginal Vault)

The usual site is the posterior or lateral fornix and cervix may be involved. The tear may be due to improper application of forceps or result from obstructed labor.

Treatment: Accessible vault tear is repaired through vaginal route. If examining finger passes completely through the tear, laparotomy is needed. In extreme cases, hysterectomy may be required for quick hemostasis.

Paravaginal Hematoma (Pelvic Hematoma)

Injuries to the vessels surrounding the wall of genital tract may lead to collection of blood anywhere in-between the pelvic peritoneum and the perineal skin and may lead to hematoma formation. The hematoma may be small or big enough to cause sudden collapse of the patient. Paravaginal hematoma should be categorized into supralevator or infralevator hematoma according to its situation either above or below the levator ani muscle (Figure 40.7).

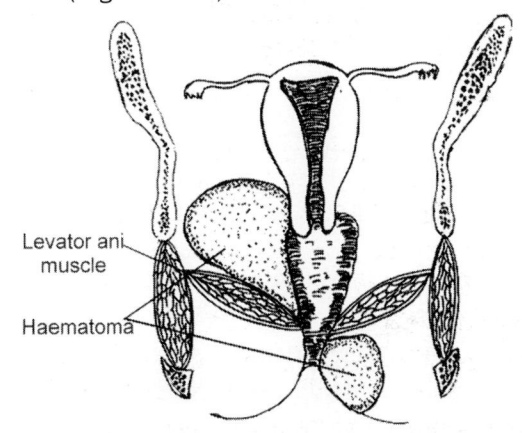

Figure 40.7: Diagrammatic representation of sites of supra and infralevator hematoma

Infralevator Hematoma

Etiology
- Disruption of paravaginal venous plexus either spontaneously following undue distention of vagina or following instrumental delivery even though the vaginal epithelium remains intact.
- Improper repair of episiotomy wound may permit bleeding from edges of vaginal epithelium or may be due to failure to obliterate dead space or improper hemostasis in the deep tissues.

The infralevater hematoma include hematoma of vulva (most common) and perineum, paravaginal hematoma or hematoma into ischiorectal fossa.

Feature: vulval swelling may be tense tender and bluish in color, usually on one side (Figure 40.8) with persistent, severe pain on perineal region. There may be retention of urine.

Treatment
- Analgesics, antibiotics and blood transfusion as required

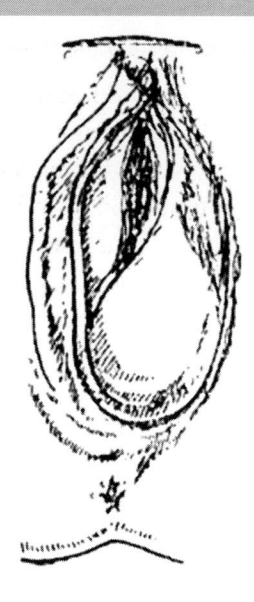

Figure 40.8: Vulval hematoma

- A surgical evacuation in operation theater by a senior obstetrician
- Usually obvious bleeding point cannot be visualized, so hemostasis is made by deep mattress suture, keeping a drain and vagina is packed for 12 to 24 hours
- A self retaining catheter is inserted for 24 hours.

Sometime a small and self limiting hematoma can be treated conservatively, but it takes long recovery time.

Supralevator Hematoma

Etiology
1. Cervical laceration extending into vaginal wall
2. Unsuspected rupture of lower uterine segment
3. Rupture of varicosities in the broad ligament.

Supralevator hematoma may lead to a grave emergency when diagnosis is missed or even with diagnosis if no proper measures have been taken in time. Supralevator hematoma may spread upward and outward beneath the broad ligament or downward to bulge into wall of the upper vagina. At times, it can be large so as to almost obliterate the vagina.

Features: Supralevator hematoma is very difficult to identify as pain is a less common feature, unless hematoma is large enough to present abdominally. A soft mass may appear in one or other iliac fossa due to collection of blood in-between layers of broad ligament. Vaginal examination will reveal a boggy swelling in the vaginal fornix with displacement of the uterus to one side. Third stage collapse may be the more characteristics feature.

Management

1. Treatment of shock.
2. Laparotomy followed by evacuation of broad ligament hematoma. Even for an experienced surgeon it is very difficult to explore that space. Blind stitches are avoided for fear of injuring ureter. A firm pressure packing for some times is very helpful.
3. Even when a pressure pack fails to control bleeding, there should not be any hesitation in ligating the internal iliac artery on the affected side.
4. Hysterectomy may be the last choice specially when there is an obvious injury to uterus and cervix.
5. Angiographic embolization of uterine and/or vaginal branch of internal pudendal artery in one or both the sides may be carried out.

INJURIES TO THE CERVIX

Minor cervical tears are invisible during labor. This causes the appearance of the parous os. It often heals spontaneously without any problem. Some times deep laceration may involve the vagina associated with profuse hemorrhage.

Etiology

1. Strong uterine contraction on rigid cervix.
2. Forceps or breech delivery through incompletely dilated cervix.

Diagnosis

1. Profuse bleeding per vagina even with firmly contracted uterus and complete delivery of placenta and membranes.
2. Inspection of cervix. Because digital examination is not adequate due to flabbiness of cervix immediately after delivery, it is best to retract the vaginal wall by right angled vaginal retractor and grasp the patulous cervix with two pairs of sponge holding forceps and apply traction on the lips of cervix along with downward suprapubic pressure on fundus by an assistant

so that cervix can be brought into view near the vulva. Sometimes several pair of sponge holding forceps can be used. Inspection has to be from 12 o'clock position and moved round the circumference of the cervix. Such proper visualization of cervix is possible and tear can be diagnosed.

Treatment

1. Minor superficial tears with no bleeding need no treatment.
2. Only deep tear requires repair
3. General or regional anesthesia will usually be necessary
4. Proper visualization as mentioned above is essential.
5. As hemorrhage usually comes from the upper angle of the tear the first suture is placed just above the angle (Figure 40.9).
6. Further interrupted or continuous sutures are applied outwards with chromic catgut or PG suture.

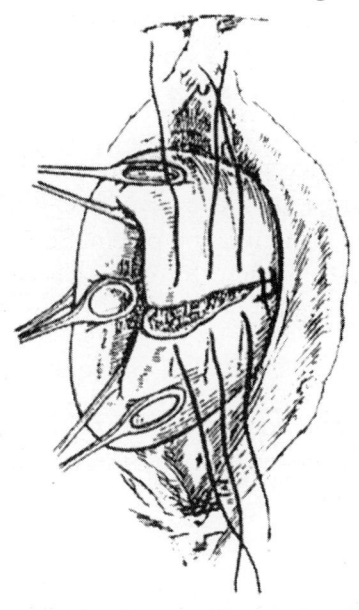

Figure 40.9: Repair of cervical tear

CERVICAL DETACHMENT

Annular or circular detachment of cervix is a very rare complication which occurs during labor. In cervical dystocia there is prolonged compression of undilating cervix by the fetal head and devitalization of the cervical cap and a ring of vaginal portion of cervix due to pressure necrosis.

Sometime during labor edematous anterior lip of the cervix may be compressed between the head and symphysis pubis. In case of severe ischemia, anterior lip of cervix may be avulsed.

Significant hemorrhage is not common in spontaneous cervical detachment

RUPTURE OF UTERUS

Rupture of the uterus is one of most dramatic and serious obstetrics emergencies and still not uncommon in developing counties.

Incidence

It is uncommon in developed countries. In India it varies from 1 in 200 to 1800 deliveries.

Etiology

1. Scar rupture:
   - Rupture of lower segment cesarean scar
   - Rupture of classical cesarean scar
   - Scar of previous operation like
   - D and C
   - Myomectomy
   - Hysterotomy
   - Metroplasty
2. Iatrogenic rupture
   - Injudicious use of oxytocics
   - Internal podalic version
   - Difficult forceps delivery
   - Manual removal of placenta
   - Destructive operation
3. Spontaneous rupture
   - Obstructed labor
   - Fundal rupture in grand multipara
   - Uterine malformation
4. Traumatic: Fall or blow on abdomen.

The most common cause of uterine rupture is separation of a previous cesarean section scar. Classical cesarean section is very rare nowadays. In developing countries obstructed labor with feto pelvic disproportion is still one of the most common causes of rupture uterus.

Types of rupture: When the uterine cavity communicates directly with the peritoneal cavity it is called *complete rupture* but when separated from it by visceral peritoneum of uterus or broad ligament it is called *incomplete rupture*. When there is separation of part of previous uterine scar with intact peritoneal coat it is called scar dehiscence. Here bleeding is minimal or absent.

Site of Rupture

Rupture due to obstructive causes and rupture of lower segment cesarean scar occur in lower segment. During pregnancy the rupture due to uterine muscular pathology or separation of other operative scars occur usually in the upper segment.

Clinical Features

Lower segment cesarean scar rupture (Figure 40.10) occur only during labor and is less dramatic in nature. Initially there is a constant dull aching pain even without any uterine contraction, in the suprapubic region. Pulse rates increase. Suprapubic bulging and tenderness are present. As the rupture is initially extraperitoneal, it is not always easily detectable. Dehiscence of lower segment scar is often diagnosed on section for delay in labor. It may cause virtually no bleeding or shock. If, however, the tear extends, there will be intraperitoneal bleeding and features of shock.

Spontaneous obstructive rupture (Figure 40.11) occurs in the patient with high parity. There is vigorous uterine contraction followed by sudden and severe bursting abdominal pain, cessation of progress of labor, fetal death and all the signs of an internal hemorrhage and an acute abdomen. Rupture begins in the lower segments often extends upward along lateral uterine wall. It involves branches of uterine artery. Rarely tear extends downward to involve vagina and cervix. Sometimes fetus is expelled out of the uterus and can be felt separately from empty contracted uterus.

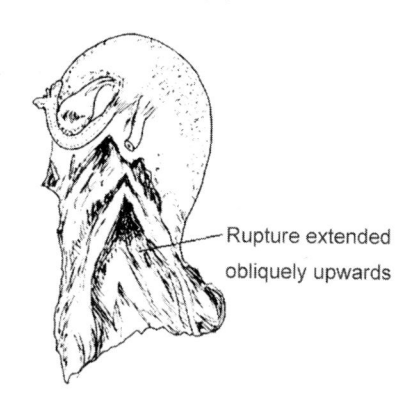

Figure 40.11: Diagrammatic representation of rupture of uterus following obstructed labor

Treatment

Once the diagnosis is reached, laparotomy must be performed along with blood transfusion. In obstructive spontaneous rupture quick subtotal hysterectomy is preferred to as patient is usually of high parity with low general condition and the anatomy is totally distorted. Total hysterectomy may be hazardous and may increase chances of ureteric injury. In case of lower segment scar rupture, hysterectomy is not always required. Repair of rupture uterus is considered in young women with no living child or those with low parity and rupture wound is clear-cut, as in lower segment scar rupture, and condition of the patient is stable.

CONCLUSION

Most of the injuries to the birth canal are undoubtedly preventable conditions. It can be prevented by proper supervision and conduction of labor followed by timely intervention. Judicious decision of cesarean section can prevent rupture of uterus. A well timed episiotomy is useful to prevent laceration of vagina and perineum. Some times such injuries may lead to a fatal condition. There is also increased morbidity. Prompt detection and appropriate management is usually necessary to avoid such complication.

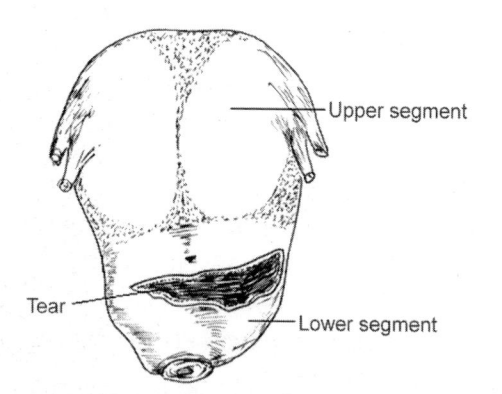

Figure 40.10: Diagrammatic representation of rupture of lower segment caesarean section scar

41.

Joydev Mukherji

Prolonged and Obstructed Labor

PART TWO — Feto-maternal Medicine

INTRODUCTION

Prolonged and obstructed labors are important causes of maternal and perinatal morbidity and mortality in developing countries. The partograph is an invaluable tool to prevent prolonged labor and to time interventions optimally. When neglected patients come with prolonged labor, as in developing countries, they require urgent management at first referral level hospitals. Clinical examination is to identify the cause and to determine the condition of the mother and baby. After excluding obstruction, augmentation may be undertaken. Obstructed labor is a desperate emergency and in majority of cases the baby is dead and the mother moribund. Active resuscitation and operative delivery are required. Destructive operations may still have a role, albeit small, in developing countries.

PROLONGED LABOR

Prolonged and obstructed labors are important causes of maternal and perinatal morbidity and mortality in developing countries. In both developed and developing countries, abnormal progress of labor or labor dystocia is one of the most frequent indications for primary cesarean sections, and proper management of the situation can lower the rates of operative delivery.

DEFINITION

Normal labor progress can be defined either in terms of the total length of labor or as the rate of progress of cervical dilatation (cm/hour). The second measure is more useful in prospective labor management when patients are admitted in early labor. The total length of labor can only be known in retrospect. The labor may be considered prolonged if the woman is not able to deliver within 18 hours of its onset.[1] The morbidity and mortality climb steeply beyond 24 hours. This definition applies mostly to neglected labors arriving late in hospitals in developing countries.

In developed countries where labor is managed prospectively, 'failure to progress' is diagnosed far earlier rather than waiting for a combined first and second stage to exceed a certain time limit. Thus, it is difficult to define prolonged labor in such a situation. Nevertheless, an active first stage of labor lasting longer than 12 hours (roughly equivalent to a rate of dilatation of 0.5 cm/hour) is commonly cited to be prolonged.[2]

Abnormal progress of labor or labor dystocia is one of the most frequent indications for primary cesarean section (CS) and proper management of labor can achieve a lower CS rate.

Role of Partography

As part of the Safe Motherhood Initiative (1987),[3] the World Health Organization (WHO) has promoted a partograph (1994) with a view to improving labor management. When implemented in South East Asia,[4] this reduced both prolonged labors and the proportion of labors requiring augmentation. The incidence of emergency CS and intrapartum stillbirths were reduced in the group who used the partograph.

With the advent of partography, a classification of labor abnormalities into three types (Figure 41.1) is possible.
1. Prolonged latent phase
2. Primary dysfunctional labor
3. Secondary arrest of dilatation

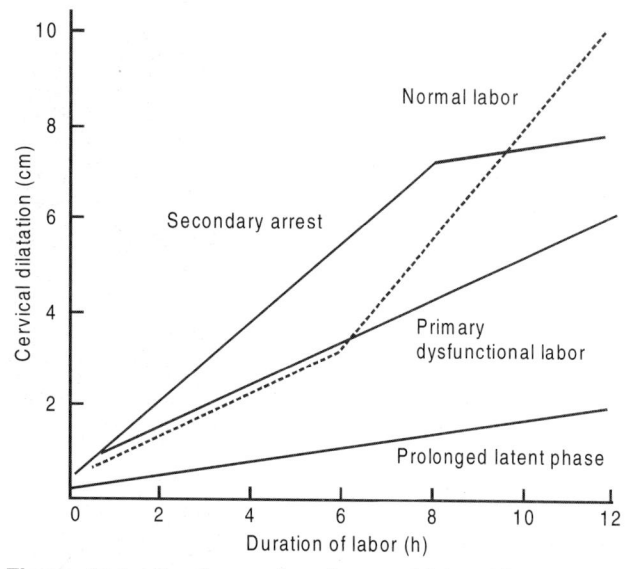

Figure 41.1: Cervicographs of normal labor (dashed line) and the three types of prolonged labor

The latent phase of labor begins with onset of painful regular uterine contractions, but can only be observed and monitored from the time that the patient gets admitted. Thus, a latent phase exceeding 8 hours in a nullipara and 6 hours in a multipara (from admission) would seem more appropriate than 20 hours and 14 hours respectively, as practised in USA, where labor is reckoned to start with maternal perception of pain, which depends on maternal memory.

The active phase is from 3 to 10 cm cervical dilatation. According to Friedman,[5] the active phase of spontaneous labor progresses at a rate of more than 1.2 cm/hour in primigravida and 1.5 cm/hour in multigravida in 95 percent of the population. Primary dysfunctional labor is one where the active phase progresses at less than 1 cm/hour from the beginning of the active phase slope (i.e. beyond 3 cm cervical dilatation). This is the most common labor abnormality. Secondary arrest describes the situation where active phase commences normally but cervical dilatation stops or slows significantly prior to full dilatation. The type of partographic abnormality, however, does not necessarily reveal its cause. Thus, secondary arrest, at one time considered to be entirely due to cephalopelvic disproportion, is often due to poor uterine contractions or malposition or deflexion of the presenting part.

The partograph cannot only be used to differentiate normal from abnormal labors; alert and action lines (Figure 41.2) can also indicate the optimum time for interventions. Progress to the right of the alert line should be used to refer patients in rural areas to the first referral units, whereas crossing the action line mandates definitive steps to augment labor or to terminate it if there are obvious signs of disproportion.

Intervention to augment labor in the latent phase is not always associated with an improvement in outcome. Pain relief, hydration, nutrition, reassurance and augmentation of labor are necessary to prevent the woman becoming exhausted and demoralised.[6] The optimum diagnosis and management of prolonged latent phase requires more research.

The timing of intrapartum interventions which may correct poor progress in active phase (especially time lag or grace period between alert and action lines) has not been subjected to rigorous evaluation. The WHO study in South East Asia used a 4-hour lag.

Prevention is better than cure and partography is useful in prospective labor management to prevent

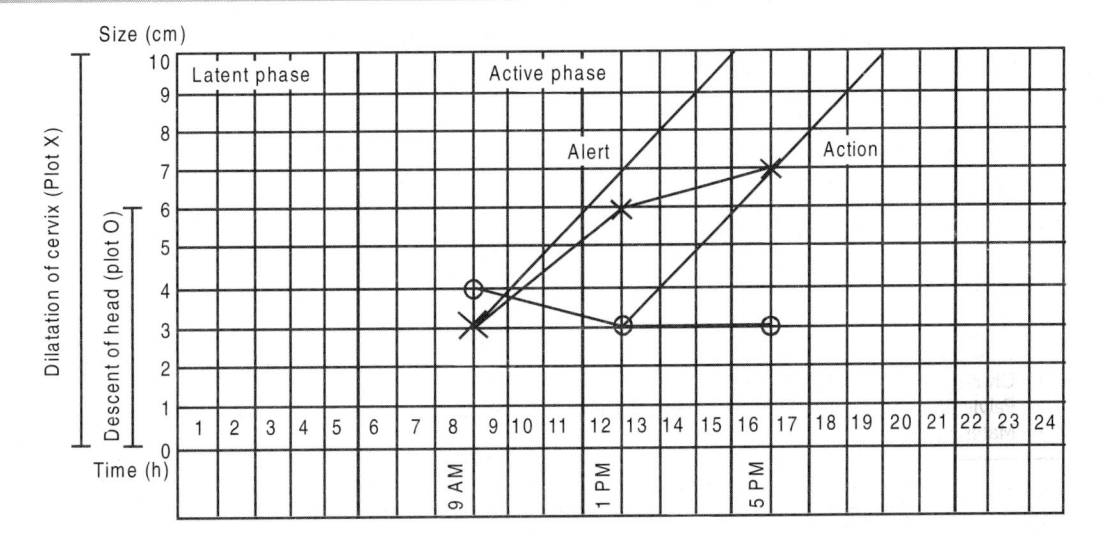

Figure 41.2: An example of the WHO partogram showing 'alert' and 'action' lines. Distinction is made between the latent phase of labor (up to 3 cm cervical dilatation) and the active phase when labor is expected to progress at a rate of at least 1 cm cervical dilatation per hour (the alert line). Action line is drawn at end of 8 hours for latent phase and 4 hours to the right of, and parallel to, the alert line in active phase. The subject's record shows progress to the right of alert line from 3 cm dilatation and WHO recommends referral from health center to hospital for this. In a central unit (FRU) conservative management is recommended until cervical dilatation crosses the action line at 5 PM

prolonged labor. However, many patients come late in labor not having had the benefit of partography. Before discussing management of neglected labors, the common causes of prolonged labor will be discussed.

Causes of Prolonged Labor

In about 70 percent of cases, *insufficient uterine contractions* is the culprit in nulliparous women; in the rest *malpositions and deflexed vertex*, *malpresentations* (transverse lie, brow, mentoposterior face) and *cephalopelvic disproportion* contribute to the delay.

Adoption of a deflexed attitude is often associated with occipitoposterior position. This causes the larger occipitofrontal diameter (11.5 cm) to come into play instead of the suboccipitobregmatic diameter (9.5 cm) with a flexed vertex. This relative increase in diameter with deflexed head is sometimes referred to as relative cephalopelvic disproportion (Figures 41.3A and B). The differentiation from absolute or genuine disproportion may be helpful in deciding a trial of labor or a repeat elective cesarean section in a subsequent pregnancy.

There is increasing recent evidence that the physical state of the cervix may also be contributory in the genesis

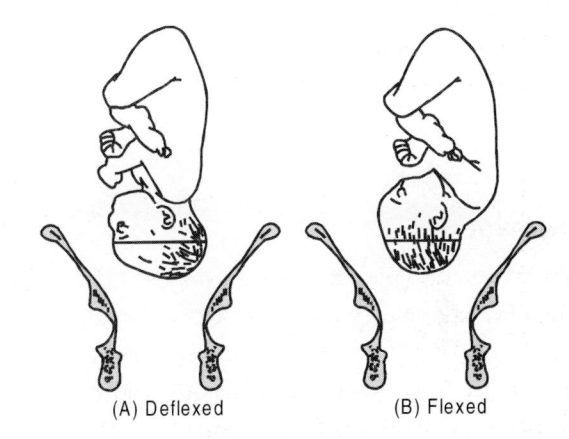

Figure 41.3: Relative cephalopelvic disproportion: A deflexed head (A) results in the larger occipito-frontal diameter (11.5 cm) to come into play in place of the smaller suboccipito-bregmatic diameter (9.5 cm) with a flexed head (B)

of prolonged labor—a *non-compliant cervix* may delay cervical effacement and dilatation (Table 41.1).

Evaluation in a Neglected Case

This is done to find the cause apart from assessing the maternal and fetal conditions. Communication with the patient and husband are important. The items to be covered are outlined in Table 41.2.

Table 41.1: Dangers of prolonged labor

Maternal
- Dehydration, acidosis, electrolyte imbalance
- Infection
- Increased operative delivery
- Postpartum hemorrhage
- Trauma to genital tract including rupture uterus
- Increased maternal mortality rate

Remote
- Vesicovaginal fistula
- Chronic pelvic infection
- Pelvic floor muscle and sphincter disturbance
- Maternal disillusionment

Fetal
- Hypoxia
- Acidosis
- Fetal distress
- Stillbirth
- Asphyxia neonatorum
- Infection
- Intracranial injuries
- Operative deliveries
- Increased perinatal mortality rate

Remote
- Delayed milestones

Table 41.2: Assessment in a neglected case of prolonged labor

History
- Past pregnancy outcome
- Present pregnancy
  - Labor onset
  - Membrane rupture
  - Interference

General examination
- Mental state
- Dehydration
- Anemia

Obstetric examination
- Abdominal
  - Uterine contractions
  - Station
  - Bladder / Bowel
  - Bandl's ring
- Fetal heart sound

Vaginal
- Malposition/malpresentation
- Caput/Moulding
- Color of liquor

Treatment

Dehydration and electrolyte disturbances are corrected. Antibiotics are given to prevent or treat infection. Gross cephalopelvic disproportion, malpresentation or fetal distress (in first stage of labor) are indications for cesarean section and must be excluded before augmentation is undertaken. Artificial rupture of membranes (ARM) should be the first step for augmentation followed by oxytocin infusion only if required. When a patient fails to respond to amniotomy in the next 3 hours, adequate oxytocin augmentation for a reasonable period (6 to 8 hours) should be carried out prior to opting for a cesarean section.

Uterine inertia is an uncommon cause of prolonged labor in the multiparous woman who responds well to amniotomy. Oxytocin infusion, if used, requires greater caution, because of the risk of hyperstimulation and rupture of the uterus.

When obstetricians talk of prolonged labor, they usually imply a prolonged first stage. Prolongation of second stage (other than in obstructed labor in developing countries) is referred to as delay in the second stage and is dealt with elsewhere.

Box 41.1: Practice points: prolonged labor

- **Causes**: Faults in power, passage or passenger. Of various maternal and fetal causes, inefficient uterine contractions is the main culprit in nulliparous women. Malpositions with deflexed head, malpresentations and cephalopelvic disproportion are the other common causes.
- **Action**: Use partography in all labors to diagnose abnormalities early and to time interventions optimally by alert and action lines.
- **Management in neglected cases**: Evaluate maternal and fetal conditions from history, general and obstetrical examination; start supportive resuscitation and, if in the periphery, refer to a first referral hospital. Augment by artificial rupture of membranes and oxytocin for inefficient uterine contractions and malpositions. Fetal distress in first stage, cephalopelvic disproportion, malpresentations and failed augmentation are indications for cesarean section.

OBSTRUCTED LABOR

Definition

Labor is said to be obstructed when in spite of good uterine contractions, the progress of labor comes to a standstill due to mechanical factors causing obstruction to delivery. The cause is either in the passage and / or the passenger. Delivery is impossible without assistance. Obstructed labors usually result from neglect and are only common in developing countries where incidence may be as high as 1-5 percent in the referral hospitals.

Causes of Obstructed Labor

The important causes are: (i) cephalopelvic disproportion and (ii) malpresentation (shoulder, brow, mentoposterior face) and malposition (impacted occipitoposterior position).

The less common causes are fetal anomalies such as hydrocephalus, fetal ascites, and conjoint twins. Soft tissue obstruction may be caused by a fibroid or ovarian tumor below the presenting part or a scarred cervix from previous amputation.

Course of Labor

During the labor uterine contractions increase in strength and frequency to overcome the obstruction. With each contraction there is some myometrial shortening (retraction) so that the upper active segment becomes progressively thicker and shorter. The passive lower uterine segment becomes progressively stretched and thinner. The junction between the two segments stands out as a pathological retraction ring or Bandl's ring. This is sometimes confused with a distended bladder, but the oblique line is diagnostic. In the primigravida, the uterus subsequently becomes secondarily inert and stops contracting. In multiparous women the uterus continues to contract vigorously, the Bandl's ring may climb upwards and rupture of the uterus is imminent unless the mother is urgently delivered.

Vaginal examination reveals an edematous vulva, a hot dry bruised vagina, fully dilated cervix, and, in vertex presentation, marked moulding and caput formation, or a hand prolapse in shoulder presentation. Since obstructed labors are prolonged labors, the complications are similar. However, all prolonged labors are not obstructed labors.

Prevention

Antenatal referral of high risk cases, such as short statured nullipara and women with bad obstetric history or malpresentations, to first referral hospitals is important. Intranatally, routine partography must be implemented.

Treatment

Treatment should be urgent and carried out in a first referral unit only. Dehydration is rapidly corrected with 1-3 liters of normal saline or Ringer's lactate infusion; broad spectrum antibiotics are given parenterally to counteract sepsis. Blood requisition is done in anticipation of atonic or traumatic postpartum hemorrhage. Oxytocin is contraindicated before delivery.

The mode of delivery depends on the state of the fetus. If alive, as it rarely is, immediate cesarean section is done. If the fetus is dead as is usual, destructive operations are an additional option. An experienced operator after excluding rupture can carry out either craniotomy (for cephalic presentations) or decapitation/ evisceration for transverse lie. Morbidity for the mother is less for operative vaginal delivery provided the pelvis is not grossly contracted, the presenting part is low down and the obstetrician is skilled. Otherwise a cesarean section is chosen even if the baby is dead. After every case of operative vaginal delivery, rupture uterus must be excluded, oxytocics given and the bladder put on continuous catheterization (10 days) to hopefully prevent vesicovaginal fistula, which can still occur due to ischemic necrosis.

Obstructed labors cause at least 10 percent of maternal deaths in India.[1] Destructive operations constituted 0.22 percent [1 in 450] deliveries; between 1988 to 1998 in the author's experience in Medical College, Calcutta [unpublished observation]. Maternal mortality in obstructed labor is due to hemorrhage, peritonitis, septic shock or rupture uterus. The perinatal mortality is close to hundred percent as the baby is mostly dead on admission.

An obstructed labor is a preventable disaster. The sad reality is that they are still rampant in developing countries, especially in the villages. While western textbooks can afford to delete this chapter, obstetricians in developing countries still need the skills to tackle the problem.

Box 41.2: Practice points: obstructed labor

- ***Causes***: Faults in passage or passenger. Cephalopelvic disproportion, malpresentations and malpositions are the principal causes.
- ***Complications***: Fetus is usually already moribund or dead. High risk of maternal mortality—from rupture in multipara and sepsis and exhaustion in nullipara.
- ***Management***: This is to be in a first referral hospital. Urgent resuscitation and operative delivery are required. Destructive operations still have a role in developing countries if experienced operator is available.

ACKNOWLEDGEMENTS

The author wishes to thank Dr. Avijit Hazra, Lecturer, Department of Pharmacology, University College of Medicine, Calcutta for preparation of the manuscript and figures.

REFERENCES

1. Rao KB: Prolonged and obstructed labor. In: Arulkumaran S, Ratnam SS, Rao KB (Eds): *The Management of Labor.* 1st ed. Chennai: Orient Longman, 301-07, 1996.
2. Prolonged labor. In: Enkin M, Kierse MJNC, Neilson J, Crowther C, Duley L, Hodnett E, *et al* (eds). *A Guide to Effective Care in Pregnancy and Childbirth.* 3rd edn. Oxford: Oxford University Press, 332-40, 2000.
3. Mahler H: The Safe motherhood initiative: A call to action. *The Lancet* **i:**168-70, 1987.
4. World Health Organization maternal health and safe motherhood programme. World Health Organization partograph in management of labor. *The Lancet* **343:**1399-1404, 1994.
5. Friedman EA: An objective approach to the diagnosis and management of abnormal labor. *Bulletin of the New York Academy of Sciences* **48:** 842-58, 1972.
6. Chamberlain G, Steer P: ABC of labor care: Labor in special circumstances. *British Medical Journal* **318:**1124-27, 1999.

Lim Chin Theam

42.

Resuscitation of the Newborn

PART TWO — Feto-maternal Medicine

INTRODUCTION

The process of birth brings the fetus from a fluid environment to an air environment. This transitional period is accompanied by a number of physiological and biochemical changes to allow the newborn infant to adapt to the new milieu. Although most infants adapt to the changes successfully and do not require any intervention, 4 to 6 percent of them may encounter problems in making this adjustment and need vigorous resuscitation. In these infants resuscitative efforts must be initiated promptly and effectively in order to prevent or minimize hypoxic insults to the infant. Although most of the fetuses at risk can be identified others cannot be predicted accurately. It is, thus, essential that labor ward personnel be well trained in neonatal resuscitation.

PATHOPHYSIOLOGY OF PERINATAL ASPHYXIA

Fetal lungs are filled with lung fluid that is derived from amniotic fluid that the fetus inhales regularly. This fluid is expelled from the lung as the fetus is squeezed through the birth canal. The remainder of the fluid is partly expelled by the initial breaths into the circulatory system and partly absorbed by the lymphatics. Infants delivered via cesarean section, thus, may have excess of lung fluid after birth and this may contribute to higher incidence of perinatal asphyxia and respiratory distress postnatally amongst infants born via this route.

The physiological response to perinatal asphyxia was well demonstrated by the classic experiment on laboratory animal fetuses conducted by Dawes *et al* in 1963 (Figure 42.1). These changes are remarkably similar to those experienced by human neonates during asphyxial insult. During the initial phase of asphyxia after breathing a few times the newborns cease to breathe heralding the onset of primary apnea lasting 1 to 2 minutes. The newborns appear cyanosed. This is accompanied by increasing blood pressure due to peripheral vasoconstriction, and a reflex bradycardia. Gasping respiration then ensues with increasing frequency and vigour and as asphyxia continues the gasping effort progressively diminishes until the newborn animals gave a last gasp (secondary or terminal apnea). The heart rate and blood pressure gradually fall and the newborns appear pale.

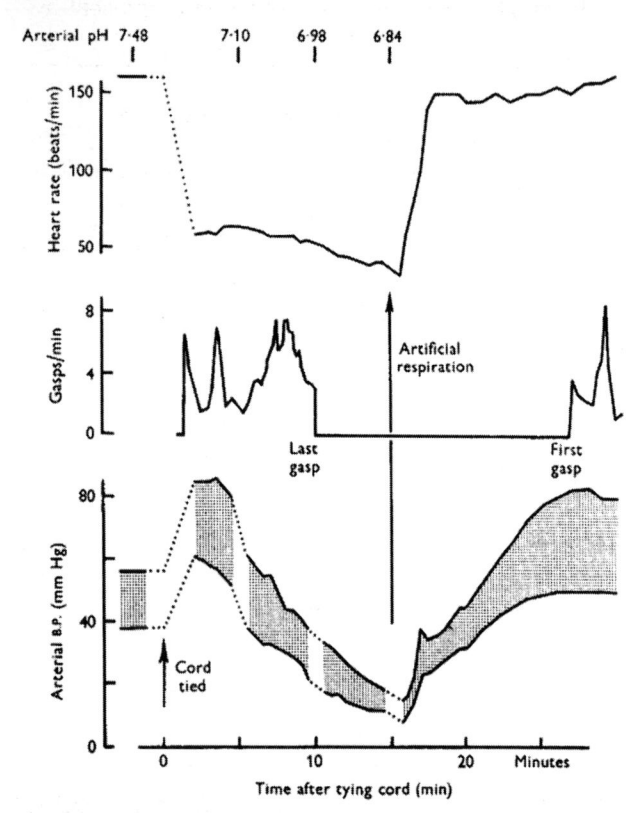

Figure 42.1: Changes in physiological parameters during perinatal asphyxia in newborns animals (Dawes GS *et al* J Physiol 1963)

It cannot be overemphasized that infants in primary apnea when given oxygen and tactile stimulation will begin to gasp and regular breathing will subsequently follow with return of normal heart rate and circulation. In secondary apnea, however, active resuscitation with intermittent positive ventilation is vital and external cardiac massage is essential if there is marked bradycardia. It is, thus, vital to differentiate secondary apnea from primary apnea.

CAUSES OF PERINATAL ASPHYXIA

Infants may suffer from asphyxia due to a number of causes such as conditions affecting the mothers (e.g. maternal diseases, maternal drug ingestion, analgesia and anesthesia), obstetric complications (such as placenta insufficiency, pregnancy-induced hypertension, vascular diseases affecting the uterus), fetal factors such as fetal distress, prematurity, lung diseases (infant respiratory distress syndrome, meconium aspiration syndrome, delayed absorption of lung fluid) and malformation of the respiratory tract and the lungs. Infants delivered following instrumentation like breech extraction, forceps, vacuum and cesarean section are also prone to asphyxia.

ASSESSMENT OF INFANTS AT BIRTH

Apgar score devised by Dr Virginia Apgar in 1953 is widely used to assess the clinical condition of the newborn (Table 42.1). Five parameters are evaluated at 1 and 5 minutes after birth. Of these five parameters, the respiratory effort, heart rate and the color of the infants are more useful and are, thus, more frequently utilized as guides in resuscitation. If an infant needs prolonged resuscitation, the assessment of Apgar scores should be extended and recorded at 5-minute intervals.

Table 42.1: Apgar score

Signs	0	1	2
Appearance (color) of trunk	White	Blue	Pink
Pulse (heart rate)	0	< 100/min	> 100/min
Grimace (Response to suction)	Absent	Facial grimace	Coughing/ crying
Activity (muscle tone)	Flaccid	Some flexion of limbs	Good activity
Respiration	Absent	Weak, gasping, irregular	Regular respiration, crying lustily

Most infants have Apgar scores between 7/10 to 10/10 at one minute and do not require resuscitation. Infants with Apgar scores of 4 to 6 require some intervention while those who have Apgar scores of ≤ 3/10 are severely compromised and warrant urgent resuscitation. Thus one minute Apgar score represents the condition of the infant at birth and subsequent scores the effectiveness of the resuscitative effort and the infant's response to resuscitation. It should be pointed out that Apgar scores are not a good indicator of the degree of asphyxial insults to the infants as they correlate poorly with long-term neurological outcomes of the infants. It is hence important to document accurately the condition of the infants at birth.

RESUSCITATION OF THE NEWBORN

The primary goal of resuscitation is to provide adequate oxygen to the vital organs especially the brain, thereby preventing hypoxia and its consequences to these organs. To achieve this, the *general principles of resuscitation* apply, viz.:
- A: Airway patency
- B: Breathing with adequate alveolar ventilation and oxygen supply
- C: Circulation—ensure good tissue perfusion
- D: Drugs—availability of appropriate drugs

While waiting for the delivery to take place always check that the necessary equipment and drugs are available at the resuscitation trolley (Table 42.2) and see that the equipment is in good functioning condition. Ensure that the radiant heater on the resuscitation trolley is switched on and is working well. It is essential to obtain maternal medical and obstetric history and information pertaining to the fetus. Note the time when the last maternal sedation was administered. If multiple gestations are expected, call for extrapairs of hands to handle the additional newborns. Observe the condition of the newborn and the state of the liquor, e.g. meconium staining. Start the stop clock as soon as the body of the infant is completely expelled from the birth canal.

After delivery of the head (before expulsion of the trunk), aspirate the oropharynx, then the nostrils, especially when there is a history of meconium-stained liquor.

After complete expulsion of the body most of the infants cry and breathe regularly with good heart rate and muscle tone. No or gentle oropharyngeal suction is required. Cut the cord and give vitamin K. Dry and swaddle the baby with a warm towel. Give the infant to the mother, encourage her to cuddle and breastfeed her newborn infant.

Overzealous suction may trigger off reflex bardycardia and apnea due to vagal stimulation.

If an infant is cyanosed, bradycardic (<100/min), and has irregular/slow respiration transfer the infant

Table 42.2: Equipment and drugs to be present at resuscitation trolley

Equipment
1. Radiant warmer (with adequate light), stop clock
2. Suction apparatus/vacuum supply
   - Maximum negative pressure 200 cm of water, usually set at 136 cm of water (100 mmHg)
   - Suction catheters FG 5,6,8
     (Mucus extractor, e.g. DeLee's suction apparatus to standby)
3. Oxygen supply, tubings
   Flow rate up to 10 L/min
   (blow off valve 40 cm of water)
4. Bag mask system
   Mask, sizes : 0,1,2
   Bag : With fitting for face mask
   Blow off valve : 40 cm of water
   Oro-pharyngeal airways: sizes : 000,00.0
6. Laryngoscopes: Straight blade preferred
   sizes: 0,1,2
7. Endotracheal tube (ETT) and adapters
   sizes: 2.5, 3, 3.5 mm
8. Macgills forceps
9. Endotracheal tube introducer:
   Nylon or metal (usually not needed)
10. Stethoscope
11. Syringes: 2.5, 5, 10 ml
    Needles: FG 21, 23, 25
    I/V cannulae: 22G, 24G
    3-way tap
    T-connector
12. Gloves, surgical spirit swabs, adhesive tapes, sterile containers for full blood counts, group-and-cross match, blood glucose, serum bilirubin.

Drugs
- Adrenaline : 1 in 10,000 (0.1 mg/mL),
- Sodium bicarbonate: 4.2 % (0.5 mmol/mL) or 8.4 % (1 mmol/L),
- Glucose : 25%
  : 10% dextrose
- Water for injection
- Naloxone 20 microgram/ml (dose 0.5 – 1mg/kg)
- Vitamin K 1 – 1 mg/ml

Equipment on standby:
- Venesection set
- Exchange transfusion set, pneumothorax drainage set

immediately to the resuscitation trolley, dry and keep warm. Position the infant in the neutral position. The airway should be cleared of fluid. The heart rate can be assessed by auscultating the heart or palpating the umbilical arterial pulsation at the base of the umbilical cord. Stimulate the infant to breathe by gentle slapping of the sole of the feet or rubbing the back of the trunk. Additional oxygen is delivered via a face mask (or funnel). Most infants will respond to stimulation. Observe the baby closely, if by 5 minutes his condition is good, treat as for healthy baby. If the baby's condition is not improving within 30 seconds or begins to deteriorate, e.g. heart rate drops below 100 per minute, bag mask ventilation (Figure 42.2, Plate 4) is indicated. With effective bag mask ventilation most infants show good response. Should the heart rate drop to less than 60 per minute external cardiac massage should be initiated.

A pulse oximeter (if available) is helpful in assessing the oxygenation status of the infant. When an infant is not responding or its condition is deteriorating despite resuscitative effort or is born in a very poor condition it should be intubated at once and intermittent positive pressure ventilation performed immediately (Figure 42.3). External cardiac massage (Figures 42.4 and 42.5, Plate 4) should be commenced when the heart rate falls below 60 per minute. The inverted pyramid concept (Figure 42.6) for the process of resuscitation proposes that the procedures that are more frequently needed be placed at the base of the pyramid. Therefore should these measures fail to bring about a satisfactory response in the infant the process should be reviewed before drugs are administered.

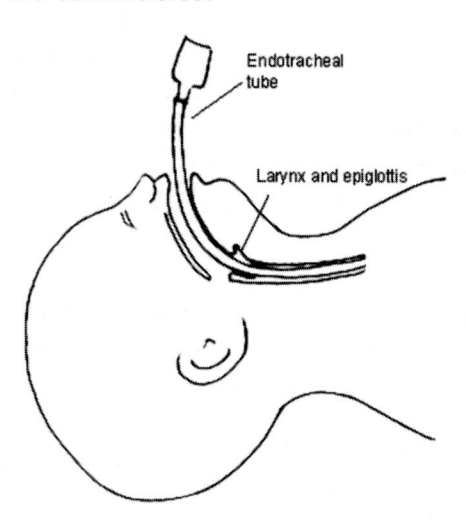

Figure 42.3: Endotracheal intubation

In the event that no response to resuscitation is observed after 15 minutes of resuscitation, further efforts should be abandoned. However, if the heart rate is still heard resuscitation should be continued until the opinion of a senior staff is sought.

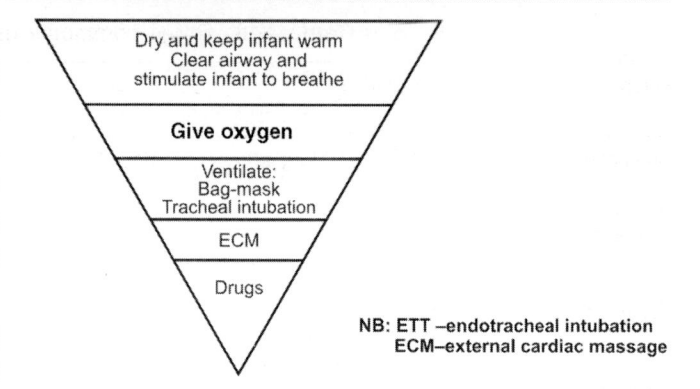

Figure 42.6: Inverted pyramid concept of neonatal resuscitation: the more commonly performed procedures are placed at the base of the pyramid

An algorithm for resuscitation of the newborn infant is depicted in Figure 42.7. The drugs frequently used in neonatal resuscitation are listed in Table 42.3.

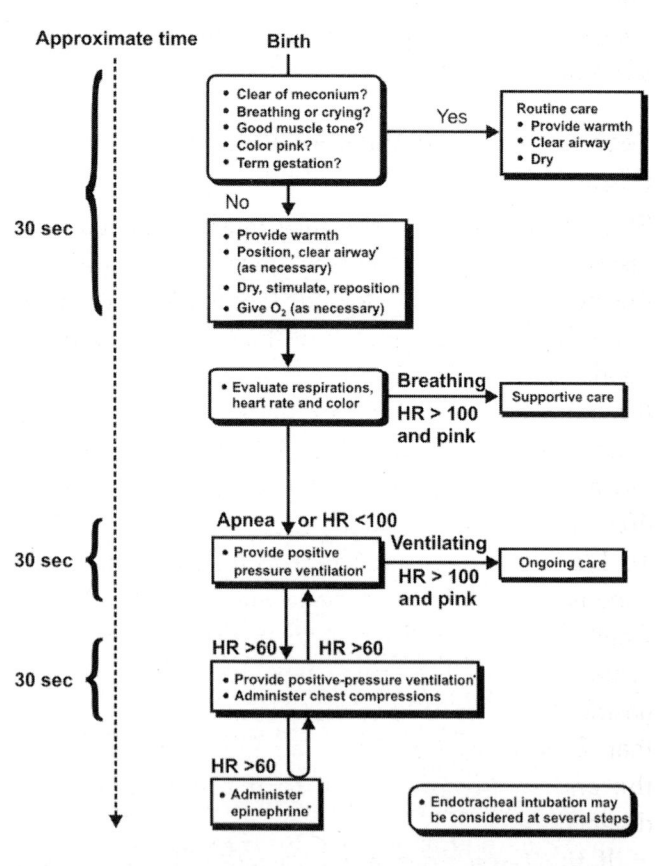

Figure 42.7: Algorithm for resuscitation of newborn infant (Circulation; 102(suppl I)) 2000

Table 42.3: Drugs commonly used in neonatal resuscitation

Drugs	Preparations	Dosages	Routes of administration	Indications
Adrenaline	1:10,000 (100 μg/ml)	10 μg/kg (0.1ml/kg)	i/v, intratracheal	Asystole, heart rate persistently < 60/minute
Naloxone hydrochloride	0.4mg/ml	0.1 mg/kg (0.25 ml/kg)	i/v, i/m, intratracheal	Depression due maternal opiates administration. Do not give to neonates born to habitual opiate users.
Volume expanders	Normal saline, Ringer's lactate, O-Rh negative blood	10-20 ml/kg	i/v	Blood loss, poor peripheral circulation
Sodium bicarbonate	4.2 percent (0.5 mmol/ml) 8.4 percent (1 mmol/ml)	1-2 mmol/kg	i/v	Severe acidosis suspected: Not responding to resuscitation, prolonged asphyxia

In the presence of thick meconium stained liquor oropharyngeal suction of the newborn should be carried out with a large bore suction catheter and the trachea sucked with endotracheal tube and a meconium aspiration device. However, if they cry vigorously at birth tracheal suctioning is not advised. Instead observe these newborns for signs of respiratory distress and manage accordingly if present.

Technique of Bag Mask Ventilation (Figure 42.2)

Place an appropriate size face mask (attached to a resuscitation bag) on the face, covering the nose and the mouth adequately. Hold the face mask between the index finger and the thumb of the left hand, with the middle finger supporting the jaw. Extend the neck of the baby slightly and lift his jaw forward. Flexing or hyperextending the neck does not help in opening the airway. Manually compress the bag at a rate of 30 to 40/minute, using FiO_2 of 100 percent (flow rate of 5 to 10 L/minute). It is important to ensure good chest expansion in order to provide adequate ventilation. Gentle pressure on the cricoids cartilage can facilitate visualization of the larynx but also help to reduce gastric distention. If bag mask ventilation lasts more than 2 minutes, aspirate the air from the stomach at the end of the procedure to prevent abdominal distention.

If the baby does not improve with bag mask ventilation in 30 seconds, proceed to endotracheal intubation.

Technique of Endotracheal Intubation (see Figure 42.3)

1. Put the baby flat or with the head slightly tilted downward and suck out the fluid from the oropharynx of the baby.
2. Extend the neck of the baby slightly.
3. Introduce an appropriate size laryngoscope with straight blade (size 0 for preterm, 1 for term infant).
4. Advance the blade to the vallecula and lift the tongue forward, exposing the epiglottis and laryngeal opening. Gentle pressure on the cricoid cartilage by the little finger or by an assistant may help to expose these structures clearly.
5. Introduce an appropriate size ETT (endotracheal tube) into the trachea, past the vocal cords, to a depth of 2 to 2.5 cm to avoid selective intubation of the right main bronchus. Hold the ETT at that position or tape it to the angle of the mouth.
6. Connect the ETT to the resuscitation bag and apply positive pressure ventilation at a rate of 30 to 40/min and FiO_2, pressure of 20 to 25 cm of water. Observe that the chest expansion is adequate following each inflation.
7. Auscultate the chest and the stomach (three-point auscultation) to confirm the position of the tip of the ETT.

External Cardiac Massage

External cardiac massage (ECM) (see Figures 42.4 and 42.5) It should be performed by the assistant, standing by the side or feet of the baby. Encircle the infant's chest with both hands such that the fingers support the back of the chest and the two thumbs placed over the lower third of the sternum. Compress the chest to a depth of one-third the anteroposterior (AP) diameter of the chest. This can also be carried out with two fingers compressing the lower sternum. The former is preferred as it gives better systolic and coronary perfusion pressure. The ratio of the ECM to lung inflation is 3:1. Look for palpable arterial pulse, the presence of which is indicative of effective external cardiac massage.

Give adrenaline if the heart rate remains less than 60 per minute despite 30 seconds of intermittent positive pressure ventilation and ECM.

Practical points

When an asphyxiated infant is not responding to resuscitation, check:
1. Oxygen source, tubing and connecting points.
2. The bag may not deliver enough pressure to inflate the lungs adequately.
3. ETT has been dislodged or esophageal intubation has occurred.
   Reintubate the baby.
4. ETT may be blocked (by blood clot or mucus) in which case the airway resistance is high. Either lavage the tube or change the ETT.
5. ETT is in the right main bronchus. Air entry will be diminished on the left side. Withdraw the ETT slightly until the air entry is equal.

After technical errors have been excluded, one should consider:
1. Tension pneumothorax.
2. Severe lung disease (hyaline membrane disease, meconium aspiration syndrome) may be developing.
3. Significant blood loss—hypotensive and pale. Give normal saline, Ringer's lactate (10-15 ml/kg body weight) or group 0-negative blood.
4. Other conditions may be present, e.g. diaphragmatic hernia, pleural effusion, pulmonary hypoplasia, congenital heart disease. Investigate accordingly.

Infants who need vigorous resuscitation should be admitted to the neonatal unit for further monitoring and management.

CONCLUSION

Although most newborn infants are born in good condition a small number may need vigorous resuscitation at birth. Unfortunately this cannot be predicted with accuracy. Thus, personnel attending to delivery should be well-versed with and be skillful at resuscitating newborn infants.

BIBLIOGRAPHY

1. Apgar V: A proposal for a new method of evaluation of the newborn infant. *Anaesth Analg* **32**:260-67, 1953.
2. Committee of Fetus and Newborn, American Academy of Pediatrics: Use and abuse of the Apgar score. *Pediatrics* **98**:141-42, 1996.
3. Dawes GS, Jacobson HN, Mott JC et al: Treatment of asphyxia in newborn lambs and monkeys. *Journal of Physiology* **169**: 167-84, 1963.
4. Hamilton P: ABC of labor care: care of the newborn in the delivery room. *British Medical Journal* **318**:1403-06, 1999.
5. Milner AD, Vyas M: Resuscitation of the newborn. In Milner AD, Martin RJ (Eds): *Neonatal and Pediatric Respiratory Medicine*, London: Butterworth, 16, 1985.
6. Neonatal Resuscitation. *Circulation* **102**:343-57.
7. Roberton NRC: Resuscitation of the newborn infant. In Yu VYH (Ed): Baillière's Clinical Paediatrics, Pulmonary problems in the perinatal period and their sequelae. WB Saunders, London, **3**:1-26, 1995.

43. Diseases of the Newborn

KK Diwakar

INTRODUCTION

The neonatal period is a phase of life where significant physiological changes occur to ensure a smooth transition of a 'maternal dependent' fetus to an independent individual. This phase of life could therefore be affected by any variations in the schedule of transition, e.g. a premature delivery enforcing an early exposure of the 'fetus' to extrauterine factors. Further, the adverse effects of the external environment could result in pathological responses unique to the neonatal period, e.g. environmental temperatures often acceptable to adults could result in hypothermia with resulting problems in the neonate.

It is necessary for all of us, more so the health care givers to appreciate and respect the abilities of the newborn infant. The steps in physiological adaptation, changes in the functions of a hitherto 'under utilized' organ system and appropriate adaptive responses to unexposed external environment, are but few of the miracles of nature the newborn teaches us. The complexities of cardiac surgery and the necessity of gradual rehabilitation of the patient, are well recognized by all. However, we fail to appreciate the equally complex changes of the cardiovascular system that take place, when an infant is delivered and placental support discontinued, with the lungs immediately taking over the functions of gas exchange. Recognizing the various physiological changes occurring in a neonate, would help us appreciate the vulnerability of the infant to diseases that are exclusive to the neonatal period.

DEFINITION[1,2]

It is essential to follow acceptable and standard definitions for standardizing and evaluating health care practices.

1. *Preterm birth*: Birth at a gestational age of less than 37 weeks
2. *Small for gestational age:* Low birth weight (LBW, <2500 g, as defined by WHO) may be due to preterm delivery or smallness for gestational age (intrauterine growth retardation), or to a combination of both. A very high proportion of infants in less developed countries are born with low birth weight.
3. *Neonatal period:* The neonatal period commences at birth and ends by 28 completed days after birth.
4. *Neonatal mortality rate:* Number of deaths among live births during the first 28 completed days of life per 1000 live births.

5. The *perinatal period* commences at 22 completed weeks of gestation (154 days) when birth weight is normally at least 500 g and ends seven completed days after birth.
6. *Perinatal mortality rate:* Number of deaths in the perinatal period during a specified period of time, per 1000 total births (live births plus fetal deaths) during the same time period.

BIRTH INJURIES

The delivery of a newborn through the maternal passages, could occasionally result in the infant sustaining some injury. Fortunately most of them are minor and require no active intervention.

Transient obstruction to the capillary and lymphatic drainage of the scalp at the point of contact with the maternal cervix results in a boggy swelling of the scalp called *caput succedaneum*. This requires no treatment and disappears over the next 24 to 48 hr. Occasionally *cephalohematoma* a subperiosteal bleed of the calvarial bone would occur over 24 to 48 hr of birth. This discrete rounded swelling is limited by the suture lines. The swelling is best left alone, and would resolve over the next few weeks. The parents must be reassured about its benign nature, lest over enthusiastic attempts to reduce it by massaging results instead in an increase in the bleed! Rarely the cephalohematoma could be associated with a fracture of the underlying bone. The treating physician should always be aware that the cephalohematoma could contribute to exaggerating the physiologic jaundice.

Subgaleal Hematoma

Bleeding into the potential space between the *galea aponeurotica* and the periosteum of the skull could spread from the orbital ridges to the occiput and laterally to the ears. It usually occurs insidiously over hours to days or may present as a hemorrhagic shock. Even the less dramatic insidious presentation could result in complications like hyperbilirubinemia. The extension beyond suture lines helps to differentiate it from cephalohematoma. The resorption occurs gradually over days.

Injury to the Bones

Injury to the bones could occur during a difficult labor. Fracture of the clavicles could present as incessant crying and pain while moving the ipsilateral arm. Radiological examination would confirm the diagnosis. It requires no treatment.

Rarely an infant could develop a fracture of the humerus or femur. Often the obstetrician would have recognized the 'snap' of the bone while conducting a difficult delivery. Decrease in spontaneous movements of the affected limb would be the earliest clue. Orthopedic intervention with immobilization by splinting is usually all that is required. If radiological examination reveals any displacement of the fractured segments, a closed reduction and cast would be required. A recovery by 2 to 4 weeks is usually the rule. An associated anemia due to hematoma must always be looked for, in all fractures of long bones.

Injury to Nerves

Facial nerve palsy: It may occur as a complication of delivery. Pressure of an extended head against the maternal sacrum, cranial fractures or trauma due to inappropriate or prolonged application of forceps could lead to damage to the facial nerve. Lower motor neuron type of facial palsy with the infant unable to close the ipsilateral eye, deviation of the angle of the mouth resulting in milk dribbling to the affected side while breastfeeding, or occasionally inability to suck well at the breast are common clinical features. Usually no treatment is required, especially in mild forms. If partial denervation has occurred, physiotherapy would be required.[3]

A facial nerve palsy should not be confused with the congenital hypoplasia or absence of the depressor anguli oris muscle. In this condition, the affected angle of the mouth does not move while crying. As the child grows and starts smiling more, the oral asymmetry would become less prominent.

Injury to the brachial plexus: It can occur when the delivery of the shoulder is difficult. Hyperextension of the neck could result in stretching the cervical roots and plexus. Injury to the C5–C6 roots resulting in 'Erb's palsy' is the most common. The affected limb would be hypotonic, adducted and internally rotated at the shoulder, extended and pronated at the elbow, with wrists flexed in the classical 'waiter's tip' posture.

Less common is the injury to the C8–T1 roots, affecting muscles supplied by them, e.g. small muscles of the hand. Total avulsion of the plexus would affect all the muscles of the arm (C5–T1).

One must remember that often these obvious neurological lesion would be associated with a significant stretch to the spinal cord, resulting in injury to the phrenic nerve (C3,4,5). Ipsilateral diaphragmatic paralysis must therefore always be looked for. The infant may be tachypneic, with the radiological evaluation revealing the elevated dome of the diaphragm.

The management is conservative, with splints to prevent the flexion deformity of the wrist and adduction of the thumb. For Erb's palsy, some therapists recommend resting the arm in an abducted and externally rotated position with the elbow flexed and in supination, while others prefer the adduction at the shoulder with the forearm resting pronated on the abdomen of the infant. Electrical stimulation of the affected muscles to prevent atrophy could be useful.[3] Recovery could be expected within 3 weeks to 3 months. Beyond this period chances of recovery becomes less with the passage of time. Surgical interventions for reconstructing the nerves have been tried by few, if recovery is not observed by 3 months.

CLINICAL EXAMINATION OF THE NEWBORN AND A FEW COMMON PROBLEMS

Examining the newborn is a skill that gets perfected with practice. As in all clinical practice good history is invaluable for examination of the newborn (Table 43.1). Needless to say, all infants must be examined only after washing ones hands and after following aseptic precautions. It must never be forgotten that health care personnel are well known to propagate cross-infection in babies. A history of passage of urine and meconium must always be asked for. The infant should have passed meconium by 24 hours of age and urine by 48 hours.

Table 43.1: Points to be considered in history

1. *Obstetric status of mother:*
   Maternal Age: Gravida   Parity
   Abortions (Trimester; spontaneous/MTP);   Preterm labor
   Living children : - i) Number, age and health status
                        ii) Details of death if any baby has died.
   Mother's blood Group (Including Rh type, h/o anti-D in previous pregnancy)

2. *Present pregnancy:*
   LMP   EDD (By maternal dates and by ultrasound)
   Antenatal care : (Booked/Unbooked)
                 Place of ANC.

3. *Fetal Well-being*
   - Foetal movements (Kick counts)
   - Ultrasound evaluation
   - Non-stress tests.
   - Others (e.g. amniocentesis/CV biopsy)

4. *Maternal problems:*
   - Hyperemesis
   - Hypertension/PIH/eclampsia
   - Diabetes
   - Infection/fever (trimester, type of infection, e.g. UTI)
   - Anemia
   - Jaundice (type)
   - Chronic maternal illness (Heart disease, seizure disorders, psychiatric, endocrinopathies)

5. *Maternal medication (Including substance abuse and tobacco):*
   - Oligo/Polyhydramnios
   - Premature labor/Post maturity
   - Prelabor rupture of membranes (PROM): (Duration; number of pervaginal examinations done after ROM)
   - Placental insufficiency/antepartum hemorrhage

6. *Intranatal period:*
   - Labor: Spontaneous/Induced;
              Duration of 1st and 2nd stage
   - Drugs:
       Pethedine/tocolytics/oxytocin
       Steroid: In premature labor (time and dosage)
       Rupture of membrane ——— Delivery Interval (RM-DI)
       Meconium staining of liquor

7. *Delivery:*
   - Place of delivery
   - Presentation: Vertex/breech/other
   - Type: Vaginal/instrumental/ceasarean section (indication, type of anesthesia)
     Apgar score/first cry
     Type of resuscitation (If required)

8. *Postnatal:*
   - Nursed with the mother (if not, where and why?)
   - Breastfeeding (Time of initiation and details)

MTP: Medical termination of pregnancy
h/o: History of
LMP: Last menstrual period
EDD: Expected date of delivery
ANC: Antenatal clinic
CV: Chorionic villus
PIH: Pregnancy-induced hypertension

Any delay in passage of urine and meconium warrants detailed evaluation.

The examination should follow a systematic pattern (Table 43.2) and must be done in a manner least distressing to the infant and the mother! While the anthropometric measurements of weight, head circumference and length are routinely done, one must not forget to examine the umbilical cord, and obtain details of the placental weight and attachment.

Table 43.2: General examination of the newborn

General	State of activity; interaction with surroundings; posture and attitude
Skin	Cutaneous stigmata; jaundice; pallor; plethora; cyanosis;
Head	Head circumference; shape; fontanelle; scalp; swellings on the head.
Eyes	Position; cornea; conjunctiva; cataract; adnexa
Ears	Position; features of pinna; developmental anomalies.
Nose	Choanal atresia
Mouth	Cleft lip and palate; sucking calosities; cysts; tongue.
Neck	Goiter; other swellings; clavicle
Chest	Shape; respiration (pattern and use of accessory muscles); nipples; cardiac apex; precordial pulsations
Abdomen	Umbilical cord; genitalia.; femoral area protrusions/ pulses
Limbs	Developmental dysplasia of the hip; congenital talipes equino varus; others.
Back and Spine	Deformities; neural tube defects; sinuses; tufts of hair.
Neonatal reflexes	—

Normal Cutaneous Stigmata

The mongolian spot, erythema toxicum, milia and pustular melanosis are commonly seen cutaneous manifestations in a neonate, and often cause concern to the parents.

1. The *mongolian spots* are greyish-blue or bluish-black pigmented lesions most commonly present in the lumbosacral region. They could be of variable sizes and shapes, but are never elevated or palpable. These spots occur due to the infiltration of melanocytes deep in the dermis. They fade as the child grows older.
2. *Erythema toxicum* appears within the 1st three days of life or upto the 2nd week of life and disappears over the next few days without any treatment. These are macular erythema, often with central clearance or clear vesicle present predominantly on the chest but may be extensive. The palms and soles are spared. The histology shows edema and perivascular eosinophilic infiltrates in the dermis. Care should be taken to differentiate these from insect bites and pyoderma
3. *Milia* are tiny cysts, 1-2 mm in size, that arise from the pilosebaceous follicles or sweat ducts. They are common on the nose and elsewhere on the face, and disappear spontaneously over a month or two.
4. *Pustular melanosis* is seen commonly in dark skinned infants. It starts with small superficial non-erythematous vesiculopustules, which progresses to a collarette of scales and finally a pigmented macule which fades and disappears over a few weeks.
5. *Cutis mormorata*, occurs due to the physiological accentuation of reticular pattern of the blood vessels of the skin. It is not uncommonly seen in chromosomal disorders like Down's syndrome. In many instances cutis mormoratus would have no definite significance. The *harlequin change* seen in the neonate is believed to be due to the immature autonomic control. This results in half of the baby's body becoming pale, while the other half remains pink. The word 'Harlequin' should not contribute to confuse this condition with 'harlequin fetus' which is a severe degree of ichthyosis.

Jaundice

Neonatal hyperbilirubinemia or neonatal jaundice is a common problem in the newborn. The hemoglobin from the physiological destruction of erythrocytes and other heme containing pigments results in the production of bilirubin. The bilirubin is conjugated in the liver and converted into water-soluble salts of glucuronic acid–thus facilitating its excretion from the body. The decreased life of the fetal red blood cells, increased hematocrit of the newborn, immaturity of the liver enzymes and increased enterohepatic circulation, contribute to the excessive accumulation of unconjugated bilirubin in the neonates, resulting in the so called physiologic jaundice of the newborn appearing by 48 to 72 hours of birth. This would normally peak by 72 to 96 hr (Day 4) in term infants and by 144 hr to 168 hrs of life (day 7) in premature infants. Jaundice occurring within the first 24 hours of life,[4] bilirubin levels rising above the expected values for the age and gestation, and jaundice persisting beyond the 'normal' period must always be considered pathological and investigated for its cause.

A significant elevation of unconjugated bilirubin should therefore be expected in the presence of Rh-isoimmunization in infants born to Rh negative mothers or "ABO" incompatibility in infants born to mothers with O group. Other causes like G6PD deficiency should always be sought if hyperbilirubinemia is accompanied by evidence of hemolysis. Congenital hypothyroidism could present as exaggerated and prolonged jaundice as its sole clinical feature.

High levels of unconjugated bilirubin seems to adversely affect the metabolism of the developing brain resulting in a chronic encepahalopathy affecting predominantly the extrapyramidal system, associated with sensory neural deafness and gaze abnormalities. While the role of elevated bilirubin has been recognized, the exact mechanisms for this encephalopathy, or the critical level for serum bilirubin to precipitate encephalopathy has not been determined. Tradition has however, recommended keeping the serum bilirubin levels below 20 mg/dl (<360 mmol/L)[5] in term infants beyond 48 hr of life. Lower values of serum bilirubin could result in encephalopathy if the infant is premature or has other associated problems like perinatal asphyxia, sepsis, acidosis, or hypoalbuminemia.

Infants with hyperbilirubinemia are treated with phototherapy at the earliest. Should the bilirubin levels approach 'encephalopathic levels' a double volume exchange transfusion is the standard modality of treatment.

Respiratory Problems

Respiratory problems are a common cause for anxiety during the neonatal period. These usually manifest as tachypnea (respiratory rate > 60/min), grunting and/or intercostal retractions. The clinical picture of a neonate with varied combination of tachypnea, retractions, nasal flaring, grunting and cyanosis constitute a familiar scenario in a neonatal intensive care unit.

Pulmonary disorders that manifest in the newborn are usually related to immaturity of the lung, events that occurred in the perinatal period, or a result of congenital malformations. While structural anomalies and pneumonia are common in both term and preterm infants, conditions like Hyaline membrane disease is almost an exclusive disease of the premature infant. Meconium aspiration on the other hand is almost always seen in term infants. A skiagram of the chest, along with history and clinical presentation is often enough to establish the diagnosis in most cases. The management of all infants presenting with respiratory distress is aimed at preventing hypoxia, hypercapnia and acidosis in the newborn. The methods adapted for this could vary from oxygen supplementation to various strategies of mechanical ventilation, and specific therapies like surfactant replacement.

Gastrointestinal Problems

Vomiting and abdominal distention are the most common gastrointestinal complaints that bring a neonate to the doctor. Vomiting could be the presentation of innocuous problems like faulty feeding and aerophagia or could represent more serious surgical or medical conditions. A detailed discussion would be beyond the purview of this chapter. A reasonable history, clinical examination and basic investigations would be adequate to differentiate most of the conditions (Table 43.3).[6] While faulty feeding and aerophagia can be managed by supportive education on feeding practices to the mother, the more complex conditions would require specialized care.

Metabolic Disturbances

The fetus is almost entirely dependent on the mother for maintaining its internal mileu. It is therefore not surprising that the neonate should be prone to metabolic disturbances in the early neonatal period. While most term infants are able to maintain their euglycemic status,[7] at risk infants, like those born to diabetic mothers or low birth weight infants often develop hypoglycemia. Monitoring the blood glucose levels of these infants constitute an essential part of newborn care. Hypocalcemia and hypomagnesemia

Table 43.4: Vomiting in newborn

	Bilious		Nonbilious		Blood stained	
Surgical	Non-surgical	Surgical	Non-surgical	Surgical	Non-surgical
With distention Malrotation	Without distention Post-ampullary duodenal obstruction	Ileus	Pyloric stenosis	Excessive/ faulty feeding	Gastric volvulus	Swallowed maternal blood
Volvulus	Perforation	Malposition of feeding tube	Pre-ampullary duodenal stenosis	Gastroesophageal reflux	Gastric duplication	Severe asphyxia
Meconium plug			Early NEC	Infection	NEC	Traumatic resuscitation
Meconium ileus				Metabolic derangement		Stress ulcers
Hirschsprung's disease				Endocrine disorders (e.g. Congenital adrenal hyperplasia)		Disseminated intravascular coagulopathy
Necrotizing Enterocolitis (NEC)						Hemorrhagic disease of the newborn
						Drugs

may manifest as seizures. The low birth weight infant on formula feeds could also develop 'late metabolic acidosis' resulting in inadequate weight gain and failure to thrive in an otherwise active infant. Anticipating these common metabolic disturbances would go a long way in preventing their occurrence.

Low Birth Weight Infant

An infant below 2500 grams have been traditionally considered to be low birth weight (LBW). Such a classification would therefore include both premature infants and growth retarded term infants. In these days of population based growth charts, an infant with birth weight below 2 SD for the specific gestation is considered small for gestational age (SGA).[8] Thus a 1400 gram infant while being low birth weight could be appropriate for 32 weeks, but is small for gestation at 36 weeks. The mere reduction in size makes an infant prone to adverse environmental effects, resulting in hypothermia with the resultant hypoglycemia. The decreased maturity of the infant makes it vulnerable to metabolic problems like hypoglycemia, hypocalcemia and hyperbilirubinemia. The inadequate maturity of the organ systems makes the preterm baby more prone for organ specific pathology, e.g. respiratory problems like surfactant deficiency syndrome (Hyaline membrane disease) and/or pulmonary hemorrhage. A vulnerable central nervous system makes the preterm infant more susceptible to intraventricular hemorrhage and an immature gastrointestinal system predisposes to necrotizing enterocolitis. Persistent ductus arteriosus and vasomotor lability are commonly encountered cardiovascular problems.

A low birth weight infant must therefore regularly be evaluated for all these problems. An anticipatory management with appropriate intervention would yield satisfactory dividends while caring for these infants.

Neonatal Seizures

Seizures are a common problem seen during the neonatal period. These could be focal or multifocal clonic, tonic, myoclonic or subtle seizures. Metabolic problems like hypoglycemia, hypocalcemia and hypomagnesemia constitute the common causes of seizures during the early neonatal period. Perinatal asphyxia and meningitis are also often associated with seizures. The general principles of proper position to ensure patent airways, prevent aspiration and ensure adequate oxygenation should never be forgotten while managing seizures. The availability of "glucostix" has ensured the bed-side detection of hypoglycemia. In the nonavailability of such facilities, therapy must always be commenced with intravenous glucose bolus (0.5 g–1 g/kg) as 10 or 25 percent solution. It is preferable to draw blood samples for glucose, calcium and magnesium levels before initiating therapy. If seizures are not controlled with glucose, 10 percent Calcium gluconate bolus (2 ml/kg) is given very slowly monitoring the heart rate to avoid bradycardia. In an unresponsive infant the presence of hypomagnesemia should be considered and 0.2 ml/kg of 50 percent magnesium sulfate is given *intramuscular*. Anticonvulsants must be given only after this stage. Intravenous phenobarbitone (10 to 20 mg/kg) as bolus is the drug of choice.

Appropriate investigations must be undertaken to confirm the etiology of the seizures.

CONCLUSION

Despite the availability of pediatric services in most hospitals, the obstetrician and obstetric nurses are often the first persons to whom the mother turns with problems regarding her baby. As the first 'care-giver' examining the baby, a reasonable awareness of the problems occurring in the newborn is a mandatory requirement for all personnel involved in obstetric practice. This chapter provides a brief insight into problems commonly encountered in the neonate during routine obstetric practice.

REFERENCES

1. Reproductive Health Programme Development: Implementing Cairo WHO/RHR/00.5.
2. Reproductive health during conflict and displacement—WHO/RHR/00.13
3. Gloria D Eng: Neuromuscular disease. In Avery GB, Fletcher MA, Macdonald MG (Eds): *Neonatology–Pathophysiology and Management of the Newborn*. 4th edn. JB Lippincott Company, Philadelphia 1164-78, 1994
4. Alpay F, Sarici SU, Tosuncuk HD, Serdar MA, Inanc N, Gokcay E: The value of first-day bilirubin measurement in predicting the development of significant hyperbilirubinemia in healthy term newborns. Pediatrics **106(2)**:E16, 2000.
5. Soorani-Lunsing I, Woltil HA, Hadders-Algra M" Are moderate degrees of hyperbilirubinemia in healthy term neonates really safe for the brain? (Pubmed) *Pediatr Res, Dec* **50(6)**:701-05, 2001.
6. Elizabeth John (Ed): *Neonatal Handbook*, Westmead NSW Australia 36-37, 2000.
7. Diwakar KK, Sasidhar MV: Plasma glucose levels in term infants who are appropriate size for gestation and exclusively breast-fed. *Arch Dis Child Fetal Neonatal* **87(July)**: F46–48, 2002.
8. Wallis MS, Harley D: Fetal growth. Intrauterine growth retardation and small for gestational age babies. In Roberton NRC (Ed): *Text book of Neonatology*. London, Churchill Livingstone; 317-24, 1992.

44. Complications of Third Stage of Labor

Thaneemalai Jeganathan
V Sivanesaratnam

ABSTRACT

Childbirth is a normal process, occasionally maternal mortality and morbidity is encountered due to problems faced in the third stage of labor. Most often, inadequately trained medical personnel manage these complications. In this chapter, definition, physiology and benefits of active management of third stage of labor are explained. Primary postpartum hemorrhage (PPH) is the leading complication. The causes, predisposing factors and management are discussed in a stepwise manner. Atonic PPH is often managed medically with simple uterotonics, but rarely it requires second line prostaglandins. Failure of medical management and morbid patient's will require various surgical interventions to arrest hemorrhage. Hysterectomy is the treatment of choice when other measures fail. Retained placenta will require manual removal of placenta under general anesthesia. Even though uterine inversion is rare, one should be competent to manage this.

INTRODUCTION

Maternal death is a tragedy and a loss to the dependants, society and the nation. About half a million women die annually across the world due to reasons related to pregnancy and childbirth. Approximately quarter of them succumb to the complications occurring at third stage of labor, primarily postpartum hemorrhage. In the United Kingdom the risk of maternal death from postpartum hemorrhage is one in 100,000 deliveries, whereas in developing countries the risk is one in 1000 deliveries. The report on the confidential enquiries into maternal deaths in Malaysia (CEMD-Malaysia) 1995-1996 showed postpartum hemorrhage as the leading cause of maternal mortality;[1] many cases of postpartum hemorrhage were managed by relatively inexperienced doctors who did not institute treatment early enough or failed to consult senior colleagues until it was too late. Therefore, to avert this tragedy, this chapter addresses the active management of third stage of labor that helps to reduce complications occurring. When complications arise, they should be managed in a stepwise manner as shown below to avert the consequences.

The third stage of labor is *defined* as a continuous process that begins with the delivery of the fetus and ends in delivery of the placenta. It usually lasts for 5 to 10 minutes, but should not last more than 30 minutes. Women are prone for various potential hazards of labor during this stage, which could result in disastrous consequences.

PHYSIOLOGY OF PLACENTAL SEPARATION

Contraction and retraction of uterine myometerium that takes place in the third stage reduces the surface area to which the placenta is attached in the upper segment, which results in the placental separation. Reduced uterine volume and continuous retraction of upper segment expels the separated placenta into the relaxed lower segment and vaginal introitus. Retraction of oblique fibers of uterine myometerium ("living ligatures") is vital in obliterating the blood vessels supplying the large placental surface and prevents blood loss.

The signs of placental separation include:
- Uterine fundal dominance that is felt as a firm globular structure due to contraction of the upper segment
- Rise in the fundal height as the separated placenta now occupies the previously collapsed lower segment
- Fresh bleeding due to separation of the placenta
- Gradual lengthening of the umbilical cord
- No retraction of the umbilical cord on displacing the fundus of uterus upwards

Management

Active management of third stage of labor has been found to have multiple benefits over the expectant management. It has halved the risk of postpartum hemorrhage, low postpartum hemoglobin and the requirement of blood transfusions. It has also reduced the duration of third stage of labor and the requirement for therapeutic oxytocis.[2]

a. Expectant management:
   - Watchful waiting for placental separation
   - No prophylactic use of oxytocin
   - No controlled cord traction or fundal pressure.
b. Active management:
   - Early clamping and division of umblical cord
   - Administration of prophylactic oxytocics—I.M syntometrine 1 ml (combination of syntocinon 5 iu and ergometrie 0.5 mg) at the delivery of the anterior shoulder
   - Brandt-Andrews technique of controlled cord traction (Figure 44.1).

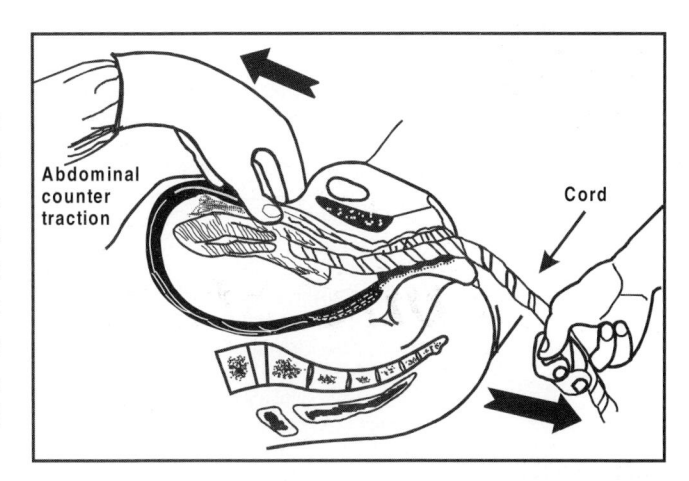

Figure 44.1: Brandt-Andrews technique of controlled cord traction

Never pull on the cord without ascertaining that the uterus is well contracted.

POSTPARTUM HEMORRHAGE

The most important complication of the third stage of labor is postpartum hemorrhage (PPH). Massive obstetric hemorrhage can lead to hypovolemic shock, disseminated intravascular coagulopathy (DIVC), renal failure, hepatic failure, and adult respiratory distress syndrome.[3] In the developing world, poor nutritional status, multiparity, lack of easy accesses to treatment, delivery by untrained birth attendants, inadequate emergency transportation, and inadequate intensive care and blood bank facilities are the additional risk factors that contribute to high maternal morbidity and mortality.[1,4]

Primary postpartum hemorrhage is defined as the blood loss of 500 ml or more from the genital tract during the first 24 hours after delivery of the baby. *Secondary postpartum hemorrhage* is defined as excessive bleeding from the genital tract occurring after 24 hours of delivery of the baby and up to 6 weeks postpartum. There is considerable controversy over the amount of 500 ml in the definition because clinical estimate of blood loss is grossly inaccurate and usually underestimated by 30 to 50 percent.[4]

The classification, causes and predisposing factors of

PPH is given in the Tables 44.1 and Table 44.2.

Table 44.1: Classification, causes and predisposing factors of primary PPH

Causes	Predisposing factors
1. Uterine atony	• Over distention of uterus (multiple pregnancy, polyhydramnios, macrosomia) • Retained products of conception • Prolonged labor • Oxytocin augmentation of labor • Grandmultiparity • Antepartum hemorrhage • Anemia • Uterine fibroids • General anesthetic drugs (halothane) • Precipitate delivery • Chorioamnionitis • Magnesium sulphate treatment of pregnancy-induced hypertension (PIH)
2. Retained placenta	• Retained placenta (placenta succenturiata, membranes, cotyeledons) • Placenta accreta (placenta previa, and situation of placenta over previous cesarean section scar, repeated uterine curettages, myomectomies)
3. Genital tract trauma (uterus, cervix, vagina, introitus)	• Perineal tear, episiotomies and ruptured vulval varicosities. Precipitate labor, macrosomic babies and instrumental deliveries can cause cervical, vaginal and vulval lacerations. • Uterine rupture (prostaglandins, oxytocis, obstructed labor and previous scar)
4. Coagulation disorders	• Amniotic fluid embolism • Abruptio placenta • Sepsis • Massive blood loss and transfusion • Severe pre-eclampsia • Chorioamnionitis • Idiopathic thrombocytopania
5. Uterine inversion	• Excessive cord traction or fundal pressure at third stage of labor • Uterine atony and uterine anomalies

Table 44.2: Causes of secondary PPH

1. Retained products of conception—this is the cause of delayed PPH in half of the cases
2. Infection
3. Breakdown of uterine wound
4. Chronic sub-involution of uterus
5. Trophoblastic disease (rare—placental site tumor, choriocarcinoma)
6. Endometrial cancer (rare)

Management of Postpartum Hemorrhage

Prophylactic Management

The primary aim of management is prevention of atonic PPH; therefore, identification of high and low risk patients based on predisposing factors is essential for instituting appropriate measures.

1. *High risk*:
   - Correct anemia during antenatal period
   - Hospital delivery by an experienced obstetric team
   - Establish intravenous line with a wide bore cannula (16G or 18G) before 2nd stage.
   - Active management in the 3rd stage of labor as mentioned above
   - Blood sent for full blood count (FBC) and group and cross match
   - Prophylactic IV Oxytocin drip 40iu for duration of 6 hours after delivery.
2. *Low risk*: Active management in the 3rd stage of labor as mentioned above.

General Management

- Realise that PPH is an obstetric emergency and call for assistance from a multidisciplinary team (anesthetist, consultant obstetrician, hematologist, theater staff, nursing staff and support staff)
- Rapid assessment of patient's general condition, establish the cause of PPH, amount of blood loss and the degree of hypovolemia.
- Retrieve 20 ml of blood (FBC, GXM 4-6 units, PT/PTT, blood urea and electrolytes)
- Resuscitate the patient (minimum 2-IV cannula-size16-14G, crystalloids or colloids infusion or plasma or blood transfusion depending upon the blood loss) It is best not to use glucose containing fluids.
- Regular monitoring of the patient's blood pressure, pulse rate, level of consciousness, pad chart, input/output chart and uterine fundal height.

Specific Management

Uterine atony: Uterine atony accounts for 80 percent of PPH and the bleeding is due to unoccluded blood vessels in the separated placental bed. Bleeding may be brisk or slow and usually intermittent and on abdominal palpation uterus will be relaxed.

Management of Atonic PPH

The following measures need to be instituted in a

stepwise manner:
- To encourage uterine contraction, uterine fundal massage needs to be performed. This is best carried out by lifting the uterus out of the pelvis by the right hand placed above the symphysis and using the left hand to massage the fundus
- Catheterize the bladder
- Re-examine the placenta and membranes to ensure that they are complete and a succenturate lobe has not been missed.
- IM syntometrine 1 ml or IV ergometrine 0.25 mg may be administered; ergometrine in higher doses given intravenously may cause headache, nausea and vomiting, and may cause elevation in the blood pressure. Syntometrine has the combined rapidly acting effect of oxytocin (within 45 sec) and the sustained action ergometrine.
- If the above measures fail, IV infusion of oxytocin (40-100 iu) in 500 ml of normal saline may be commenced. A much higher dose of upto 200 iu may be needed in some instances.
- If the uterus remains atonic IM Carboprost/Hemabate (15 methyl-prostaglandin F2α) 250 μ gms can be administered. This can be repeated after 15 minutes for a maximum of 3 doses. This could also be given into the myometrium. Misoprostol 800 μgm given rectally is an alternative.[4]
- If the bleeding persists despite having achieved a well contracted uterus, suspect a cervical or vaginal tear being present. A careful examination under anesthesia needs to be done.
- If there is a torrential hemorrhage, immediate bimanual compression of the uterus (internal or external) or aortic compression is performed to reduce the blood loss until the patient could be transported to an operation theater and appropriate surgical treatment is carried out (Figures 44.2 and 44.3).

Surgical Management of Atonic PPH

Operative intervention is a last resort.

Examination under anesthesia
Patient is placed in the lithotomy position, and systematic examination of the genital tract is carried out

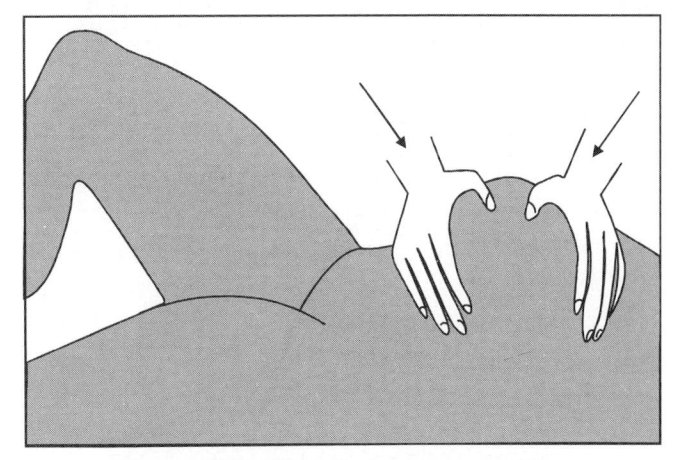

Figure 44.2: External uterine compression

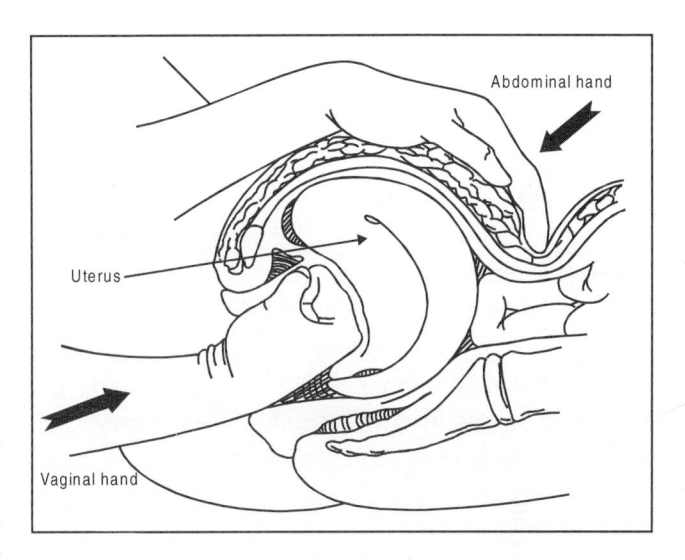

Figure 44.3: Bimanual uterine compression

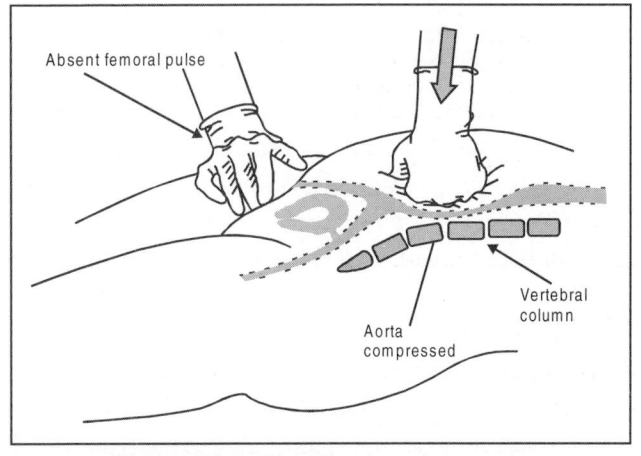

Figure 44.4: Compression of the aorta

under a good light source with proper vaginal retractors and able assistants. Look for tears in the vagina, cervix and endocervix that will require suturing. Tears extending into the uterus needs laparotomy. If the above causes are excluded, then manual exploration of the uterus should be performed. Look for any remnants of retained placenta or pieces of membrane or cotyledons; these when present can be freed digitally and removed with sponge forceps. Curettage is best avoided. If it is necessary then a light curettage may be performed using a large blunt curette, taking care to avoid perforation of soft postpartum uterus. Uterine cavity needs to be empty for uterus to contract.

Coagulopathy should also be corrected before proceeding to further surgical management.[5,6]

Tamponade test: This test provides a means of selecting those patients that require further surgery. The Sengstaken-Blakemore tube, stomach balloon is inserted into the uterine cavity and balloon is inflated with 75-150 ml of warm saline. The warm saline may speed up the coagulation cascade and the aspiration channel in the tube allows the collected blood to be drained. Intravenous oxytocin infusion is supplemented to maintain the uterine contraction. The tamponade test is deemed successful if the bleeding is decreased and no further surgery is then required. If, however, the bleeding persists, the test is unsuccessful and laparotomy is required to control the hemorrhage.[7]

Uterine compression sutures
Uterine conservation procedures are performed in women where future fertility is desired.
1. *B- Lynch suture and modifications:* B-Lynch suturing technique involves insertion of a pair of vertical brace sutures around the uterus, essentially to appose the anterior and posterior walls and apply continuous compression pressure on the bleeding placental bed. Complete hemostasis is secured, while preserving the uterus and fertility. It is commonly performed following a cesarean section; if after a vaginal delivery, uterus needs to be opened to insert a brace suture. The suturing is shown in the Figure 44.5. The modified B-Lynch suture as shown in the Figure 44.6 does not require opening the uterus following vaginal

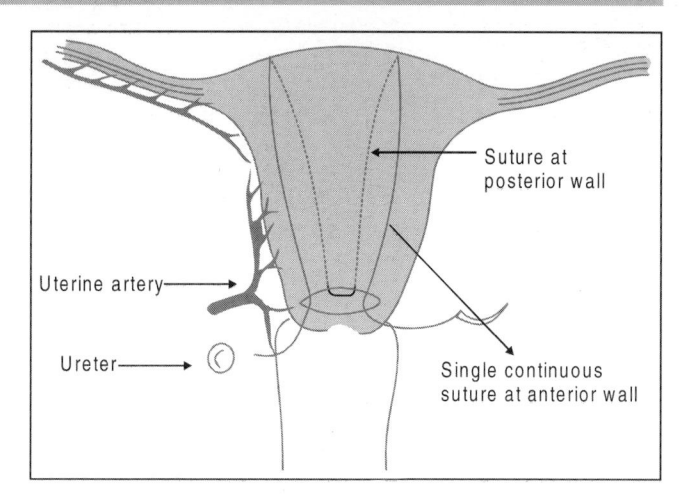

Figure 44.5: B-Lynch suture

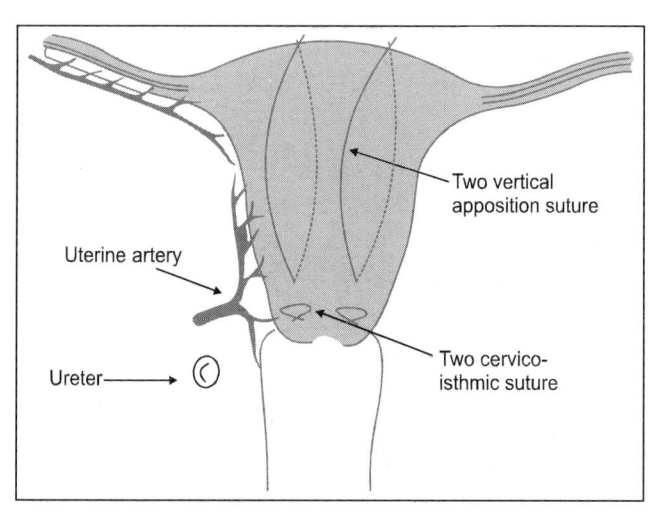

Figure 44.6: Vertical and horizontal compression suture

delivery or cesarean section and is simpler to perform. More tension is required in compressing the uterus, and this is easily achieved with two separate sutures in the modified technique compared with single brace suture in B-Lynch suture. The horizontal additional sutures in the modifications are very effective in controlling bleeding from the lower segment.[7]

2. *Hemostatic suturing technique (Multiple square):* It is to approximate the anterior and posterior uterine wall until no space is left in the uterine cavity. It is very useful in securing hemostasis secondary to uterine atony or placental site hemorrhage. The

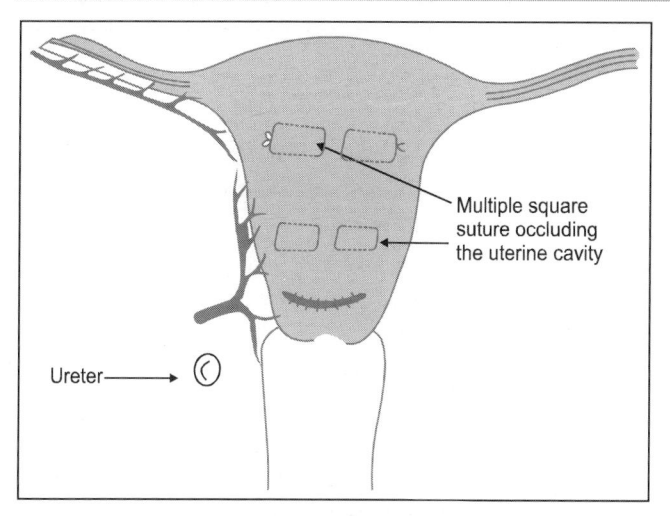

Figure 44.7: Multiple square sutures

technique is shown in the Figure 44.7. It is easy to perform; it is a procedure that is safe as no important structures such as ureters or great vessels could be injured.

The senior author has been performing a simpler procedure of *"plication of the uterine wall"* as shown in Figures 44.8A and B; aimed at occluding only the placental bed with interrupted square sutures and has found this to be effective. The uterine cavity is not

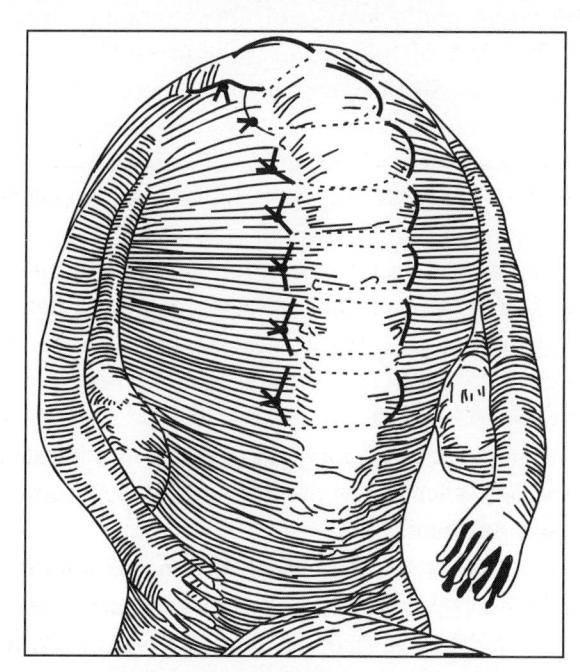

Figure 44.8A: Plication of uterine wall

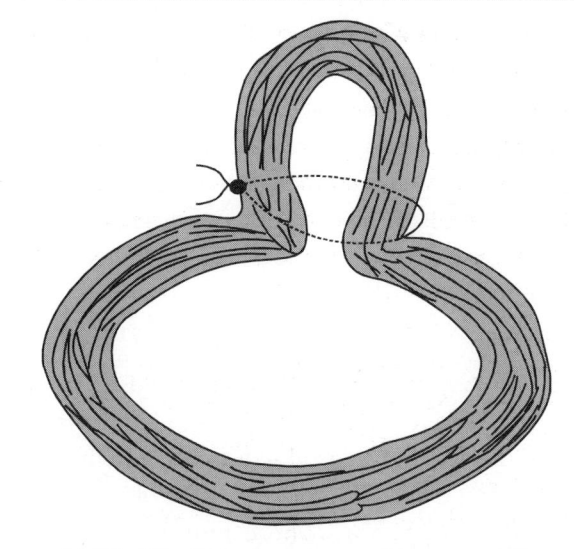

Figure 44.8B: Plication of uterine wall—cross-section view

occluded.

Devascularization procedures

These procedures can be performed on their own or in addition to the above.

1. *Bilateral uterine artery ligation:* It is easier and safer than internal iliac artery ligation; with this technique 90 percent of uterine blood supply is reduced. A large atraumatic needle is used to traverse in the avascular space of the broad ligament and 2 to 3 cm of myometerium to ligate the ascending branch of uterine artery. The suture is placed below vesico-uterine fold of peritoneum, carefully avoiding injury to the ureters, bladder and bowel.

2. *Bilateral internal iliac artery ligation:* It reduces the uterine and vaginal bleeding. The success rate of the procedure is 40 percent, it reduces the blood flow in the internal iliac vessels by converting arterial pressure system into venous, promoting the coagulation cascade. It is difficult to perform by the less experienced due to the edematous tissues in pregnancy. Moreover, an accurate understanding of anatomy is required to identify retroperitoneal structures such as ureters and iliac vessels.

3. *Utero-ovarian artery anastomosis ligation:* An avascular area in the meso-ovarium is chosen to place a ligature around the utero-ovarian anastomosis (between the ovary and fundus of uterus)

without jeopardizing the vascularity of the ovaries.

4. *Arterial embolization:* An interventional radiologist usually performs it. Femoral artery cathetrization is performed to identify the uterine vessels, which are then embolized with thrombogenic material.[3,7] It achieves the similar effect as the uterine artery ligation described above.

Hysterectomy

This is the last step in achieving hemostasis, when all other steps have failed. But in grand multiparous women, in severely shocked women and in those with coagulopathy where no replacement of blood products is available or in those where future fertility is not desired this step should be considered early.

1. *Total hysterectomy* should be the aim in all cases. However, the soft and effaced cervix may be difficult to identify during the procedure and this requires experience.
2. *Subtotal hysterectomy* is quicker, simpler and safe procedure and is associated with less blood loss. However, it is inadequate in cases where bleeding is from the lower segment, such as bleeding placenta previa with accreta and tears in the lower segment. Further, the subsequent development of cervical stump carcinoma poses a dilema in treatment.

GENITAL TRACT TRAUMA

Bleeding from or into genital tract in the presence of a contracted uterus can be profuse; it is important that the above cause be excluded. Patient is examined under general anesthesia with the aid of a good light source, adequate exposure (optimal positioning, extension of episiotomy or use of special vaginal retractors) and appropriate assistants to identify the injury. Excessive bleeding may obscure the view, which could be overcome with vaginal packs to reduce bleeding and adequate suction for good visualization. *Vaginal tears* are sutured; starting above the apex of the tear to arrest the upper most bleeding point using long needle holders and polyglycolic absorbable suture materials. If the apex cannot be identified, temporary suture is inserted as high as possible and traction on this will enable access to the apex. The suturing can be continuous or interrupted. If tearing of vaginal wall is encountered, the two ends are sutured individually and the raw area is left to re-epithelialize without scarring and the vagina is packed for 12 to 24 hours and bladder is continuously drained. The broad-spectrum antibiotic is administered and the deranged coagulopathy is corrected.

1. *Cervical laceration* occurs commonly at 3 o' clock and 9 o' clock positions and can result in profuse vaginal bleeding. It will require immediate resuscitation and suturing in the theater as mentioned above. Sponge-holding forceps may be applied to the anterior and posterior lips of the cervix to pull down the cervix to the introitus to facilitate inspection and suturing. Cervical lacerations need not be sutured unless they are bleeding.
2. *Uterine ruptures* are rare, life-threatening emergency requiring laparotomy. Simple scar dehiscence and small tears could be repaired in two layers. Major tears and uncontrolled hemorrhage will require a hysterectomy.
3. *Vaginal wall hematomas* are encountered occasionally. These may be superficial or deep. Large expanding hematomas can cause distention of perineum and severe pain; these require surgical evacuation of hematoma followed by securing hemostasis. Stable hemotomas can be observed and treated conservatively. Lateral vaginal wall hematoma due to collection of blood above the insertion of levator ani are deep. These will require exploration under anesthesia to identify the bleeding point and securing hemostasis. If bleeding cannot be controlled by the vaginal route, a laparotomy and internal iliac artery ligation may be necessary.

RETAINED PLACENTA

Retained placenta is *defined* as failure of the placenta to be expelled within 30 minutes after delivery of the fetus. Empty the bladder and apply controlled cord traction. If this is unsuccessful, a gentle vaginal examination is performed. If the placenta has partially extruded through the cervix, then it is grasped with fingers and steadily withdrawn from the cervix.

If the placenta is retained, there may or may not

be profuse bleeding. If there is profuse bleeding, then it is due to a partially separated placenta and inadequately contracted and retracted uterus. Patient should be resuscitated to prevent shock and the dose of oxytocic should be repeated to promote uterine contraction and retraction, and placental separation; controlled cord traction is then applied to deliver the placenta. If the placenta continues to retain or is entrapped, manual removal of placenta in the theater under general anesthesia should be considered immediately.

Manual removal of placenta
Patient is placed in lithotomy position. The bladder should be catheterized, if this has not been done previously, one hand is placed on the abdomen to exert counter pressure at the fundus of the uterus and the other hand adequately lubricated with chlorhexidine cream is placed in the vagina. The right hand is apposed at the tip of all five fingers to form a cone and inserted into the cervical os. To identify the retained placenta in the upper segment, cord is followed through the cervical os. The placenta is separated at the edge of the placenta by sliding the fingers held flat together between the placenta and the uterine wall. The abdominal hand gives counter-pressure on the uterus against the shearing force of the finger within the uterus and prevents perforation of the thin myometrium (Figure 44.9). The placenta is removed only, when it is totally separated. The uterine cavity is explored for retained cotyledons and membranes, before the vaginal hand is removed. The removed placenta needs to be examined carefully for missing cotyledons and membranes. Oxytocin infusion is commenced to promote uterine contraction and broad-spectrum antibiotic is given intravenously at the onset of the procedure.[9]

PLACENTA ACCRETA

In this condition the placental villi become directly attached to the myometerium, due to the absence of the decidual basalis layer or imperfect development of the fibrinoid layer. Placenta *increta* is said to occur if the chorionic villi penetrates the myometerium. When the villi reaches the outer serosal layer it is called placenta *percreta*.

During manual removal of placenta, if one is unable to identify the plane between uterus and the placenta then the above should be suspected. Extensive placenta accreta usually requires a hysterectomy. Due to the risk of massive obstetric hemorrhage, no attempt should be made to remove the placenta piecemeal. There is a limited role for conservative management.[7]

UTERINE INVERSION

Uterine inversion, a rare complication of *turning inside out of the uterus* most commonly occurs due to mismanagement of third stage of labor, especially when controlled cord traction is applied when the uterus is not contracted. It is often not associated with massive hemorrhage, and the shock is often out of proportion to the blood loss; this is the result of neurogenic shock due to traction on the uterine supports. If the placenta is completely or partially separated profuse bleeding can occur.

When this is diagnosed immediate replacement of the inverted uterus manually should be carried out. Summon the anesthetist immediately. If initial manual replacement fails, immediate intravascular crystalloids are administered to expand the intravascular volume. When the patient's condition is stable the uterine inversion is

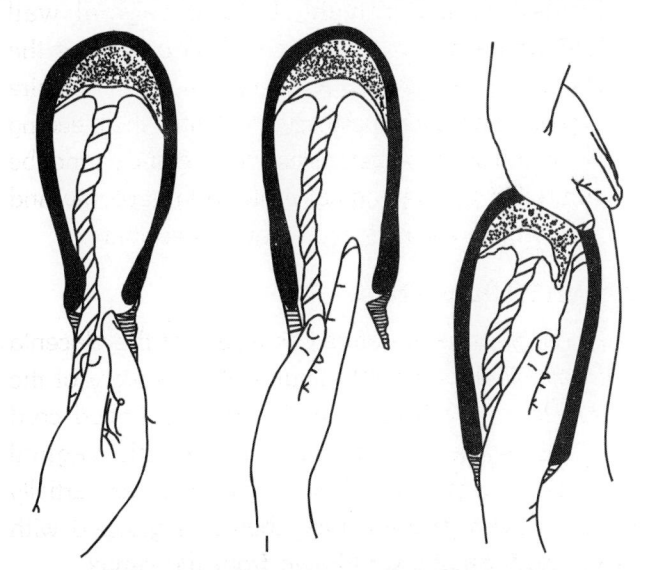

Figure 44.9: Manual removal of placenta

corrected by *O'Sullivan hydrostatic method* under general anesthesia. This is carried out by rapid infusion of warm saline 2 to 3 liters into the vagina and the introitus is sealed with both hands or with silastic vacuum cup. *If the placenta is intact, then it is manually removed only when the uterus has been restored in the pelvic cavity* and oxytocin infusion is commenced immediately to promote uterine contraction. This simple method is successful in majority of cases. If the hydrostatic method fails then an attempt should be made to *manually replace* the inversion by placing the 'cupped' hand around the fundus and elevating it along the long axis of the vagina. Halothane anesthsia is helpful in this procedure; alternatively IV terbutaline to relax the uterine muscle can be used. *It is important that the attached placenta be not removed prior to complete replacement of the fundus has been achieved to prevent bleeding from the placental site.*

Rarely replacement of the uterus may not be achieved from below. In these situations a *laparotomy* is performed; a vertical *incision* placed posteriorly in the cervix to divide the constriction ring and the fundus "hoisted" up to be replaced in the normal position in the pelvic cavity. This incision is subsequently sutured.

REFERENCES

1. Ministry of Health Malaysia. Report on the confidential enquiries into maternal deaths in Malaysia 1995-1996, 2000.
2. Murray E, Marc J N C, James Neilson *et al:* The third stage of labor. In A guide to effective care in pregnancy and childbirth. 3rd edn, Oxford University press, 300-09, 2000.
3. Bonnar J, 2000. Massive Obstetric Hemorrhage. Bailliers Best pract Res Cli Obstet Gynecol; 14:1-18.
4. Mousa, Hatem A, Walkinshaw et al, 2001. Major Postpartum hemorrhage. Current Opinion in Obstetrics and Gynecology; 13(6): 595-603.
5. Kuldip Singh, Arulkumaran S, 1996. The Third Stage of Labor. In Arulkumaran S, Ratnam S S, Bhasker Rao S (eds). The Management of Labor Orient Longman: 170-182.
6. Arulkumaran S, Haththotuwa R, Chua S, 1996. The Management of Postpartum Hemorrhage. In Arulkumaran S, Ratnam S S, Bhasker Rao S (eds). The Management of Labor. Orient Longman: 183-196.
7. Tamizian O, Arulkumaran S, 2002. The Surgical Management of Post-partum Hemorrhage. Bailliers Best pract Res Cli Obstet Gynecol; 16:81-98.
8. Liu DTY, Fairweather DVI, 1991. Emergencies in the Immediate Puerperium. In Labor Ward Manual. 2nd edn. Butterworth Heinemann. 95-99.

45.
Normal Puerperium

Jyothi Shetty

DEFINITION

The puerperium refers to the six-week period, which follows childbirth. During this time, the pelvic organs return to the non-pregnant state, the physiological changes of pregnancy are reversed and lactation is established.

Good postnatal care is based upon a sound understanding of the physiological changes in the puerperium.

PHYSIOLOGICAL CHANGES

Involution of the Uterus

Immediately after placental expulsion, the fundus of the uterus is slightly below the umbilicus. During the puerperium, the uterus begins to shrink so that within two weeks the fundus will have descended below the symphysis pubis. By the end of six weeks, uterus regains its previous non-pregnant size. The process by which the postpartum uterus returns almost to its pre-pregnancy state is known as involution.

During involution, the number of muscle fibers is not decreased; instead, the individual cells decrease in size. Autolysis of the cytoplasm occurs by the proteolytic enzyme with liberation of peptones, which enter the bloodstream. These are excreted through the kidneys as urea and creatinine.

Changes in the Cervix and Vagina

The cervix is very flaccid after delivery. The cervical opening gradually contracts and for the first few days admits two fingers. It involutes along with the uterus, so that by 2 to 3 weeks the internal os is closed.

Vagina gradually diminishes in size. The hymen disappears and is represented by several small tags of tissue which cicatrize and are known as carunculae myrtiformes. This is a characteristic sign of parity.

Lochia

Lochia is the vaginal discharge for the first 2 to 3 weeks during puerperium. It is comprised of blood and necrotic decidua.

After delivery, the remaining decidua becomes differentiated into two layers. The superficial layer becomes necrotic and it is sloughed off in the lochia. The basal layer remains and is the source of new endometrium. The endometrium arises from proliferation of the endometrial glandular remnants and the stroma of the interglandular connective tissue.

Types of lochia

1. *Lochia rubra:* For the first 4 days, lochia is red in color. It contains blood as well as decidual debris.
2. *Lochia serosa:* From 5th to 9th day, lochia becomes pale in color. It contains still some red cells, but predominantly leucocytes and necrotic decidua.
3. *Lochia alba:* After the 10th day, the lochia changes to yellowish white color. It consists now principally of serous fluid and leucocytes.

Urinary Tract

The puerperal bladder has increased capacity and is insensitive to the raised intravesical pressure. Therefore, the bladder can be overdistended and incomplete emptying is common in the puerperium. The insensitivity of the bladder is due to trauma sustained by the nerve plexus during delivery. Stagnation of urine predisposes to bacterial multiplication and to ascending infection of the urinary tract.

Normal pregnancy is associated with an increase in extracellular water and puerperal diuresis is a reversal of this process. Diuresis occurs between the second and fifth days.

Dilated ureters and renal pelves return to their prepregnant state within 8 weeks.

Blood

Cardiac output rises soon after delivery and remains elevated for at least 48 hours postpartum. By the 2nd week, these changes have returned to nonpregnant values. Thus the early puerperium is a time which requires close surveillance in any woman at risk of cardiac compromise from conditions such as rheumatic heart disease.

During postpartum period there is an outpouring of fresh platelets with increased adhesiveness and a rapid rise in platelet count. Fibrinogen level remains elevated upto the second week of puerperium. The hypercoagulable state persists until about 6 weeks. This has implication when planning prophylactic anticoagulant regimens for women at risk from thromboembolic disease.

Return of Menstruation and Ovulation

The onset of the first menstrual period following delivery is variable and depends on lactation. Mothers who do not breastfeed have an early resumption of menstruation by 6 to 8 weeks. In contrast, breastfeeding women experience a period of lactational amenorrhea and reduced fertility. With full or nearly full breastfeeding approximately 70 percent of women remain amenorrheic till 6 months. During the greatest part of lactational amenorrhea, ovulation is suppressed and conception cannot occur. However, in the 4 weeks prior to the end of lactational amenorrhea, ovarian activity will return and 30 percent of these cycles will be ovulatory. Hence, total protection is achieved by the exclusively breastfeeding woman for a duration of only 10 weeks.

Mechanism of Lactational Amenorrhea

Suckling induces changes in the sensitivity of the hypothalamic-pituitary axis to estrogen, making it more sensitive to the negative feedback effects of ovarian steroids and less sensitive to positive feedback. As a result, there is inhibition of GnRH, leading to diminished secretion of LH. High levels of prolactin reduces gonadotropin secretion from the pituitary.

The dominant physiological event is lactation, which will be discussed later in this chapter.

MANAGEMENT OF NORMAL PUERPERIUM

Vital Signs

During the patient's stay in hospital, regular checks are made of her pulse, blood pressure and temperature. There may be slight reactionary rise in temperature following delivery by 0.5°F but comes down to normal within 12 hours.

Involution of the Uterus

The rate of involution of the uterus can be assessed clinically by noting the height of the fundus in relation to the symphysis pubis. On the first day following delivery, the height of the fundus is about 12 cm above the symphysis. The measurement should be taken after emptying the bladder. It decreases in height by 1 cm per day, so that by the end of second week the uterus becomes a pelvic organ. The rate of involution thereafter slows down and by 6 weeks, the uterus becomes almost normal in size.

Lochia

The color and amount of the lochia is recorded. It has a sweetish mawkish odor.

Offensive lochia, which may be accompanied by pyrexia and a tender uterus, suggests endometritis. Persistent red lochia suggests delayed involution that is usually associated with infection or retained bits of placental tissue.

Care of the Bladder

If the woman has not voided within 4 to 6 hours of delivery, it is likely that her bladder is in danger of overdistention. This is particularly common in women who have undergone epidural analgesia, a traumatic delivery such as a difficult instrumental delivery, multiple lacerations or a vulvovaginal hematoma. The distended bladder should either be palpable as a suprapubic cystic mass or it may elevate the uterine fundus above the umbilicus. She should be encouraged to walk to the toilet or an analgesic is administered to reduce pain. If these measures fail, an indwelling catheter should be left *in situ* for 24 to 72 hours, or until the bladder tone is regained.

Care of the Bowel

Constipation is a common problem in the puerperium. Mother should be encouraged to increase the fluid intake and roughage content in her diet. If this is inadequate, bulk forming drugs should be prescribed such as ispaghula husk.

Advice

1. *Rest and sleep*: The mother is in need of rest. She is encouraged to have good sleep and should be protected against undue fatigue. "Rooming in" means keeping baby in a cot with mother. This improves breastfeeding and mother-baby bondage.
2. *Early ambulation*: Women can move out of bed within a few hours after delivery. Early ambulation has reduced the frequency of venous thrombosis and pulmonary embolism. For at least the first ambulation, an attendant should be present to help prevent injury if the woman becomes syncopal.
3. *Diet:* Normal diet is given soon after the delivery. Adequate amount of fluid intake is important for successful breastfeeding. Mother is encouraged to drink about a liter of milk everyday. For the lactating mother the calories and protein intake should be increased. Fresh fruits and vegetables will provide the necessary vitamins. Most women from the developing world will benefit from oral iron therapy (ferrous sulfate 200 mg) for a period of 6 weeks.
4. *Care of the vulva*: The episiotomy wound should be cleaned with antiseptic solution at least twice a day. If the woman complains of pain at the episiotomy site, moist heat can be provided with warm sitz bath. Analgesics such as ibuprofen 400 mg orally thrice daily may be prescribed to relieve the perineal discomfort. Any signs of infection should be treated with antibiotics.
5. *Immunization*: Anti-D gammaglobulin is administered within 72 hours to Rh negative mother bearing Rh positive baby. Women who are susceptible to rubella can be vaccinated with live attenuated rubella vaccine.
6. *Contraception:* Postpartum sterilization can be offered to mothers who are certain that they have completed their family and are unlikely to come for an interval procedure a few months later. Tubal ligation is performed early in the puerperium between 48 and 72 hours. During the hospital stay, a concerted effort should be made to provide family planning education.
7. *Time of discharge*: Following vaginal delivery, if there are no complications, the woman is discharged after 48 hours and at times after 5 days in those who have perineal sutures.
8. *Postnatal exercise*: The woman should be encouraged to start exercise to tone up the abdominal and

pelvic floor muscles. These exercises should be continued for at least 3 months.

Management of Ailments

After pain: It is the spasmodic pain felt in the lower abdomen particularly when the infant suckles. They are caused by strong uterine contractions, which are in turn caused by oxytocin liberated in response to suckling. Occasionally analgesics have to be prescribed to relieve the pain.

Pain on the perineum: When a patient complains of severe perineal pain, the first step is to reexamine the perineum to detect if there is a hematoma or infection.

Puerperal mental disorders: It is fairly common for a mother to exhibit some degree of depression during the first week after delivery. This transient depression or postpartum 'blues' is a self limiting condition. The mother is reassured that it is likely to last only a few days.

Puerperal psychosis may arise during the puerperium. The warning features are restlessness, insomnia, hallucinations and delirium. This is a serious condition and requires expert psychiatric evaluation and treatment.

POSTNATAL EXAMINATION

Postnatal examination is carried out at the end of 6 weeks. Any problems that the mother may present are discussed. The doctor enquires about her general health, whether the lochia has ceased and about infant feeding problems. The abdomen is examined and the state of the musculature noted. Pelvic examination is performed to check if episiotomy has healed and that the uterus has involuted.

Practical contraceptive advice should be given to women to space their next pregnancy. Although breastfeeding has contraceptive effect, it is not absolutely reliable, especially after menstruation returns. Hence, all women should accept contraceptive method by at least 3 months postdelivery. If an intrauterine device like copper T is preferred, the insertion is performed 6 weeks after delivery. Injectable contraception such as Depot medroxy progesterone acetate (Depo-provera) IM every 3 months is also effective. The most annoying side effect is unpredictable spotting and bleeding. Contraceptive pills containing estrogen are not prescribed during breastfeeding as they inhibit lactation. Progestogen only pill can be prescribed.

MANAGEMENT OF LACTATION

Anatomy and Physiology of Breast

Breast has 15 to 20 lobes, each containing many lobules. The mammary gland lobule consist of clusters of rounded alveoli opening into ductules which unite to form lactiferous duct. The lactiferous duct dilate to form a lactiferous sinus before converging to open in the nipple. Contractile myoepithelial cells surround the ducts as well as the alveoli.

Pregnancy is associated with remarkable growth of both the ductal and lobuloalveolar structures. Estrogen stimulates proliferation of the lactiferous ducts while progesterone is responsible for the development of the mammary lobules. During early pregnancy lactiferous ducts and alveoli proliferate, while in later pregnancy the alveolar cells exhibit secretory activity. The lactogenic hormones, prolactin and human placental lactogen modulate these changes during pregnancy.

During pregnancy only minimal amounts of milk are formed in the breast despite high levels of lactogenic hormones, prolactin and placental lactogen. This is because the actions of these lactogenic hormones are inhibited by the secretion of high levels of estrogen and progesterone from the placenta. When the estrogen and progesterone are withdrawn following delivery, prolactin begins its milk secretory activity in previously fully developed mammary glands.

Physiology of Lactation

Two mechanisms are involved in the establishment of lactation (Figure 45.1).

Production of milk

Prolactin is secreted from the anterior pituitary in response to suckling and is essential for successful lactation. The suckling stimulus of the baby sends afferent impulses to the hypothalamic-pituitary axis,

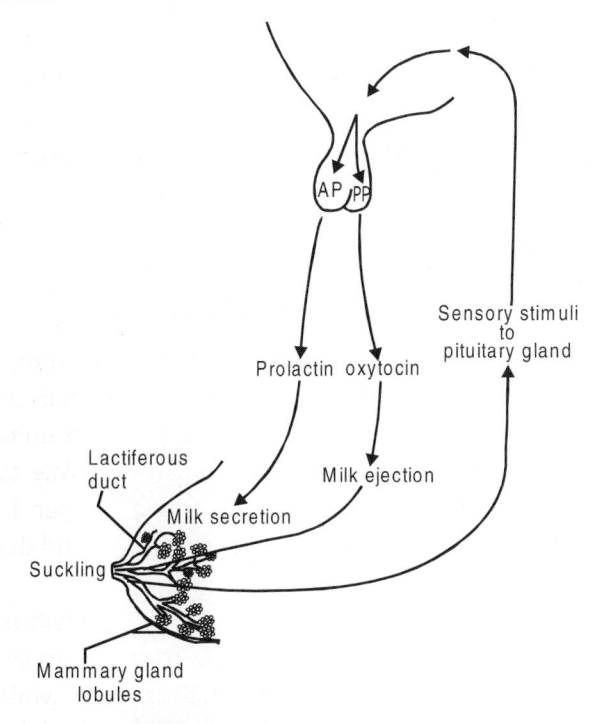

Figure 45.1: Physiology of lactation

leading to a surge of prolactin release. It acts on secretory cells of the alveoli and stimulates the synthesis of milk proteins.

Prolactin release is controlled by prolactin inhibitory factor, e.g. dopamine.

Milk Ejection Reflex

The milk ejection reflex is initiated by suckling which stimulates the release of oxytocin from the posterior pituitary. Oxytocin contracts the myoepithelial cells surrounding the alveoli and the lactiferous ducts thereby aiding expulsion of milk. This is recognized by the mother as the milk let down. The milk ejection reflex is inhibited by emotional stress and this may explain why maternal anxiety leads to failure of lactation.

Stimulation of Lactation

Women should be advised that breastfeeding confers advantages to mother and infant. Early suckling helps to promote breastfeeding. For the first 2 days following delivery, colostrum which starts during pregnancy becomes more abundant. Milk secretion actually starts on the 3rd or 4th postpartum day. If milk production is inadequate, dopamine receptor blockers, e.g. metoclopramide, domperidone can be used to augment lactation.

Suppression of Lactation

There may be several reasons for suppression of lactation, e.g. may be stillbirth or woman infected with HIV.

Drugs

Dopamine receptor agonist such as bromocriptine inhibits prolactin secretion and thus suppresses lactation. The dosage of bromocriptine is 2.5 mg orally twice daily for 14 days.

Mechanical

Tight brassiere is used in conjunction with the drugs to inhibit lactation. The mother should not express the milk from the breast.

BIBLIOGRAPHY

1. Glazener CMA, Mac Arthur C and Garcia J: Postnatal care: time for a change. Contemp. *Rev Obstet Gynaecol* 130-36, 1993.
2. Kennedy KI, Visness CM: Contraceptive efficiency of lactational amenorrhea. *Lancet* **339:** 227-30, 1992.
3. Robson SC, Dunlop W, Hunter S: Hemodynamic changes during the early puerperium. *British Medical Journal* **294:**1065, 1987.

46. Abnormalities of Puerperium

Krishnendu Gupta
Sajal Datta
Sudip Chakravarti

INTRODUCTION

The puerperium is indeed a time of great importance for both the mother and her baby, and yet it is an aspect of maternity care that has received relatively far less attention than pregnancy and delivery.

The problems of the puerperium are diverse and can be conveniently discussed under the following broad headings:
1. Secondary postpartum hemorrhage.
2. Puerperal sepsis.
3. Breast.
4. Venous system.
5. Urinary tract.
6. Chest.
7. Mental health.
8. Genital tract.

Since the first two aspects of puerperal problems (secondary postpartum hemorrhage and puerperal sepsis) have already been adequately covered in the previous chapter, this communication will briefly address the other encountered problems, both common and uncommon, during the puerperium.

PROBLEMS OF PUERPERIUM

Breast Problems

Engorgement

Breast engorgement (synonymous with: congestive mastitis), is common in primigravidae than in multiparae, and usually occurs on the second or third postpartum day.
1. *Diagnosis:*
   - Breasts are swollen, tender, tense and warm
   - Patient's temperature may be mildly elevated (15%); rarely exceeds 39°C and characteristically lasts no longer than 24 hours
   - Axillary adenopathy is usually seen
2. *Treatment:* The form of treatment depends on whether or not the patient wants to breastfeed.

- Wants to breastfeed
  - Manual emptying the breasts following breastfeeding
  - Supportive brassiere
- Does *not* want to breastfeed
  - Ice packs
  - Restriction of breast stimulation
  - Analgesics
  - Supportive brassiere.

Mastitis

Infection of the breast (synonymous with: infectious mastitis) occurs almost exclusively in lactating women in two forms:

1. *Epidemic:* Often acquired in hospital and caused by *Staphylococcus aureus.*
2. *Non-epidemic:* Usually acquired outside the hospital and caused by host flora, including *Staphylococcus* species, and most often the result of incomplete evacuation of the breast.

1. *Diagnosis:*
   - Epidemic: Fever and localized tenderness occur 2 to 4 days postpartum; Abscess is common
   - Nonepidemic: Fever, tenderness and malaise; Abscess is uncommon
2. *Treatment:*
   - Oral or parenteral broad spectrum antibiotics.
   - Supportive brassiere
   - Continue nursing of the affected breast.
3. *Prevention:*
   - Nipple hygiene.
   - Active care of cracks and fissures. Lanolin is most helpful
   - Early diagnosis and prompt antibiotic therapy can prevent most abscesses.

Abscess

This infection usually enters through a break in the skin (cracked nipple). It is usually confined to one quadrant of the breast. The most common organism identified is *Staphylococcus aureus*, mostly from the infant's nose/throat. The infant is usually infected from the nursery personnel.

1. *Diagnosis:*
   - *History*
     - Time of appearance: Usually in the third or fourth week postpartum; Rarely, before the end of the first week
     - Fever with or without chills
     - Painful area of one breast.
   - *Examination*
     - Raised temperature
     - Tachycardia
     - Erythematous segment of the breast
     - Brawny swelling or even fluctuation.
2. *Investigation:*
   - Expressed breast milk from the affected side for bacteriological examination
   - Ultrasound of the affected breast.
3. *Management:*
   - Broad spectrum antibiotic coverage: cloxacillin; cephalexin; cefuroxime
   - Incise under a general anesthetic: Circumareola incision followed by drainage; Leave a drain through dependent part
   - Adequate supportive brassiere
   - Continue breastfeeding from the normal breast
   - Empty the affected breast by means of a breast pump (manual expression is such cases is not possible due to the extreme tenderness and resultant pain).

Venous System Complications

Thromboembolism

The postpartum period is the most common time in pregnancy for a thromboembolism, as the puerperium fills all the criteria for Virchow's triad which are as follows:

A. *Increased coagulation:* The increase in clotting factors that occur in pregnancy remains although plasma volume returns to normal within a few hours of delivery.
B. *Stasis:* Many women have been immobilized during labor or in the immediate puerperium.
C. *Damage to venous endothelium*
   - Uterine veins: When the placenta separates

- Deep leg veins: When weight of the legs continues to compress veins, if the woman is immobilized in bed

1. *Diagnosis:*
   - *History*
     - Calf pain
     - Unilateral edema
   - *Examination*
     - A low-grade postpartum pyrexia
     - An unexplained maternal tachycardia
     - Tenderness over the deep veins of the calf
     - A positive Homan's sign (calf tenderness on dorsifexion of the foot).

2. *Investigations:*
   - Simple continuous wave real-time Doppler ultrasound
   - Color flow Doppler
   - Venography
   - Radioisotope scanning (with ^{125}Iodine): Contraindicated antenatally but may be performed, only if indicated, during the puerperium.

3. *Management:*
   - *Prevention*
     - Early mobilization
     - High dose estrogens are no longer given to suppress breast milk
     - Prophylaxis: Compression stockings (Subcutaneous heparin for high-risk group).
   - *Treatment*
     - Bed rest
     - Analgesics
     - Immediate anticoagulation therapy with intravenous (IV) heparin by means of a continuous infusion pump to prevent further extension of the venous thrombosis, for a period of 10 days
     - After 10 days, warfarin therapy is instituted for a period of 12 weeks
     - Graded ambulation later, when the symptoms subside.

Phlegmasia alba dolens

- Synonymous with: White leg; Milk leg
- Uncommon complication nowadays
- A clinico-pathological condition usually caused by retrograde extension of pelvic thrombophlebitis to involve the iliofemoral vein. The femoral vein may be directly affected from adjacent cellulitis.

1. *Diagnosis:*
   - Usually develops in the second week postpartum
   - Initially, mild fever
   - Later, high fever with chills and rigor
   - Constitutional disturbances: Headache; malaise; tachycardia
   - Patient looks toxic
   - The affected leg is swollen, painful (due to arterial spasm), white and cold (the left leg is more commonly involved than the right)
   - Tenderness and induration along the femoral vein

2. *Investigations:*
   - Blood counts: Leucocytosis

3. *Prevention and treatment:*
   - On similar lines as that of thromboembolism.

Pulmonary Embolism

The most common resting place of a clot embolus from the soleal or pelvic veins is in the pulmonary circulation.

A. Mild cases follow microemboli
   - Dyspnea and slight pleural pain may be followed by poor localization and the condition resolves in a few days with no specific treatment.

B. Severe cases arise from the:
   - Soleal veins: Clot extends to popliteal vein and breaks off (30%)
   - Uterine and ovarian veins: A thrombophlebitis with a friable clot following mid pelvic sepsis (20%).

In 50 percent of cases, no clinical evidence of peripheral vein thrombosis exists before the pulmonary embolism.

1. *Incidence:* The estimated average is about 1:6400 pregnancies.

2. *Diagnosis:*
   - *History*
     - Pre-existing deep vein thrombosis (50%)
       - History of unexplained pyrexia
     - Initially, dyspnea and faintness, followed by chest pain, cough and hemoptysis.

- *Examination*
  - Initially, tachypnea, tachycardia and dyspnea
  - Later, cyanosis develops followed by local signs of pulmonary underperfusion leading to right heart failure
  - Hypotension
  - Increased jugular venous pressure
  - Later still, pleural signs and collapse of a pulmonary lobe.
3. *Investigations*
   - Chest X-ray
   - ECG
   - Spiral computed tomography[1]
   - Ventilation-perfusion scintigraphy with radioactive technetium (^{99m}Tc) macroaggregated albumin[1]
   - Pulmonary angiography
   - Left and right heart catheterization.
4. *Management:* Two-thirds of those who die do so within 2 hours, so the point of greatest importance is to act quickly on suspicion, not waiting for the sophisticated tests unless they are very easily available.
   - Resuscitation, if required
     - External cardiac massage
     - Positive pressure oxygen by intubation, if necessary
     - Heparin 40,000 units IV daily
     - Emergency embolectomy (only in thoracic units with by-pass facilities)
   - Definitive treatment, if resuscitation is successful
     - Anticoagulants: Heparin
     - Thrombolytics: Streptokinase
     - Embolectomy, when there is either no response, failure or contraindication to thrombolytic therapy (Mortality rate: 25%).

Urinary Problems

Infection

About 2 to 4 percent of women develop urinary tract infection (UTI) postpartum. Following delivery, the bladder and lower urinary tract remain somewhat hypotonic, and residual urine and reflux result. This altered physiologic state, in conjunction with catheterization, birth trauma, conduction anesthesia, frequent pelvic examinations, and nearly continuous contamination of the perineum, is sufficient to explain the high incidence of lower UTIs postpartum. In many women, pre-existing asymptomatic bacteria, chronic UTIs, and anatomic disorders of the bladder, urethra and kidneys contribute to UTI postpartum.

1. *Diagnosis:*
   - Dysuria, frequency, urgency
   - Low-grade fever with or without chills
   - Tenderness: Suprapubic or renal angle
   - Urinary retention.
2. *Investigations:*
   - Blood counts: Leucocytosis
   - Urine microscopy: Pus cells usually in abundance
   - Urine culture: *Escherichia coli* is the most common organism isolated (75% cases); *Proteus, Klebsiella* are also isolated in some women.
3. *Treatment:*
   - High fluid intake
   - Urospecific spasmolytics: flavoxate; phenazopyridine
   - Broad spectrum urospecific antibiotics: Norfloxacin; Ciprofloxacin.

Untreated UTIs postpartum can lead to pyelonephritis which requires treatment with higher grade IV antibiotics (Third/fourth generation cephalosporins and aminoglycosides).

Retention

Common complication of early puerperium

1. *Etiology:*
   - Bruising and edema of the bladder base
   - Due to referred pain from perineal injury.
2. *Treatment:*
   - Counseling and encouragement to void via naturalis
   - If simple measures (like hot compress) fail, then continuous catheterization is done till the bladder regains its normal tone (usually for a period of 2 to 5 days)
   - After catheter removal, check the amount of residual urine; If more than 100 ml, then recatheterization is done
   - Analgesics and urospecific spasmolytics

- Antibiotics (after urine culture and sensitivity)
3. *Prevention:*
    - Great care to protect the perineum and paraurethral area during delivery is mandatory
    - Early ambulation and encouraging women to void early after delivery.

Incontinence

Uncommon complication of the puerperium; Approximately, 20 percent of women suffer from this problem, three months postpartum.
1. *Etiology:*
    - Disruption of pelvic floor supports
      - Large baby
      - Prolonged second stage
      - Operative vaginal delivery, particularly after a large episiotomy or following tear/lacerations on the perineum, paravaginal and paraurethral tissues.
2. *Types:*
    - Overflow incontinence
    - Stress incontinence
    - True incontinence (Genitourinary fistula: Vesicovaginal, urethrovaginal, ureterovaginal).
3. *Treatment:*
    - Stress incontinence following childbirth usually resolves with physiotherapy and improving tone of the pelvic floor[2]
    - Urinary fistulae, unless very small, usually require an operative closure. If small, continuous drainage for few weeks may help to bring about closure.
4. *Prevention:*
    - Great care to protect the perineum and paraurethral area during delivery is mandatory.

Chest Complications

Pneumonia

Women with obstructive lung disease, smokers, and those undergoing general anesthesia are at increased risk of developing pneumonia postpartum. The most common organisms are *Streptococcus pneumoniae* and *Mycoplasma pneumoniae*.

1. *Diagnosis:*
    - Productive cough, rales
    - Chest pain
    - Fever, chills
2. *Investigation:*
    - Chest X-ray: Infiltrates will be seen
    - Sputum for Gram stain and culture
3. *Treatment:*
    - Broad spectrum antibiotics: Amoxycillin; Cephalexin; Roxithromycin
    - Oxygen (if the patient is hypoxic)
    - Pulmonary toilet

Mental Health Problems

Puerperal Blues

- Syn: "The baby blues"; "4th day blues"
- Many women feel weepy and depressed 3 to 5 days after delivery but this is usually short-lived, settles within 48 hours

1. *Factors that prolong "the baby blues" are:*
    - Postpartum pyrexia
    - Anemia (Hb <8 gm/dl)
    - Inadequate sleep
    - Delayed healing of the episiotomy or cesarean section wound
    - Delay in establishment of breastfeeding
    - Decline in sympathy, congratulations and attention of friends and family as childbirth is past
2. *Treatment:*
    - Adequate explanation of what is happening to the baby
    - Night sedation
    - Pain relief
    - Visiting by husband and family and encouragement for motherhood
    - Getting home early; Very early discharge schemes: **DOMINO** (**DOM**estic **IN** and **O**ut)

Puerperal Depression

- Gradual onset over the first two months postpartum
- "The baby blues" may merge imperceptibly with serious depression

Evidence suggests that there is no specific form of depression that is related solely to pregnancy and childbirth.
1. *Factors that aggravate depression are:*
    - The swings in hormone changes around the time of childbirth acting on a predisposition to depression
    - An unconscious conflict in the responsibilities of looking after a new baby
    - Guilt
    - Anxiety
    - Fantasies
    - A background disposition due to previous history or family history
2. *Treatment:*
    - Involve a psychiatrist
    - In the presence of psychotic delusions, suicidal tendencies and aversion to food and drink, such women should be admitted and treated accordingly
    - Oral antidepressants: Lofepramine[3] (a tricyclic antidepressant) is the present drug of choice, may be continued for 6 months
    - Refractory cases may need definitive treatment such as electroconvulsive therapy (ECT).

Puerperal Psychosis

- Rare condition; Incidence: 1-2/1000 women
- Potentially life-threatening to both mother and the baby
1. *Diagnosis:*
    - Abrupt onset (20%) between 3rd to 14th day
    - Search for risk factors in the family
    - Detailed personal history
    - Rejection of baby
    - Delusion; hallucination
    - Confusion; restlessness; insomnia; no interest in food or drink.
2. *Management:*
    - Admit the mother and baby ideally to a mother-baby unit in a well manned psychiatry ward
    - Ensure 24-hour supervision
    - Give appropriate psychotherapy drug/s, in conjunction with a psychiatrist.

3. *Prognosis:*
    - Ninety-five percent of women improve within 2 to 3 months
    - Postpartum psychosis is recurrent (20-50%), but the chances are decreased by a 2-year or more gap between pregnancies.

Genital Tract Problems

Episiotomy Wound Infection

It is surprising that infected episiotomies do not occur more often, since contamination at the time of delivery is almost universal. Subsequent contamination during the healing phase must also be common, yet infection and disruption of the wound are infrequent (0.5-3%). The excellent local blood supply is suggested as an explanation for this phenomenon.

In general, the more extensive the laceration or episiotomy, the greater the chances for infection and breakdown of the wound. More tissue is devitalized in a large episiotomy, thereby providing greater opportunity for contamination. Women with infections elsewhere in the genital area are probably at a greater risk for infection of the episiotomy.
1. *Diagnosis:*
    - Pain at the episiotomy site
    - Purulent discharge[4]
    - Spontaneous drainage is frequent, so a mass rarely forms
    - Dysuria, with or without urinary retention
    - Incontinence of flatus and stool should warrant a careful inspection of the anal sphincter and rule out a rectovaginal fistula
2. *Investigations:*
    - Laboratory findings: Mixed aerobic and anaerobic organisms
3. *Treatment:*
    - Cleaning the wound, freeing the wound of infection and promoting formation of granulation tissue
    - Broad spectrum antibiotics
    - Warm sitz baths or Hubbard tank treatments help the debridement process
    - Surgical closure, if necessary

4. *Complications:*
   - Necrotizing fasciitis[5]
   - Very rarely, life-threatening septic shock[6]

Pelvic Abscess

Pelvic abscess (synonymous with: cul-de-sac abscess) may occur as a sequelae to acute pelvic inflammation and/or lower uterine, cervical or paravaginal injuries postpartum. The commonly isolated organisms are anaerobic, especially *Bacteriodes*.

1. *Diagnosis:*
   - Painful defecation, severe back pain or both (the severity of symptoms is often directly proportionate to the size of the abscess)
   - High fever
   - Patient looks toxic.
2. *Investigations:*
   - Blood counts: Leucocytosis
   - Ultrasound of the lower abdomen and pelvis
3. *Treatment:*
   - IV hydration
   - Broad spectrum antibiotics IV
   - Although with early treatment, the prognosis for a woman with a well-localized abscess is generally good, should her general condition deteriorate despite vigorous IV multidrug antibiotic therapy, colpotomy to drain out the pus/exploratory laparotomy may also be required
   - Blood transfusion, if required.
4. *Complications:*
   - Life-threatening peritonitis
   - Very rarely, psoas abscess[7]

Inversion of the Uterus

Uterine inversion is the prolapse of the fundus to or through the cervix, so that the uterus is in effect turned inside out. Almost all cases of inversion occur after delivery and may be worsened by excess traction on the cord before placental separation.

Puerperal inversion has been classified on the basis of its duration:

A. *Acute inversion:* Occurs immediately after delivery and before the cervix constricts (most common: >95%); Occurs within 24 hours.
B. *Subacute inversion:* Occurs after the cervix constricts, after 24 hours but before 4 weeks.
C. *Chronic inversion:* Inversion noted 4 weeks after delivery; Rare incidence: 1:20,000 deliveries.

The morbidity and mortality associated uterine inversion correlate with the degree of hemorrhage, the rapidity of diagnosis, and the effectiveness of treatment.

1. *Etiology:*
   - Mismanaged third stage of labor
     - Faulty cord traction on a fundally implanted placenta
     - Injudicious use of oxytocin
     - Crede's maneuver (never performed nowadays)
2. *Problems:*
   - Acute inversion: Postpartum hemorrhage (90%); Injury to intestines and appendages entrapped by the prolapsed uterine fundus; Shock
   - Chronic inversion: Problems of acute inversion + Endomyometritis.
3. *Diagnosis:*
   - Uterine fundus seen turned inside out at the vulva
   - Shock and hemorrhage is prominent.
4. *Treatment:*
   - Management of shock
     - Antibiotics; IV hydration; Blood transfusion, if required
   - Perineal toilet
   - Acute inversion: Manual repositioning of the uterus
     - If simple repositioning fails, O'Sullivan's technique[8] (intravaginal hydrostatic pressure application or douche with warm antiseptic solution) may be attempted
     - If the placenta is not removed prior to the inversion, do not attempt to remove the placenta till reposition is complete.
   - Chronic inversion: Operative treatment
     - Conservative approach
       a. Abdominal route: Haultain's procedure (when fertility is no longer desired)

b. Vaginal route: Spinelli's procedure; Kustner's procedure
- Hysterectomy (vaginal/abdominal), if necessary

CONCLUSION

When compared with the dramatic events of delivery, the puerperium may seem rather uneventful. Nevertheless, significant physiological changes occur during this interval, and these influence many of the problems that often arise without warning.

Although a humble attempt has been made to touch upon some of the important problems that are encountered postpartum, there are yet many more uncommon problems related to the pulmonary circulation, cardiovascular, respiratory and nervous systems, thyroid, the postpartum hemolytic-uremic syndrome and the toxic shock syndrome, which have been left uncovered.

REFERENCES

1. Cunningham FG, Gant NF, Leveno JK, et al: Pulmonary disorders. In Cunningham FG et al (Rds): *William's Obstetrics*, 21st edn, McGraw Hill, New York; 1237, 2001.
2. Howie PW: The puerperium. In Edmonds DK (Ed): *Dewhurst's Textbook of Obstetrics and Gynecology for Postgraduates*, 6th edn, Blackwell Science, London; 344-46, 1999.
3. Nicholls KR, Cox JL: Antidepressants and breastfeeding (letter). *Psych Bull* **20**:309, 1996.
4. Ramin SM, Gilstrap LC: Episiotomy and early repair of dehiscence. *Clin Obstet Gynecol* **37**:816, 1994.
5. Urschel JD: Necrotizing soft tissue infections. *Postgrad Med J* **75**: 645, 1999.
6. Soltesz S, Biedler A, Ohlmann P et al: Puerperal sepsis due to infected episiotomy wound. *Zentralbl Gynakol* **121**:441, 1999.
7. Segal S, Gemer O, Sestopal-Epelman M et al: Retroperitoneal abscess after normal delivery. A report of two cases. *J Reprod Med* **41**:276, 1996.
8. O'Sullivan JV: *J Obstet Gynec Brit Emp* **53**:210, 1946.

Index

A

3-dimensional ultrasound 135
A pregnant mother 72
  examination 75
    attitude 77
    auscultation 78
    estimation of fetal weight 78
    inspection 76
    lie and presentation 77
    palpation 76
    pelvic examination 79
    percussion 79
    position and station 77
  history 72
    family history 73
    first trimester 74
    history of present pregnancy 73
    history of the presenting complaint 75
    obstetric history 72
    past medical and surgical history 73
    past obstetric and gynecological history 73
    second trimester 74
    social history 73
    third trimester 75
Abdominal circumference 121, 266
Abruptio placenta 181
  investigations 182
  management 182
  postnatal care 183
  risk factors associated 181
  signs 181
  symptoms 181
Abscess of breast 379
Accoustic stimulation test 269
Acrosome reaction 13
Acute abdomen 258
  differential diagnosis 259
    complications of pregnancy 261
    conditions associated with pregnancy 260
    conditions unrelated to pregnancy 259
  effect of physiological changes 258
  management of the fetus 263
Agents of infections in pregnancy 165, 166
Amniocentesis 129
Amnion and umbilical cord 67
  clinical correlation 69
  composition of the amniotic fluid 68
  development of membranes 67
Amniotic fluid fibroblast 241
Amniotic fluid index 266
Amniotomy 278
Analgesia for labor 301
  parenteral and inhalational 302
  regional 302
    combined spinal epidural 302
    epidural 302
    spinal 303
Anemia in pregnancy 138
  classification 140
    dimorphic 144
    iron deficiency 140
    megaloblastic 143
  iron dynamics 138
  management 145
  physiological considerations 138
Anesthesia for cesarean section 304
  general 304
  regional 305
Antenatal care 102
  aims 102
  general advice about lifestyle 103
    first trimester 104
    second trimester 106
    third trimester 107
  preconception counseling 102
Antepartum hemorrhage 176
  etiology 176

Antibody 58
Antigen 57
Antihypertensives 192
Antinuclear antibodies 61
Apt's test 184
Atonic PPH 366
Atrial natriuretic peptide 53

B

Baby blues 382
Bacterial vaginosis 170
Bag mask ventilation 355
Bag of membranes 295
Balloon catheters 277
Ballotment 37
Barker's hypothesis 233
Biochemical testing 272
Biophysical tests 267
Biparietal diameter 120, 265
Birth injuries 358
  clinical examination 359
  common problems 359
    cutaneous stigmata 360
    gastrointestinal problems 361
    jaundice 360
    low birth weight infant 362
    metabolic disturbances 361
    neonatal seizures 362
    respiratory problems 361
Bony pelvis 25
Braxton Hick contractions 37
Breech extraction 325

C

Candidial vaginitis 171
Capacitation 12
Carcinoma of cervix 201
Cardiac diseases in pregnancy 244
  clinical features 245
  functional classification system 245
  incidence 245

management 245
  antenatal 246
  cardiac failure 246
  labor 246
  termination of pregnancy 246
  risk factors 245
Carpal tunnel syndrome 116
Cervical detachment 343
Cervical dilatation curve 296
Cervix 22
Cesarean section 334
  technical clues 334
    cesarean hysterectomy 335
    classical cesarean section 335
    lower segment vertical section 335
  vaginal birth after 336
Chadwick's sign 34
Chorionic adreno-corticotrophin 53
Chorionic thyrotrophin 53
Chorionic villous sampling 241, 130
Chronic hypertension pregnancy 196
  causes 196
  management 196
Circumvallate placenta 184
Clitoris 24
Coccygeus 28
Color Doppler 270
Colporrhexis (rupture of vaginal vault) 341
Common iliac artery 29
  external 30
  internal 30
Comparative genome hybridization 136
Complement 58
Congenital heart defects 131
Congenital heart disease 245
Contraction stress test 268
Cord prolapse 326
  diagnosis 327
  etiology 327
  management 328
Cordocentesis or fetal blood sampling 130
Cowper's (Bulbourethral) and urethral glands 11
Crown-rump length 119
Crowning of head 298
Cutaneous stigmata 360
Cutis mormorata 360
Cystic fibrosis 134
Cystic ovarian tumor 39
Cytogenetic analysis 136
Cytokines 58

D

Day care unit 190
Diabetes in pregnancy 147
  complications 150
    fetal and neonatal 150
    maternal 150-
  investigations 152
  management 152
  pregnancy as a diabetogenic state 148
  screening for diabetes 148
    diagnostic test 149
    screening test 149
  treatment 153
Diagnosis of pregnancy 33
  first trimester 33
    breast changes 34
    breast discomfort 34
    cessation of menstruation (amenorrhea) 33
    fatigue 34
    hormonal tests
    nausea with or without vomiting 33
    pelvic organ changes 34
    ultrasound 36
    urinary symptoms 34
  second trimester 36
    abdominal examination 37
    general examination 36
    subjective symptoms 36
    ultrasonography 38
    vaginal examination 38
  third trimester 38
    investigation 39
    objective signs 39
    subjective symptoms 38
Diagnostic ultrasound 129
Dilatation of cervix 294
Distended urinary bladder 39
DNA (Deoxyribonucleic acid) analysis 136
Down syndrome 128, 132
Dystocia 291

E

Eclampsia 194
  principles of treatment 194
    general measures 194
    obstetric management 195
    treatment of complications 196
Ectopic pregnancy 88
  Arias-Stella reaction 89
  etiology and risk factors 90
    assisted reproduction 90
    intrauterine contraceptive devices 90
    tubal damage 90
  incidence 88
  investigation 91
    βhCG measurement 91
    discriminatory zone 92
    laparoscopy 92
    ultrasound 91
  management 93
    expectant 93
    medical 93
    surgical 93
  pathophysiology 88
  presentation 90
  sites of implantation 89
    abdominal 89
    cervical site 89
    ovarian 89
    tubal 89
Effacement of cervix 294
Egg release and transport 11
Embryo hatching 15
Embryo-endometrial contact 16
Embryogenesis of gonads and gametes 2
Endocrinology of labor 55
Endocrinology of pregnancy 50
  peptide hormone synthesis in placenta 53
  placental steroid hormones 50
  protein hormones 50
    chorionic adreno-corticotrophin 53
    chorionic thyrotrophin 53
    corticotrophic relaxing hormone 53
    growth hormone variant 53
    human chorionic gonadotropin 51
    human placental lactogen 52
    thyrotrophin releasing hormone 53
Endotracheal intubation 354, 355
Engorgement 378
Epididymis 10
Episiotomy wound infection 383
Erythema toxicum 360
Estimated fetal weight 266
Estrogen 54
Estrogen biosynthesis 53
Eutocia 291
External cardiac massage 355
External cephalic version 321

F

Fallopian tube 20
  structure 21

INDEX

Father of modern embryology 1
Female external genitalia 23
Female reproductive organs 9
Femur length 121
Femur to abdomen ratio 266
Fertilization 13
Fetal abnormalities 131
   chromosomal 132
   congenital viral and parasitic
      infections 134
   genetic 132
   structural 131
Fetal adrenal 54
Fetal axis pressure 295
Fetal biometry 265
Fetal biophysical profile 268
Fetal blood sampling 241
Fetal DNA in maternal circulation 136
Fetal fibronectin 217
Fetal nuchal translucency 128
Fetal ponderal index 266
Fetal surveillance 265
Fetal tissue biopsies 131
Fetal wellbeing 264
Fetoscopy 130
Fetus 69
   circulation 69
   fetal blood 70
   gastrointestinal tract 70
   growth and development 69
   immune system 70
   respiratory system 70
   urinary system 70
FISH (Fluorescent in situ hybridization) 137
Follicle formation 3
   at puberty and during reproductive years 4
   early intrauterine period 3
   late intrauterine period 4
   neonatal and childhood period 4
Folliculogenesis 6
Forceps delivery 330
   classification 331
   instrument 331
   tips for success 331
Fragile X syndrome 132

G

Gametes 2
Gemellology 203
Genital tract disorders 199
Genital tract trauma 370
Gestational diabetes mellitus 147
Glucose challenge test 149
Goodell's sign 34

H

Head to abdomen circumference ratio 266
Hegar's sign 35
Hematoma
   infralevator 341
   paravaginal (pelvic) 341
   supralevator 342
Hemoglobinopathies 132, 239
Human chorionic gonadotropin 41, 51
   human placental lactogen 42
   other placental hormones production 42
Human placental lactogen 42, 52
Human spermatozoa 7
Hydatidiform mole 62
Hygroscopic mechanical dilator 277
Hymen 23
Hyperactivation 12
Hypertensive disorders in pregnancy 186
   clarifications 187
   classification 186
Hyperthyroidism 248
Hypothyroidism 248
Hysterectomy 370

I

Immunization in pregnancy 174
Immunology 57
Immunoregulation 58, 59
Implantation 15
Indeterminate antepartum hemorrhage 183
Induction of labor 274
   contraindications 275
   indications 274
      elective or non-urgent 275
      post-term pregnancy 275
      semi-urgent 275
      urgent 274
   induction in special circumstances 280
      intrauterine fetal death 280
      prelabor rupture of membranes 280
      previous cesarean section 280
      twin pregnancies 280
   methods 275
      cervical ripening 276
      labor induction 278
   risks of induction 279
Infant mortality rate 214
Infections in pregnancy 165
   intra-amniotic 166
   STDs 168
      chlamydia trachomatis infection 169
      cytomegalovirus infection 173
      gonorrhea 169
      herpes simplex virus (HSV) infection 172
      Human papilloma virus infection 170
      rubella infection 172
      syphilis 168
      toxoplasmosis 171
      trichomoniasis 171
      vaginitis 170
   tuberculosis 167
   urinary tract 165
Inferior mesenteric artery 29
Injuries to birth canal 338
   cervical detachment 343
   injuries to the cervix 342
      diagnosis 342
      etiology 342
      treatment 343
   injury to vulva 340
   perineal injuries 338
      causes 338
      postoperative care 340
      prevention 339
      repair 339
      types 338
   rupture of uterus 343
      clinical features 344
      etiology 343
      site of rupture 344
      treatment 344
   vaginal injury 341
      management 342
      types 341
Intrauterine growth restriction 227
   complications 229
   etiology 228
   management 232
   pathogenesis 229
   screening and identification 230
      newer screening tools 232
   types 228
Intrauterine growth restriction 62
Inversion of the uterus 384
Iron cycle 139
Iron deficiency anemia in pregnancy 140
   clinical features 140
   diagnosis 141
   maternal and fetal consequences 140
   treatment 141
      blood transfusion 143
      management during labor and puerperium 143

oral iron therapy 142
parenteral iron therapy 142

J

Jaundice 360

K

Karyotyping 136

L

Labia majora 23
Labia minora 24
Lactation 376
  anatomy of breast 376
  physiology 376
    milk ejection reflex 377
    production of milk 376
    stimulation of lactation 377
    suppression of lactation 377
Lactational amenorrhea 374
Leiomyoma of uterus 39
Levator ani 28
Linea nigra 37
Lochia 373
Low birth weight infant 362
Lymphocytes
  B 58
  T 57

M

Macrophages 58
Magnetic resonance imaging 135
Male reproductive organs 9
Malpresentations 312
  breech presentation 318
    clinical types 319
    diagnosis 320
    etiology 319
    intranatal management 323
    mode of delivery 323
    types of breech 319
  brow presentation 314
    diagnosis 315
    etiology 315
    mechanism of labor 316
  face presentation 312
    diagnosis 312
    etiology 312
    management options 314
    mechanism of labor 314
  transverse lie 316
    diagnosis 317
    etiology 316
    management options 318
    mechanism of labor 317

Mastitis 379
Maternal death 364
Maternal mortality ratio 96
Medication in pregnancy 250
  breastfeeding 252
  drugs used in 252
    analgesics 254
    anti-inflammatory drugs 254
    antibiotics 252
    anticoagulants 253
    anticonvulsants 253
    antihypertensive drugs 254
    antiretroviral agents 255
    corticosteroids 254
    immunosuppressants 254
    psychotropic drugs 254
  pharmacokinetics 251
  prescribing principles 251
  timing of exposure and pregnancy outcome 250
  treatment of minor ailments 255
Megaloblastic anemia 143
  clinical features 144
  diagnosis 144
  etiology 144
  management 144
  pathophysiology 144
Metoclopramide 113
Milia 360
Milk ejection reflex 377
Minor disorders of pregnancy 115
  backache 116
  carpal tunnel syndrome 116
  constipation 116
  heartburn 116
  nausea and vomiting 115
  pubic symphysis diastasis/pelvic osteoarthropathy 117
  urinary problems 116
  varicosities 117
Miscarriage
  classification 81
    complete 82
    incomplete 81
    inevitable 81
    missed 82
    recurrent 82
    septic 82
    threatened 81
  clinical features 83
  complications 87
  etiology 82
    fetal factors 82
    immunological factors 83
    luteal phase defect 82
    maternal factors 82

    paternal factors 83
    uterine abnormalities 83
  incidence 80
  management 83
    complete 84
    incomplete 84
    induced 85
    inevitable 84
    missed 84
    preabortion 86
    recurrent 85
    septic 84
  methods of termination 86
  pathology 80
Misoprostol 277
Mongolian spots 360
Mosaicism 136
Moulding 289
Multicolor FISH 135
Multiple pregnancy 203
  antenatal management 207
  diagnosis 204
  fetal complications 205
    cardiac twinning 207
    congenital anomalies 207
    discordant growth 206
    monoamniotic twin pregnancies 206
    preterm labor 205
    single fetal demise 206
    twin to twin transfusion syndrome 206
    umbilical cord problems 207
  genesis of twins 204
  incidence 203
  management during labor 207
    cesarean section delivery 208
    delivery of the first twin 207
    delivery of the second twin 208
    locking of twins 209
    management of the third stage of labor 208
  maternal complications 205

N

Nagele's rule 74
Natural killer cells 58
Nausea and vomiting during pregnancy 108
  complications 111
  diagnosis and clinical features 110
  investigations 111
  management 111
    hyperemesis gravidarum 112
    simple nausea and vomiting 111
  pathogenesis 108
  pathology 110

Index

Neonatal mortality 214
Neonatal mortality rate 357
Neonatal period 357
Neonatal seizures 362
Neural tube defects 131
Nitric oxide synthase expression 56
Non-stress test 267
Normal hemoglobin 239
Normal labor 283, 293
   components 283
      passage 284
      passenger 285
      powers 283
   management 297
      fourth stage 299
      second stage 298
      third stage 299
   mechanism 286
      descent 287
      engagement 286
      extension 288
      external rotation 289
      flexion 287
      internal rotation 287
      lateral flexion 289
      restitution 288
   physiology 293
      bag of membranes 295
      dilatation of cervix 294
      effacement of cervix 294
      events in first stage of labor 294
      events in second stage of labor 297
      events in third stage of labor 297
      fetal axis pressure 295
      metabolic changes 294
      primary forces 293
      secondary forces 294
      uterine contractions 294
Normal position and malposition 306

O

Obstetrical use of ultrasonography 118
   Doppler ultrasound technology 124
   indications 119
      assessment of amniotic fluid 122
      assessment of early pregnancy 119
      complications of early pregnancy 119
      determination of gestational age 119
      fetal-malformation 122
      multiple pregnancies 122
      placental localization 122
   issue of safety 118
   methods 119
   the schedule 123

Obstructed labor 349
   causes 349
   course of labor 349
   prevention 349
   treatment 349
Obturator internus 26
Occiput posterior position 306
   causes 307
   diagnosis 307
   management of labor 311
   mechanism of labor 307
   outcome of labor 309
Onset of labor 291
   endocrinology 291
      date of onset of labor 292
      fetoplacental contribution 291
      nervous factor 292
      oxytocin 291
      prostaglandins 292
   stages 292
      first stage (cervical stage) 292
      fourth stage 293
      prelabor period 292
      second stage 293
      third stage 293
Oocyte maturation 3, 13
Operative obstetrics 330
Oral glucose tolerance test 149
Osiander's sign 34
Ovarian artery 29
Ovarian cysts 201
Ovary 19
   blood supply 20
   changes with age 20
   embryological remnants 20
   lymph drainage 20
   nerve supply 20
   structure 19
Ovulatory menstrual cycle 5
Oxytocin 278

P

Pain pathways 301
Palmer's sign 34
Paracervical block 304
Pelvic floor 28
Pelvic lymphatic drainage 32
Pelvic nerves 30
   autonomic 32
   somatic 30
      lumbar plexus 30
      sacral plexus 31
Pelvic vessels 28
Pelvic walls 26
Penis 11
Perinatal asphyxia 331
   assessment of infants at birth 352
   causes 352
   pathophysiology 331
   resuscitation of the newborn 353
      drugs commonly used 354
Perinatal mortality rate 213, 358
Perinatal period 358
Pernicious vomiting of pregnancy 108
Phenothiazines 113
Phlegmasia alba dolens 380
Physiological changes in pregnancy 41
   cardiovascular system 43
      blood pressure 43
      cardiac output 43
      peripheral resistance 43
      plasma volume 43
      pulse rate 43
      stroke volume 43
   endocrine systems 47
      adrenal gland 48
      hypothalamic-pituitary axis 47
      pancreas 48
      parathyroid gland 48
      thyroid gland 48
   gastrointestinal system 47
   hematology 43
      erythropoiesis 44
      other blood constituents 44
      red cell volume 43
      redistribution of blood flow in pregnancy 44
   placental hormone secretion 41
      human chorionic gonadotropin 41
      human placental lactogen 42
      other placental hormones 42
   renal system 46
   respiratory system 45
Placenta 64
   circulation 66
   development 64
   function 67
   structure 66
Placenta accreta 371
Placenta accreta/increta/percreta 180
   postnatal care 180
Placenta previa 177
   complications associated 177
   etiology 177
   investigations 178
   management 178
   signs 178
   symptoms 178
Placental separation 365
Plication of the uterine 369
Pneumonia 382
Polyhydramnios 209
   acute versus chronic 210

complications 211
diagnosis 210
etiopathology 210
incidence 210
management 211
intrapartum management 212
Polymerase chain reaction 137
Postpartum hemorrhage 365
management 366
Pre-eclampsia 62, 188
diagnosis 189
etiology 188
management 190
intrapartum management 193
intrapartum monitoring 191
obstetric management 194
preventive therapy 190
systemic changes associated with 189
Pregestational diabetes mellitus 147
Pregnancy immunology 60
Preimplantation 14
Preimplantation genetic diagnosis 136
Prenatal diagnostic tests 129
Prenatal screening 125
criteria for screening 126
second trimester biochemical screening 126
Preterm birth 357
Preterm labor 213
assessment of gestational age 216
etiology 214
incidence 214
management 218
corticosteroids for fetal benefits 218
mode of delivery in preterm labor 221
neonatal facilities and in utero transfer 218
rescue cervical cerclage 221
physical examination and investigations 217
survival and mortality 215
pediatric morbidity 216
symptoms and signs 216
Preterm prelabor rupture of membranes 221
etiology 222
incidence 222
management 223
amniotic fluid infusion 224
antenatal corticosteroids 224
induction of labor 224
mode of delivery 224
prophylactic antibiotics 224
tocolysis 224

physical examination and investigations 223
presentation 223
Prolapse of the pregnant uterus 200
Prolonged labor 345
causes 347
evaluation in a neglected case 347
role of partography 346
treatment 348
Prolonged pregnancy 234
practice points 238
predictors 235
principles of management 235
confirmation of length of pregnancy 235
monitoring in labor 237
preparing the cervix for induction 237
stripping/sweeping the membranes 237
to deliver or not to deliver 236
problems associated 235
Pronucleus formation-syngamy-embryonic cleavage 14
Prostaglandins 276, 279, 292
Prostate 10
Pseudocyesis 39
Pudendal block 304
Puerperal psychosis 383
Puerperium 373, 378
management 374
care of the bladder 375
care of the bowel 375
involution of the uterus 374
lochia 375
vital signs 374
management of ailments 376
physiological changes 373
blood 374
changes in the cervix and vagina 373
involution of the uterus 373
Lochia 373
return of menstruation and ovulation 374
urinary tract 374
postnatal examination 376
problems 378
breast 378
chest 382
genital tract 383
mental health 382
puerperal blues 382
puerperal depression 382
puerperal psychosis 383
urinary 381
venous system 379

Pulmonary embolism 380
Pulmonary hypoplasia 223
Pustular melanosis 360
Pyriformis 26

R

Recurrent spontaneous abortion 61
Reproduction 1
Respiratory diseases in pregnancy 246
acute bronchitis 247
asthma 247
bronchiectasis 247
chronic bronchitis 247
pulmonary Koch's infection 247
Retained placenta 370
Retroversion of uterus 199
Rhesus isoimmunization 242
management 242
pathophysiology 242
prevention 243
Rheumatic heart disease 245
Role of partography 346
Rupture of uterus 343

S

Safe motherhood initiative 95
road ahead 99
integrated management of pregnancy and childbirth 100
making pregnancy safer 99
strategies 97
early detection of complication 98
emergency obstetric care 98
protocol for essential obstetric care for all 97
Seminal vesicles 11
Seminiferous tubules 9
Sertoli cells 9
Shoulder dystocia 336
drill or plan of action in the event of emergency 337
Sickle cell disorder 133
Small for gestational age 357
Sperm release and transport 12
Sperm-egg interaction 13
Spermatogenesis 7, 8
Stillbirth 213
Subgaleal hematoma 358
Sweeping of membranes 278
Symphysiofundal height 37

T

Tamponade test 368
Teratogenesis 256
Testes 9

Thalassemia 133
Thalassemia syndromes 239
  alpha thalassemia 240
    investigations 240
    management 240
  beta thalassemia 240
    management 241
    prenatal diagnosis 241
Thromboembolism 379
Thyroid disorders 248
Thyroid nodule 248
Tocolysis 219
Toxoplasmosis 171
Trichomoniasis 171
Trophoblastic disease and tumors 62
Tropical disease in pregnancy 156
  acute viral hepatitis 160
  chickenpox 162
  hepatitis 159
    treatment 161
  hypoglycemia 159
  malaria 157
    clinical features 158
    drug treatment 159
    incidence 157
    management 158

U

Ureter 27
Uterine compression sutures 368
Uterine contractions 294
Uterine fibroids 200
Uterine inversion 371
Uterine rupture 183
Uterine segment formation 296

Uterus 21
  blood supply 22
  lymphatic drainage 22
  nerve supply 22
  structure 21

V

Vacuum delivery 332
  soft vacuum extractions cups 333
  tips for safe vacuum delivery 333
  vacuum versus forceps 334
Vacuum extraction 311
Vagina 23
Vaginitis 170
Vas deferens 10
Vasa previa 183
Vestibule 24
Vulva 23